vitamins etc.

Nicola Reavley

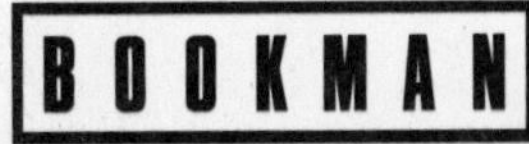

Published in Australia by Bookman Press Pty Ltd
227 Collins St
Melbourne, VIC 3000
Ph (03) 9654 2000
Fax (03) 9654 2290

Email bookman@bookman.com.au

National Library of Australia
Cataloguing in Publication entry

Reavley, Nicola
Vitamins etc.

ISBN 1 86395 121 0

1. Dietary supplements. 2. Vitamins in human nutrition. 3. Food - Vitamin content. 4. Nutrition. 5. Minerals in nutrition. I. Title

612.399

PUBLISHER'S NOTE
The information contained in this book is not intended as a substitute for consulting your physician. All matters regarding your health require medical supervision.

Contents

Contents

Contents

We are all familiar with the saying, 'You are what you eat', and more than ever, people are focusing on nutrition to help them live healthier, longer and happier lives. Growing evidence suggests that many people suffer from diseases that can be controlled or prevented through diet and lifestyle, and the last fifteen years has seen an explosion of research into the links between nutrition and health. Along with the interest in diet has come a focus on nutritional supplements as people search for ways to feel better and stay healthy.

Supplements are a $6 billion-a-year business. As many as 70 per cent of people take them at least occasionally, and almost every mall has a health food store filled with products that promise to relieve pain, help you sleep better and boost your health, vitality and virility.

But many people still have questions. What do vitamins and minerals do? Am I getting enough from the food I eat? Should I take supplements? Which ones should I take and how much? Can supplements make me look and feel healthier? Can they prevent diseases? Can they slow the aging process?

The answers to these questions are not always clear-cut. There is an almost daily barrage of media reports on new studies, some suggesting that a supplement does you good, others indicating that it may be harmful. The scientific and medical community are divided on many issues, making it even harder to sort out truth from media hype. And then there are the advertisements....

So how do you sort out fact from fiction?

The official line is that a healthy adult can get adequate amounts of nutrients from a balanced diet. Adequate to prevent deficiency disease – yes, but adequate for optimum health? That is a more complex question to answer.

Many people don't get all the nutrients they need from their diets because they don't eat well. Only one person in ten regularly eats the recommended five servings a day of fruits and vegetables. Many people are on weight loss diets, regularly skip meals or eat a lot of foods high in sugar and fat. People also have varying nutritional needs and ways of meeting those needs. And then there are those with clearly increased needs such as pregnant women, the elderly, those taking long-term medications, and those who are chronically ill. Such people probably all have needs greater than their diet can meet. This is where the 'nutritional insurance' of supplements can help.

Many experts prefer not to recommend supplements because they worry that this may lead people to believe that they can eat all the fatty, sugary, processed foods they like as long as they remember to pop their vitamin pills every morning. But supplements don't turn a poor diet into a healthy one. Foods contain thousands of nutrients over and above those contained in a supplement bottle. If you depend on supplements rather than trying to eat a variety of whole foods, you miss out on possible health benefits from these phytochemicals.

If you are trying to sort your way through the maze of information and decide which foods to eat; whether to take supplements, and if so, which ones, how often and how much; it helps to have a good understanding of the roles played by vitamins and minerals in health and disease. You also need to understand how their functions are affected by your age, sex, state of health and lifestyle. In some situations, taking supplements can be harmful; for example, an iron supplement that stops a teenage girl from becoming anemic may increase the risk of heart disease in an older man.

Of all the major factors affecting our health, we have the greatest control over the food we eat. Most of us, therefore, have the power to dramatically affect our health and quality of life. It is human nature to deny the possibility of disease until it occurs, and as diet has a huge role to play in the *prevention* of disease, eating well and consuming adequate amounts of vitamins and minerals are vital for both present and future health. The aim of this book is to give you the necessary knowledge to make informed choices about the food you eat and the supplements you take.

Vitamins, minerals and diet: the basics

What are vitamins?

Vitamins are substances which, in small amounts, are necessary to sustain life. They must be obtained from food as they are either not made in the body at all, or are not made in sufficient quantities for growth, vitality and wellbeing. Lack of a particular vitamin or mineral can lead to incomplete metabolism, fatigue and other health problems; and in severe cases, to deficiency disease. A deficiency of a particular vitamin causes disease symptoms which can only be cured by that vitamin.

Vitamins are chemically unrelated substances and all are organic. Organic substances are those that contain carbon and come from materials that are living, such as plants and animals; or that were once living, for example, petroleum or coal. It is impossible to sustain life without all the essential vitamins.

What do vitamins do?

Vitamins have many functions and influence the health of nearly every organ in your body. Their combination with other substances such as minerals, proteins and enzymes brings about certain chemical reactions. Individual vitamins have specific functions which vary widely and can overlap. They are involved in growth, the ability to produce healthy offspring, and the maintenance of health. They play a role in metabolism, enabling your body to use other essential nutrients such as carbohydrates, fats, proteins and minerals. Vitamins are important for a normal appetite, in digestion, mental alertness, and resistance to bacterial infections.

In addition to their basic roles in metabolism, some vitamins have specific preventive and therapeutic effects when taken in larger amounts. For example, niacin can be used to lower cholesterol and vitamin B6 can be used to treat premenstrual syndrome. Large doses of vitamins may slow, or even reverse many diseases previously thought an inevitable part of aging; such as cancer, heart disease, osteoporosis, impaired immunity, nerve degeneration and other chronic health problems. Many experts consider that taking larger doses of some vitamins is necessary for optimum health.

Vitamins are not substitutes for food. They cannot be assimilated without taking in food. They have no energy value of their own and are not components of body structures.

Where does the word vitamin come from?

In 1912, a Polish biochemist called Casimir Funk suggested that disease might be caused by a lack of something in the diet and cured by adding it. He thought this substance was necessary for life (*vita*) and contained nitrogen (*amine*) thus '*vitamine*'. Later research showed that few of these substances contained nitrogen so the final 'e' was dropped giving us the word 'vitamin'.

How were vitamins discovered?

Diseases such as scurvy, rickets and pellagra have been known for centuries. It is only this century that the vitamins necessary for preventing them have been identified and isolated. Vitamins were originally discovered through animal experiments. Scientists fed animals diets known to cause certain diseases in man and then treated those animals with the nutrient missing from the diet. If the nutrient was found to cure or prevent the disease, it was identified as a vitamin.

How many vitamins are there?

In the USA the following are officially listed as vitamins: vitamin A; vitamin C; vitamin D; vitamin E; vitamin K; and the B vitamin complex containing: vitamin B1 (thiamin), vitamin B2 (riboflavin), vitamin B3 (niacin), vitamin B6 (pyridoxine), folic acid, vitamin B12 (cobalamin), biotin and pantothenic acid.

There are other substances whose vitamin status has not been established. Some researchers consider these to be vitamins but this is not generally accepted. Such substances include choline, inositol, para-aminobenzoic acid (PABA) and coenzyme Q10.

Vitamins are usually divided into two categories: fat soluble and water soluble. Vitamins A, D, E and K are fat soluble. They require an adequate supply of minerals and fats to be absorbed in the digestive system and are stored in the liver. The remaining vitamins are water soluble with any excess being excreted in the urine. These need to be replenished frequently.

What are minerals?

Minerals are naturally occurring inorganic (noncarbon containing) elements which play a part in many biochemical and physiological processes necessary for body maintenance. They are important structural components of several body tissues; for example, calcium, phosphorus and magnesium make up an important part of bone tissue. Minerals are as important as vitamins for your body to function properly.

As the body cannot make any minerals, they must be obtained from plant and animal foods and from water, which may contain dissolved minerals. Minerals can be grouped into those required in the diet in amounts greater than 100 mg a day, known as major minerals; and those required in amounts less than 100 mg a day, which are known as minor or trace minerals.

Which are the essential minerals?

About 20 minerals are known to be necessary for body maintenance and regulatory functions. The major minerals are calcium, phosphorus, potassium, sodium, chloride, magnesium and sulfur. Trace minerals are boron, chromium, copper, iodine, iron, manganese, molybdenum, selenium, silicon, vanadium and zinc. Other minerals which may be necessary for humans include fluorine, cobalt and nickel.

How do vitamins and minerals work?

In order to be effective, vitamins and minerals work with the other nutrients found in food. They are known as micronutrients because they are required in very small quantities. Macronutrients, which include oxygen, water, carbohydrates, proteins and fats are needed in large quantities.

What are the functions of macronutrients?

Macronutrients provide energy and help maintain and repair the body.

Oxygen

Cells burn fuel for energy by combining it with oxygen.

Water

Your cells and organs depend on the involvement of water in all processes, including digestion, absorption, circulation and excretion. Water surrounds and fills cells and tissues, forms the basis of body fluids, acts as a lubricant, transports oxygen and nutrients, keeps food moving through your gut, helps to regulate your body temperature and keeps your skin moist. Without food you could probably survive for several weeks; without water you would die in a few days.

Water makes up around 60 per cent of body weight and the average person needs two to three quarts (liters) of water per day to replace what is lost through the skin, urine, bowels and lungs. You obtain water from food, as a by-product of metabolism, and from drinking. Making sure you drink enough water is vital to maintaining good health. Many people do not drink enough.

Protein

Proteins are organic molecules containing carbon, oxygen, hydrogen, nitrogen and in some cases, sulfur. They are made of linked chains of smaller molecules known as amino acids. These amino acids can combine in an infinite number of ways, and thousands of different proteins have been identified. Each protein has a unique sequence of amino acids which gives it a specific structure, shape and chemical characteristics.

The proteins in your body are made up of 20 main naturally occurring amino acids and some other minor ones. Some of these amino acids are essential constituents of your diet as your body cannot make them, whereas others are nonessential as your body can make them. Some amino acids can be considered semi-essential as they are only essential in your diet at certain times in your life, such as during childhood and in high growth demand states such as pregnancy. The essential amino acids are tryptophan, lysine, methionine, phenylalanine, threonine, valine, leucine and isoleucine. Arginine and histidine are considered semi-essential. The nonessential amino acids are tyrosine, glycine, serine, glutamic acid, aspartic acid, taurine, cystine, proline, and alanine.

Proteins are involved in growth, repair and maintenance of body tissues. Enzymes are protein molecules which act as catalysts to stimulate biochemical reactions. There are literally thousands of different enzymes within a single cell that have many functions including the breaking down, joining together or separation of a wide variety of substances. Many hormones are proteins, including insulin, which regulates your blood sugar levels; and thyroid hormone, which controls your metabolic rate. Proteins also play a vital role in the functioning of your immune system, help to keep the correct amount of water in the cells, help to normalize the acid-base balance by acting as buffers, and can also be used as a source of energy for your body. One gram of protein provides 4 calories (17 kJ) of energy.

Carbohydrates

Carbohydrates are organic molecules which contain the elements carbon (C), hydrogen (H), and oxygen (O) in a ratio of 1:2:1. They come in several different types; including simple carbohydrates such as glucose, sucrose and fructose, which are found in refined sugar, fruits and honey; and complex carbohydrates, which are mainly starches and are found in grains, legumes and vegetables. Fiber is also a carbohydrate. Glucose is the end product of most carbohydrate metabolism in the body.

The most important function of dietary carbohydrates is to provide you with energy for all your body functions, including heat production and muscle exertion. Glucose is converted to carbon dioxide and water and energy is released. Each gram of carbohydrate releases four calories of energy for use by the body. Carbohydrates also help in the digestion and assimilation of foods and in the regulation of protein and fat metabolism.

Glucose is the most common source of energy in the body and is particularly important for the brain and red cells as it is the sole source of energy for these body structures. Glucose is important in pregnancy for the formation of structural carbohydrates and lactose for lactation. Excess glucose is stored in the liver

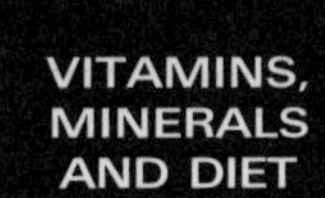

and muscles as glycogen, and when these reserves are filled to capacity, excess glucose is converted to, and stored as, fat.

Some carbohydrates cannot be digested by your body. These include cellulose, which therefore acts as a dietary fiber. Eating plenty of fiber helps to move food through your intestines, which contributes to the elimination of waste products.

Fats

Fats, which are also known as lipids, are compounds that are not soluble in water but are soluble in organic solvents. Like carbohydrates, they contain carbon, hydrogen and oxygen; and some contain nitrogen and phosphorus. The main type of dietary fat is triglycerides; others include phospholipids such as lecithin, and sterols such as cholesterol.

Fats have several vital functions including protecting internal organs from damage, providing insulation, helping to regulate body temperature, and transporting fat soluble substances such as vitamins A, D, E and K. Fats are also a source of energy. One gram of fat provides 9 calories (38 kJ) of energy after absorption. Fats also add flavor to food and help you feel full.

Fats are part of every cell membrane, organ and tissue. The type of fat you eat influences the characteristics of your cell membranes and organs, keeping them healthy or making them susceptible to disease. Fats are also important for the function of the nervous system and are involved in the manufacture of hormones and hormone-like compounds known as prostaglandins.

There are several different types of fats, which affect your health in varying ways. These include saturated, polyunsaturated and monounsaturated fats. All fats contain a mixture of these three types of fat, and one type predominates in a particular food.

Fats that are solid at room temperature are mostly saturated fat. Animal products, such as beef, pork, poultry, whole milk, cheese, sour cream, and yoghurt, as well as coconut, palm and palm kernel oils, contain mostly saturated fats. These fats can increase blood cholesterol levels and therefore raise the risk of heart disease. Eating foods high in saturated fats can also increase the risk of some cancers, including bowel cancer. Trans fats are produced from polyunsaturated fats, typically in margarine manufacture. Due to their adverse effects on health, they are usually grouped with saturated fats.

Fats and oils that are liquid at room temperature are mostly unsaturated, either monounsaturated or polyunsaturated. Canola, olive, and peanut oils are high in monounsaturated fats while corn, soybean, and sunflower oils are high in polyunsaturated fats. Two polyunsaturated fats are necessary for healthy body function. These are the essential fatty acids, linoleic and alpha linolenic acid.

For a few years, people were advised to eat polyunsaturated fats because they lower total blood cholesterol. However it is now known that polyunsaturated fats are susceptible to damage by free radicals and lower levels of beneficial HDL cholesterol. This increases damage to tissues and also the build-up of atherosclerotic plaque in the arteries. High intake of polyunsaturated fats has also been linked to cancer.

Monounsaturated fats can also help to lower levels of harmful LDL cholesterol and raise levels of beneficial HDL cholesterol. As they are less susceptible to oxidation, they do not increase the risk of disease. People who live in countries where the most commonly used type of fat is olive oil tend to have lower risk of diseases such as heart disease and cancer.

How much of each vitamin and mineral do we need?

For every person who asks this question, the answer will be slightly different. Each one of us has different needs and different ways of meeting those needs – a unique combination of stress and biochemical individuality. Genetic factors play an important part in this. For example, recent research indicates that as many as 5 to 15 per cent of people may have a particular type of genetic mutation in the DNA which codes for an enzyme involved in the metabolism of an amino acid known as homocysteine. This leads to higher homocysteine concentrations and therefore an increased risk of heart disease, and in women, of having babies with neural tube defects. Because folate and other B vitamins are involved in homocysteine metabolism, such people have higher folate requirements than those who do not have this type of genetic mutation, and may need supplements. Future research may show the presence of other common genetic variations, which throws doubt on the concept of assuming normality for nutrient requirements in any population.

Lifestyle factors also play a part. Someone who smokes or has a history of illness will have greater vitamin and mineral needs than someone who does not. The nutrient needs of an Olympic athlete are different to those of someone who sits on the couch and watches TV all day. Needs also vary according to sex, age and specific life events; a pregnant woman needs more iron than an elderly woman. Stress, disease, prescription drugs, environmental factors and intense physical activity can also raise requirements.

People vary in their ability to absorb and metabolize different nutrients. One person's genetic make up may mean they get enough vitamin C from an average diet whereas another would benefit from taking a supplement. The amounts and types of food people eat and the way they cook also affects the ability to obtain enough nutritional value from food.

What about Recommended Dietary Allowances?

In an effort to answer the question of how much people should aim to eat of the major nutrients, recommended dietary allowances (RDAs) were established by the Food and Nutrition Board of the US National Academy of Sciences National Research Council. RDAs were originally developed in the 1940s for food production in the military, and since their publication in 1943, they have been recognized as the most authoritative source of information on nutrient levels for healthy people. They are regularly updated, and since publication of the 10th edition in 1989, there has been an enormous amount of new research on the impact of nutrition on chronic disease.

In order to try and take this research into account, the expert panel responsible for setting the RDAs has reviewed and revised its approach and have published a new set of guidelines known as the Dietary References Intakes (DRI).

This new series of references includes what is known about how the nutrient functions in the human body; which factors may affect how it works; and how the nutrient may be related to chronic disease. Scientific research on nutrient metabolism and data on intakes in the US population, are used to set intakes for each age group, from babies to elderly people. Recommendations for pregnancy, lactation and maximum intake are also made.

The DRI provides sets of measures for each nutrient. The first of these is the Estimated Average Requirement (EAR), the intake value that is estimated to meet the requirement in 50 per cent of people in a specific group, usually defined by age and sex. At this level of intake, the remaining 50 per cent of the group would not have its needs met. The Recommended Dietary Allowance (RDA) is the dietary intake level that is sufficient to meet the nutrient requirements of nearly all the people in the group. These values refer to average daily intake over one or more weeks. The Tolerable Upper Intake Level (UL) is the upper limit of intake associated with a low risk of adverse effects in most people. It applies to long-term daily use.

For some essential vitamins and minerals, there is not enough information to come up with RDAs; and even for those nutrients for which they have been established, the lack of enough basic data means that they may be less accurate than they ideally should be. Where the experts consider that there is not enough evidence to come up with RDAs, they have established adequate intake (AI) values. DRIs have been published for the B vitamins, calcium, phosphorus, vitamin D, fluoride and magnesium. Others will follow in the near future.

RDAs are designed for those of average height, weight, nutrient absorption ability and stress levels; and those who do not fit into those categories may need more. RDAs contain a margin of safety to make allowances for individual differences in absorption and metabolism. The RDA can be used as a goal for planning individual dietary intake. It is not intended to be used for assessing the diets of either individuals or groups or for planning diets for groups. The EAR may be more suitable for that purpose.

A separate set of recommendations called Reference Daily Intakes (RDIs) (previously known as the US RDAs) has been developed by the Food and Drug Administration (FDA). These do not vary with age or gender, but take the highest recommended dietary allowance value. On food labels you may see these referred to as Daily Values (DVs), listed for people who eat 2000 to 2500 calories each day.

Other countries use slightly different terms to refer to the RDAs. In Australia, the term Recommended Dietary Intakes (RDI) is used and in the UK, Recommended Nutrient Intakes (RNI).

The RDIs set by the FDA are:

Vitamin A	5,000 iu
Vitamin C	60 mg
Vitamin D	400 IU
Vitamin E	30 IU
Vitamin K	80 mcg
Thiamin (B-1)	1.5 mg
Riboflavin (B-2)	1.7 mg
Niacin (B-3)	20 mg
Vitamin (B-6)	2 mg
Folate	400 mcg
Vitamin B-12	6 mcg
Biotin	300 mcg
Pantothenic Acid (B-5)	10 mg
Calcium	1,000 mg
Magnesium	400 mg
Phosphorous	1,000 mg
Chloride	3,400 mg
Chromium	120 mcg
Copper	2 mg
Iodine	150 mcg
Iron	18 mg
Manganese	2 mg
Molybdenum	75 mcg
Selenium	70 mcg
Zinc	15 mg

RDAs can be used as a basis for planning daily intakes. Many nutritionists advise aiming for 100 per cent of the RDA for all nutrients including vitamins and minerals. Greater intakes of vitamin C, beta carotene (which the body can convert to vitamin A) and vitamin E might be beneficial; but intakes of vitamins and minerals which may be toxic in large doses, such as vitamin A and vitamin D, should be limited to no more than 300 per cent of the RDA.

RDAs are calculated to meet the needs of healthy people, rather than the needs of those who are ill, stressed, taking medications or living in environments which cause nutrient requirements to be raised. They are also designed for people who are not particularly active, and those who exercise a lot may have greater needs. In recognition of the fact that older people usually require much higher levels of nutrients than those covered by the old RDAs, the new DRIs are, in some cases, higher for older people.

The state of optimum health

The answer to the question of how much of each vitamin and mineral a person needs also depends on how healthy a person wants to be. Health can be looked at as a variable state which ranges from severe illness to optimum health. It may be that a person feels healthy, but increasing the intake of vitamins and minerals could improve fitness, mental alertness and recovery time from injury. That person would then move further towards the state of optimum health.

An increasing amount of research suggests that for certain nutrients, particularly the antioxidant vitamins and minerals, the RDA level may not be enough to protect against some of the most prevalent diseases in developed countries, including cancer and heart disease.

While it is not possible to make *accurate* recommendations for the intakes necessary for optimum health, there has been a large amount of research into this issue. The following recommendations are made on the basis of studies which have looked at the therapeutic effects of vitamins and minerals.

Recommended dietary allowances and suggested optimal intakes

	Men	Women	Suggested intake
Vitamin A	1000 mcg RE	800 mcg RE	1500 mcg RE
Beta carotene			10 to 30 mg
Thiamin	1.2 mg	1.1 mg	5 to 10 mg
Riboflavin	1.3 mg	1.1 mg	5 to 10 mg
Niacin	16 mg	14 mg	10 to 100 mg
Vitamin B6	1.3 mg	1.3 mg	2 to 50 mg
(over 50)	1.7 mg	1.5 mg	

Vitamin B12	2.4 mcg	2.4 mcg	11 to 100 mcg
Pantothenic acid	5 mg	5 mg	10 mg
Biotin	30 mcg	30 mcg	30 to 300 mcg
Folic acid	400 mcg	400 mcg	400 mcg
Vitamin C	60 mg	60 mg	100 to 1000 mg
Vitamin D (under 50)	200 IU	200 IU	100 to 600 IU
(over 50)	400 IU	400 IU	
(over 70)	600 IU	600 IU	
Vitamin E	10 mg alpha TE	8 mg alpha TE	67 to 500 mg alpha TE
Vitamin K	80 mcg	65 mcg	60 to 300 mcg
Boron			2 to 7 mg
Calcium (under 50)	1000 mg	1000 mg	1200 to 1500 mg
(over 50)	1200 mg	1200 mg	
Chromium	50 to 200 mcg	50 to 200 mcg	200 to 400 mcg
Copper	1.5 to 3 mg	1.5 to 3 mg	3 mg
Fluoride	3.8 mg	3.1 mg	
Iodine	150 mcg	150 mcg	200 mcg
Iron	10 mg	15 mg	15 to 30 mg
Magnesium	420 mg	320 mg	350 to 500 mg
Manganese	2 to 5 mg	2 to 5 mg	10 mg
Molybdenum	75 to 250 mcg	75 to 250 mcg	250 mcg
Phosphorus	700 mg	700 mg	700 mg
Potassium	2000 mg	2000 mg	2000 to 5000 mg
Selenium	70 mcg	55 mcg	100 to 200 mcg
Vanadium	10 to 60 mcg	10 to 60 mcg	50 to 100 mcg
Zinc	15 mg	12 mg	15 to 30 mg

Is it possible to get enough vitamins and minerals from food?

People living in Western cultures usually have all the nutritional advantages and disadvantages of an affluent lifestyle. By choosing the right types and amounts of food from the wide range of fresh, processed, mixed or pre-prepared food available, it should be possible for the average person to meet the RDAs for vitamins and minerals. However, the food available in Western cultures provides more fats, sugars, sodium and alcohol than is consistent with a healthy diet.

Many, although by no means all, nutrition experts agree that a balanced diet can supply all the vitamins and minerals that a healthy person needs. This line is most often taken by government organizations such as the American

Dietitians Association and the American Heart Association. However, this view may be changing. In the light of recent research on folate and the prevention of neural tube defects, Godfrey Oakley, MD of the Centers for Disease Control in Atlanta, commented in an editorial in the *New England Journal of Medicine,* that "anyone who chooses to counsel a woman to consume 400 mcg of food-derived folate rather than 400 mcg of supplemental folic acid will be recommending a strategy that has not been proved to prevent birth defects and that leads to lower blood folate concentrations."

Leaving aside the fact that opinions differ as to exactly what constitutes a balanced diet, not everyone is able to, or wants to, eat such a diet all the time. Individual vitamin and mineral requirements may vary as much as 200-fold due to differences in genetic make up, lifestyle, physical and emotional stress, and other factors. Some people are able to meet their nutritional requirements with an average diet and no supplements, while others have needs which are greater than their diet can meet.

The issue of the quality of the food we eat is also relevant. Modern methods of food production and manufacturing can adversely affect the nutritional value of food. Soil quality has been lowered through farming methods and the use of fertilizers. Many chemicals are added to food during the growing and processing stages and several of these, including pesticides, can accumulate in the body and have toxic effects. Fruit and vegetables are often picked before they are ripe, in some cases before they have developed their full content of vitamins and minerals. When food is stored for later use, some of the content may decay during storage. Processing of foods removes many valuable nutrients, and a person whose diet is high in these foods may be at risk of nutrient deficiencies.

The basics of a healthy diet

Ideas about what comprises healthy eating behaviour vary from one culture to another. For several generations, America has been a meat and milk country with the daily consumption of dairy products and beef seen as a healthy luxury. However, growing evidence suggests that the typical American diet is too high in protein, fat and salt and too low in fruit, vegetables and complex carbohydrates.

People choose to eat foods for many reasons, not just for their nutritional value. Habit, tradition, economy, convenience, availability, emotional comfort, religious beliefs and environmental concerns play an important part in food choices. It seems that there is no right way for everybody to eat. However, there are some general guidelines to help you eat a healthy diet. It is important to remember that it is the food eaten over a number of days which is important rather than individual meals or days. This allows more flexibility in choosing foods, and fits the theme of consuming a variety of foods with room for the occasional treat.

- Eat a wide variety of different types of foods. This ensures you get all the nutrients you need and limits your intake of the ones which may cause you harm. Eating fresh foods, preferably simple ones that are in season, is vital to make the most of what your food has to offer. Processed and prepared foods should be avoided as much as possible, as they are often high in sugar, salt, fat and additives.
- Try to eat plenty of different types of fruit and vegetables, particularly greens and those that are brightly coloured. They should be raw or lightly cooked and should not be coated in fatty dressings or cream sauces. If possible, eat organic to minimise consumption of pesticides.
- Legumes and whole grains should be regularly included in your diet . They are great sources of carbohydrate, and they contain healthy levels of protein and many other beneficial substances.
- Complex carbohydrates should account for around 40 to 50 per cent of total calories consumed; more if you exercise a lot. Whole grain products are better than refined ones because they still contain the vitamins and minerals lost in the refining process.
- Try to limit your sugar intake, particularly if you suffer mood swings, depression and fluctuating energy levels. If you do eat sugar, try not to combine it with fat, particularly if you are trying to lose weight.
- The latest research on fat suggests that it is not just how much you eat but what type that increases the risk of obesity and disease. Try to cut down on foods high in saturated fat such as meat, whole milk, butter, palm oil and coconut oil. Polyunsaturated fats found in margarine and some vegetable oils are linked to an increased risk of cancer, autoimmune diseases and lowered immunity. Replace these fats with olive oil, preferably extra virgin or virgin. It is consistently associated with lower disease levels. Beneficial omega-3 fatty acids are found in oily fish and oils such as flaxseed oil, and these should be included in your diet as often as possible.
- Limit your protein intake. A 110 g serving of meat, chicken, fish or tofu once a day is likely to be enough unless you are pregnant, breastfeeding or ill. Too much protein may contribute to fatigue, lowered immunity, lack of energy and liver and kidney problems. It also leaches minerals such as calcium out of your body, and increases the risk of osteoporosis.
- Limit intake of dairy products as they can aggravate mucus production and lower immunity.

- Limit salt intake, particularly if you are salt-sensitive.
- How your body processes the food you eat is as important as the food you put into it. Try to eat with full attention and chew your food properly. Eating with care and attention helps your body to digest food more efficiently than if you eat when you are angry or stressed. And last but by no means least, learn to trust your body and understand its needs and signals. Eating should be a pleasurable experience and eating foods you don't like because you think they are good for you is not listening to your body.
- Drink alcohol in moderation if at all. Children, adolescents and pregnant women should not drink alcohol.

How does food preparation affect vitamins and minerals?

The way food is prepared also affects its nutritional value. For example, fried chicken contains twice the calories of grilled chicken but the same amount of protein, vitamins and minerals. The way food is stored and cooked affects the vitamin and mineral content. Some vitamins are easily affected by exposure to light, heat and air.

- Vitamins A, D, E and K, riboflavin and beta carotene are destroyed when exposed to light.
- Vitamins C, A, B12, folic acid and thiamin are destroyed by heat.
- Vitamins C, A, D, E, K, B12 and folic acid are destroyed by exposure to air.
- Vitamins C, B6, thiamin, riboflavin, niacin, selenium, potassium and magnesium leach into cooking water.
- Vitamins C, B12, folic acid, thiamin and riboflavin are destroyed when combined with acid or alkaline substances.

To make the most of the vitamins and minerals in food, there are several guidelines to follow.

Food storage

- Eat fruit and vegetables as fresh as possible.
- Store refrigerated foods at less than 40°F, frozen foods below 0°F and canned and dry food in a cool, dry place.
- Store canned and frozen food for no longer than the use by date.
- Store grains, flour and dried beans and peas in dark containers or in the refrigerator.

Food preparation

- Cook food in a minimal amount of water for the shortest possible time. Vegetables should be just tender rather than soggy and overcooked. Frozen vegetables should be cooked without thawing and fresh vegetables should be chopped just before cooking or serving.
- Use low to moderate heat when cooking meat, eggs and milk.
- Use the leftover liquid for sauces, stews or juices.

What about enriched and fortified foods?

Adding vitamins and minerals to certain foods is common practice in developed countries. Enrichment involves putting back nutrients lost during processing, while a fortified food will have a nutrient added to levels not present in its natural state. For example, flour is usually enriched with thiamin, riboflavin and niacin, and milk is fortified with vitamin D. Since January 1998, commercial grain products in the USA have also been enriched with 140 mcg of folic acid per 100 g of grain product. It is estimated that this will deliver an average increase in intake of 100 mcg per day. Breakfast cereals may contain up to a daily dose of folic acid.

For many people, these foods are very important sources of vitamins and minerals and may be responsible for the low levels of deficiency diseases seen today. However, enriched foods often contain much lower levels of nutrients than those which are present in the unprocessed versions. For example, almost all the B vitamins are removed from the cereals and grains used in baking and only a few are put back synthetically during enriching. Eating a diet that includes, but is not limited to, enriched foods is one way to get essential nutrients.

When choosing foods, it is important to read the labels carefully as these contain information on the fat, sugar, salt and vitamin and mineral content of food. In general, the more processed a food is, the higher the salt, sugar and fat content and the lower the vitamin, mineral and fiber content.

How good is the average diet?

Surveys suggest that most people do not consume a balanced diet. Results of nutrition surveys show a large gap between the dietary guidelines and what people actually eat. The US National Health and Nutrition Examination Survey (NHANES II) shows that sugar intake makes up 25 per cent of total calories and fat intake approaches 34 per cent. This means that foods which have poor nutritional value make up over half the daily calories.

Other results show that:

- On any one day, an estimated 45 per cent of people don't consume any fruit or juice and 22 per cent don't eat any vegetables. Less than 10 per cent of people consume the recommended five or more servings of fruit and vegetables.
- Only a third of the population consumes foods from all the food groups on a typical day, with less than 3 per cent consuming foods from all food groups in at least the recommended amount.
- Many diets contain half the recommended amount of magnesium and folic acid; as many as 80 per cent of women who exercise may be iron-deficient; and the average calcium intake is 636 mg per day (two-thirds the RDA).
- Seventy-one per cent of males and 90 per cent of females consumed less than the 1980 recommended dietary allowance (RDA) of vitamin B6.
- The average calcium intake of teenage girls resembles that necessary for 3–5 year olds.

How common are nutrient deficiencies?

It is often difficult to link one vitamin with a particular disease except in severe cases where a deficiency results in well-documented physical symptoms. For example, bleeding gums are a sign of scurvy which is caused by lack of vitamin C, and goiter is caused by an iodine deficiency.

Nutrient deficiencies occur for several reasons; including inadequate intake, inadequate absorption, inadequate utilization, increased requirement, increased excretion and increased breakdown. Anyone in whom these situations are found is at risk of deficiency. In developed countries, where the food supply is good, there are relatively few cases of severe deficiency. However, the statistics given above suggest that marginal deficiencies may be common.

Nutrient deficiencies can be classified into five stages:

1. A preliminary deficiency.
2. A biochemical deficiency where the nutrient concentration in the tissues becomes lower.
3. A physiological stage where the critical body processes, such as enzymes and hormones that depend on the nutrient are slowly lost. The first three stages are sub-clinical or marginal stages.
4. A clinical stage where the signs of the deficiency are obvious and can be detected by the eye.
5. An anatomical stage which can lead to death.

Marginal deficiency symptoms are nonspecific and can often go unnoticed or be attributed to other causes. When combined with other factors such as disease, prescription drugs, stress, smoking and pollution, they can increase susceptibility to illness or lead to clinical deficiencies. It is possible that marginal nutrient deficiencies play a role in many of the diseases of old age such as osteoporosis, arthritis, heart disease and high blood pressure. Ensuring optimal intakes of vitamins and minerals is therefore vital for present and future health.

What are the signs of marginal nutrient deficiencies?

There are many signs of marginal nutrient deficiencies and these can often be similar for different nutrients. In many cases, the only signs of a marginal deficiency will be vague symptoms such as fatigue, lethargy, difficulty concentrating or just feeling that things are not quite right. Diagnosing marginal deficiencies is difficult as many laboratory tests are expensive and time-consuming, if they are available at all. Marginal deficiencies of single nutrients are rare as it is likely that a person whose diet is deficient in one vitamin or mineral is deficient in others too. Some marginal deficiency symptoms include:

- Bruising easily may be linked to vitamin C and K deficiency.
- High cholesterol may be due to antioxidant vitamin and B complex deficiencies.
- Reduced taste sensation may be due to zinc deficiency.
- Fatigue may be due to iron, vitamin B12, folic acid or iodine deficiency.
- High blood pressure may be due to potassium and calcium deficiencies.
- Muscle cramps and pains may be due to calcium and magnesium deficiencies.
- Osteoporosis may be linked to calcium deficiency.

There is increasing evidence to suggest that long-term marginal intake of certain nutrients can increase the risk of developing degenerative diseases such as cancer, diabetes and heart disease.

Can cravings be a sign of vitamin or mineral deficiencies?

It is possible that nutrient deficiencies may result in cravings for certain foods; for example, potassium deficiency might result in a craving for bananas or potatoes; calcium deficiency might result in a craving for cheese, milk; and B vitamin deficiency in a craving for nuts. There are, however, many other factors such as food allergies and hormonal influences which may play a role in food cravings. There is evidence to suggest that inadequate vitamins and minerals in the diet may result in cravings which cause people to fill up on foods that are high in calories and low in nutrients, causing the increasingly common problem of obesity.

Are there tests for vitamin and mineral deficiencies?

There are many tests for assessing vitamin and mineral status. They vary widely in availability, credibility and accuracy. A detailed medical history and physical examination can detect clinical vitamin and mineral deficiencies in more advanced stages. Such an examination would involve looking carefully at weight, height, the condition of skin, hair, fingernails, tongue, eyes and the mucous membranes inside the mouth and eyes.

Laboratory tests of blood, urine or tissues can detect vitamin or mineral deficiencies at an earlier stage than a physical examination. Blood levels of various enzymes are also indicators of nutritional status. However, many laboratory tests are too expensive and complicated to conduct on a routine basis.

There are many alternative tests to determine nutritional status. However, there is no proof that these tests can provide a complete analysis of a person's nutritional state. They may be useful in certain cases. Hair analysis, as a test for nutritional status, is considered unreliable as results can be affected by shampoo, dyes, tobacco smoke and other environmental factors. Hair growth can also slow down in malnourished people, increasing nutrient concentrations in hair while body stores drop. It can be a useful test for toxic metal concentrations.

Are vitamin and mineral supplements necessary?

Whether or not vitamin and mineral supplements are necessary is the most controversial topic in nutrition. The question of a need for supplements is central to the debate about the levels of vitamins and minerals required to promote optimal health. Given that people vary so much in their requirements and that very few people eat really well-balanced diets, vitamin and mineral supplements can be viewed as a relatively inexpensive form of 'nutritional insurance'. Increasing evidence suggests that the amounts of nutrients adequate to prevent deficiencies are not the same as those necessary for optimal health.

Who takes supplements?

Data from the second National Health and Nutrition Examination Survey (NHANES II) suggest that almost 35 per cent of Americans between 18 and

74 years of age take vitamin and mineral supplements regularly. Other surveys put the figure much higher. In 1988, Americans spent approximately $2-2.5 billion on vitamin and mineral supplements. The total amount spent on foods and pill supplements for health benefits was $6 billion. Nutritional supplements are big business and marketing hype often starts where the scientific evidence ends.

Those who use supplements tend to be older, have higher income and higher education levels. However, statistics also show that those with higher nutrient intakes are more likely to take vitamin supplements. This means that, in many cases, supplements are taken most often by those who need them least.

The most popular supplements are multivitamins, vitamin C, vitamin E, B complex, calcium and magnesium. Recent media coverage of the benefits of herbs such as Echinacea, St John's wort and Ginkgo means that these are also very popular. Women are more likely to use supplements than men, and most people who take them tend to do so because they feel that their food is of poor quality and contains toxic chemicals. Some people see supplements as health insurance and some take them for what they see as their specific benefits; for example, vitamin C for colds.

Who might need supplements?

Many people may benefit from a balanced vitamin and mineral supplement, including those who have irregular eating habits, skip meals, or eat large amounts of processed and refined foods. There are also certain groups of people who are at particular risk of nutrient deficiencies because of other lifestyle, environmental or disease factors. The following are some examples of those at risk.

- Older people often have higher nutrient needs than younger ones due to lower dietary intake, reduced absorption and metabolism, and illness. Lack of appetite, loss of taste and smell, and denture problems can all contribute to a poor diet. Older people who eat alone or are depressed may also not eat enough to get all the nutrients you need from food. Those age 65 or older are likely to need to increase intake of several nutrients, particularly vitamin B6, vitamin B12 and vitamin D because of reduced absorption. They may benefit from supplements (See page 454 for more information.) There's also evidence that a multivitamin may improve immune function and decrease the risk of infections in older people.
- Premenopausal women may benefit from iron supplements as their diets are often low in this mineral and iron deficiency anemia is relatively common.

However, there is evidence that too much iron can increase the risk of heart disease in those who are susceptible, and certain people should avoid iron supplements (See page 258 for more information.)

- Postmenopausal women have high calcium needs (up to 1500 mg per day in those not taking hormone replacement therapy). This amount is not usually found in multivitamin supplements as it is too bulky and separate supplements may be useful (See page 197 for more information.) Higher vitamin D intake is also necessary.
- It is worth considering taking extra vitamin C, vitamin E and beta carotene as several studies show that these vitamins in large doses may help protect against aging-related disorders such as cancer, heart disease, diabetes and cataracts. This may be particularly important in those who have a family history of such diseases.
- Pregnant women are routinely prescribed folic acid supplements to prevent neural tube defects; and calcium, iron and zinc requirements also substantially increase. (See page 104 for more information.)
- Someone who is chronically ill has higher nutrient needs and may find vitamin and mineral supplements useful, particularly if they are taking long- term medications.
- Supplements may also be beneficial for those on weight loss diets. Many people, particularly women, eat low calorie diets which are inadequate in iron, calcium and zinc.
- If your diet has limited variety due to intolerance or allergy, you may benefit from a vitamin-mineral supplement.
- Diseases of the liver, gallbladder, intestine and pancreas, or digestive tract surgery, may interfere with normal digestion and absorption of nutrients. Anyone with one of these conditions may be advised to supplement with vitamins and minerals.
- Strict vegetarians who avoid meat and dairy products must obtain vitamin B12 from supplements. They may also benefit from extra iron, calcium and zinc (See page 448 for more information.)
- Those who smoke may benefit from vitamin C supplements. Smoking reduces vitamin C levels and causes production of harmful free radicals.
- Those who drink a large amount of alcohol may need supplements. Alcohol affects the absorption, metabolism and excretion of vitamins.
- Those under physical or emotional stress may also benefit from supplements.

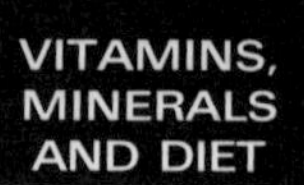

Where do the vitamins in supplements come from?

Most vitamins are extracted from the food sources in which they naturally occur. For example, vitamin A is often extracted from fish liver oil. Vitamin B comes from yeast or liver, vitamin C from rose hips, and vitamin E from soybeans, wheatgerm or corn.

Supplements are available from many sources but most supplement manufacturers get the raw materials from the same small group of suppliers. They are then packaged and labeled before being sent to distributors or retail outlets.

What types of supplements are available?

There is a vast range of vitamin, mineral and other nutritional supplements available in supermarkets, health food stores and drugstores. Products vary widely in quality and effectiveness, and evidence to support some of the claims made by those who sell them is inconclusive at best.

Most supplement manufacturers follow good manufacturing practices, which ensure that the product contains what it says on the label; that it breaks down to a form which is available for absorption; and does not contain toxic chemicals. If in doubt, it is worth checking with the supplier. Good quality supplements are available from medical practitioners, health food stores, drugstores and supermarkets. Many experts recommend buying name brands or own brand supplements from large national stores with a reputation for quality.

Vitamin and mineral supplements come in various forms. The most common are tablets which are convenient to store and carry and have the longest shelf life. Capsules are also easy to store, but may not be as good at protecting the contents from oxidation. Enteric-coated capsules, which are also known as timed release supplements, are another form. They are designed to pass through the stomach to dissolve in the intestine. Fat soluble vitamins and other oil supplements often come in the form of gelatin capsules. Powder forms do not contain fillers, binders or additives. Liquids are suitable for people who have difficulty swallowing capsules.

Vitamin supplements contain many other substances such as fillers, binders, lubricants, disintegrators, colors, flavors and sweeteners, coating materials and drying agents. A person who is prone to allergies should check the ingredients of a particular type of supplement.

When buying supplements, it is helpful to have a clear idea of what nutrients are necessary, and in what amounts. This should be based on dietary strengths and weaknesses and particular needs. Reading the labels carefully should provide enough information to match the product with a person's individual needs.

Supplement labeling

The US government has recently announced new rules on the labeling of dietary supplements. The new rules are designed to give consumers more complete information regarding the ingredients in dietary supplements. They apply to vitamins, minerals, herbs and amino acids. The rules require the products to be labeled as dietary supplements and to carry a 'Supplement Facts' panel that lists how much of the RDI of nutrients are in the product. For ingredients that have no RDI, such as herbs, the package will list the ingredients. Herbal products must identify the part of the plant used to make the substance.

Supplements could only claim to be 'high potency' if a nutrient is present at 100 per cent or more of the RDI. For multivitamin supplements to carry the 'high potency' labeling, at least two-thirds of the nutrients must be present at levels that are more than 100 per cent of the RDI.

The term, antioxidant, may be used to describe a nutrient where scientific evidence shows that if it is absorbed in sufficient quantity, the nutrient (such as vitamin C) will inactivate free radicals or prevent free radical-initiated chemical reactions in the body.

The amounts of vitamins and minerals in supplements are indicated in a number of ways:

- A milligram (mg) is 1/1000th of a gram (g); there are 1000 mg in a gram.
- A microgram (abbreviated mcg or mg) is 1/1000th of a milligram; there are 1,000,000 micrograms in a gram.
- The international unit (IU) is an arbitrary measure used for vitamin A (and beta carotene), vitamin D and vitamin E.
- Retinol equivalents (RE) are now being used to measure vitamin A (and beta carotene activity) and tocopherol equivalents (TE) to measure vitamin E. This is because vitamins A and E are found in several different forms in the body and these measurement units make it possible to compare the various forms (See pages 39 and 163 for more information.)

Types of supplements

There are various types of supplements. Different preparations suit different people and it is a good idea to experiment with different types to find the best combination.

Water solubilized fat soluble vitamins

The oil soluble vitamins A, D, E and K are available in dry or water soluble form for people who cannot, or do not want to consume oil, for example acne sufferers or people with fat malabsorption disorders such as celiac disease.

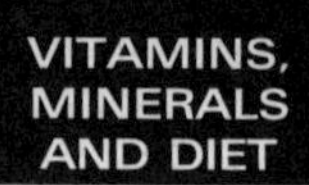

Natural vs synthetic

In most cases, natural vitamins have not been shown to be more beneficial than synthetic vitamins. However, vitamin E seems to be the exception and the natural form of vitamin E, d-alpha tocopherol is more potent than the synthetic form, dl-alpha tocopherol. Sometimes vitamin supplements contain other compounds which may enhance the effectiveness of the vitamin, although this is a much debated issue. For example, natural vitamin C contains compounds known as bioflavonoids which, although they may or may not enhance absorption, possibly have anticancer properties of their own. Yeast grown on chromium and selenium-rich media form organic compounds which may be better absorbed by the body than inorganic salts.

Chelated minerals

Some minerals in supplements are combined with other compounds to make organic forms. This process is known as chelation and may make the minerals more digestible as it is similar to the form in which they occur in nature. For example, ferrous fumarate is a chelated form of iron. Chelated mineral supplements may be absorbed better than nonchelated minerals. Some people, particularly those who are older, often have low stomach acid; and minerals are often chelated with acidic compounds, for example calcium citrate. In some cases, chelated minerals may be less irritating to the stomach than nonchelated minerals.

Timed release supplements

Timed release or sustained release vitamins are designed to dissolve and be absorbed slowly. The theory behind this is that the vitamins have maximum effectiveness when blood levels are stable, and losses through excretion are minimal. However, some experts believe that timed release supplements are not necessarily better. It is possible that by the time some of these tablets have dissolved, they have passed the particular part of the intestine where they would be absorbed. High blood levels of some vitamins may also be useful in treating some conditions.

General guidelines for buying and taking supplements

- A well-balanced multivitamin supplement is usually better than several single supplements. Such supplements contain approximately 100 per cent to 300 per cent of the RDA for those vitamins and minerals which may have protective effects or are often lacking in the diets of many people. These include vitamins A (preferably in the form of beta carotene), E, C, thiamin, riboflavin, niacin, B6, folic acid, pantothenic acid, biotin, calcium, copper, iron, magnesium and zinc. However, many multivitamin and mineral supplements do not contain sufficient calcium or magnesium, and additional single supplements may be useful for those who need higher doses, such as postmenopausal women.

- Some supplements group vitamin A and beta carotene together, making it difficult to tell how much of each is present. A supplement which provides vitamin A as beta carotene only may be best. Most multivitamin supplements contain only small amounts of beta carotene so it may be worth taking a separate supplement; although probably not if you are a smoker.
- It may be beneficial to choose a supplement that provides minerals in the following amounts: chromium 50 to 200 mcg, manganese 2.5 to 5.0 mg, selenium 50 to 200 mcg. Amounts much higher than this may be toxic.
- Supplements which contain useless or potentially harmful substances should be avoided. Most experts feel that ingredients which have not been shown to be necessary in the diet may merely increase the price of a supplement. It is also best to avoid products which contain artificial flavor, preservatives and color.
- Expensive supplements are not necessarily better. It is more important to check the nutrient content of the supplement. Supplements with the same ingredients which are priced much lower than various reliable brands may not be high quality and those which are priced considerably higher may be too expensive.
- Avoid expensive supplements sold through multilevel marketing (MLM). These include multimineral and spray vitamins. There is almost no scientific evidence to support the claims that are often made, and the products are over-priced.
- Vitamins should be stored in a cool dry place away from direct sunlight in a closed container. If they are kept sealed, in these conditions they should last for two or three years. Once they are opened, they usually have a 12-month shelf life.
- If you are unsure whether the products you are buying will break down in your stomach in time to be absorbed, try dropping the tablet into a glass of vinegar. If it dissolves in 30 minutes it is likely you will be able to absorb the nutrients it contains.

Supplements are no substitute for a balanced diet

The most important thing to remember is that supplements are no substitute for a balanced diet. Even the best vitamin studies only show a partial reduction in the risk of disease. No supplement allows a person to smoke, drink a lot of alcohol, eat whatever they want and still stay healthy. There are many substances, other than vitamins and minerals, which play an essential role in protecting against disease and improving health. Many studies show that people whose diets are high in fruit and vegetables live longer. For example, eating broccoli, carrots and leafy green vegetables does appear to be more protective than taking beta carotene and vitamin C supplements. As well as being a good source of beta carotene and vitamin C, broccoli contains compounds known as indoles that may protect against certain forms of cancer. It is also high in fiber.

When should you take supplements?

Vitamins work with food so supplements should usually be taken with meals. This also helps to minimize the nausea, heartburn and other gastric disturbances that some supplements can cause if taken on an empty stomach. The digestive juices can help to break down supplements so they are better absorbed. Supplements can be easier to swallow if taken with thicker liquids such as juices. It may be better to take supplements in smaller doses several times per day.

Some experts feel that, if vitamins are taken once a day it should be after the largest meal, which is usually dinner. Others feel that the body is in the best state to absorb nutrients earlier in the day.

Some vitamins and minerals compete for absorption or antagonize each other. In these cases, it may be best to take the supplements at different times; although if a person is taking large doses of supplements, these interactions may not matter.

Can large doses of vitamins be harmful?

For the majority of people who take a daily multivitamin supplement with no more than 100 per cent of the RDA, the risks of side effects are probably small. However, high doses of some vitamins can have serious side effects.

Fat soluble vitamins stay in the body longer than water soluble ones, and there have been cases where large doses of vitamin A and vitamin D have had toxic effects. These cases are rare and symptoms disappear when the large doses are stopped. Research has suggested that temporary and even permanent damage can be caused by overdosing on B vitamins. People at risk of developing kidney stones should avoid large doses of vitamin C (see sections on individual vitamins for cautions).

Interactions between different nutrients are very complex. Minerals work in critical ratios to one another. Too high an intake of one mineral may result in a deficiency of another so minerals should be taken in one-to-one RDA ratios. For example, excessive zinc intakes can result in iron and copper losses, so if daily zinc intake is doubled from 15 mg to 30 mg, then daily iron intake should be doubled from 10 mg to 20 mg to maintain the ratio.

Are large doses of vitamins beneficial for certain conditions?

Megavitamin or megadose therapy is the use of vitamins and minerals in amounts greater than ten times the RDA. Vitamins exert their natural physiological functions by binding to compounds such as enzymes. The amount of a particular enzyme that a cell can make is limited, and when the vitamin has bound to all the available enzymes, it may not exert any greater physiological effect. Vitamins and minerals in doses larger than those needed for these effects exert pharmacological or drug-like effects. An example of this is the use of niacin at 40 times the RDA to lower cholesterol.

The use of vitamins and minerals in this way is relatively new and in most cases, extremely controversial. Many of these treatments are not accepted by mainstream medical doctors for the reason that there is a lot of ambiguity, incomplete information and hypothesis.

Orthomolecular medicine

Orthomolecular medicine is defined as "the preservation of good health and the treatment of disease by varying the concentrations of substances in the human body that are normally present and required for health." This definition was given by the Nobel Prize winning chemist, Linus Pauling, who believed that many diseases can be treated or prevented by finding the optimal amounts of nutrients required for each person's health.

Orthomolecular medicine is concerned not only with maintaining optimal health but with the prevention and treatment of disease. Experiments using large doses of vitamins have included niacin therapy for schizophrenia, vitamin C for cancer and viral illnesses, and vitamin B6 for carpal tunnel syndrome. The results of these and other nutrition studies have generated a lot of media attention. One of the main criticisms of those who use orthomolecular medicine is that their research has little support from clinical trials.

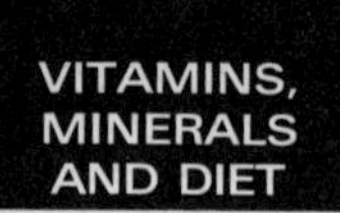

Clinical trials

Much of the information we have about the effects of vitamins comes from clinical trials. A clinical trial is an experiment conducted with patients as subjects. The strongest experimental design is the randomized design in which subjects (patients) are randomly assigned to treatment groups. Some clinical trials compare treatment methods and others assess the affect of a particular treatment on prevention of disease.

Controlled trial

A controlled trial is a study in which researchers actively produce a treatment and deliberately assign people to the treatments.

Randomized trial

In a randomized clinical trial, there are two or more therapeutic treatment groups. One treatment may be a placebo control in which a biologically inert substance is used. Often, the 'control' condition is compared to experimental treatments.

Single-blind trial

A trial in which the treatment is given in such a way that the subject cannot tell what it is. This helps to minimize other effects of the treatment, such as the placebo effect.

Double-blind trial

A double-blind trial is a completely random design where there is one real treatment and a placebo. Not only are the subjects assigned to the two groups at random, but neither the subjects nor those administering the treatments knows which treatment a subject is getting.

Observational study

Researchers observe what happens but do not actively intervene with the assignment of people to treatment groups.

Crossover trial

A trial in which participants receive two or more treatments one after the other and act as their own controls for comparison of drug treatments

Anecdotal evidence

Evidence based upon haphazard observations which come to attention because they are striking in some way.

Confounding factor

A factor that is not taken into account that gets mixed up with the treatment factors and has a marked effect on the response.

Bias

The favoring of certain outcomes not due to the treatments.

Epidemiological studies

The study of the occurrence, distribution and causes of disease in man.

Prospective cohort study

In this type of epidemiological study two groups (cohorts) of subjects are identified, one of which is exposed to a treatment, an environmental condition, or health risk factor, and the other group is not. The subjects are then followed over time and the effects assessed.

Case-control study

In an epidemiological case-control study a group of patients who already have a disease or other outcome (the cases) is compared to another group of controls who do not. These studies are done retrospectively.

Meta analysis

A systematic review of studies that pools the results of two or more studies to obtain the answer to an overall question of interest.

How reliable are scientific studies reported in the news?

Media reporting of nutritional issues can often add to the confusion that most people feel. Sometimes news stories about health seem to contradict one another, one says something is good for you, and another says that the same thing is bad for you. Conflicting medical reports can make even the most educated consumer confused about what to believe and what to do.

Nutrition stories regularly make headlines in newspapers and magazines and often seem credible because they claim to report 'scientific research.' Due to the pressure to report whatever is new, some stories get more media attention than they deserve and can become distorted in the process. News stories, particularly those on TV and radio, must often be condensed because of space limitations. It is worth analyzing the whole article to find out more about the research. Studies tend to carry more weight if they are done in large academic institutions, by well-qualified researchers and reported in reputable scientific journals which have been reviewed by other scientists. Studies done on humans rather than animals and on large groups of people are also more significant.

No single scientific study, however well done, can change the totality of evidence. There are many links in the process of drawing conclusions about the course of a disease and the ability of vitamins and minerals to affect it. A new

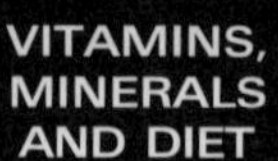

study may move current thinking a little bit more in one direction than another, but a large number of studies from different places are necessary to understand a disease process. Science requires repeatable experiments. If a nutrient is useful, the effects will be seen time and again if the experiments are done properly.

Vitamins

Vitamin A and carotenes

For thousands of years, liver has been used as a cure for night blindness but it was only in the early part of the 20th century that researchers discovered that it is a rich source of vitamin A, which is essential for healthy eyes. The first vitamin to be discovered, vitamin A was identified in 1913 when two American scientists showed that butter and egg yolk contained a substance which was necessary for healthy growth in rats. They called this substance 'fat soluble A'.

In 1930 the structure of vitamin A was determined, and five years later it was found to be necessary for normal vision. In the years that followed, researchers started to study the vital role vitamin A plays in growth, development and reproduction.

Vitamin A is the name given to a group of compounds which have certain actions in the body. One of these compounds is called retinol and it is used as a standard against which the activity of other compounds can be measured.

While the vitamin A we obtain from food comes in many different forms, these can be divided into two main types - pre-formed vitamin A and provitamin A. Pre-formed vitamin A which is often in the form of retinol or retinal, is found in foods of animal origin such as liver and butter. Provitamin A is the name given to around 50 compounds in a group of plant pigments known as carotenes (or carotenoids), with beta carotene being the best known of these. This is because these compounds can be turned into vitamin A in the body. Both pre-formed vitamin A and provitamin A are fat soluble.

Vitamin A

QUICK GUIDE

Essential for

- healthy eyes and vision
- growth, repair and cell differentiation
- health of epithelial cells
- protection against infection
- a healthy reproductive system

Absorption and metabolism

Fat is necessary for vitamin A absorption.

Deficiency

Symptoms include night blindness, xerophthalmia, dry skin, retarded growth, increased susceptibility to infection and cancer.

Sources

Good sources of pre-formed vitamin A include liver, butter, whole milk and egg yolks.

Daily recommended dietary intakes

Men	1000 mcg RE (3333 IU)
Women	800 mcg RE (2666 IU)
Pregnancy	800 mcg RE (2666 IU)
Lactation	+500 mcg RE (1666 IU)

1 mcg RE is equivalent to 3.33 International Units (IU).

Toxic effects of excess intake

Symptoms include headaches; bone and joint pain; dry, itchy skin; and liver damage. High daily doses of vitamin A (above 3000 mcg RE) in pregnancy may cause birth deformities.

Interactions

Mineral oil laxatives, cholestyramine, colchicine and alcohol decrease vitamin A absorption.

Therapeutic uses of supplements

Supplements are used to boost immunity; prevent cancer; treat skin disorders such as acne and psoriasis; and treat eye problems.

Cautions

Supplements should not be taken with vitamin A-derivative acne drugs or broad spectrum antibiotics. Pregnant women should avoid doses of vitamin A above 3000 mcg RE.

What it does in the body

Vitamin A is essential, either directly or indirectly, for the function of all the organs in your body and is particularly important for growth and development. Despite the fact that vitamin A was the first vitamin to be discovered, its actions in the cells of our bodies are not well understood at a chemical level.

Maintenance of normal vision

Our eyes need vitamin A to function effectively as vitamin A is involved in the production of a chemical called visual purple, which helps us to see in dim light.

Growth, repair and cell differentiation

Vitamin A is necessary for the growth and repair of many body cells including those of bones, teeth, collagen and cartilage. It is also essential for a process known as cell differentiation in which unspecialized cells are modified so that they can perform specific functions. Thus vitamin A plays a central role in tissue development and maintenance.

Health of epithelial cells

Vitamin A is vital for the formation of healthy epithelial cells. These cells cover the internal and external surfaces of the body and are found in the skin, lungs, developing teeth, inner ear, cornea of the eye, sex organs, glands and their ducts, gums, nose, cervix and other areas. Many epithelial cells produce mucus which is necessary to lubricate body surfaces and protect against invading micro-organisms. For example, the good health of the digestive tract lining is important in protecting against ulcers, and maintenance of the lining of the vagina and uterus is important in fertility.

Pregnancy and fetal development

Because of its vital role in cell development and differentiation, adequate vitamin A helps to ensure that the changes which occur in the cells and tissues during fetal development take place normally. It may be involved in cell to cell communication.

Protection against infection

Known as 'the anti-infective vitamin', vitamin A plays an essential role in protecting your body from infection. It keeps body surfaces healthy so they can act as barriers to invading micro-organisms. Vitamin A stimulates and enhances many immune functions including antibody response and the activity of various white blood cells such as T helper cells and phagocytes. This immune-enhancing function promotes healing of infected tissues and increases resistance to infection.

Other actions

Laboratory experiments have shown vitamin A to have antiviral activity. Vitamin A also has antioxidant activity and has a role in protecting against free radical damage which contributes to many common diseases. (See page 417 for more information.) Vitamin A is involved in iron metabolism and storage.

Absorption and metabolism

The presence of fat and bile in the intestines is necessary for vitamin A absorption. Around 80 to 90 per cent of vitamin A in the diet is absorbed, although this is reduced in older people and those who have trouble absorbing fat, such as pancreatitis, celiac disease and cystic fibrosis sufferers, who may run the risk of vitamin A deficiency.

Vitamin A is joined to fatty acids in the intestinal lining, combined with other substances and transported to the liver, which stores 90 per cent of the body's vitamin A.

Deficiency

The World Health Organization estimates that as many as 250 million children worldwide are threatened by vitamin A deficiency. However, it is relatively rare in developed countries and is usually limited to those who have absorption difficulties, liver disease or who drink a lot of alcohol. Vitamin A deficiency is common in alcoholics and contributes to some of the disorders of alcoholism such as night blindness, skin problems, cirrhosis of the liver and susceptibility to infections.

Eyes

One of the first symptoms of deficiency is night blindness due to lack of visual purple. Prolonged deficiency leads to xerophthalmia, a condition in which eyes become dry, ulcers appear on the cornea, the eyelids become swollen and sticky, and which eventually leads to blindness. Vitamin A deficiency is the leading preventable cause of blindness in developing countries.

Skin

Prolonged deficiency leads to thickened dry skin which is prone to infections. Small hardened bumps of a protein known as keratin may develop around the hair follicles.

Growth

Deficiency causes growth retardation; weight loss; diarrhea, thickening of bone shafts; congenital malformations; impaired hearing, taste and smell; wasting of testicles; and reduced sperm count. Inadequate vitamin A intake can lead to improper tooth formation in children and to gum disease.

Immune system

Epithelial surfaces are adversely affected by vitamin A deficiency, causing increased susceptibility to skin and respiratory infections. Immune cells and antibody functions are also affected which may lead to an increase in pre-cancerous cells in the epithelial tissues of the mouth, throat and lungs.

Many studies have shown that vitamin A deficiency is associated with increased risk of infection in developing countries. This may also be the case in developed countries. A 1992 study involving 20 children with measles in Long Beach, California found that half of them were vitamin A deficient.[1]

Vitamin A deficiency is often seen in HIV-positive people and this may be due to metabolic changes associated with HIV infection. A 1995 study done on HIV-infected drug users in the US found that there was a higher risk of death in those with vitamin A deficiency. Vitamin A deficiency is often seen in HIV-positive pregnant women and severe deficiency increases infant mortality and the risk of mother-to-child transmission of HIV.

Thyroid gland

A deficiency of vitamin A can contribute to lower levels of active thyroid hormone with symptoms of low body temperature, depression, difficulty with weight loss, headaches and lethargy.

Cancer

Several population studies suggest links between low vitamin A intakes and various types of cancer, particularly those of the lungs, head and neck. Vitamin A deficiency may also increase the risk of breast cancer. In a study published in 1997, researchers at Harvard School of Public Health compared the concentrations of various forms of vitamin A in the breast fat tissue from 46 cancer patients and 63 women with benign breast lumps. They found an increased risk of disease in those with low levels of vitamin A.[2]

Other disorders

Low blood levels of vitamin A may be associated with the development of heart disease. Researchers involved in a 1997 study done in Madrid, Spain looked at vitamin A levels in 62 heart attack patients and compared these with levels in 62 people free of heart disease. The results showed that vitamin A levels in heart attack patients were almost 25 per cent lower.[3] Vitamin A levels have also been found to be low in rheumatoid arthritis and systemic lupus erythematosus sufferers. Vitamin A metabolism may be altered in diabetics.

Sources

Pre-formed vitamin A occurs in foods of animal origin such as cod liver oil, beef liver, some seafood, butter, whole milk and egg yolks. It is sometimes added to milk.

Food	Amount	Vitamin A (mcg RE)
Liver, fried	100g	10729
Cod liver oil	1 tbsp	4080
Liverwurst	28g	2353
Carrot, raw, peeled	½ cup, slices	1715
Squash	1 cup	1435
Kale, boiled	1 cup	962
Mangoes, raw, peeled	1 fruit	805
Vegetable soup, canned	1 cup	588
Cantaloupe melon, raw, peeled	1 cup, diced	502
Apricots, canned in syrup	1 cup	412
Mixed vegetables, frozen, boiled	½ cup	389
Canned vegetable juice	1 cup	283
Sardines	1 can	259
Tomato sauce, canned	1 cup	240
All Bran	½ cup	225
Apricot juice drink, canned	1 cup	145

Milk, vitamin A-fortified	1 cup	139
Pumpkin, peeled, boiled	½ cup, mashed	132
Paté	1 tbsp	130
Kidney, lamb, simmered	85g	116
Margarine	1 tbsp	112
Broccoli	½ cup	108
Butter	1 tbsp	107
Sweet potatoes, peeled, boiled	½ cup, mashed	96
Green peppers, raw	1 cup	93
Apricots	1 fruit	91
Egg, boiled	1 large	84
Cheeseburger	1 serve	79
Milk	1 cup	75
Cream cheese	1 tbsp	55

Recommended dietary allowances

Vitamin A is the name for a group of compounds which have the biological activity of retinol. Vitamin A is measured in retinol equivalents (RE) which allows the different forms of vitamin A to be compared. One retinol equivalent equals 1 mcg of retinol or 6 mcg of beta carotene. Vitamin A is also measured in international units (IU) with 1 mcg RE equivalent to 3.33 IU.

	Men	*Women*	*Pregnancy*	*Lactation*
USA	1000 mcg RE (3333 IU)	800 mcg RE (2666 IU)	800 mcg RE (2666 IU)	+500 mcg RE (+1666 IU)
UK	700 mcg RE (2333 IU)	600 mcg RE (1999 IU)	700 mcg RE (2333 IU)	950 mcg RE (3166 IU)
Australia	750 mcg RE (2499 IU)	750 mcg RE (2499 IU)	750 mcg RE (2499 IU)	+450 mcg RE (+1499 IU)

The RDA for vitamin A is based on the amount needed to prevent the eye disease xerophthalmia with an added margin of safety.

Supplements

Cod liver oil is a rich source of vitamin A and is sometimes used to make supplements. Vitamin A palmitate and vitamin A acetate are synthetic forms of vitamin A found in supplements and fortified foods. Vitamin A palmitate can be absorbed in the absence of dietary fat.

Low dose supplementary vitamin A may be beneficial in the elderly and in those who cannot absorb fats. Vitamin A needs may be increased in cases of trauma, anxiety, stress, alcohol use and smoking.

Toxic effects of excess intake

As vitamin A is fat soluble and can be stored in the liver for long periods of time, it has a high potential for toxicity. The first sign of vitamin A overdose is usually headache, followed by chapped lips, dry skin, fatigue, emotional instability and bone and joint pain. There may also be hair loss, vertigo, vision problems, poor appetite, loss of weight, vomiting, liver damage and amenorrhea (cessation of menstrual periods). Individual tolerance to vitamin A varies widely and these effects can occur at doses over 7500 mcg RE (25 000 IU) although in most adults signs of toxicity occur with single doses over 75 000 mcg RE (250 000 IU) or smaller doses of 15 000 mcg RE (50 000 IU) taken for long periods. It is recommended that regular daily intake of vitamin A does not exceed 7500 mcg RE (25 000 IU) for adults and 3000 mcg RE (10 000 IU) in children.

Pregnant women who take above 3000 mcg RE (10 000 IU) per day have a greater chance of giving birth to malformed babies. Vitamin A acne cream has been known to cause birth deformities and is now available only on prescription.

In a study published in 1995, researchers at Boston University School of Medicine assessed the links between vitamin A from food and supplements in 22,748 women who were pregnant between October 1984 and June 1987. Women who consumed more than 4500 mcg RE (15,000 IU) of pre-formed vitamin A per day from food and supplements were over three times more likely to have a baby with a birth defect than women who consumed 1500 mcg RE (5000 IU) or less per day. For vitamin A from supplements alone, women who consumed more than 3000 mcg RE (10 000 IU) per day had almost five times the risk of birth defects than women who consumed less than 1500 mcg RE (5000 IU) per day. The increased frequency of defects was concentrated among the babies born to women who had consumed high levels of vitamin A before the seventh week of pregnancy. The researchers estimated that among the babies born to women who took more than 3000 mcg RE (10,000 IU) of pre-formed vitamin A per day in the form of supplements, about one infant in 57 had a malformation attributable to the supplement.[4]

However, a 1997 study conducted by researchers at the National Institute of Child Health and Human Development did not find a link between vitamin A consumption and birth defects. Their results showed that the proportion of women consuming doses of vitamin A between 2400 mcg RE (8000 IU) and 7500 mcg RE (25,000 IU) was no higher in those with birth defects than in the normal control group.[5]

Overdose is reasonably common with as many as 5 per cent of people taking vitamin A suffering from the toxicity symptoms. Stopping the large doses usually reverses the symptoms with no lasting damage, although in children damage can be permanent.

Therapeutic uses of supplements

The main use of vitamin A supplements the prevention and treatment of deficiency. They are often used in developing countries to protect against or treat measles and other viral infections.

Immunity

Adequate vitamin A intake, either from diet or supplements, is very important in boosting immunity and preventing sickness and death in children. Many studies have found that vitamin A supplementation reduces the risk of infectious diseases in areas where vitamin A deficiency is widespread. A recent research review analyzing the results of several studies found that adequate vitamin A intake in children resulted in a 30 per cent decrease in deaths from all causes. Children in developing countries are often at high risk of vitamin A deficiency. In developed countries, ensuring adequate vitamin A intake is particularly important in those with life threatening infections such as measles and in those at risk of relative deficiency, such as premature infants.[6]

In a 1995 double-blind, randomized trial done in South Africa, vitamin A supplements were shown to reduce sickness rates in children born to HIV-infected women. The patients in this study were not in a population at high risk for vitamin A deficiency and the effect was particularly noticeable in those children who were HIV-positive.[7]

Cancer

Many studies suggest that high blood levels of vitamin A can help prevent certain forms of cancer, particularly cancers of epithelial tissue. This may be due to the importance of vitamin A in maintaining healthy epithelial cells, strengthening the immune system and stimulating the response to abnormal cells.

A 1993 Italian study tested the effects of vitamin A on cancer recurrence in smokers who had undergone surgery for lung cancer. The 307 patients took daily doses of 90 000 mcg RE (300 000 IU) for one year. After a follow-up period of 46 months, the number of patients with either recurrence or new tumors was 56 (37 per cent) in the vitamin A group and 75 (48 per cent) in the control group. Eighteen patients in the treated group developed a second primary tumor, and 29 patients in the control group developed 33 second primary tumors.[8]

Results from the recent large scale Beta Carotene and Retinol Efficacy Trial (CARET) involving a total of 18 314 smokers, former smokers, and workers exposed to asbestos failed to show any benefit of vitamin A supplementation on lung cancer. This may be due to the adverse effects of cigarette smoke on beta carotene. (See page 54 for more information.)

In a 1998 study done in Western Australia, 1024 blue asbestos workers known to be at high risk of diseases such as mesothelioma and lung cancer, were enrolled in a cancer prevention program using vitamin A. Half the subjects were given 30 mg per day of beta carotene and the other half 7500 mcg (25,000 IU) of retinol. The workers were followed up from the start of the study in June 1990 until May 1995. Four cases of lung cancer and three cases of mesothelioma were observed in those in the vitamin A group, and six cases of lung cancer and 12 cases of mesothelioma in the beta carotene group. In the retinol group, there was also a significantly lower rate of death from all causes.[9] When the researchers compared these results with those workers who had not taken part in the study they found that those taking part in the study had significantly lower death rates than non-participants.[10]

Vitamin A has also been shown to exert protective effects against leukoplakia, a pre-cancerous change in mucous membranes. It often occurs in the mouth and throat and is related to smoking. In a study done in 1997 researchers tested the effects of the retinyl palmitate form of vitamin A on leukoplakia of the larynx. The treatment period was five weeks and the doses used ranged from 90 000 mcg RE per day (300 000 IU) to 270 000 mcg (1 500 000 IU) per day. Complete remission was observed in 15 out of 20 patients and partial response was seen in the remaining five patients.[11]

Results of a US study reported in the *Journal of the National Cancer Institute* in 1997 suggest that the development of lung cancer may be due to a decreased ability of cells to respond to vitamin A-related compounds known as retinoids. When researchers at the University of Texas looked at the lung tissue from 79 patients with lung cancer and 17 without lung cancer they found that all the healthy cells carried receptors that bound retinoids. However, only 42 to 76 per cent of the cancerous cells had this ability. Of the six different types of retinoid receptors, three were found at lower levels in cancer cells.[12] Retinoids play an important role in the growth and differentiation of cells. This study raises the possibility that increasing dietary intake of vitamin A or taking supplements can be used to reduce the risk of lung cancer.

Lung function

Vitamin A supplements may be useful in treating chronic obstructive pulmonary disease. Researchers involved in a Brazilian study published in 1996 examined vitamin A levels in healthy non-smokers, healthy smokers, those with mild chronic obstructive pulmonary disease, and those with more severe symptoms. Patients in the last group had low vitamin A levels. Supplements of 1000 mcg RE (3330 IU) per day improved lung function.[13]

In a study reported in *Nature Medicine* in 1997, researchers at Georgetown University in Washington investigating the treatment of emphysema in rats found that the retinoic acid form of vitamin A reversed the lung abnormalities seen in the disease. The researchers induced emphysema in the rats and then gave them injections of retinoic acid for 12 days. The condition of the lungs improved almost to pre-disease levels.[14]

Skin disorders

Because of its important role in the formation of healthy skin, vitamin A is used to treat skin disorders including rashes, ulcers and wounds.

Acne

Vitamin A may have some benefit in the treatment of acne although most of the studies that support the effectiveness of vitamin A have involved the use of very large doses. Synthetic vitamin A derivative drugs known as retinoids are used to treat cases of severe acne which have not responded to other treatment or which have only shown partial response to antibiotic therapy. These drugs, including tretinoin, isotretinoin and etretinate are prescription medications which are used under the supervision of a doctor. Side effects are relatively common and are similar to the symptoms of vitamin A toxicity. These drugs can cause birth defects if taken during pregnancy and should also be avoided by breastfeeding women. A 1995 study by National Cancer Institute researchers suggests that long-term therapy with etretinate may increase the risk of osteoporosis.[15]

Psoriasis

Vitamin A derivative drugs are also used to treat psoriasis, particularly pustular psoriasis. These drugs help to normalize skin development by reducing the increased growth, turnover and keratinization of skin which occurs in the disorder. Similar cautions apply to the use of these drugs in the treatment of psoriasis.

Skin aging

According to a 1997 report in the *New England Journal of Medicine*, creams that contain the vitamin A derivative tretinoin, may help to combat premature skin aging. Researchers studied the activity of enzymes known as metalloproteinases which break down collagen and found that exposure to ultraviolet light increased the activity of these enzymes. Even a small amount of ultraviolet light, although not sufficient to cause redness, was enough to increase enzyme activity. This suggests that exposure to a few minutes of sunlight periodically over several years may lead to premature skin aging.

This increase in enzyme activity was blocked by treatment with tretinoin before radiation. The researchers conclude that tretinoin may be useful in treating patients with signs of premature skin aging but note that careful monitoring of tretinoin use is essential as over-treatment can cause irritation and reddening of skin. The results of this study may lead to the development of new sunscreens and anti-aging creams containing vitamin A derivatives.[16]

Other uses

Vitamin A eye drops have been used to treat eye problems including blurred vision, cataracts, glaucoma, conjunctivitis and dry eyes. Other disorders for which vitamin A has been tried include asthma, sebaceous cysts, fibrocystic breast disease and premenstrual syndrome.

Vitamin A may also be useful in the prevention of ulcers. In a study involving almost 48 000 men reported in 1997 in the *American Journal of Epidemiology* researchers found a lower risk of ulcer in those with high intakes of vitamin A, either from food or supplements.[17]

Interactions with other nutrients

Vitamin E plays a role in the absorption, storage and utilization of vitamin A and protects it from oxidation. Vitamin E may protect against some of the effects of excess vitamin A.

Vitamin A is necessary for calcium metabolism and is also necessary for the absorption, metabolism and storage of iron. Vitamin A deficiency lowers blood levels of hemoglobin. When iron supplements are given it is important to ensure that vitamin A levels are high enough to protect against the exacerbation of bacterial activity that iron may cause.[18] With zinc deficiency, levels of vitamin A in the liver rise and blood levels fall.

Interactions with drugs

Vitamin A absorption is reduced by mineral oil laxatives. Antacids; the anti-gout drug, colchicine; and the cholesterol-reducing drug, cholestyramine also inhibit vitamin A absorption. Broad spectrum antibiotics should not be taken with high doses of vitamin A.

Alcohol irritates the digestive tract and inhibits the absorption of vitamin A. It also depletes the body's tissue stores.

Cautions

Vitamin A supplements in doses of more than 3000 mcg RE (10 000 IU) should not be taken by women who may become pregnant.

Vitamin A supplements should not be taken with vitamin A derivative drugs or by anyone with impaired liver or kidney function. If vitamin A supplements are taken with large amounts of alcohol, liver damage may occur.

Carotenes

QUICK GUIDE

Carotenes are substances found in food which can be converted to vitamin A as the body requires. Beta carotene is the best known of the carotenes as it is readily converted to vitamin A and is abundant in many foods. Other carotenes include lycopene, alpha carotene, lutein and zeaxanthin.

Carotenes are also beneficial because they act as antioxidants and help to protect the body against heart disease, cancer, eye damage and other disorders.

Absorption and metabolism

Carotenes require fat and bile acids for absorption.

Deficiency

Diets low in carotenes may lead to increased risk of cancer and heart disease.

Sources

Good sources include yellow, orange and dark green fruits and vegetables such as sweet potatoes, carrots, broccoli, spinach and apricots. Some carotenes are used by the food industry as yellow food colouring.

Daily recommended dietary intakes

There is no RDA for beta carotene. Some experts recommend a daily intake of 10 to 30 mg.

Toxic effects of excess intake

Beta carotene is safe even at high doses. Some areas of skin may become orange/yellow in colour if high doses are taken for long periods. This clears when intake is reduced. There is the possibility of menstrual abnormalities with long-term excessive intake.

Therapeutic uses of supplements

Beta carotene supplements have been used to prevent cancer, heart disease, autoimmune diseases and eye damage; and to boost immune function. Lycopene may help to prevent prostate cancer and lutein may help to prevent macular degeneration.

Cautions

Recent research suggests that large doses of beta carotene may actually increase the risk of cancer in those who drink alcohol and smoke heavily.

Carotenes are a group of highly colored plant compounds, some of which can be converted into vitamin A in the intestinal wall and liver, as the body requires. They are also referred to as carotenoids. Beta carotene is the best known of the carotenes as it has high pro-vitamin A activity and is abundant in many foods. Other carotenoids include lutein, zeaxanthin, beta cryptoxanthin, lycopene and alpha carotene. Carotenoids interact with each other during intestinal absorption, metabolism, and clearance from the body.

What they do in the body

Antioxidant action

The beneficial effects of some carotenoids are partly due to their conversion to vitamin A. They also have potent activity of their own due to their ability to act as antioxidants and protect against free radical damage. This type of damage may lead to several medical problems, such as inflammatory damage and tissue injury after trauma; and chronic conditions, such as cardiovascular disease, eye disorders, autoimmune diseases and cancer. (See page 417 for more information.) Carotenoids also affect cell growth regulation and gene expression.

Protection against cancer

High levels of dietary carotenoids have been linked to decreases in the risks of several types of cancer.

Colon cancer

In a small study of cancer patients done in 1997, Italian researchers assessed carotenoid levels in four healthy patients, seven patients with pre-cancerous lesions and seven patients with colon cancer. They found significantly lower carotenoid levels in the cancer patients.[1]

Breast cancer

In a study published in the *Journal of the National Cancer Institute* in 1996, researchers examined the links between dietary intake of carotenoids (including nonfood supplements) and premenopausal breast cancer risk. The study involved 297 premenopausal women 40 years of age or older who were diagnosed with breast cancer from November 1986 to April 1991. These were compared with 311 women without cancer. The results showed a reduction in risk associated with high intake of several nutrients including beta carotene, lutein and zeaxanthin.[2]

In a study published in 1998, researchers in Missouri examined blood levels of various nutrients in women who developed breast cancer after donating blood to a bank over a ten-year period. They then compared these levels to women who were free of cancer. They found lower levels of the carotenoids beta cryptoxanthin, lycopene, lutein and zeaxanthin in patients who developed breast cancer.[3]

In a 1997 study reported in the *American Journal of Clinical Nutrition*, researchers at Harvard School of Public Health compared carotenoid concentrations in the breast fat tissue from 46 cancer patients and 63 women with benign breast lumps. They found an increased risk in those with low levels of beta carotene, lycopene, lutein and zeaxanthin.[4]

Lung cancer

Several population studies have shown lower levels of carotenoids in lung cancer cases. In a study published in 1998, researchers at Johns Hopkins University measured nutrient levels in blood samples from 258 patients with lung cancer and compared these with those in samples from 515 people free of cancer. Blood concentrations of cryptoxanthin, beta carotene, lutein and zeaxanthin were significantly lower among the cancer patients. Small differences were noticed for alpha carotene and lycopene.[5]

Protection against cardiovascular disease

Population studies have shown that diets high in carotenoids can protect against cardiovascular diseases. They may do this by preventing the oxidation of LDL cholesterol and reducing free radical damage at sites of atherosclerotic plaque formation.

Researchers involved in the Massachusetts Health Care Panel Study examined the links between consumption of carotene-containing fruits and vegetables and death from cardiovascular disease among 1299 elderly people. The results of the study, which were published in the *Annals of Epidemiology* in 1995 showed that during the follow-up period of almost five years, there were 161 deaths from cardiovascular disease. The risk of death in the group who ate the most carotene-containing foods was almost half that of those people whose carotene consumption was low.[6]

In a 1996 study UK researchers compared blood levels of antioxidant vitamins in Belfast, Northern Ireland with those of people in Toulouse, France where the incidence of coronary heart disease is much lower. The results showed that levels of carotenoids such as lutein, cryptoxanthin and alpha carotene were much higher in people from Toulouse.[7]

Protection against eye disorders

Oxidative damage is also implicated in the development of eye disorders such as cataracts and macular degeneration.

Researchers at Harvard Medical School examined the link between cataract development and intake of various foods and antioxidant vitamins in over 50 000 women. The results of their studies showed that those with high beta carotene and vitamin A intakes were less likely to develop cataracts. Those whose diets contained spinach also seemed to have a lower risk. The researchers concluded that dietary carotenoids, although not necessarily beta carotene, can decrease the risk of cataracts severe enough to require extraction.[8]

Absorption and metabolism

Carotenoids need bile acids for absorption and unless they are converted to vitamin A in the wall of the small intestine, they are absorbed unchanged. Conversion appears to depend on several factors including protein, thyroid hormone action, zinc and vitamin C. Around 40 to 60 per cent of dietary beta carotene is absorbed, although this appears to be reduced in the presence of low stomach acid. Beta carotene can be stored in the lung, liver, kidneys, skin and fat.

Sources

Good sources of beta carotene include carrots, sweet potatoes, pumpkin and other orange winter squashes, cantaloupe, pink grapefruit, spinach, apricots, broccoli, and most dark green leafy vegetables. The more intense the green, yellow or orange color the more beta carotene the vegetable or fruit contains. These foods are also good sources of alpha carotene. Beta carotene is not destroyed by cooking which, in fact, may make it easier to absorb.

Good sources of lycopene include tomatoes, carrots, green peppers and apricots. Spinach, paprika, corn and fruits are high in zeaxanthin; and green plants, corn, potatoes, spinach, carrots and tomatoes are high in lutein.

Beta carotene

As an antioxidant, beta carotene has beneficial effects in protecting against oxidative damage including that caused by ultraviolet light.[9] Beta carotene has been shown to stimulate and enhance many immune system processes. It increases the numbers of immune cells such as B and T lymphocytes and natural killer cells. T cells play a very important role in determining immune status and are produced by the thymus gland, which is particularly sensitive to free radical and oxidative damage. Beta carotene protect macrophages, white blood cells which engulf and destroy foreign substances. It also facilitates communication between immune cells and makes the stimulatory action of interferon on the immune system more powerful.

Protection against cancer

As with other carotenoids, research suggests that low levels of beta carotene increase the risk of certain types of cancer, including those of the lung, stomach, breast, prostate, colon, ovary and cervix. Several population studies have shown that cancer victims have lower dietary and/or blood beta carotene levels than healthy people. The evidence from these studies is strongest for lung cancer.

In a study done in Wellington, New Zealand researchers investigated the links between beta carotene and cancer. They compared levels in 389 people with cancer to those in 391 hospital patients without cancer. They also assessed the family members of the study participants to compensate for the fact that changes in beta carotene levels may have occurred after the cancer developed. Low levels of beta carotene were found in people with a number of cancers, including those of the lung, stomach, esophagus, small intestine, cervix, and uterus. Low levels were also found in the relatives of these cancer patients and the links were strongest in those with lung cancer. In this study patients with cancers of the breast, colon, prostate, and skin did not have lower levels of beta carotene and neither did their families. These results suggest that the cancer sites associated with beta carotene levels are, in general, sites for which smoking is a strong risk factor.[10]

Lung cancer

Researchers at Yale University School of Medicine compared diets in 413 nonsmokers suffering from lung cancer and compared these with 413 people without cancer. The results of the study, which were published in 1994, showed that high dietary intake of fruit and vegetables and beta carotene was linked to a decreased risk of lung cancer in both men and women.[11]

Breast cancer

In a study published in 1996, Italian researchers investigated the relationship between selected nutrients and breast cancer risk in 2569 women with the disease and 2588 women with no history of cancer. The results showed significantly less risk in women with high beta carotene intakes.[12]

In another recent study published in the *British Journal of Cancer,* West Australian researchers investigated the effect of increased intake of beta carotene on survival in breast cancer patients. Over a six-year period only one death occurred in the group with the highest consumption of beta carotene, while there were eight and 12 deaths in the intermediate and lowest groups of consumption respectively.[13]

Prostate cancer

Results from the Chicago Western Electric Study published in 1996, suggest that surviving prostate cancer is more likely in men with higher beta carotene intakes. The study involved 1899 middle-aged men who were followed for a total of 30 years. During that time 132 men developed prostate cancer and survival was found to be less likely in those with low beta carotene intakes.[14]

Cervical cancer

Research suggests that women with low beta carotene levels in their cervical tissues may be at increased risk of cervical cancer. Laboratory studies show that beta carotene can slow the growth of cervical cancer cells.[15] Increasing intake of beta carotene may help to overcome this tissue-specific deficiency.[16]

Protection against heart disease and stroke

Several studies suggest high dietary beta carotene intake can protect against cardiovascular disease. As an antioxidant, beta carotene has been shown to inhibit oxidative damage to cholesterol and protect against atherosclerotic plaque formation.

The relationship between intake of dietary antioxidants and risk of stroke was investigated as part of the Chicago Western Electric Study. The researchers found a moderately reduced risk in those with high beta carotene intakes.[17]

In a 1997 study, researchers in Italy investigated the relationship between non-fatal heart attacks and dietary intake of beta carotene. The study involved 433 heart attack patients and 869 women without cardiovascular disease. The results showed that women with high beta carotene intakes had around half the risk of heart attack of those with low intakes.[18]

Autoimmune diseases

Free radical damage may also contribute to the development of autoimmune diseases such as arthritis. Increasing dietary levels of antioxidants may help to prevent this damage. Researchers at Johns Hopkins University examined the links between dietary intake of beta carotene and rheumatoid arthritis and systemic lupus erythematosus. The study involved people with the disorders that developed two to 15 years after donating blood for a serum bank in 1974. The results showed that disease sufferers had significantly lower blood concentrations of beta carotene than those without the disorders.[19]

Wound-healing

Oxidative stress is linked to inflammation and may contribute to secondary tissue damage and impaired immunc function after burns and other kinds of injuries. As beta carotene has antioxidant and anti-inflammatory properties it may help to promote wound-healing.

Eyes

Free radical damage is implicated in the formation of cataracts and as an antioxidant, beta carotene may exert protective effects by reducing this damage. It may also act as a filter and protect against light-induced damage to the fiber portion of the eye lens. Beta carotene may also protect against macular degeneration, a disease of the retina to which older people are particularly susceptible.

Finnish researchers recently compared the differences between beta carotene levels in patients admitted to eye wards for senile cataract with those without eye disorders. The results showed that those with low concentrations of beta carotene were 1.7 times as likely to suffer from cataract.[20]

Mental function

In a study reported in 1996, Dutch researchers looking at the effect of foods rich in beta carotene on memory impairment and mental function found that these had protective effects. The researchers studied 5182 people aged 55 to 95 from 1990 to 1993. They found that those with intakes of less than 0.9 milligrams of beta carotene per day were almost twice as likely to have impaired memory, disorientation and problem solving difficulty as those with intakes of 2.1 milligrams of beta carotene.[21]

Researchers involved in a 1997 Swiss study found similar results. The study which was reported in the *Journal of the American Geriatrics Society*, involved 442 men and women, aged from 65 to 94 in 1993. Antioxidant levels were originally tested in 1971 and then again in 1993, when the participants were also given memory related tests. Higher vitamin C and beta carotene levels were associated with higher scores on free recall, recognition and vocabulary tests.[22]

Candidiasis

Lower levels of beta carotene have been seen in the cells of women with vaginal candidiasis (thrush). In an American study done in 1994, researchers compared beta carotene levels in vaginal cells from women with candidiasis to those in women without the infection. They found significantly lower levels in women with candidiasis. Women are more susceptible to candida infection when the immune response is suppressed and as beta carotene has been shown to boost immune response the high levels may protect against the overgrowth of candida.[23]

Recommended dietary allowances

There is no RDA for beta carotene. An intake of 6 mg beta carotene is needed in order to meet the vitamin A RDA of 1000 mcg RE. 1 RE is equivalent to 6 mcg beta carotene. Some experts recommend a daily intake of 10 to 30 mg.

The RDA for vitamin A for women who are breastfeeding increases from 800 mcg RE to 1300 mcg RE. This can be met by increasing the intake of beta carotene-rich foods.

Supplements

Beta carotene supplements are available in various forms, including synthetic forms and those extracted from algae and palm oil. Some studies suggest that those extracted from palm oil are absorbed more efficiently. Natural beta carotene may have greater beneficial effects than synthetic forms.[24]

Toxic effects of excess intake

Unlike vitamin A, beta carotene is not toxic in large amounts although it may cause the skin of the hands, feet and face to become yellow. This disappears when large intakes are stopped and does not appear to have any ill effects. Research in animals suggests the possibility of menstrual problems with long-term excessive intake.

Therapeutic uses of supplements

Beta carotene supplements have been used in cancer and cardiovascular disease prevention trials, including the Finnish Alpha Tocopherol Beta Carotene Cancer (ATBC) Prevention Study, the US Carotene and Retinol Efficacy Trial (CARET) and the US Physicians Health Study. In 1996, these studies reported results which received wide publicity.

ATBC study

The ATBC Prevention group studied 29 000 men who smoked and drank alcohol. The results showed an 18 per cent increase in lung cancer deaths and an 11 per cent increase in ischemic heart disease deaths in men who took daily supplements of 20 mg beta carotene.[25]

CARET study

The CARET study was stopped 21 months early. This study was examining the effect of beta carotene (30 mg daily) and retinol (7500 mcg RE daily) supplementation on the prevention of cancer and heart disease in over 18 000 smokers and people who had been exposed to asbestos. The trial was stopped when the results showed a 28 per cent increased risk of lung cancer, a 26 per cent increase in the risk of death from cardiovascular disease, and a 17 per cent increase in overall deaths in the group receiving the supplements.[26]

Physicians Health Study

This study examined the effect on over 22 000 male doctors of 50 mg beta carotene taken every other day for 12 years. The results suggest that beta carotene has no effect, either positive or negative, on the risk of cardiovascular disease or cancer. Analysis of a subgroup of 333 men in the study with a prior history of heart disease suggested that beta carotene supplements reduced the risk of heart attacks and death by a small amount.[27]

There are a number of possible explanations for the adverse effects of beta carotene supplements found in these studies and for the failure of supplements to show the protective effects suggested by epidemiological studies.

Beta carotene is susceptible to oxidative damage from alcohol and the gases in cigarette smoke which may lead to the formation of harmful by-products.[28] Beta carotene may be dependent on other antioxidants, such as vitamins C and E to exert protective effects. An individual's total dietary intake of antioxidants may therefore need to be considered when assessing protection by beta carotene.

Further analyses of results from the ATBC trial support the suggestion that smoking and alcohol consumption may contribute to the adverse effects of beta carotene. The adverse effects appeared stronger in men who drank alcohol and in those who smoked 20 cigarettes a day than in those who smoked less. This is confirmed by the CARET results which showed greater risk in current smokers than former smokers and also in those who drank alcohol.

Another aspect to be considered is the fact that beta carotene exists in many possible forms and some research suggests that the specific form chosen for use in these clinical trials was not the most active. A mixture of various forms of beta carotene, similar to that which occurs naturally, may have the most beneficial effect. It is also possible that the large dose of the particular form of beta carotene used in the trials competed with other, possibly more beneficial forms at vital sites in the body.

The results of these trials point to the importance of considering total diet and a balanced mixture of nutrients when studying protection against cancer risk. High blood levels of carotene seem to predict lower risk and these high blood levels of beta carotene may be accompanied by high levels of other carotenoids, and even other nutrients, which may also play a vital part in cancer protection. Both the ATBC and CARET studies found that those with higher blood beta carotene levels on entering the trials had a lower risk of lung cancer.

Laboratory research suggests that vitamin C protects against the harmful effects of beta carotene in smokers. Smokers tend to have low levels of vitamin C and this may allow a build-up of a harmful form of beta carotene called the carotene free radical which is formed when beta carotene acts to regenerate vitamin E. These results suggest that in smokers, dietary vitamin C supplementation should accompany beta carotene supplementation.[29]

Double-blind placebo-controlled studies may be more useful for evaluating a specific drug for one condition in one population group and less suitable for investigating multifactorial agents in complex, mixed population studies. These studies do not invalidate hundreds of other studies showing that diets high in fruits and vegetables protect against a variety of diseases.

Immune system support

In a 1997 double-blind, placebo-controlled study done in the UK, researchers tested the effects of daily doses of 15 mg of beta carotene in 25 healthy, adult male nonsmokers. Their findings showed improvement in function in various parts of the immune system, including white blood cells known as monocytes which are involved in surveillance of tumors.[30]

Large doses of beta carotene may boost immune function in AIDS patients. In a Yale University study done in 1995, researchers found that daily supplements of 60 mg beta carotene given to seven AIDS patients for a period of four weeks increased CD4+ lymphocyte cell counts.[31]

Other uses

In addition to exerting protective effects against a wide range of diseases, beta carotene may slow the rate of aging in the skin and other organs by protecting against free radical damage caused by smoking, pollution, ultraviolet light and other chemicals. Beta carotene is also used to treat oral leukoplakia, a pre-cancerous condition of mucous membranes.

Beta carotene may also be beneficial in pre-eclampsia.[32] Other results from the CARET study suggest that beta carotene supplements can help to improve lung function in men that have been exposed to asbestos.[33]

Beta carotene is used to decrease light sensitivity reactions in sufferers of the disease, erythropoietic protoporphyria. Beta carotene supplements have been shown to have beneficial effects in cystic fibrosis by decreasing harmful lipid peroxidation. Fibrocystic breast disease, a painful cystic swelling of the breast which affects 20 to 40 per cent of premenopausal women, may be helped by vitamin A and beta carotene.

Interactions with other nutrients

The conversion of beta carotene to vitamin A depends on vitamin C, zinc and thyroid hormones. The function of beta carotene is enhanced by the levels of the other antioxidants, vitamin C, vitamin E and selenium. Large doses of beta carotene may increase the requirements for vitamin E. Beta carotene improves iron absorption.[34]

Interactions with drugs

Oral contraceptive use may decrease beta carotene levels.[35] Drinking large amounts of alcohol and smoking lowers blood levels of carotenoids.[36]

Cautions

People with hypothyroidism or liver disease have trouble converting beta carotene to vitamin A and should not rely solely on beta carotene to meet their vitamin A requirements. Diabetics may also have trouble converting beta carotene to vitamin A, although recent research suggests that this may not be the case.[37]

Large doses of beta carotene may increase the risk of cancer in those who drink alcohol and smoke heavily. Vitamin C supplements may be useful in protecting against the damaging effects of large doses of beta carotene.

Lycopene

Lycopene is the carotenoid which gives tomatoes their red color and is one of the major carotenoids in the diet of North Americans and Europeans. It is found in high concentration in testes, adrenal gland and prostate. Levels of lycopene seem to decrease with age. Several studies suggest that lycopene may help to prevent cardiovascular disease and cancers of the prostate, pancreas and gastrointestinal tract.[38] According to the results of a 1997 study done in Germany, lycopene from tomato paste is more bio-available than lycopene from fresh tomatoes.[39]

Prostate cancer

Tomato-based foods, which are rich in lycopene, seem to be linked with a lower risk of prostate cancer. In a study published in 1995, researchers at Harvard Medical School assessed the links between diet during a one-year period and prostate cancer in almost 48 000 men taking part in the Health Professionals Follow-up Study. They found that men who ate more foods such as tomatoes, pizza and tomato sauce which are high in lycopene, were less likely to be at risk of prostate cancer.[40]

Heart attack

Researchers involved in the EURAMIC study assessed the links between antioxidants and heart attacks. They studied people from ten European countries and analyzed for levels of carotenoids in those who had suffered heart attacks and those who had not. They found protective effects of alpha carotene, beta carotene, and lycopene. Lycopene was particularly protective with those in the highest intake group, having around half the risk of heart attack of those in the lowest intake group.[41]

Lutein

Like the other carotenoids, lutein has been shown to have antioxidant effects. Lutein and zeaxanthin are constituents of the pigment of the eye. A low density of this pigment in the macula of the eye may increase the risk of the disorder macular degeneration, possibly because it permits greater blue light damage.

In a study published in 1997, researchers at Florida International University in Miami tested the effects of 30 mg of lutein on eye pigment in two people for a period of 140 days.The results showed that 20 to 40 days after the people started taking the lutein supplement, the density of the pigment in their eyes started to increase. This amount of blue light reaching the vulnerable eye tissues that are damaged in macular degeneration was reduced by around 30 to 40 per cent.[42]

Oxidative damage to the lens of the eye is also implicated in the development of cataract, in which the eye lens becomes clouded. (See page 603 for more information.) In a 1997 study, researchers at Arizona State University assessed the relationship between carotenoid pigments in the retina of the eye and the density of clouding in the lens. The study involved younger people (ages 24 to 36 years) and older people (aged 48 to 82 years). The results showed that lens density increased with age, and that the increase was related to lower macular pigment carotenoids. These findings open up the possibility that lutein and zeaxanthin may be used to slow down age-related increases in lens density.[43]

Vitamin B complex

Vitamin B is a complex of eight water soluble vitamins including thiamin, riboflavin, niacin, vitamin B6, pantothenic acid, folic acid, biotin and vitamin B12. These vitamins act together in the body and if they are taken as supplements, they should be consumed in the proper ratios. Choline, inositol and PABA are part of the B complex in food but are regarded as factors rather than vitamins. As the B vitamins are water soluble, excesses are excreted in the urine rather than stored, and a daily intake is necessary to maintain health.

What it does in the body

B vitamins are necessary for the metabolism of carbohydrates, fats and proteins essential for growth. They are involved in maintaining the health of the hair, skin, nerves, blood cells, immune system, hormone-producing glands and digestive system.

Deficiency

B vitamin deficiencies cause a variety of disorders ranging from the severe deficiency diseases, beriberi and pellagra, to dermatitis and anemia. Marginal deficiencies of B vitamins may be relatively common in some population groups, such as elderly people, and may result in reduced mental functioning. B vitamin deficiencies are often found in psychiatric patients and may contribute to depression and other symptoms. Prolonged ingestion of large doses of one B vitamin can result in depletion of the others.

Sources

B vitamins are present in liver, kidney, whole grains, all seeds, nuts, dairy products, eggs, bran, wheatgerm, brewer's yeast, lentils, beans, peas, soybeans and leafy green vegetables.

Therapeutic uses of supplements

B complex supplements may be useful for anyone who is ill or under stress. Those who smoke, drink alcohol or use recreational drugs may also benefit.

Thiamin

QUICK GUIDE

Essential for

- releasing energy from food
- carbohydrate and fatty acid metabolism
- healthy growth
- healthy skin, blood, hair and muscles
- a healthy brain and nervous system
- alcohol metabolism

Absorption and metabolism

Daily intake is necessary.

Deficiency

Symptoms include fatigue, depression, reduced mental functioning, muscle cramps, nausea, heart enlargement and eventually beriberi, which can cause paralysis. Alcoholics are at particular risk of thiamin deficiency.

Sources

These include meat, whole grains, fish and nuts.

Daily recommended dietary intakes

Men	1.2 mg
Women	1.1 mg
Pregnancy	1.4 mg
Lactation	1.5 mg

Toxic effects of excess intake

Toxicity is rare. Symptoms include headache, irritability, hyperthyroidism and insomnia.

Interactions

Alcohol reduces thiamin absorption and conversion to the biologically active form. Digoxin, indomethacin, anticonvulsants, antacids and diuretics increase the risk of deficiency.

Therapeutic uses of supplements

Thiamin supplements have been used to improve mental function in alcoholics and the elderly. They may be useful in times of stress and have also been used to treat fatigue, irritability, depression, to aid digestion, and to promote healing.

Thiamin, which is also known as vitamin B1, was the first B vitamin to be discovered. Scientists in the late 19th century noticed that animals fed a diet of polished rice developed the thiamin deficiency disease, beriberi, and that this could be cured by adding rice husks to the feed. In 1926, two Dutch scientists isolated pure thiamin, the active anti-beriberi agent in the rice. In the human body, thiamin is found in high concentrations in the muscles, heart, liver, kidneys and brain.

What it does in the body

Metabolism

Thiamin is part of an enzyme system known as thiamin pyrophosphate which is essential for nearly every cellular reaction in the body. It is involved in energy production and carbohydrate and fatty acid metabolism. It is vital for normal development, growth, reproduction, healthy skin and hair, blood production and immune function. Thiamin is also necessary for the metabolism of alcohol.

Brain and nerve function

Thiamin is particularly important for the normal functioning of nerves. It is necessary for the synthesis of acetylcholine, a neurotransmitter which affects several brain functions including memory, and also maintains muscle tone of the stomach, intestines and heart.

Absorption and metabolism

Digestive diseases such as colitis, diverticulosis, celiac disease and chronic diarrhea reduce thiamin absorption as do protein and folate deficiencies. Some thiamin is stored in the heart, liver and kidneys but these stores do not last long and a continuous intake is necessary to prevent deficiency.

Raw freshwater fish and shellfish contain an enzyme which breaks down thiamin. This can happen during food storage and preparation or as food passes through the gut. Thus large intakes of raw fish and shellfish can increase the risk of thiamin deficiency. Drinking large quantities of tea and coffee may reduce thiamin absorption.

Deficiency

Thiamin deficiency is rare in developed countries as refined flours and cereals are often fortified with this vitamin. However, deficiency symptoms are still seen in parts of the world where white rice makes up a major part of the daily diet.

Those at greatest risk of deficiency include some young children and teenagers, stressed adults, those who exercise very heavily, alcoholics, pregnant women, those on fad diets and people suffering from malabsorption diseases. Marginal deficiencies without clinical symptoms may be quite common among these groups. Elderly people are also at risk of thiamin deficiency and this may lead to reduced mental functioning, depression, weakness, suppressed immunity and gastrointestinal problems. Early thiamin deficiency may be easily overlooked as the symptoms are generalized and can include fatigue, depression and stress-induced headaches. There is some evidence to suggest that recurring mouth ulcers are due to thiamin deficiency.[1]

Thiamin deficiency affects every cell in the body. Deficiency symptoms may be due to the interference of nerve functions dependent on thiamin and the build-up of toxic compounds as carbohydrates are incompletely metabolized. Factors which increase the demand for the conversion of carbohydrate to energy; for example, exercise, alcohol and sugary foods; may aggravate thiamin deficiency. Severe thiamin deficiency causes beriberi. Beriberi can affect the cardiovascular system (wet beriberi) and the nervous system (dry beriberi).

Brain and nervous system

One of the earliest signs of thiamin deficiency is reduced stamina. Depression, irritability and reduced ability to concentrate are later followed by fatigue, muscle cramps and various pains. Dry beriberi symptoms include numbness and tingling in the toes and feet, stiffness of the ankles, cramping pains in the legs, difficulty walking, and finally, paralysis of the legs with wasting of the muscles. Permanent damage to the nervous system can occur if the deficiency is not corrected in time. Thiamin deficiency may also be associated with reduced tolerance to pain.

Gastrointestinal system

Thiamin deficiency can also lead to nausea, lack of appetite, weight loss and constipation. Carbohydrate digestion and the metabolism of glucose are diminished.

Cardiovascular system

In the advanced stages of thiamin deficiency, the symptoms of wet beriberi include heart enlargement. Symptoms of cardiac failure such as breathlessness, ankle swelling and fatigue may follow. Marginal thiamin deficiency may contribute to heart disease.

Alcoholics

Alcoholics and binge drinkers are especially prone to thiamin deficiency as alcohol reduces absorption, alters metabolism and depletes body stores. Alcoholics also tend to have poor diets. Thiamin deficiency is associated with some of the symptoms of alcoholism such as mental confusion, visual disturbances and staggering gait. If thiamin deficiency is not corrected, permanent brain damage may result. This condition is known as Wernicke Korsakoff syndrome and is usually seen in people who have been addicted to alcohol for many years.

Sources

Good natural sources of thiamin include brewer's yeast, organ meats, wheatgerm, oatmeal, whole grains, pork, fish, poultry, nuts, dried beans and peas, avocado, vegetables such as spinach and cauliflower, and thiamin-enriched flours and cereals.

Thiamin is found in the germ and bran of wheat and in the outer covering of rice grains, so refining grains removes much of the thiamin. The vitamin is easily destroyed by cooking heat and is lost in the water used to cook food. It is also destroyed when food becomes alkaline, thus adding bicarbonate of soda to thiamin-rich foods causes losses. Sulfite food additives also destroy thiamin.

Food	Amount	Thiamin (mg)
Pork	1 chop	1.23
Oats	1 cup	1.19
Wheatgerm	1 cup	1.08
Pecans	1 cup	0.91
Past, fresh	100g	0.71
Pistachios	½ cup	0.53
Special K	1 cup	0.52

All Bran	½ cup	0.39
Green peas	1 cup	0.39
Kidney beans	100g	0.36
Brazil nuts	6-8 nuts	0.28
Ham	1 slice	0.25
Liver, fried	100g	0.21
Scallops, fried	6 pieces	0.20
Chickpeas, cooked	1 cup	0.19
Cod	1 fillet	0.16
Cashews	½ cup	0.14
Kidney, simmered	100g	0.13
Pearl barley, boiled	1 cup	0.13
Whole grain bread	1 slice	0.11
Bulgur, boiled	1 cup	0.10
Beef steak	100g	0.09

Recommended daily intakes

The RDAs for thiamin in the USA were revised in 1998.

	Men	*Women*	*Pregnancy*	*Lactation*
USA	1.2 mg	1.1 mg	1.4 mg	1.5 mg
UK	1.0 mg	0.8 mg	0.9 mg	1.0 mg
Australia	1.1 mg	0.8 mg	1.0 mg	1.2 mg

Women who are carrying or breastfeeding more than one baby would have a greater thiamin requirement.

Supplements

Thiamin supplements may be useful during times of stress, fever, diarrhea and during and after surgery. Many experts recommend 100 mg of thiamin per day for those who drink alcohol.

Toxic effects of excess intake

Toxicity is very rare as excess thiamin is excreted in the urine. Long-term excessive use can produce symptoms of hyperthyroidism: headache, irritability, trembling, rapid pulse and insomnia. With injected thiamin, reactions of itching, weakness, gastrointestinal bleeding, low blood pressure, pain, sweating, nausea, tingling and faintness can sometimes occur. The lowest daily dose known to cause side effects is 5 mg, but many people can tolerate much larger doses.

Therapeutic uses of supplements

Thiamin supplements are used to prevent and correct the heart and nerve problems caused by thiamin deficiency. Thiamin also has a mild diuretic effect and may be beneficial to heart function. Restoring normal thiamin levels in diabetics who are deficient leads to improvements in blood sugar metabolism.

Elderly people

The results of a trial reported in the *American Journal of Clinical Nutrition* in 1997 suggest that thiamin supplements may help to improve quality of life in many elderly people. Researchers from hospitals in Christchurch, New Zealand measured red blood cell concentrations of thiamin pyrophosphate (TPP) in 222 people aged over 65 years. This measurement was done twice in three months. Thirty-five people had low levels at both measurement times. These people were divided into two groups and were given either a thiamin supplement of 10 mg per day or a placebo for three months. The researchers then assessed blood pressure, body weight, height, body mass index, hand grip strength and cognitive function in the subjects. The results showed that the supplements decreased blood pressure and weight and improved quality of life. There was a trend towards improved sleep and energy.[2]

Fatigue

Like the other B vitamins, thiamin is used to treat fatigue. High-dose thiamin supplementation may be helpful in preventing or accelerating recovery from exercise-induced fatigue. In a small Japanese study done in 1996, the effects of 100 mg per day of thiamin was assessed in 16 male athletes. The athletes exercised on bicycles and changes in blood, heart and lung functioning were measured. In the thiamin supplement group, changes in blood glucose were suppressed and the athletes felt less fatigued.[3]

Mental function

Thiamin supplements have been shown to improve mood and mental function, possibly via effects on the neurotransmitter, acetylcholine. Thiamin supplements also appear to improve mental function in epileptics treated with the anticonvulsant drug, phenytoin.

In a study done in Wales in 1997, researchers gave 120 young adult women either a placebo or 50 mg thiamin, each day for two months. The women were not thiamin-deficient. Before and after taking the tablets, mood, memory and reaction times were assessed. The women taking the thiamin reported that they felt more clearheaded, composed and energetic. Tests showed no influence on memory but reaction times were faster following supplementation.[4]

Alcohol and drugs

Thiamin has been used to treat some of the symptoms of alcohol abuse, such as the reduction in brain chemicals associated with memory and thought processes.

In a study done in the US in 1997, thiamin supplements improved memory in cocaine-dependent patients. The patients were not taking cocaine during the study and were given 5 g of thiamin or a placebo. They were then asked to perform memory scanning tasks. The results showed that the patients taking the thiamin supplements performed significantly better than those taking the placebo.[5]

Alzheimer's disease

Thiamin metabolism appears to be altered in Alzheimer's with lower levels of thiamin and enzymes which metabolize thiamin found in the brains of Alzheimer's disease patients. Clinical data suggest that high dose thiamin may have a mild beneficial effect in some patients with Alzheimer's disease but it does not appear to halt the progress of the disease.[6]

Other uses

Thiamin supplements have been used to treat other problems that affect the nerves, including multiple sclerosis. Bell's palsy, neuritis and diabetic neuropathy. Thiamin may stimulate digestion by improving hydrochloric acid production and intestinal muscle tone. As with the other B vitamins, thiamin is used to relieve stress and muscle tension and to speed healing after surgery. Some people use thiamin supplements in doses of up to 100 mg to help repel mosquitoes and other biting insects, and it may take several weeks of supplement use before beneficial effects appear.

Interactions with other nutrients

Magnesium is necessary for the conversion of thiamin to its active form. Vitamin C helps improve thiamin absorption.

Interactions with drugs

Alcohol reduces thiamin absorption and conversion to the biologically active form. Digoxin, indomethacin, anticonvulsants, antacids and some diuretics may lead to the risk of deficiency. Smoking, caffeine, sulfa drugs and estrogen may also raise thiamin requirements.

Riboflavin

QUICK GUIDE

Essential for

- the production of energy from food
- normal growth and development
- a healthy immune system
- healthy skin, hair and blood cells
- iron, pyridoxine and niacin functions
- hormone function
- a healthy nervous system and brain

Absorption and metabolism

Daily intake is necessary.

Deficiency

Symptoms include red, swollen, cracked mouth and tongue; fatigue; depression; anemia; and greasy, scaly skin on the face, body and limbs. Deficiency may also contribute to cataract formation.

Sources

Good sources include meat, dairy products and fortified grains.

Daily recommended dietary intakes

Men	1.3 mg
Women	1.1 mg
Pregnancy	1.4 mg
Lactation	1.6 mg

Toxic effects of excess intake

Riboflavin toxicity is very rare. Possible symptoms include itching, numbness, sensations of burning or pricking, and a sensitivity to light.

Interactions

Sulfa drugs, estrogen, alcohol, major tranquilizers and some antidepressants may increase riboflavin requirements.

Therapeutic uses of supplements

Supplements have been used to treat anemia, skin problems, carpal tunnel syndrome, migraine, stress and fatigue.

Also known as vitamin B2, riboflavin was the second B complex vitamin to be discovered. In pure form it is a yellow-orange, water soluble compound.

What it does in the body

Metabolism

Riboflavin is part of two coenzymes known as flavin adenine dinucleotide (FAD) and flavin mononucleotide (FMN) which are essential for tissue respiration and the generation of energy from the metabolism of carbohydrates, amino acids and fats. Riboflavin is vital for normal reproduction, growth, repair and development of body tissues including the skin, hair, nails, connective tissue and immune system. Riboflavin is mainly converted into FAD and FMN in the small intestine, liver, heart and kidney.

Brain and nerve function

Nerve development and the metabolism of brain neurotransmitters require riboflavin.

Blood cells

Blood cells require riboflavin for their development and for iron metabolism.

Hormones and glands

Riboflavin is involved in adrenal gland function and in the production and regulation of certain hormones.

Absorption and metabolism

Riboflavin is easily absorbed from food. A small amount is stored in the liver and kidneys, but amounts above about 25 mg are excreted in the urine so a regular dietary intake of is it necessary. Excess riboflavin excreted in the urine causes it to become bright yellow in color, which many people notice when they take B vitamin supplements.

Deficiency

Severe riboflavin deficiency is rare and often occurs with other B vitamin deficiencies. Symptoms include red, swollen, cracked lips, mouth and tongue; aversion to bright light; loss of appetite; weakness; fatigue; depression; anemia; loss of vision; burning and itching of the eyes; and dermatitis. Decreased sensitivity to touch, temperature, vibration and position may occur in the hands and feet. Riboflavin deficiency may be associated with an increase in throat and esophageal cancers. Cancer, cardiac disease and diabetes may lead to or exacerbate riboflavin deficiency.

People who are lactose intolerant and who cannot drink milk (which is a good source of riboflavin) may be at risk of deficiency. Those with malabsorption disorders, diarrhea and irritable bowel syndrome may also be at risk. Mild riboflavin deficiency may be quite common in elderly people whose diets are low in red meat and dairy products. Systemic infections, even without gastrointestinal tract involvement, may increase riboflavin requirements.

Cataract

Riboflavin deficiency may be associated with the development of cataracts. Researchers involved in the New York State Lens Opacities Case-Control Study assessed the risk factors for various types of cataract among 1380 participants aged 40 to 79 years. They found an increased risk with low levels of several nutrient including riboflavin.[1] Riboflavin is necessary for the activity of an enzyme which exerts protective effects on the eye.

Rheumatoid arthritis

In a 1996 study UK researchers assessed the links between riboflavin status and rheumatoid arthritis in patients and in those without the disease. The results showed that biochemical riboflavin deficiency was more frequent in patients with active disease. Riboflavin is necessary for the action of an enzyme which has anti-inflammatory activity and deficiency could reduce the activity and beneficial effect of that enzyme.[2]

Sources

The richest sources of riboflavin include organ meats such as liver, kidney and heart. Milk, yeast, cheese, oily fish, eggs and dark green leafy vegetables are also rich sources. Flour and cereals are enriched with riboflavin.

Riboflavin is stable when heated but will leach into cooking water. It is easily destroyed by light, and foods stored in clear containers will lose their riboflavin content in a short period of time. Alkalis, such as baking soda, also destroy riboflavin.

Food	Amount	Riboflavin (mg)
Lambs liver, fried	100g	4.03
Almonds, blanched	½ cup	0.98
Scallops, fried	6 pieces	0.85
Pink salmon, canned	1 can	0.84
Malted milk powder	4-5 tsp	0.75
All Bran	½ cup	0.42
Spinach, cooked	1 cup	0.42
Milk, whole and skim	1 cup	0.40
Mackerel, cooked	1 fillet	0.36
Veal, cooked	100g	0.35
Wheatgerm	½ cup	0.29
Lamb, cooked	100g	0.27
Pork sausages, grilled	100g	0.25
Eggs, boiled	1 medium	0.25
Milk chocolate	100g	0.24
Fruit yoghurt	1 tub	0.23
Feta cheese	1 cup	0.23
Oats	1 cup	0.21
Beef steak, grilled	100g	0.21
Green peas	1 cup	0.19
Soy milk	1 cup	0.17
Pork, cooked	100g	0.11

Cheddar cheese	1 slice	0.11
Brazil nuts	¼ cup	0.17

Recommended dietary allowances

The RDAs for riboflavin in the USA were revised in 1998.

	Men	*Women*	*Pregnancy*	*Lactation*
USA	1.3 mg	1.1 mg	1.4 mg	1.6 mg
UK	1.3 mg	1.1 mg	1.4 mg	1.6 mg
Australia	1.7 mg	1.2 mg	1.5 mg	1.7 mg

The Australian recommended daily intake is based on a requirement of 0.15 mg for every 1000 kJ of food taken in. Women pregnant with or breastfeeding more than one baby have higher riboflavin requirements.

Supplements

Supplements may be of benefit for those at risk of deficiency, particularly for elderly people, alcoholics or those with absorption difficulties. Stress and heavy exercise may increase riboflavin needs.

Toxic effects of excess intake

High doses of riboflavin are not well absorbed so the risk of toxicity is very low. Possible reactions to excess intakes include itching, numbness, sensations of burning or pricking, and sensitivity to sunlight.

Therapeutic uses of supplements

Riboflavin supplements are used to treat or prevent riboflavin deficiency.

Anemia

Riboflavin supplements may be of benefit in the treatment of sickle cell anemia and may also enhance the effectiveness of iron supplements when these are used to treat anemia.

Migraine

High doses of riboflavin may be effective in the treatment of migraine. In a 1998 study done in Belgium, researchers tested the effects of either 400 mg of riboflavin or a placebo on 55 patients with migraine in a randomized trial lasting three months. The results showed reductions in attack frequency and headache days. Fifty nine per cent of patients in the riboflavin group improved compared to 15 per cent in the placebo group. No serious side effects occurred. The researchers felt that because of its effectiveness, excellent tolerability, and low cost, riboflavin is a valuable option for migraine prevention.[3]

Carpal tunnel syndrome

Riboflavin may help to relieve the symptoms of carpal tunnel syndrome, a neurological disorder of the wrists and hands which causes pain and stiffness.Riboflavin is usually combined with vitamin B6 to treat this disorder and treatment with both vitamins may be more effective than treatment with B6 alone.[4,5] This is possibly due to the fact that riboflavin is involved in the conversion of vitamin B6 to its active form.

Other uses

Skin problems such as acne, dermatitis, eczema and ulcers; eye problems such as cataracts; and muscle cramps, may be improved by treatment with riboflavin supplements. Like the other B vitamins, riboflavin can be used to treat stress.

Interactions with other nutrients

Riboflavin is necessary for the activation of vitamin B6 and is also necessary for the conversion of tryptophan to niacin.

Interactions with drugs

Sulfa drugs, anti-malarial drugs, estrogen, cathartic agents and alcohol may interfere with riboflavin metabolism. High doses of riboflavin can reduce the effectiveness of the anticancer drug methotrexate. Some antibiotics and phenothiazine drugs may increase riboflavin excretion.

Riboflavin must be activated in the liver. This activation may be inhibited by major tranquilizers, and some antidepressants. Long-term use of barbiturates may adversely affect riboflavin status.

Cautions

High doses of riboflavin can produce urine discoloration which can affect urine analysis results.

QUICK GUIDE

Essential for

- the release of energy from food
- healthy skin, blood cells and digestive system
- normal growth and development
- hormone production
- a healthy brain and nervous system
- repair of genetic material

Absorption and metabolism

Niacin is the common name for nicotinic acid and nicotinamide (niacinamide). Daily intake is necessary and needs are partly met by the conversion of the amino acid, tryptophan, to niacin.

Deficiency

Deficiency eventually leads to pellagra, with symptoms of dermatitis on the hands and face, weakness, appetite loss, sore mouth, diarrhea, anxiety, depression, and dementia.

Sources

These include meat, fish, pulses and whole grains.

Daily recommended dietary intakes

Men	16 mg
Women	14 mg
Pregnancy	18 mg
Lactation	17 mg

Toxic effects of excess intake

High doses of the nicotinic acid form of niacin can cause skin flushing, headaches, tingling and burning. Larger doses can cause liver damage.

Interactions

Niacin may enhance anticonvulsant drug action.

Therapeutic uses of supplements

Niacin is used to treat diabetes, mental problems, high cholesterol, digestive problems, headaches, skin ailments and fatigue.

Cautions

People who have diabetes, gout, asthma, liver disease, an active peptic ulcer, and those taking high blood pressure medication should avoid high doses of niacin.

Niacin, which is also known as vitamin B3, is the common name for both nicotinic acid and nicotinamide (or niacinamide). The niacin deficiency disease, pellagra, was first recognized in the early 18th century but it was not until the 1930s that niacin was found to cure the disease. Niacin is a water soluble white powder and is more resistant to destruction than other B complex vitamins. The body can convert the amino acid tryptophan into niacin.

What it does in the body

Metabolism

Like other B vitamins, niacin is essential for the manufacture of enzymes that provide cells with energy through tissue respiration and carbohydrate, protein and fat metabolism. These enzymes are nicotinamide adenine dinucleotide (NAD) and nicotinamide adenine dinucleotide phosphate (NADP). Niacin is involved in over 200 enzyme reactions and is essential for healthy skin, tongue and digestive tract tissues and the formation of red blood cells.

Hormones

Niacin is essential for the synthesis of various hormones including sex hormones, cortisone, thyroxin and insulin. Nicotinic acid is part of the glucose tolerance factor, a compound which enhances the body's response to insulin (the hormone responsible for transporting glucose into cells and storing it in the liver and muscles).

Protection of genetic material

The repair of the genetic damage that occurs when cells are exposed to viruses, drugs or other toxic substances requires niacin-dependent coenzymes.

Nervous system

Niacin is essential for the normal functioning of the brain and nervous system.

Absorption and metabolism

Niacin is absorbed in the small intestine, mostly in the form of NAD or NADP. These compounds are then broken down to form nicotinamide which can be converted by bacteria to nicotinic acid. As niacin is water soluble, excess is excreted in the urine, although small amounts may be stored in the liver.

The amino acid, tryptophan, is converted to niacin in the body if sufficient iron, riboflavin and vitamin B6 are present. More than half the RDA for niacin can be obtained through the conversion of tryptophan.

Deficiency

Severe niacin deficiency causes the disease known as pellagra. Symptoms include the 'three Ds': diarrhea, dementia and dermatitis. The most characteristic sign is a reddish skin rash on the face, hands and feet which becomes rough and dark when exposed to sunlight. Other symptoms include weakness, loss of appetite, lethargy, a sore mouth and tongue, inflamed membranes in the intestinal tract and diarrhea. Nervous system effects include dementia, tremors, irritability, anxiety, confusion and depression. Pellagra may actually be a complex disorder involving thiamin, riboflavin and other nutrients. Niacin deficiency was originally observed in cultures whose diets relied heavily on corn prepared in a way which left the niacin unavailable for absorption.

Large amounts of tryptophan can overcome a niacin-poor diet and deficiency is usually seen in those whose diets are low in both niacin and protein. People at risk of deficiency include those with absorption difficulties, alcoholics, the elderly who neglect their diet, some infants and pregnant women.

Sources

Most niacin in food is in the form of NAD or NADP. The richest sources of niacin and tryptophan are chicken, fish, cooked dried beans and peas, brewer's yeast, wheat bran, peanuts, beef, and whole grain wheat products. Niacin in grain foods is bound to other compounds and only around 30 per cent is available for absorption. Fruits, vegetables and dairy products all contain some niacin as do dates, figs and prunes. Milk and eggs are good sources of tryptophan. Processing of grains removes most of their niacin content so flour is enriched with the vitamin. Niacin is relatively stable to heat and light, and little is lost during cooking. Treating corn with lime water, a procedure which is common in Central America and Mexico, increases the availability of niacin.

Under normal conditions, tryptophan obtained in the diet is first used for the maintenance of protein levels and then for the manufacture of niacin. Although it appears to vary widely, an average conversion rate is 60 mg tryptophan to 1 mg niacin.

Food	Amount	Niacin (mg)
Tuna, canned	1 can	41.8
Salmon, canned	½ cup	29.7
Special K	1 cup	22.6
All Bran	½ cup	16.7
Lamb liver, fried	100g	12.2
Swordfish	100g	11.8
Veal, cooked	100g	10.5
Peanuts, salted	½ cup	8.8
Trout	1 fillet	8.3
Chicken, roast	100g	7.9
Lamb, cooked	100g	6.6
Lamb kidney, simmered	100g	6.0
Mackerel	1 fillet	6.0
Beef, cooked, lean and fat	100g	3.9
Wheatgerm	½ cup	3.9
Plain hamburger	1 serve	3.7
Pork, cooked, lean and fat	100g	2.5
Pork sausage	100g	4.5
Kidney beans	1 cup	3.0
Corn	1 cup	2.6
Spaghetti, cooked	1 cup	2.3

Recommended dietary allowances

The RDAs for niacin in the USA were revised in 1998.

	Men	*Women*	*Pregnancy*	*Lactation*
USA	16 mg	14 mg	18 mg	17 mg
UK	17 mg	13 mg	13 mg	15 mg
Australia	19 mg	13 mg	15 mg	18 mg

As for the other B vitamins, niacin requirements are greater in women pregnant with or breastfeeding more than one child.

Supplements

Niacin supplements are available in nicotinic acid and niacinamide forms, both separately and combined. These have different applications. Sustained release niacin supplements are available and although these may reduce the skin flushing reaction caused by large doses of niacin, they may be more toxic to the liver.

A newer form of niacin known as inositol bound niacin or inositol hexanicotinate is now available, and may be safer than other forms as it does not cause liver damage or flushing.

Toxic effects of excess intake

Doses in excess of 1000 mg of nicotinic acid can produce flushing of the skin, intense itching, headaches, tingling and burning, severe heartburn, nausea, vomiting, abnormalities of glucose metabolism, and eye problems such as blurred vision. The flushing is caused by the action of hormone-like compounds called prostaglandins which dilate blood vessels. Doses in the thousands of milligrams can cause liver damage and jaundice (a yellowing of the skin and eyes). The flushing can be minimized by taking nicotinic acid with meals or by taking an aspirin 30 minutes before each dose. The nicotinamide form of niacin does not cause flushing.

Therapeutic uses of supplements

Cardiovascular disease

Niacin has been used for many years to treat high blood lipid levels. It reduces total cholesterol, harmful LDL cholesterol and triglycerides, and increases beneficial HDL cholesterol levels. It has been shown to reduce the incidence of heart attacks and deaths from heart disease. Niacin also favorably influences other lipid levels including lipoprotein (a). (See page 559 for more information.) Doses used range from 1500 to 2500 mg. Sustained-release niacin may be associated with more dramatic changes in LDL cholesterol and triglyceride, whereas the short-acting preparation may cause greater increases in HDL cholesterol. The increase of HDL cholesterol seems to occur at a lower dose (1500 mg per day) than the reduction of LDL cholesterol. In general it is usual to start taking lower doses (around 50 to 100 mg) and then gradually increase to the higher doses over a period of two to three weeks.

Researchers involved in a 1997 study done in Minneapolis compared blood lipid levels in 244 patients treated with niacin and 160 treated with lovastatin, a widely used cholesterol-lowering drug. The results showed that both lovastatin and niacin effectively reduced LDL cholesterol levels with a greater drop seen in those taking lovastatin. Niacin use was associated with a 16.3 per cent improvement in HDL cholesterol, while HDL cholesterol levels in the lovastatin group improved 1.5 per cent. The improvement in triglyceride levels was also much greater in the niacin group.[1]

Nicotinic acid can also enhance the effects of other cholesterol-lowering medications. This may mean that the doses of these drugs can be reduced, thus lessening the possibility of undesirable side effects. In a recent US study, researchers found that combination therapy with niacin and low dose lovastatin was as effective as high dose lovastatin.[2]

In a 1997 US study, researchers assessed the effect of 1.5 mg of niacin per day in 23 diabetic patients who were unable to achieve desirable blood lipid levels with low-dose pravastatin treatment. The results showed significant reductions in LDL cholesterol with niacin treatment.[3] Taking vitamins A and E with nicotinic acid may reduce the dose of niacin necessary to produce beneficial effects.

Nicotinic acid has also been shown to have favorable effects on the blood clotting system which can reduce the build-up of atherosclerotic plaque.[4] It has also been used to treat peripheral vascular disease and circulatory disorders such as Raynaud's disease as it dilates blood vessels, thereby increasing blood flow to certain areas of the body.

Type I diabetes

Nicotinamide has been shown to prevent the development of Type I (insulin dependent) diabetes in animals, possibly by helping insulin to act more efficiently and by preventing the immune system from attacking the pancreatic beta cells which produce insulin. Because it has a protective effect on beta cells it needs to be given early in the course of the disease while there are beta cells still remaining. Several small scale studies in humans suggest that nicotinamide may have a role to play in preventing the onset of Type I diabetes.

Researchers in New Zealand carried out a controlled trial of oral nicotinamide in the prevention of the onset of diabetes mellitus in a group of high risk children. All eight of the untreated children developed diabetes during the follow-up period of the study whereas only one of 14 treated children did.[5] In 1996, the same researchers published the findings of a population-based diabetes prevention trial involving nicotinamide treatment of 173 children aged 5 to 8 at risk for Type I diabetes. The results showed a 50 per cent reduction in the development of diabetes in a five-year period and suggest a protective effect of nicotinamide.[6]

Mental disorders

Both tryptophan and niacin have been used to treat depression, anxiety and insomnia. The psychiatric symptoms of niacin deficiency disease resemble the symptoms of schizophrenia and large doses of niacin have been used to treat this disorder. In some cases, the results of such studies have been promising, while in others niacin has failed to show any beneficial effect.

Other uses

Niacin has been used to stimulate tooth eruption, to treat fatigue, irritability, digestive disorders, headaches, migraines, arthritis, cramps and nerve problems such as Bell's Palsy and trigeminal neuralgia.

Interactions with other nutrients

Vitamin B6, riboflavin and iron are necessary for the conversion of tryptophan to niacin. Niacin works with other B vitamins to perform its functions in the body. The amino acid, leucine, competes with tryptophan for absorption and diets low in niacin and high in leucine may lead to niacin deficiency disease. Niacin may also enhance the utilization of zinc and iron.[7]

Interactions with drugs

Niacin may reduce the toxic side effects on heart tissue of the anticancer drug adriamycin without reducing its effectiveness in the treatment of cancer. It may also enhance the effectiveness of anticonvulsant drugs such as phenobarbital. Antibiotics may cause niacin flushes to become more severe. The drug, isoniazid, may cause niacin deficiency disease as it reduces the conversion of tryptophan to niacin. Oral contraceptives appear to increase the conversion efficiency of tryptophan to niacin.

Alcohol may increase niacin needs and nicotinamide has been shown to protect against the damage to liver cells caused by drinking a large quantity of alcohol.[8]

Cautions

High doses of nicotinic acid should be avoided in those with impaired liver function, gall bladder disease, gout, asthma, cardiac arrhythmias, inflammatory bowel disease, migraine, or an active peptic ulcer. Nicotinic acid in high doses can reduce blood pressure and should be avoided by those taking drugs to control high blood pressure. Niacin in high doses can affect glucose metabolism and should be used cautiously by diabetics.

QUICK GUIDE

Essential for

- the release of energy from food
- healthy cardiovascular, nervous and immune systems
- protein metabolism and hormone production
- healthy skin, hair and red blood cells
- manufacture of the genetic material of the cell
- the conversion of tryptophan to niacin

Absorption and metabolism

Daily intake is necessary.

Deficiency

Symptoms include weakness, poor appetite, dermatitis, a sore mouth, susceptibility to infection, and eventually, convulsions and anemia. Deficiency may play a role in heart disease, kidney stone formation, carpal tunnel syndrome and depression.

Sources

These include meat, fish, eggs, milk and whole grains.

Daily recommended dietary intakes

Men	1.3 mg
Men (over 50)	1.7 mg
Women	1.3 mg
Women (over 50)	1.5 mg
Pregnancy	1.9 mg
Lactation	2.0 mg

Toxic effects of excess intake

High doses for long periods may cause nerve damage.

Interactions

Alcohol, smoking, estrogen, some antibiotics and antidepressants may increase requirements.

Therapeutic uses of supplements

These include asthma, cardiovascular disease, mood disorders, PMS, stress, carpal tunnel syndrome, fatigue, nausea of pregnancy, skin problems and kidney stones.

Cautions

Those taking the anti-Parkinsonian drug, levodopa, or anticonvulsant drugs should consult a doctor before taking supplements.

Vitamin B6 is a family of chemically-related compounds including pyridoxamine and pyridoxal which are found in animal products, and pyridoxine which is found in plants. The form most commonly used in fortified foods and supplements is pyridoxine.

What it does in the body

Metabolism

Like the other B complex vitamins, vitamin B6 is involved in the functioning of enzymes involved in the release of energy from food. The coenzyme forms of vitamin B6 are pyridoxal 5' phosphate and pyridoxamine 5' phosphate, and these are necessary for nearly 100 enzymatic reactions. These include the synthesis and breakdown of amino acids, the conversion of amino acids to carbohydrate or fat, and the conversion of one type of fat to another. Thus, it is involved in the manufacture of most protein-related compounds and plays a role in almost all bodily processes.

Cardiovascular system

Vitamin B6 is essential for the manufacture of fat-derived substances known as prostaglandins which are involved in processes such as blood pressure regulation and heart function. Vitamin B6 is also necessary for red blood cell formation.

Immune system

Vitamin B6 plays a vital role in maintaining a healthy immune system by affecting functions such as cell multiplication and antibody production.

Nervous system and brain

Adequate vitamin B6 is vital to the healthy development and function of the nervous system. It is involved in the manufacture of several neurotransmitters including serotonin, GABA, dopamine and noradrenaline, and plays an important role in regulating mental processes and mood. Concentrations of vitamin B6 are up to 25 to 50 times higher in the brain than in the blood.

Skin and hair

Vitamin B6 is important in maintaining healthy hair and skin.

Hormones

Vitamin B6 plays a role in modulating the effects of hormones, including male and female sex hormones and adrenal hormones.

Other functions

Vitamin B6 is also involved in the manufacture of the genetic material of the cell, sodium-potassium balance, histamine metabolism, the conversion of tryptophan to niacin, absorption of vitamin B12 and the production of hydrochloric acid.

Absorption and metabolism

Vitamin B6 is readily absorbed in the small intestine. Excess vitamin B6 is excreted in the urine so adequate daily intake is essential. The forms of vitamin B6 found in food are converted to active forms in the liver. Zinc and riboflavin are necessary for this process.

Deficiency

Adolescents, the elderly, people with heart disease, those on restricted diets and alcoholics are at risk of vitamin B6 deficiency. Others at risk include women on oral contraceptives, those under stress, those whose diets are high in sugar and fat and those taking certain medications. (See page 95) People who exercise heavily and athletes often have low vitamin B6 levels. Exercise causes vitamin B6 blood levels to increase during an exercise session possibly because of the release of vitamin B6-dependent enzymes from muscle storage or the transfer of the vitamin from the liver to the muscles. As vitamin B6 is involved in a wide range of body functions, the symptoms of deficiency are widespread.

Elderly people

Low vitamin B6 levels are common among elderly people and may lead to increased risk of several disorders including heart disease. In a study published in 1996 Dutch researchers studied the vitamin B6 intake and blood levels in 546 elderly Europeans, aged from 74 to 76, with no known vitamin B6 supplement use. They also examined links with other dietary and lifestyle factors, including indicators of physical health. The results showed that 27 per cent of the men and 42 per cent of the women had dietary vitamin B6 intakes below the mean minimum requirements. Twenty-two per cent of both men and women had low blood levels.[8]

In a French study published in 1997, researchers assessed vitamin B6 levels in elderly patients with infections during hospitalization. During infection, vitamin B6 levels were much lower than in healthy patients.[9]

Brain and nervous system

Vitamin B6 deficiency can cause the mental symptoms of irritability, weakness, drowsiness, depression and poor appetite. Even a marginal deficiency can affect enzymes involved in the metabolism of several brain neurotransmitters. Vitamin B6 deficiency causes convulsions in young children.

In a study published in 1996, US Department of Agriculture researchers investigated the effects of blood levels of the amino acid, homocysteine and vitamins B12 and B6 and folate, on performance in cognitive tests of 70 men, aged 54 to 81 years. The results showed that higher concentrations of vitamin B6 were related to better performance on memory tests.[1]

Pregnancy

Low levels of vitamin B6 in pregnant women can affect the development of a baby's nervous system. Deficiency may also contribute to water retention, morning sickness, pre-eclampsia and birthing difficulties. It may also lead to diabetic and blood sugar problems in pregnancy.

Skin

Vitamin B6 deficiency can lead to greasy inflammation of the skin around the nose, eyebrows and hairline, and cracking of the lips and tongue.

Immune system

Immune response is adversely affected by vitamin B6 deficiency. Many different aspects of the immune system are affected, including the quality and quantity of antibodies and the number of infection-fighting white blood cells. Some immunosuppressive drugs affect the activity of a vitamin B6-dependent enzyme and vitamin B6 supplements may help to counter some of the side-effects of these drugs.

HIV/AIDS

Vitamin B6 deficiency is common in HIV-infected people. In a 1991 study, University of Miami researchers examined the relationship between deficiency and immune dysfunction. The results showed that while CD4+ and CD8+ cell numbers were not affected, other measures of immune system function were.[2]

Kidney

Vitamin B6 deficiency may also play a role in the development of some kinds of kidney stones.

Cardiovascular disease

Vitamin B6 deficiency can raise the risk of developing cardiovascular disease. One theory of the development of atherosclerosis links high levels of a compound known as homocysteine to damage of the cells lining the arteries. A deficiency of vitamin B6 leads to an accumulation of homocysteine and may also lead to defects in artery wall formation. Several studies, including the Framingham Heart Study, have confirmed the link between low pyridoxine levels and high homocysteine levels Researchers analyzed blood samples from the study participants to assess levels of homocysteine and the relationship between B vitamins and carotid artery narrowing, which increases the risk of heart attack. The results showed that low intakes of folate and vitamin B6 were associated with high homocysteine levels. Those with the highest homocysteine levels were twice as likely to have carotid artery narrowing when compared with those in the lowest homocysteine group.[3]

Another study, published in 1998 in the American Heart Association journal *Circulation* provides further evidence of the importance of vitamin B6 in preventing heart disease. Researchers involved in a study done in several centers in Europe compared 750 patients with vascular disease and 800 control subjects of the same ages and sex. They measured blood levels of homocysteine, folate, vitamin B12, and vitamin B6. The results showed that those with high blood homocysteine concentrations had a high risk of vascular disease. In addition, low concentrations of folate and vitamin B6 were also associated with increased risk. In this study, the relationship between vitamin B6 and atherosclerosis did not appear to be solely due to increased homocysteine levels, suggesting that vitamin B6 may have other important roles in heart disease prevention.[4]

Intake of folate and vitamin B6 above the current recommended dietary allowance seems to be important in the prevention of coronary heart disease among women. Researchers from the Harvard School of Public Health investigated the links between intakes of folate and vitamin B6 and the incidence of heart attacks in 80 082 women taking part in the Nurses' Health Study. The women had no previous history of cardiovascular disease, cancer, high cholesterol levels or diabetes when they entered the study. During the 14 years of follow-up, there were 658 nonfatal heart attacks and 281 fatal ones. The results showed that those with the highest intakes of vitamin B6 had just over 30 per cent less risk of heart attack than those in the low intake group. Women in the group with the highest intakes of both folate and vitamin has just less than half the risk of women in the lowest intake group. Risk of coronary heart disease was reduced among women who regularly used multiple vitamins, the major source of folate and vitamin B6.[5]

Low vitamin B6 levels are linked to an increased risk of heart attack. In a study published in 1996, researchers studied the links between homocysteine, vitamins B12, B6 and folate levels, and the risk of heart attack. The cases were 130 hospitalized heart attack patients and 118 healthy people. The results showed that average homocysteine levels were 11 per cent higher in cases compared with health people. Dietary and blood levels of vitamin B6 and folate were lower in cases than in controls.[6]

Carpal tunnel syndrome

Several small studies have found low vitamin B6 levels in sufferers of the carpal tunnel syndrome, a neurological disorder of the wrists and hands which causes pain and stiffness.[7]

Other symptoms

Vitamin B6 deficiency also leads to anemia and may play a part in the accelerated joint degeneration seen in osteoarthritis. It may also be linked to an increased risk of osteoporosis, arthritis, recurrent yeast infections, the worsening of some types of seizure disorders, the development of diabetes associated cataracts, and certain forms of cancer including cervical cancer.

Sources

The richest sources of vitamin B6 are chicken, fish, liver, kidney, pork, eggs, milk, wheatgerm and brewer's yeast. Other good sources include brown rice, soybeans, oats, whole wheat products, peanuts and walnuts.

Long-term storage, canning, roasting or stewing of meat and food processing techniques can destroy vitamin B6. Cooking reduces the vitamin B6 content of food because of losses into the water.

Food	Amount	Vitamin B6 (mg)
Wheatgerm	1 cup	1.42
Beef liver, fried	85g	1.22
Wheat bran	1 cup	0.72
Bananas	1 medium	0.68
Chicken, roast	1 cup, chopped	0.63
Avocado	1 medium	0.56
Ham, cooked	1 cup	0.51
Tuna, canned in water	1 cup	0.51
Spinach, cooked	1 cup	0.42
Kidneys, cooked	85g	0.44
Soybeans, cooked	1 cup	0.38
Mackerel, cooked	1 cup	0.38
Raisins	1 cup	0.34
Beef, sirloin, grilled	85g	0.35
Green peas, cooked	1 cup	0.33
Pork chop, grilled	85g	0.32
Pink salmon, cooked	½ fillet	0.29
Brown rice, cooked	1 cup	0.27
Peanuts	½ cup	0.25
Pearl barley, cooked	1 cup	0.17
Potatoes, flesh, baked	½ cup	0.17
White rice, cooked	1 cup	0.14
Brussels sprouts, cooked	½ cup	0.13
Lamb, sirloin, roasted	85g	0.12

Recommended dietary allowances

The RDAs for vitamin B6 have recently been revised.

	Men	Women	Pregnancy	Lactation
USA	1.3 mg	1.3 mg	1.9 mg	2.0 mg
(over 50)	1.7 mg	1.5 mg		
UK	1.4mg	1.6 mg		
Australia	1.3-1.9 mg	0.9-1.4 mg	+0.1 mg	+0.7-0.8 mg

The tolerable upper intake limit has been set at 100 mg per day.

The RDA for vitamin B6 is based on protein intake. Those with high protein intakes may need higher levels of vitamin B6. A 1998 study published in the *American Journal of Clinical Nutrition* suggests that the US RDA for women is not adequate. The researchers found that the amount of vitamin B6 necessary to normalize body levels of vitamin B6 metabolites after depletion was 1.94 mg.[10]

Supplements

Vitamin B6 is available as pyridoxine hydrochloride and pyridoxal-5'-phosphate. The latter is the more active form and may be best for those with liver disease who cannot convert pyridoxine to pyridoxal-5-phosphate. Anyone at risk of deficiency or who is suffering from a condition possibly linked to vitamin B6 deficiency is likely to benefit from supplements.

Toxic effects of excess intake

Large doses of vitamin B6 (over 2000 mg) can cause nerve damage. Symptoms include tingling in the hands and feet, a stumbling gait and lack of muscle coordination. Daily doses of 300 mg taken for many months or years may also lead to damage which can be permanent even when high doses are discontinued. Night restlessness, vivid dreams, sun sensitivity and an acne-like rash may also occur with high doses.

Therapeutic uses of supplements

Vitamin B6 supplements are used to treat deficiency symptoms. They have also been widely used in the treatment of a number of other health conditions.

Asthma

Limited research suggests that some children with asthma have a partial defect in tryptophan metabolism. An increased intake of vitamin B6 may reduce the symptoms of asthma in these patients. A study done in the 1970s looked at the effect of five months of pyridoxine therapy (200 mg daily) in asthmatic children and found significant improvement in symptoms and decreased need for anti-asthma medications.[11] Researchers involved in a 1985 study found a dramatic decrease in frequency and severity of wheezing or asthmatic attacks in those taking vitamin B6 supplements.[12] However, not all studies have found beneficial effects.[13]

Long-term therapy with theophylline, a drug often given to asthmatic patients, lowers vitamin B6 levels. Vitamin B6 supplements may be useful in preventing the side effects of the drug which include headaches, nausea, sleep disorders and convulsions.[14]

Cardiovascular disease

Low vitamin B6 levels increase the risk of cardiovascular disease and there is some evidence that supplements may be beneficial in preventing this. The results of the 1998 Harvard Study mentioned on page 87 showed that risk of coronary heart disease was reduced among women who regularly used multiple vitamins, the major source of folate and vitamin B6.

In a study done in 1993, South African researchers measured vitamin B6, vitamin B12, and folic acid levels in a group of healthy men with moderately high homocysteine levels. They found these levels to be low. In a placebo-controlled follow-up study, they found that a daily vitamin supplement containing 10 mg vitamin B6, 1.0 mg folic acid and 0.4 mg of vitamin B12 normalized elevated plasma homocysteine concentrations within six weeks.[15]

In a study published in 1998 Irish researchers screened a group of clinically healthy working men aged 30 to 49 years and selected 132 with mildly raised homocysteine concentrations. They then assessed the effects of eight weeks of supplementation with B group vitamins and antioxidant vitamins on homocysteine concentrations. The men were randomly assigned to one of four groups: supplementation with B group vitamins alone (1 mg folic acid, 7.2 mg pyridoxine, and 0.02 mg vitamin B12), antioxidant vitamins alone, B-group vitamins with antioxidant vitamins, or placebo. The results showed significant decreases in both groups receiving B group vitamins either with or without antioxidants. The effect of the B group vitamins alone was a reduction in homocysteine concentrations of almost 30 per cent.[16]

Vitamin B6 may also exert beneficial effects on the cardiovascular system by protecting against the aggregation of blood platelets. This prolongs clotting time and helps to reduce atherosclerotic plaque build-up.[17] Vitamin B6 has also been shown to lower blood pressure and blood cholesterol levels. In a Swedish study published in 1990, researchers assessed the effect of 120 mg a day of vitamin B6 on seventeen 88 year old men with low vitamin B6 levels. After supplementation for eight weeks, the average plasma total cholesterol and LDL cholesterol concentrations were decreased by 10 per cent and 17 per cent respectively.[18]

Mood disorders

Vitamin B6 deficiency is often found in depressed people and some studies have shown that supplements can improve mood. Vitamin B6 is involved in the metabolism of serotonin, a neurotransmitter which is involved in the regulation of mood. Vitamin B6 is also used to treat stress conditions.

In a randomized placebo-controlled study published in 1992, researchers at Harvard Medical School assessed the effects of 10 mg each of vitamins B1, B2, and B6 in 14 geriatric inpatients with depression who were taking antidepressant drugs. The results showed that those patients taking the vitamins showed greater improvement in scores on ratings of depression and cognitive function when compared with placebo-treated patients.[19]

Premenstrual syndrome and estrogen therapy

Vitamin B6 has also been used in the treatment of premenstrual syndrome symptoms including water retention, acne and mood changes. Many experts recommend doses of 50 mg to 150 mg per day started on day ten of the menstrual cycle and continued until day three of the next cycle.

Researchers in Oxford, UK conducted a double-blind trial to study the effects of 50 mg of vitamin B6 per day on premenstrual syndrome symptoms. The trial involved 63 women aged 18 to 49 years old who had noticed moderate to severe premenstrual symptoms during the previous year. Thirty-two women completed the full seven months of the study and the results showed a significant beneficial effect of vitamin B6 on emotional-type symptoms such as depression, irritability and tiredness.[20]

As estrogen may suppress vitamin B6 metabolism, supplements may be beneficial for pregnant women, those on the contraceptive pill or hormone replacement therapy (HRT) who suffer from mood swings and depression. Vitamin B6 is sometimes known as the women's vitamin.

Nausea of pregnancy

Vitamin B6 has been shown to provide relief from nausea and vomiting during pregnancy. Researchers at the University of Iowa studied the effects of vitamin B6 in doses of 25 mg every eight hours in a randomized, double-blind placebo-controlled study. Thirty-one patients received vitamin B6 for 72 hours, and 28 patients received placebo. At the completion of therapy, only eight of 31 patients in the vitamin B6 group had any vomiting, compared with 15 of 28 patients in the placebo group.[21]

Carpal tunnel syndrome

Vitamin B6 has been used to treat nerve compression including that seen in carpal tunnel syndrome. Some research suggests that treatment with supplements in doses of around 50 mg to 200 mg can improve symptoms.[22] However not all studies have reported positive results. In a 1996 study of 125 randomly selected industrial plant workers, researchers did not find a link between vitamin B6 and carpal tunnel syndrome.[23] Vitamin B6 has been shown to change pain thresholds in clinical and laboratory studies which may explain studies which have shown significant improvements in pain scores when nerve conduction test results showed only mild improvements. A 1998 study suggests that a high ratio of vitamin C to vitamin B6 may worsen the symptoms of the disorder.[24]

Vitamin B6 supplements may be useful in the treatment of carpal tunnel syndrome but intake should not exceed 100 mg per day as large doses can cause nerve damage. Higher doses should only be used under supervision. Some experts believe that a therapeutic effect may take at least three months to become apparent.

Convulsions

Some babies are born with a metabolic defect which means that they are unable to metabolize pyridoxine efficiently. This results in convulsions which must be treated with large doses of pyridoxine in order to avoid mental retardation.

Immune system

Vitamin B6 supplementation may boost the immune system in older people, thus reducing the risk of infection and possibly even cancer. Recent research from Johns Hopkins University suggests that vitamin B supplements may help HIV-positive people live longer. In an eight-year study of 281 HIV-positive, people vitamin B6 supplementation at twice the RDA was shown to be particularly effective in prolonging survival time.[25]

Other uses

Vitamin B6 has been used to treat kidney stones; muscle pain; skin problems such as eczema, dermatitis and psoriasis; migraines; fatigue; prostatitis; headaches; nerve disorders such as diabetic neuropathy; and low blood sugar. Vitamin B6 is also reputed to stimulate dream activity.

Interactions with other nutrients

Vitamin B6 requires riboflavin, zinc and magnesium for its normal function in the body. Vitamin B6 deficiency may result in low blood levels of vitamin C, increased excretion of calcium, zinc and magnesium, and reduced copper absorption.

Interactions with drugs

Alcohol increases breakdown of the biologically active form of vitamin B6 and long-term use may cause liver damage which interferes with the conversion of vitamin B6 to the active form. Amphetamines, levodopa, some antidepressants, isoniazid, penicillamine and hydralazine may alter vitamin B6 requirements. Oral contraceptives may also affect vitamin B6 metabolism and increase needs.[26] Large doses of vitamin B6 may interfere with the action of anticonvulsant drugs.

Cautions

Vitamin B6 supplements should not be taken by those taking anticonvulsants or levodopa for Parkinson's disease as they may alter the effectiveness of these medications. Vitamin B6 may lower blood sugar and should be used with caution by diabetics.

QUICK GUIDE

Essential for

- the synthesis of genetic material
- protein metabolism
- a healthy pregnancy
- healthy red blood cells, bones and hair
- healthy nervous, digestive and immune systems

Absorption and metabolism

Some folic acid is stored in the liver.

Deficiency

Symptoms include anemia, mood disorders and gastrointestinal disorders. Deficiency in pregnancy causes neural tube defects in babies. Low levels may increase the risk of heart disease and cancer.

Sources

Good sources include liver, pulses and dark green leafy vegetables.

Daily recommended dietary intakes

Men	400 mcg
Women	400 mcg
Pregnancy	600 mcg
Lactation	500 mcg

Toxic effects of excess intake

These are rare and include gastrointestinal problems and sleep disturbances.

Interactions

Tobacco, alcohol, estrogen, anticonvulsants and several other drugs may raise requirements.

Therapeutic uses of supplements

Uses include prevention of neural tube defects in pregnancy, treatment of anemia, fatigue, mental problems, skin disorders and prevention of heart disease and cancer.

Cautions

Large doses can mask vitamin B12 deficiency which may lead to permanent nerve damage. Folic acid can interfere with the action of anticonvulsant drugs.

Folate is the name used for any compound which has vitamin-like activity similar to that of folic acid, the form of this vitamin most commonly used in supplements and fortified foods. Folic acid takes its name from the Latin word for foliage as it was originally isolated from leafy green vegetables. The terms folic acid and folate are generally used to refer to the same substance.

What it does in the body

Genetic material

Folic acid is essential for the synthesis of DNA and RNA, the genetic material of cells. It plays a vital role in the growth and reproduction of all body cells, maintaining the genetic code, regulating cell division and transferring inherited characteristics from one cell to another.

Metabolism

Folic acid is essential for protein metabolism. As part of its role in protein metabolism, folate converts the amino acid known as homocysteine to methionine. High levels of homocysteine have been linked to an increased risk of cardiovascular disease.

Blood

The formation of healthy red and white blood cells requires folic acid.

Brain and nervous system

Folic acid is involved in the production of neurotransmitters such as serotonin and dopamine, which regulate brain functions including mood, sleep and appetite. Folic acid is essential for the development of the brain, spinal cord and skeleton in the fetus.

Absorption and metabolism

Folic acid is absorbed from the small intestine. The amount of folic acid absorbed from food depends on the source but the average is around 50 per cent. Research shows that synthetic forms of folic acid are absorbed better than natural food forms with around 85 per cent of supplemental folic acid being absorbed if it is taken with a small amount of food.[1]

Around 50 per cent of body stores are in the liver. The amount stored may last for about four months before symptoms of deficiency develop.

Deficiency

Folate deficiency is the most common nutritional deficiency in the world. Diets low in vegetables, frequent alcohol and prescription drug use and the sensitivity of folate to light and heat contribute to this widespread deficiency. The elderly, alcoholics, psychiatric patients, people taking certain medications and women taking the contraceptive pill may be at greatest risk of folate deficiency. Prolonged stress, viral infections and chronic liver disease are also risk factors.

When folate intake is inadequate, levels in serum fall, levels in red blood cells also fall, homocysteine concentration rises and finally, changes in the blood cell-producing bone marrow and other rapidly dividing cells occur. Ultimately, folate acid deficiency affects the growth and repair of all the cells and tissues of the body.

Because red blood cells have a lifespan of 120 days, folate levels in the blood can be lowered for many weeks before symptoms of anemia become apparent. Tests which rely on anemia to diagnose folate deficiency may therefore not be appropriate.

As many as 5 to 15 per cent of people may have a particular type of genetic mutation in the DNA which codes for an enzyme involved in homocysteine metabolism. This leads to higher homocysteine concentrations and therefore an increased risk of heart disease; and in women, of having babies with neural tube defects. Such people have higher folate requirements than those who do not have this type of genetic mutation, and may need supplements.[2]

Elderly people

Many elderly people are at risk of folate deficiency. In a study published in 1996, Canadian researchers investigated folate and vitamin B12 intakes and body levels in 28 men and 30 women aged over 65 years. The results showed that 57 per cent of men and 67 per cent of women were at risk of deficiency.[3]

Folate deficiency may cause or worsen the mental difficulties which older people often experience. In a 1996 study, Spanish researchers analyzed the relationship between mental and functional capacities and folate status in a group of 177 elderly people. In this study, almost 50 per cent of the people had folate intakes below recommended values. Those with poor test results had significantly lower folate levels.[4]

Blood

Folic acid deficiency causes macrocytic anemia in which the red blood cells are fewer in number, larger in size and contain less oxygen-carrying hemoglobin than normal cells. The symptoms of anemia are lethargy, apathy, breathlessness, poor body temperature regulation, pallor, forgetfulness, irritability and stomach disorders.

Cardiovascular disease

Many studies have shown that low folic acid levels are linked to an increased risk of atherosclerosis and heart disease. Folic acid may exert its protective effects on the cardiovascular system by reducing the levels of homocysteine in the blood. Homocysteine is a product of protein breakdown which can damage the cells which line the arteries and promote the clumping together of platelets which increases clot formation. Homocysteine levels are influenced by dietary intakes of folate, vitamin B6 and vitamin B12. They also vary according to race, gender, age and certain disease conditions.

Evidence from the Framingham Heart Study, an ongoing analysis of the risk factors for heart disease which began almost 50 years ago and involves over 1000 men and women, supports the links between folate, homocysteine and heart disease. During the study, researchers examined the relationship between intake of folate from foods and supplements with blood plasma folate and homocysteine concentrations among 885 elderly people. The results showed that plasma folate was significantly greater and homocysteine lower in women than in men. Users of supplements, breakfast cereals, or green leafy vegetables had significantly greater plasma folate and lower homocysteine levels than non-users. Plasma folate concentration was also greater in those who drank orange juice.[5]

In a study published in 1998, researchers at the Cleveland Clinic conducted a study to investigate the relationships between homocysteine, B vitamins, and vascular diseases. The study involved 750 patients with documented vascular disease and 800 control patients matched for age and sex. The results showed that those in the top 20 per cent for homocysteine concentrations had a greater risk of vascular disease. Those in the lowest 10 per cent of folate intakes also had an increased risk of disease.[6]

A 1996 Canadian study of the relationship between fatal coronary heart disease and folic acid levels in 5000 men and women found that the risk of coronary heart disease increased as folic acid levels decreased. Those in the lowest intake group were 69 per cent more likely to die of heart disease than those with the highest intakes.[7]

Low blood folic acid levels also seem to increase heart attack risk in young women. In a 1997 study, researchers at the University of Washington measured the homocysteine, folic acid and vitamin B12 levels in 79 heart attack survivors under 45 and compared these with levels in 386 healthy control subjects. Those with the highest homocysteine levels had 2.3 times the risk of heart attack compared to those with the lowest levels. Those with the highest levels of folic acid had around half the risk of heart attack compared with those with the lowest levels.[8]

Results from the US Physicians Health Study published in 1996 found a small link between low folate levels and risk of heart attack, but this was not statistically significant.[9]

Nervous system

Folic acid deficiency causes mood disorders with symptoms of irritability, forgetfulness and hostility. Low levels may play a role in depression, possibly due to a reduction in neurotransmitter levels.

In a study published in 1996, USDA researchers investigated the relationships between plasma concentrations of homocysteine and vitamins B12 and B6 and folate, and cognitive test scores in 70 men, aged 54 to 81 years old. Lower concentrations of vitamin B12 and folate and higher concentrations of homocysteine were associated with poorer results on the tests.[10]

Folate deficiency may also be linked to depression. Borderline low or deficient folate levels have been detected in as many as 38 per cent of adults diagnosed with depressive disorders.[11] Low folate levels have also been linked to poorer response to the antidepressant drug Prozac. In a study published in 1997, researchers examined the relationships between levels of folate, vitamin B12, and homocysteine in 213 depressed patients taking Prozac. The results showed that people with low folate levels were more likely to have melancholic depression and were significantly less likely to respond to the drug.[12]

Gastrointestinal system

Symptoms of folic acid deficiency also include loss of appetite, inflamed tongue, gastrointestinal problems and diarrhea. Folic acid deficiency can damage the lining of the gut and reduce absorption of other nutrients which can lead to malnutrition.

Neural tube defects

Folic acid deficiency may affect up to a third of all pregnant women and is associated with birth defects. Pregnant women who are folic acid-deficient risk having babies with neural tube defects, such as anencephaly (failure of the brain to develop) and spina bifida (failure of the spinal column to close). The risk of neural tube defects in the US is around one per 1000 pregnancies. The high risk period for folate deficiency-related birth defects is around one month before conception until around one month after. Many women are unaware that they are pregnant during this time so maintaining adequate folic acid levels is vital for any woman who might become pregnant. (See page 104)

Cancer

Folate deficiency may play a role in cancer development, particularly cancers of the cervix, lung and colon. It may be that folate deficiency itself is not carcinogenic but may contribute to an increased risk of cancer as deficiency may affect the repair of DNA and increase chromosome fragility. It may also diminish the ability of the immune system to fight cancer cells and viruses. Deficiency has been shown to affect a gene involved in suppressing tumor formation.[13]

Colorectal cancer

In a study published in 1996, researchers examined the relationship between folate status and colorectal cancer in male smokers aged 50 to 69 involved in the Alpha-Tocopherol Beta carotene (ATBC) Study. The researchers measured folate levels in 144 cases of colorectal cancer and 276 healthy people. Those with higher dietary folate intakes had a reduced risk of colon cancer. Men with a high-alcohol, low-folate, low-protein diet were at higher risk for colon cancer than men who consumed a low-alcohol, high-folate, high-protein diet.[14]

Cervical dysplasia

Low blood levels of folic acid may increase the risk of cervical dysplasia (precancerous changes in the cells lining the cervix), possibly by enhancing the effect of other risk factors. Researchers from the University of Alabama in Birmingham investigated the links between folate deficiency and cervical dysplasia in 294 young women with the disorder and 170 healthy women. They also assessed the impact of factors such as smoking, oral contraceptive use, human papillomavirus (HPV) infection, and number of sexual partners. The results showed that at low folate levels the risk of dysplasia caused by HPV infection was increased.[15]

Other symptoms

Low folic acid may also contribute to rheumatoid arthritis and osteoporosis, constipation, cataracts, headaches and infertility.

Sources

The best sources of folate are liver, brewer's yeast and dark green leafy vegetables such as spinach and kale. Dried beans, green vegetables, oranges, avocados and whole wheat products are also good sources.

Food processing such as boiling and heating can destroy folic acid. It can also be destroyed by being stored unprotected at room temperature for long periods.

Food fortification with folic acid

Since January, 1998, commercial grain products in the USA have been enriched with 140 mcg of folic acid per 100 g of grain product. It is estimated that this will deliver an average increase in intake of 100 mcg per day. Breakfast cereals may contain up to a daily dose of folic acid.

There has been concern that fortifying foods with folic acid would increase the risk of permanent damage from vitamin B12 deficiency due to the fact that high folic acid intakes can mask this deficiency. However, a study published in the *Journal of the American Medical Association* in 1996 suggests that the benefits of folic acid fortification, which include reduced risk of stroke and heart disease, outweigh the risk of masked vitamin B12 deficiency. Researchers at Tufts University, Boston, looked at the food intakes and blood folate and homocysteine concentrations of almost 750 people aged 67 to 96 years. From these results they predicted the value of adding folic acid to grain products and the effect on cardiovascular disease and vitamin B12-related disorders. Their results suggest that fortification at a level of 140 mcg per 100 g of grain product would reduce the risk of coronary artery disease by 5 per cent.[16]

A 1998 study reported in the *New England Journal of Medicine* provides further support for the possibility of reducing homocysteine levels by fortifying foods with folic acid. Researchers assessed the effects of breakfast cereals fortified with three levels of folic acid in a randomized, double-blind, placebo-controlled, crossover trial in 75 men and women with coronary artery disease. The results showed that folic acid increased and plasma homocysteine decreased in proportion to the folic acid content of the cereal. Cereal providing 127 mcg of folic acid daily, (which is about the amount that would result from the FDA's enrichment policy) decreased plasma homocysteine by only 3.7 per cent. However, cereals providing 499 and 665 mcg of folic acid daily decreased plasma homocysteine by 11 per cent and 14 per cent respectively.

These results suggest that folic acid fortification at levels higher than that recommended by the FDA may be necessary to effectively reduce homocysteine levels and reduce the risk of cardiovascular disease.[17]

Food	Amount	Folate (mcg)
Chicken liver, cooked	½ cup, chopped	512
Lentils, cooked	1 cup	340
Black-eyed peas, cooked	1 cup	200
Beef liver, fried	85g	187
Spinach, cooked	1 cup	249
Navy beans, cooked	1 cup	242
Kidney beans	1 cup	218
Peanuts	½ cup	166
Turnip greens, cooked	1 cup	162
Lima beans, cooked	1 cup	148
Fortified oats, ready to eat	1 cup	142
Avocado	1 fruit	124
Peas, cooked	1 cup	96.0
Asparagus, cooked	4 spears	87.6
Yellow corn	1 cup	72.3
Orange juice	1 cup	71.3
Papaya	1 cup, cubes	50.4
Brussels sprouts	½ cup	44.7
Wheat bran	1 cup	43.5
Almonds	½ cup, whole	39.6
Cos lettuce	½ cup, shredded	38.0
Oranges	1 medium	39.7
Walnuts	½ cup, chopped	37.6
Broccoli	½ cup, chopped	37.0

Recommended dietary allowances

In 1989, the government lowered the RDAs from 400 mcg to 200 mcg for men and 180 mcg for women. Increasing awareness of the importance of folic acid in preventing birth defects and cardiovascular disease led in 1998 to the raising of RDAs to 400 mcg. The tolerable upper intake level has been set at 1000 mcg per day.

	Men	*Women*	*Pregnancy*	*Lactation*
USA	400 mcg	400 mcg	600 mcg	500 mcg
UK	200 mcg	200 mcg	300 mcg	260 mcg
Australia	200 mcg	200 mcg	400 mcg	350 mcg

The RDA for pregnant women doubles due to the role of folic acid in cell growth in the baby and for increased blood volume and expanding tissues in the mother. Folic acid is the vitamin most closely related to pregnancy outcome.

Supplements

Folic acid is the type of folate usually found in supplements and fortified foods, as it is the most stable. Some supplements contain folinic acid, the most active form of folate.

Pregnant women, the elderly, and those with absorption difficulties are likely to benefit from supplements. Any condition that increases metabolic rate, such as infection and hyperthyroidism; and any condition that increases cell turnover, such as rapid tissue growth or hemolytic anemia, increases folate requirements. Anyone taking medications that increase folate requirements may also benefit from supplements.

Surveys show that for the last 25 years, around a quarter of Americans have regularly taken a multivitamin containing 400 mcg of folic acid. It is becoming clear that those who do so have a reduced risk of disease, particularly cardiovascular disease. A woman who takes a folate supplement reduces the risk that her child will be born with a birth defect. However, research shows that only one third of women of childbearing age consume a supplement containing the recommended amount of folic acid daily.[18]

According to a 1996 study of prescription multivitamins reported in the *Journal of The American Pharmaceutical Association*, US researchers found that several brands did not deliver the expected amount of folic acid because the tablets did not dissolve quickly enough. The researchers examined nine multivitamin products to see if they released 75 per cent of the folic acid within one hour, as required by the United States Pharmacopoeia Convention's dissolution standard. Only three of the products did so and most of the products missed the standard by a wide margin. Folic acid is best absorbed in the area of the intestine that lies just beyond the stomach. If the multivitamins do not dissolve within about an hour, the folic acid may pass this area and the amount available for optimal absorption is not adequate.[19]

Toxic effects of excess intake

Toxicity is considered rare. Symptoms are gastrointestinal disturbances, sleep problems and possible allergic skin reactions. These effects can occur at doses above 15 mg.

Therapeutic effects of supplements

Pregnancy

In 1992, the US Public Health Service issued a recommendation that all women capable of becoming pregnant should consume 400 mcg of folic acid daily in order to avoid the risk of neural tube defects in their babies. Around 50 per cent of neural tube defects may be preventable by increasing folate intakes. Eating foods naturally high in folic acid, eating fortified foods and taking supplements are good ways of increasing folic acid intake to recommended levels. Adequate consumption of folic acid should begin before and continue during at least the first four weeks after conception when the fetal neural tube is being formed.

Research suggests that in women who have previously had a child with a neural tube defect, folic acid in doses of up to 4 mg daily can reduce the risk of recurrence by about 70 per cent. This is something to be discussed with a doctor as such large amounts of folic acid are only available on prescription.

Studies suggest that the levels of folate necessary to prevent neural tube defects are more easily derived from fortified foods or supplements than from natural food sources alone. In an editorial in the *New England Journal of Medicine,* Godfrey Oakley MD of the Centers for Disease Control in Atlanta commented that "anyone who chooses to counsel a woman to consume 400 mcg of food-derived folate rather than 400 mcg of supplemental folic acid will be recommending a strategy that has not been proved to prevent birth defects and that leads to lower blood folate concentrations." Many experts recommend folic acid supplements and a diet rich in folates for women who are hoping to become pregnant.

In a study published in *The Lancet* in 1996, Irish researchers tested the effectiveness of different ways of raising folic acid levels. Participants in the three month trial included 62 women randomly assigned to one of the following five groups: folic acid supplement (400 mcg per day); folic-acid-fortified foods (an additional 400 mcg per day); dietary folate (an additional 400 mcg per day); dietary advice, and control. The results showed that red blood cell folate concentrations increased significantly in the groups taking folic acid supplements or food fortified with folic acid. The researchers concluded that advice to women to consume folate-rich foods as the only way to boost folate levels is misleading.[20]

In another study also published in *The Lancet*, researchers studied blood folic acid levels in 95 women in order to determine the minimum effective dose of folic acid for food fortification necessary to prevent neural tube defects. The women in the study were divided into four groups. One group received no folic acid while the other groups got doses of 100, 200 and 400 mcg daily. After six months, the researchers found that women taking 100 mcg daily had blood folic acid levels sufficient to prevent 22 per cent of neural tube defects. Those taking 200 mcg had a 41 prevention level and 400 mcg gave a 47 per cent prevention level. The researchers felt that as between 50 and 70 per cent of neural tube defects are thought to be preventable by folic acid, the reduction achieved by an additional 100 mcg per day would be substantial.[21]

A trial of the effects of vitamin supplements containing folate supplements on the incidence of neural tube defects involving over 4700 women was carried out in Hungary. In the women who did not receive folic acid there were six babies born with neural tube defects. In the group receiving the supplements, there were none.[22]

Cardiovascular disease

Folic acid supplements may reduce the risk of coronary heart disease by reducing homocysteine levels. In a paper published in the *British Medical Journal* in 1998, researchers analyzed the results of randomized controlled trials that assessed the effects of folic acid-based supplements on blood homocysteine concentrations. The data included that from 1114 people in 12 trials. They found that 0.5 to 5 mg folic acid daily reduced blood homocysteine concentrations by 25 per cent.[23]

In 1998, researchers at the Harvard School of Public Health published data from the Nurses Health Study which showed that intake of folate and vitamin B6 above the current recommended dietary allowance is important in the prevention of coronary heart disease among women. The study involved 80 082 women with no cardiovascular disease, cancer, high cholesterol or diabetes on entry to the study. During a 14 year period there were 658 cases of non-fatal heart attack and 281 cases of fatal coronary heart disease. Women in the highest folate intake group had around a 30 per cent reduced risk of disease. The risk of coronary heart disease was reduced by about 25 per cent in women who regularly used multiple vitamins.[24]

Those with the highest homocysteine levels may respond best to increases in folic acid intake, and above a certain level of intake, increasing folic acid may not affect homocysteine levels. In a 1997 Irish study, researchers assessed the effects of various doses of supplements on homocysteine levels. Of the three folic acid doses, 200 mcg appeared to be as effective as 400 mcg, while 100 did not lower levels sufficiently.[25]

Cancer

Several studies suggest that folic acid supplements can help to reduce the risk of cancerous changes in several areas such as the cervix, lung and gastrointestinal tract.

Colorectal cancer

In a study published in 1997, researchers at the Cleveland Clinic investigated the links between folate and cancerous changes in 98 patients with ulcerative colitis. Patients taking folic acid supplements had a 30 per cent lower risk of developing cancerous changes in the bowel. The lower the folate levels, the more advanced the degree of cancerous changes in the cells.[26] In a 1997 Italian study, researchers also studied the effects of folate supplements on pre-cancerous cell changes in ulcerative colitis. The results showed that folate reduced these changes.[27] Folic acid may also help to prevent the pre-cancerous changes in lung tissue caused by smoking.[28]

Cervical dysplasia

Folic acid supplementation may protect abnormal cells from becoming cancerous and may reverse cervical dysplasia in some cases. A 1996 study done at the

University of Alabama at Birmingham suggests that supplements may be useful in preventing the initial changes but do not appear to affect the progress of established disease.[29] Some researchers have found a higher risk of abnormalities in cervical tissue in women using oral contraceptives and suggest that folic acid supplements are beneficial in preventing cervical dysplasia in these women.[30]

Anemia

Folic acid is used to treat folic acid deficiency anemia and for supplementation in those suffering from sickle cell disease.

Mental function

Many psychiatric patients show folic acid deficiency, especially those suffering from depression. Supplements may be particularly beneficial in elderly people suffering from impaired mental function. This may be due to effects on neurotransmitters such as serotonin and dopamine.

Other uses

Folic acid supplements are given to those taking the drug, methotrexate, to prevent toxic side effects.[31] Folic acid may be of value in the treatment of gout and may also shorten the recovery time from hepatitis. Supplements may be useful in the treatment of osteoporosis as increased homocysteine levels may lead to defective bone formation. Folic acid may also be useful in improving skin condition in vitiligo.[32] Folic acid mouthwash may be useful in the treatment of periodontal disease and gum inflammation.

Interactions with other nutrients

Folic acid requires vitamin B12, niacin and vitamin C to be converted to its biologically active form. Vitamin C helps to reduce folic acid excretion. High folic acid intakes may reduce zinc absorption, although the effect is likely to be a subtle one.

Interactions with drugs

NSAIDs such as aspirin, ibuprofen and acetaminophen can increase folate requirements if taken for long periods. Anticonvulsant drugs such as phenytoin and phenobarbital also raise folate requirements which may be of particular concern as these drugs are often taken for long periods. Methotrexate increases requirements and it is recommended that people taking this drug for long periods also take folic acid supplements. Cholestyramine, chloramphenicol, estrogen, colchicine, antacids, antituberculosis drugs, trimethoprim, sulfasalazine, corticosteroid drugs and tobacco can raise folic acid requirements. Chronic alcohol use leads to folic acid deficiency.

Cautions

Large amounts of folic acid can mask anemia caused by vitamin B12 deficiency. Although this is rare, in some cases it may lead to permanent nerve damage. Amounts greater than 400 mcg per day should not be taken by anyone with anemia unless a diagnosis of pernicious anemia is ruled out.

Folic acid can interfere with the effectiveness of anticonvulsant drugs such as phenytoin and can result in an increase in seizure activity if large doses are taken.

QUICK GUIDE

Essential for

- energy release from food
- amino acid and fatty acid metabolism
- healthy nerves, blood cells, skin and hair
- production of genetic material
- growth and development

Absorption and metabolism

Vitamin B12 requires a compound known as intrinsic factor for absorption.

Deficiency

Deficiency leads to pernicious anemia with symptoms of fatigue, lightheadedness, headache and irritability. Other symptoms include nausea, loss of appetite, sore mouth, diarrhea, abnormal gait, loss of sensation in hands and feet, confusion, memory loss and depression.

Sources

These include meats, fish, eggs and dairy products.

Daily recommended dietary intakes

Men	2.4 mcg
Women	2.4 mcg
Pregnancy	2.6 mcg
Lactation	2.8 mcg

Toxic effects of excess intake

There have been no reports of toxic effects.

Interactions

Antacids, laxatives, alcohol, estrogen, sleeping pills, cholestyramine and colchicine may raise requirements.

Therapeutic uses of supplements

Supplements are used to treat pernicious anemia, immune deficiency, some psychiatric disorders, fatigue, allergies and sleep disorders. Some people use vitamin B12 injections as a general tonic.

Cautions

Large doses of vitamin B12 should not be used by those with low potassium levels.

Vitamin B12, which is also known as cobalamin, was the last B vitamin to be identified. It is water soluble, bright red in color and has an atom of cobalt at its center. The average adult body contains 2 to 5 mg of vitamin B12, with 80 per cent of this stored in the liver.

What it does in the body

Metabolism

Vitamin B12 is essential for metabolism of fats and carbohydrates and the synthesis of proteins. Vitamin B12 is also essential for the transport and storage of folate in cells and for conversion to its active form. Rapidly dividing cells, such as those in the epithelium and bone marrow, have the greatest need for vitamin B12.

Brain and nervous system

Vitamin B12 is involved in the manufacture of the myelin sheath, a fatty layer which insulates nerves. It is also essential in the formation of neurotransmitters.

Blood cells

The manufacture and normal functioning of blood cells requires vitamin B12.

Genetic material

Vitamin B12 is necessary for the production of nucleic acids, which make up DNA, the genetic material of the cell.

Absorption and metabolism

A compound known as intrinsic factor which is secreted by the cells lining the stomach is necessary for absorption of vitamin B12 from the small intestine. Those with malabsorption problems; such as celiac disease, low stomach acid, or who have had stomach or intestinal surgery; may have problems absorbing vitamin B12. Calcium and iron assist with vitamin B12 absorption.

Vitamin B12 is bound to proteins known as transcobalamins in the blood. It is excreted in the bile and re-absorbed. Those on diets which are low in vitamin B12 may obtain more from re-absorption than from food. Because of this re-absorption, vitamin B12 deficiency can take many years to become apparent.

The Schilling test, which uses a small dose of radioactive vitamin B12 and then a larger dose of normal B12 to flush this out, is used to measure the ability of a person to absorb vitamin B12.

Deficiency

As the body stores vitamin B12, symptoms of deficiency can take up to four to five years of poor dietary intake or lack of intrinsic factor production to appear. Deficiency is more commonly linked to the inability to absorb the vitamin due to lack of intrinsic factor than to insufficient dietary intake.

Elderly people

Vitamin B12 deficiency is more common in the elderly than in younger people, with around 15 per cent of elderly men and women affected. This is usually because of decreased absorption due to reduced production of intrinsic factor or to a stomach disorder known as atrophic gastritis. Supplementation can prevent irreversible neurological damage if started early. Elderly people with vitamin B12 deficiency may show psychiatric or metabolic deficiency symptoms even before anemia is diagnosed. Screening for low vitamin B12 levels is necessary in elderly people with mental impairment, although it has also been found that deficiency states can still exist even when blood levels are higher than the traditional lower reference limit for vitamin B12. Patients who are most at risk of vitamin B12 deficiency include those with gastrointestinal disorders, autoimmune disorders, Type I diabetes mellitus and thyroid disorders, and those receiving long-term therapy with gastric acid inhibitors.[1]

Blood

Vitamin B12 deficiency causes pernicious anemia with symptoms of tiredness, pallor, lightheadedness, breathlessness, headache and irritability. Red blood cells become abnormally enlarged and reduced blood platelet formation causes poor clotting and bruising. A high intake of folic acid can prevent the red blood cell changes caused by vitamin B12 deficiency. It does not, however, prevent the nerve damage which may only become apparent in later stages and which may not be reversible. Strict vegetarians, whose folic acid intakes are high while their vitamin B12 intakes are low, may be at particular risk of nerve damage.

Immune system

Vitamin B12 deficiency leads to reduced numbers of white blood cells which causes increased susceptibility to infection. Recent research has shown that elderly patients with low vitamin B12 levels have impaired antibody response to bacterial vaccine, even when there are no clinical signs of deficiency.[2]

Brain and nervous system

Vitamin B12 deficiency eventually leads to a deterioration in mental functioning, to neurological damage and to a number of psychological disturbances including memory loss, disorientation, dementia, moodiness, confusion and delusions. Alzheimer's disease sufferers are often found to have low vitamin B12 levels, although it is unclear whether these are a contributing factor or a result of the disease.

Vitamin B12 deficiency leads to a loss of nerve-insulating myelin which begins at the peripheral nerves and eventually moves up to the spine causing decreased reflexes, abnormal gait, weakness, fatigue, poor vision and impaired touch or pain sensation. Other signs include tingling or loss of sensation and weakness in hands and feet, and diminished sensitivity to vibration and position sense.

Gastrointestinal system

Vitamin B12 deficiency causes poor cell formation in the digestive tract and leads to nausea, vomiting, loss of appetite, poor absorption of food, soreness of the mouth and tongue, and diarrhea.

Heart disease

Vitamin B12 deficiency may lead to increased levels of an amino acid called homocysteine, which has been linked to an increased risk of heart disease. (See page 560 for more information.)[3]

Other symptoms

Vitamin B12 is involved in production of the genetic material of the cell and deficiency may cause defective production which could lead to cancer. A 1997 Australian study found that low levels of vitamin B12 could contribute to chromosome damage in white blood cells.[4] Low levels of Vitamin B12 may also contribute to diabetic neuropathy, poor vision, recurrent yeast infections and infertility. Vitamin B12 affects bone cells, and deficiency may be risk factor for osteoporosis.[5]

Sources

Good sources of vitamin B12 include liver and organ meats, muscle meats, fish, eggs, shellfish, milk and most dairy products. Sea vegetables and fermented soybean products such as miso also contain forms of vitamin B12, although some research suggests that the human body may not be able to absorb these forms and they may even block true vitamin B12 absorption. Many vegetarian and vegan products are fortified with vitamin B12, including yeast extract, vegetable stock and soya milk. Cooking has little effect on vitamin B12 although some may be lost when food is cooked to temperatures above 212 °F.

Food	Amount	Vitamin B12 (mcg)
Beef liver, cooked	85g	95.0
Beef kidney, cooked	85g	43.6
Trout, cooked	1 fillet	4.64
Tuna, canned,	1 cup	4.38
Pink salmon, cooked	½ fillet	4.29
Beef steak, grilled	100g	2.11
Haddock, cooked	1 fillet	2.08
Tempeh	1 cup	1.58
Cottage cheese	1 cup	1.36
Clams	¾ cup	1.05
Oysters	6 oysters	1.02
Cheeseburger	1 serve	0.97
Skim milk	1 cup	0.88
Whole milk plain yoghurt	1 cup	0.86
Whole milk	1 cup	0.83
Feta cheese	1 wedge	0.64
Miso	1 cup	0.54
Eggs, hard boiled	1 large	0.56
Eggs, scrambled	1 large	0.47
Chicken, roast	1 cup, chopped	0.44

Eggs, omelette	1 large	0.43
Breaded fried chicken	6 pieces	0.31
Cheddar cheese	1 slice	0.23
Ham	1 slice	0.23

Recommended dietary allowances

The RDAs for vitamin B12 have recently been raised in the US.

	Men	*Women*	*Pregnancy*	*Lactation*
USA	2.4 mcg	2.4 mcg	2.6 mcg	2.8 mcg
UK	1.5 mcg	1.5 mcg		2.0 mcg
Australia	2.0 mcg	2.0 mcg	3.0 mcg	2.5 mcg

Supplements

Vitamin B12 is available in several supplemental forms, both oral and injectable. Cyanocobalamin is the main synthetic form and has a cyanide molecule attached. Methylcobalamin is one of two active forms of vitamin B12 and may be a more effective supplement.

Vegans are at particular risk of vitamin B12 deficiency and may need supplements. Vitamin B12 tablets should be taken one hour before food for optimal absorption.

Toxic effects of excess intake

There have been no reports of toxic effects even at high doses.

Therapeutic uses of supplements

Pernicious anemia

Both oral and injectable vitamin B12 supplements are used to treat pernicious anemia. In those who lack sufficient intrinsic factor and cannot absorb vitamin B12, it is usually given by injection, although there is evidence that oral administration in high enough doses is effective.[6] An intranasal gel is also available.

HIV/AIDS

Lower than normal serum vitamin B12 levels are common in those infected with HIV and may help predict those patients in whom the disease will progress most rapidly.[7] AIDS patients often show signs of nerve damage including numbness and tingling in the hands and toes, and vitamin B12 may be useful in treating these symptoms. Recent studies have found that deficiency of vitamin B12 is associated with lower measures of immune system effectiveness in HIV-positive people and that increasing vitamin B12 levels increases these counts.[8,9]

Sleep

Some research suggests that vitamin B12 might affect sleep quality and performance. In a 1996 study, researchers explored the effects of 3 mg of vitamin B12 on the quality of sleep and work performance of ten healthy, male staff members of an Austrian industrial plant. The results showed better sleep quality and shorter total sleep time in those taking supplements.[10]

Other uses

Vitamin B12 therapy has also been used to treat Alzheimer's disease, childhood asthma in those sensitive to sulfites, insomnia, diabetic neuropathy, some psychiatric disorders including depression, and some forms of dermatitis.

Vitamin B12 injections are used by some people as a general tonic and many people report feelings of increased energy and improved health after these injections. Between 70 and 90 per cent of any dose over 1 mg is excreted into the urine.

Interactions with other nutrients

Vitamin B12 works closely with folic acid and vitamin B6 in a number of body functions. Vitamin B6 deficiency reduces vitamin B12 absorption.

Interactions with drugs

Acids and alkalis, water, sunlight, alcohol, estrogen and sleeping pills can destroy vitamin B12. Antacids, anti-epileptic drugs, cholestyramine and colchicine may decrease vitamin B12 absorption. Chloramphenicol and other bone marrow suppressant drugs may interfere with the red blood cell functions of vitamin B12. Smoking affects vitamin B12 metabolism.

Cautions

The clinically available cyanocobalamin form of vitamin B12 should not be used in patients with hereditary optic nerve atrophy or suspected cobalt hypersensitivity. Large doses of vitamin B12 should be used with caution in those with low blood levels of potassium (due to diuretic drugs or other causes).

QUICK GUIDE

Essential for

- the release of energy from food
- protein metabolism
- the manufacture of genetic material
- healthy hair
- a healthy immune system

Absorption and metabolism

Biotin is absorbed from food and from intestinal bacteria.

Deficiency

Biotin deficiency leads to hair loss, dermatitis, anemia, muscle pain, loss of appetite, lethargy, depression, hallucinations and lowered immunity.

Sources

Liver, kidney, brewer's yeast, egg yolks, fish, nuts, oatmeal and beans are all good sources of biotin.

Daily recommended dietary intakes

The adequate intake for biotin is set at 30 mcg per day. This increases to 35 mcg per day for breastfeeding women.

Toxic effects of excess intake

No toxic effects have been reported.

Interactions

Biotin works closely with pantothenic acid, folic acid and vitamin B12. Sulfa drugs, estrogen and alcohol raise biotin requirements. Long-term use of antibiotics can reduce the manufacture of biotin in the intestines. Prolonged use of anticonvulsant drugs may lead to biotin deficiency.

Therapeutic uses of supplements

Biotin supplements are used to treat biotin deficiency; dermatitis and other skin disorders; hair problems; to improve blood sugar control and treat neuropathy in diabetes; to improve fat metabolism in weight loss programs; and to treat Duchenne muscular dystrophy.

Biotin is a water soluble vitamin which was first isolated in 1936. As well as being obtained from dietary sources, biotin is also produced by gut bacteria.

What it does in the body

Biotin functions as an essential cofactor for several enzymes.

Metabolism

Biotin is essential for carbohydrate metabolism and in the synthesis of fatty acids. It also helps incorporate amino acids into protein.

Genetic material

Biotin is essential for cell growth and replication through its role in the manufacture of DNA and RNA, which make up the genetic material of the cell.

Hair

Healthy hair and nails require biotin.

Absorption and metabolism

Biotin is absorbed in the small intestine and any excess is excreted in the urine. Normally, the amount of biotin excreted in the urine and feces is up to six times greater than the amount eaten in food. This is due to the large quantities produced by gut bacteria.

Deficiency

Biotin deficiency is rare due to bacterial synthesis in the gut. Those at risk include infants with inherited deficiency disorders, babies fed biotin-deficient formula diets, those who eat large amounts of raw egg whites which inactivate biotin, and those who are fed intravenously.

Symptoms include hair loss, a scaly red rash around the nose, mouth and other body openings, conjunctivitis, anemia, high cholesterol, loss of appetite, nausea, lethargy, muscle pain, and tingling and numbness in the hands and feet. Mental symptoms include intense depression, sleeplessness and hallucinations. In infants, symptoms include seborrheic dermatitis (cradle cap), developmental delay and a lack of muscle tone. Biotin deficiency also affects the functioning of the immune system. A recent animal study showed a decrease in white blood cell function with biotin deficiency.[1]

Sources

Liver, kidney, brewer's yeast, egg yolks, whole grains, breads, fish, nuts, beans, meat and dairy products are all good sources of biotin. Food processing techniques can destroy biotin.

Food	Amount	Biotin (mcg)
Beef liver	100g	100
Peanuts, roasted	100g	39
Chocolate	100g	32
Eggs	100g	25
Peas, dried	100g	18
Cauliflower	100g	17
Mushrooms	100g	16
Hazelnuts	100g	14
Lima beans, dried	100g	10
Molasses	100g	9
Oysters	100g	9
Halibut	100g	8
Bacon	100g	7
Corn	100g	6
Chicken	100g	5-10
Milk	100g	5
Whole wheat	100g	5
Salmon	100g	5
Bananas	100g	4
Beef	100g	4
Onions, dry	100g	4
Grapefruit	100g	3

Carrots	100g	2
Cheese	100g	2

Recommended dietary allowances

The adequate intake for biotin has been set at around 30 mcg per day. This increases to 35 mcg per day during breastfeeding. Average daily biotin intake in the American diet is estimated to be around 28 to 42 mcg.

Supplements

Biotin is available commercially as isolated biotin or as a complex in brewer's yeast.

Toxic effects of excess intake

There have been no reported toxic effects even at large doses.

Therapeutic uses of supplements

Large doses of biotin are used to treat infants with a potentially fatal genetic abnormality which leads to an inability to use biotin in the body.

Skin disorders

Biotin supplements are used to treat some skin disorders such as seborrheic dermatitis, which in infants appears to be caused by a biotin deficiency. Supplements are given either directly to the infant or to the mother if she is breastfeeding.

Diabetes

Biotin supplements may help to improve blood glucose control in diabetics by enhancing insulin sensitivity and increasing the activity of enzymes involved in glucose metabolism.[2] Biotin in high doses may also be useful in the treatment of diabetic neuropathy.[3]

Other uses

Biotin can be used to treat frail, splitting or thin fingernails and to improve hair condition.[4] It is also used to treat gray hair, although this is only likely to be useful in cases where there is deficiency. Biotin may improve hair health through its action on the metabolism of scalp oils. Biotin has also been used to treat metabolic abnormalities in sufferers of Duchenne muscular dystrophy [5], to normalize fat metabolism in weight loss programs, and to treat intestinal candidiasis.

Interactions with other nutrients

Biotin works closely with folic acid, pantothenic acid and vitamin B12. It can lessen the symptoms of pantothenic acid and zinc deficiencies. Raw egg white contains a protein called avidin that prevents biotin absorption.

Interactions with drugs

Sulfa drugs, estrogen, and alcohol may raise biotin requirements. Prolonged use of anticonvulsant drugs may lead to biotin deficiency. Long-term use of antibiotics can affect the balance of the digestive system and reduce or stop the manufacture of biotin by bacteria.

Pantothenic acid

QUICK GUIDE

Essential for

- the release of energy from food
- cholesterol and fatty acid metabolism
- healthy red blood cells
- a healthy immune system
- healthy adrenal gland function
- a healthy nervous system

Absorption and metabolism

Some pantothenic acid may be stored in the liver.

Deficiency

Deficiency is rare in humans except in cases of general malnutrition. Symptoms in animals include graying of hair, decreased growth and adrenal gland abnormalities.

Sources

Good sources include yeast, liver, eggs, wheatgerm, milk, meat, poultry and whole grains. It is also produced by bacteria in the gut.

Daily recommended dietary intakes

The adequate intake for pantothenic acid has been set at 5 mg per day.

Toxic effects of excess intake

The risk of toxicity is very low. Symptoms may include diarrhea, fluid retention, drowsiness and depression.

Interactions

Sulfa drugs, sleeping pills, estrogen and alcohol may raise pantothenic acid requirements.

Therapeutic uses of supplements

Supplements have been used to treat fatigue, stress, allergies, headaches, arthritis and nerve disorders. Pantetheine has been used to lower high cholesterol and blood fats.

Pantothenic acid, which is also known as vitamin B5, takes its name from the Greek word "panto" meaning "everywhere" as it is found in a wide range of foods. It is also synthesized by intestinal bacteria.

What it does in the body

Metabolism

Pantothenic acid is essential for the release of energy from food. It is used in the manufacture of a compound called coenzyme A which plays a vital role in the breakdown of fats and carbohydrates. It is also necessary for building cell membranes.

Brain and nervous system

Pantothenic acid is necessary for the production of some neurotransmitters, such as acetylcholine, and is essential for normal nervous system function.

Immune system

Antibody synthesis requires pantothenic acid and it is also involved in wound-healing.

Hormones and glands

Normal adrenal gland function requires pantothenic acid as it is essential for production of adrenal hormones, such as cortisone, which play an essential part in the body's reaction to stress. Pantothenic acid is also necessary for the production of other steroid hormones and cholesterol, as well as vitamin A, vitamin D and vitamin B12.

Red blood cells

The formation of healthy red blood cells requires pantothenic acid as it is involved in the production of compounds needed to make hemoglobin.

Absorption and metabolism

Pantothenic acid is absorbed from the intestine and excesses are excreted in the urine. The body has a limited ability to store pantothenic acid.

Deficiency

A deficiency of pantothenic acid has not been found naturally in human beings but has been induced under experimental conditions. It causes the adrenal glands to shrink and leads to symptoms of fatigue, headache, depression, sleep disturbances, personality changes, nausea and abdominal distress. Other symptoms of deficiency include numbness and tingling of the hands and feet, muscle cramps, impaired coordination, immune problems, dermatitis and itching.

Sources

Good sources of pantothenic acid include yeast, liver, eggs, wheatgerm, bran, peanuts, peas, meat, milk, poultry, whole grains, broccoli, mushrooms and sweet potatoes. Most vegetables and fruits contain small amounts. Heat, food processing techniques and canning destroy pantothenic acid.

Food	Amount	Pantothenic acid (mg)
Beef liver, cooked	85g	5.03
Avocado	1 avocado	1.95
Chicken, roast	1 cup, chopped	1.47
Mushrooms, raw	1 cup, pieces	1.46
Beef kidney, cooked	85g	1.44
Trout, cooked	1 fillet	1.39
Wheatgerm	½ cup	1.24
Peanuts	½ cup	1.23
Wheat bran	1 cup	1.21
Lentils, cooked	1 cup	1.20
Pink salmon, cooked	½ fillet	1.07
Oysters	6 oysters	1.06
Baked potatoes, flesh	1 medium	0.87
Milk, skim	1 cup	0.77
Lima beans, cooked	1 cup	0.76
Whole milk	1 cup	0.73
Tomato sauce, canned	1 cup	0.72

Eggs, hard boiled	1 large	0.70
Bulgur	1 cup	0.60
Brown rice, cooked	1 cup	0.53
Cottage cheese	1 cup	0.47
Broccoli	½ cup, chopped	0.38
Oranges	1 medium	0.33
Almonds	½ cup	0.33

Recommended dietary allowances

The adequate intake for pantothenic acid is set at 5 mg per day. The pantothenic acid content of the average American diet is 4 to 10 mg per day.

Supplements

Pantothenic acid is usually present in oral supplements as calcium pantothenate. Pantetheine is the most stable active form of pantothenic acid.

Toxic effects of excess intake

The risk of toxicity is very low. At high doses the side effects are mild diarrhea, fluid retention, memory loss, drowsiness, depression and nausea.

Therapeutic effects of supplements

High blood lipids

The pantetheine form of pantothenic acid lowers harmful LDL cholesterol and triglyceride levels and raises beneficial HDL cholesterol levels. Pantetheine may act by inhibiting cholesterol synthesis and accelerating the use of fats as an energy source. Diabetics have been shown to benefit from pantetheine supplements.

In a 1990 Italian study, researchers gave 900 mg per day of pantetheine to 24 women aged from 45 to 55 years who had cholesterol levels. After 16 weeks of treatment, significant reductions of total cholesterol, LDL cholesterol

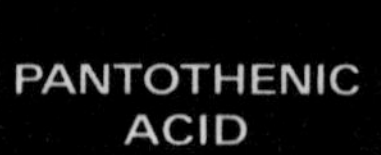

and LDL/HDL cholesterol ratio were seen. The treatment was about 80 per cent effective and none of the patients complained of adverse reactions.[1]

Other uses

Pantothenic acid supplements have been used in the support of adrenal function; to alleviate the symptoms of rheumatoid arthritis; in weight loss programs; to boost immunity during viral infections;[2] and to speed up wound-healing. Supplements have also been reported to enhance athletic performance by improving endurance and aerobic capacity. Not all studies have shown beneficial effects.

Interactions with other nutrients

Pantothenic acid interacts with carnitine and coenzyme Q10 in body functions.

Interactions with drugs

Sulfa drugs, sleeping pills, estrogen and alcohol may raise pantothenic acid requirements.

QUICK GUIDE

Essential for

- the manufacture of collagen, a protein which forms the basis of connective tissues such as bones, teeth and cartilage
- wound-healing
- healthy immune and nervous systems
- adrenal hormone production
- as an antioxidant to help prevent disease

Absorption and metabolism

Daily intake is necessary.

Deficiency

Severe deficiency leads to scurvy with symptoms of bleeding gums, joint pain, easy bruising, dry skin, fluid retention, and depression. Marginal deficiencies may play a role in the development of cancer, cardiovascular disease, high blood pressure, lowered immunity, diabetes and cataracts.

Sources

Good sources include fruits and vegetables.

Daily recommended dietary intakes

Men	60 mg
Women	60 mg
Pregnancy	70 mg
Lactation	95 mg

Toxic effects of excess intake

These include diarrhea, nausea, stomach cramps and skin rashes.

Interactions

It aids iron absorption and acts with other antioxidant vitamins. Smoking, pollutants, aspirin, alcohol, estrogen, antibiotics and steroids raise requirements.

Therapeutic uses of supplements

These include the treatment and prevention of many disorders including cardiovascular disease, high blood pressure, cancer, gallstones, cataracts, diabetes, asthma and infections.

Cautions

Large doses may cause kidney stones in kidney disease sufferers and may also affect blood and urine test results.

The vitamin C deficiency disease, scurvy, was recognized at least 3000 years ago but it was not until the 16th century that people realized that certain fruits and vegetables could prevent or cure the disease. In the late 18th century, English sailors carried limes on long voyages to ward off scurvy, causing them to be nicknamed "limeys". In 1928 vitamin C was isolated and shown to be the substance necessary to prevent and cure scurvy. In its pure form, vitamin C, which is also known as ascorbic acid, is a water soluble white powder. Humans are among the few species that cannot manufacture vitamin C and must obtain it from food.

What it does in the body

Vitamin C is involved in hundreds of vital biological processes in the body.

Collagen and connective tissue

The main role of vitamin C is in the manufacture of collagen. This protein forms the basis of connective tissue, the most abundant tissue in the body, and acts as a cementing substance between cells. It helps support and protect blood vessels, bones, joints, organs and muscles, and forms a sizable proportion of skin, tendons, the cornea of the eye, ligaments, cartilage, teeth and bone. Collagen forms a protective barrier against infection and disease, and promotes healing of wounds, fractures and bruises.

Immune system

Vitamin C is critical to immune function as it is involved in antibody production and white blood cell function and activity. Other functions include the production of interferon, an antiviral and anticancer substance. Vitamin C requirements are raised when the immune system is under stress.

Antioxidant properties

Vitamin C is a powerful water soluble antioxidant and plays a vital role in protecting against oxidative damage. It neutralizes potentially harmful reactions in the watery parts of the body, such as the blood and the fluid inside and surrounding cells. It also helps protect LDL cholesterol against free radical damage. This antioxidant action helps to protect against cancer, the effects of aging, heart disease, and an array of other health problems (See page 417 for more information.)

Hormones

Vitamin C is important in the synthesis of adrenal hormones and is depleted from the adrenal glands in times of stress.

Nervous system

Vitamin C plays a role in the manufacture of neurotransmitters. It is necessary for the conversion of tryptophan to serotonin, and of tyrosine to dopamine and adrenaline.

Other functions

Vitamin C is involved in the manufacture of carnitine, a substance necessary for the production of energy from fatty acids in cells, especially cardiac and skeletal muscle cells. (See page 374 for more information.) Vitamin C is necessary for the activity of the enzyme system which metabolizes drugs in the body. It is also necessary for iron absorption and plays a role in the conversion of cholesterol to bile acids for excretion. Vitamin C may also affect prostaglandin metabolism.

Absorption and metabolism

Absorption of vitamin C occurs in the intestine. The amount absorbed depends on the dose as the absorption mechanism is saturable and any excess excreted in the urine in two to three hours. As vitamin C is water soluble, only a small amount (about 4 to 5 g) is stored in the body. Vitamin C levels in the body are regulated by absorption and kidney excretion mechanisms.

Deficiency

A lack of vitamin C leads eventually to scurvy. The symptoms are mainly due to poorly formed collagen and include the breaking open of small blood vessels, the reddening and bleeding of gums, loose teeth, joint pains, dry scaly skin and blood vessel damage. Other symptoms include general weakness, fluid retention, depression and anemia. Vitamin C deficiency can also cause slower wound-healing, increased susceptibility to infections, male infertility and increased genetic damage to sperm cells, which may lead to birth defects.

Scurvy and severe vitamin C deficiency are rare in developing countries but marginal deficiencies may be relatively common and may play a role in the development of diseases such as cancer and heart disease. The first National

Health and Nutrition Examination Survey (NHANES I) looked at the vitamin C intake of over 11 000 people during a five-year period. Results showed that men whose intakes of vitamin C were greater than 50 mg daily had a 34 per cent lower chance of death from all causes than those whose intakes were lower than 50 mg daily.[1]

In a 1998 study, researchers at the Arizona State University assessed the vitamin C status of 494 healthy middle-class people. The results showed that 6 per cent of subjects had plasma vitamin C concentrations that indicated vitamin C deficiency, and 30.4 per cent of people were vitamin C depleted. Participants in the study with diabetes were more likely to be vitamin C-depleted.[2]

Men, the elderly, smokers, diabetics, those with high blood pressure and perhaps oral estrogen-containing contraceptive users have lowered plasma vitamin C levels and are at greatest risk of deficiency-related diseases.

Cardiovascular disease

Many population studies have linked low vitamin C intakes to an increased risk of cardiovascular disease. These include a study reported in 1996 in the *American Journal of Epidemiology.* During the study, which was begun in 1981, USDA researchers assessed the health and nutrition status of 747 people aged 60 years and over. Particular attention was paid to the foods the participants usually ate and the levels in their blood of the antioxidant vitamins C, E and beta carotene. The researchers following up the subjects from nine to 12 years later found that among people who ate lots of dark green and orange vegetables, there were fewer deaths from heart disease and other causes. The results showed that a daily intake of more than 400 mg and higher blood levels of vitamin C were linked to reduced risk of death from heart disease.[3] In a study published in 1993, Swiss researchers found an increased risk of death from ischemic heart disease in people with low vitamin C levels.[4]

In a study published in the *British Medical Journal* in 1995, UK researchers assessed the links between dietary intake and blood levels of vitamin C, and death from stroke and coronary heart disease in people aged 65 and over. The study involved 730 men and women who were followed up for a 20-year period. The results showed that those with the highest intakes had around half the risk of death from stroke when compared with those with the lowest intakes. However in this study, no link was found between vitamin C status and risk of death from coronary heart disease.[5]

Low vitamin C levels are also associated with an increased risk of heart attack. In a 1997 study, Finnish researchers examined this link in 1605 men aged between 42 and 60 who were free from heart disease when they entered the study. During the follow-up period there were 70 heart attacks. The results showed that men with vitamin C deficiency were three-and-a-half times more likely to have a heart attack than those who were not deficient.[6]

However, not all studies have shown protective effects of vitamin C. These include the large Nurses and Health Professionals Studies.[7,8]

Researchers from Cambridge University in the UK examined the relationship between blood levels of vitamin C status and angina in women aged from 45 to 74. Forty-two women with previously undiagnosed angina were compared with 877 women with no disease. Those with higher vitamin C levels had a 66 per cent reduced risk of angina.[9] The same researchers examined the link between blood levels of vitamin C and blood fat levels. Their results showed that a high intake of vitamin C from food raises beneficial HDL cholesterol and lowers serum triglyceride.[10]

Other studies suggest that people with low vitamin C levels have higher total and harmful LDL cholesterol levels and lower beneficial HDL cholesterol levels. In a study reported in the *American Journal of Clinical Nutrition,* USDA researchers found that high blood levels of vitamin C were associated with high levels of HDL cholesterol in 316 women and 511 men aged from 19 to 95.[11] Vitamin C also helps to protect blood fats and artery walls against oxidative damage by free radicals, and seems to have beneficial effects on clotting.

High blood pressure

Vitamin C deficiency also appears to be linked to an increased risk of high blood pressure. In a study done in Cambridge, UK researchers examined the relationship between blood pressure and vitamin C levels in the blood in 835 men and 1025 women aged from 45 to75. The results showed that low vitamin C levels were associated with higher systolic and diastolic blood pressures.[12]

Cancer

Low intake of vitamin C appears to be a risk factor for many forms of cancer. Diets high in fruit and vegetables, and therefore high in vitamin C, have been found to be associated with lower risk for cancers of the oral cavity, esophagus, stomach, colon, and lung. Many studies have found a reduced risk of cancer in people who have high vitamin C intakes. The protective effect seems to be strongest for cancers of the esophagus, larynx, mouth and pancreas. Vitamin C also seems to provide some protection against cancers of the cervix, liver, stomach, rectum, breast and lungs.[13] However, in many of these studies it is not possible to tell whether the protective effect is due to vitamin C, vitamin E, or carotene, to a combined effect of these nutrients, or even due to additional substances found in food.

Results from the Western Electric Study published in 1995 suggest a link between low vitamin C levels and death from cancer. The researchers obtained information on diet and other factors from 1556 employed, middle-aged men. During the follow-up period 231 men died from cancer. The results showed that those with the highest vitamin C and beta carotene intakes were 40 per cent less likely to die of cancer than those with the lowest intakes.[14]

Prostate cancer

Further results from the Western Electric Study reported in 1996, suggest that vitamin C improves survival in those with prostate cancer. Researchers examined the links between dietary beta carotene and vitamin C and the risk of prostate cancer in 1899 middle-aged men over a 30-year period. During this time, prostate cancer developed in 132 men. The results showed that associations between vitamin C intake and risk of prostate cancer differed depending on whether the cancer was diagnosed during the first 19 years of follow-up or the next 11 years of follow-up. Overall, higher intakes of vitamin C and beta carotene were linked to improved survival.[15]

Stomach cancer

Results from the Seven Countries Study published in 1995 suggest that low vitamin C intake is linked to an increased risk of stomach cancer. In the 1960s, researchers collected detailed dietary information and in 1987, they assessed average food intakes. They then examined the links between this information and death from stomach cancer. The results showed that the average intake of vitamin C was strongly related to the risk of stomach cancer. However, vitamin C intake was not related to the risk of lung and colorectal cancer in this study.[16] Other studies have shown similar results.[17]

Lung Cancer

Results from a Dutch study published in 1997 suggest a weak protective effect of vitamin C against lung cancer. Researchers obtained dietary information from 561 men from the town of Zutphen, in 1960, 1965, and 1970. During the period from 1971 to 1990, 54 new cases of lung cancer were identified and analysis of the diets of the men showed an increased risk of lung cancer in those with lower fruit and vegetable and vitamin C intakes.[18]

Colon cancer

Researchers at the University of Southern California assessed the links between fruits and vegetables and vitamin C intake in 11 580 residents of a retirement community who entered the study free from cancer. During the period from 1981 to 1989 a total of 1335 cases of cancer were diagnosed. The results showed a decreased risk of colon cancer in women with higher vitamin C intakes. Supplemental use of vitamins A and C also showed a protective effect on colon cancer risk in women.[19]

Italian researchers investigated the relationship between estimated intake of selected micronutrients, including vitamin C, and the risk of disease in 828 patients with colon cancer, 498 with rectal cancer and 2024 people without cancer. Those in the highest intake group for vitamin C had a 60 per cent lower risk of cancer than those in the low intake group.[20]

Breast cancer

In a study published in 1994, researchers examined the effect of diet before diagnosis on the risk of dying of breast cancer in 678 women who were diagnosed with the disease from January 1982 through June 1992. The results showed that those women with the highest vitamin C intakes had a 57 per cent lower chance of dying of breast cancer than those with the lowest intakes.[21] However, results from the Nurses Health Study did not show a protective effect against the disease.[22]

Cataracts

The vitamin C content of the eye is 20 times greater than that in the blood. Results from some studies including the Beaver Dam Eye Study, suggest that people with high levels of vitamin C are at less risk of cataracts than those with low levels of vitamin C.[23]

Diabetes

Diabetics often have lower levels of antioxidants, which can increase the risk of diabetic complications such as cardiovascular disease. The cellular uptake of vitamin C is promoted by insulin and inhibited by high blood sugar; and as diabetics have low insulin levels, they are at greater risk of vitamin C deficiency. Most studies have found people with diabetes to have at least 30 per cent lower vitamin C concentrations than people without the disease. Levels seem to be lower in diabetic people as a result of the disease rather than as a result of poor dietary intake.[24]

Elevated fasting insulin concentrations and insulin resistance have been associated with non-insulin-dependent diabetes mellitus (NIDDM), obesity, atherosclerosis, and hypertension; and some research suggests that antioxidant vitamins may help to reduce insulin resistance. However, a study reported in the *American Journal of Clinical Nutrition* in 1997 suggests that vitamin E and vitamin C intakes are not linked to improved insulin sensitivity. Researchers working on the Insulin Resistance and Atherosclerosis Study (IRAS) assessed insulin concentrations and insulin sensitivity in 1151 African American, Hispanic, and non-Hispanic white men and women with a wide spectrum of glucose tolerance. They also assessed the intake of vitamins E and C in the subjects. They did not find a link between vitamin intake and insulin resistance.[25]

Lung function and asthma

Low vitamin C levels seem to impair lung function. Researchers in Cambridge, UK examined the links between vitamin C levels in the blood and respiratory function in 835 men and 1025 women aged 45 to 75. The results showed that vitamin C was protective for lung function.[26]

Vitamin C intake in the general population appears to be linked to the incidence of asthma, suggesting that a diet low in vitamin C is a risk factor for asthma. Symptoms of ongoing asthma in adults may be decreased by vitamin C supplementation, although not all studies show positive results. Vitamin C is the major antioxidant substance present in the airway surface liquid of the lung, where it could be important in protecting against both damage from toxic chemicals and free radicals, which may worsen the symptoms of asthma.[27] Low vitamin C levels are associated with increased bronchial reactivity.[28]

Immunity

Vitamin C is important for the functioning of the immune system, and deficiency can increase susceptibility to infection. In a study published in 1997, French researchers assessed vitamin C levels in 18 elderly patients in hospital. The patients were divided into three groups: those with acute infection, those who were malnourished, and a control group. Those with acute infection had considerably lower vitamin C levels than those in the other groups.[29]

Other disorders

Vitamin C deficiency may also play a role in macular degeneration of the eye, arthritis, Parkinson's disease, pre-eclampsia of pregnancy, the common cold, low sperm counts and skin ulcers.

Sources

Good sources of vitamin C include citrus fruits such as oranges and grapefruits. Other sources include strawberries, kiwifruit, blackcurrants, papaya; and vegetables such as red peppers, broccoli and brussels sprouts. Vitamin C from natural sources such as these is associated with bioflavonoids which enhance the beneficial effects of vitamin C (See page 364 for more information.)

Vitamin C is easily lost during storage and cooking. Aging, bruising, overcooking and re-heating all destroy vitamin C. Slicing vegetables exposes a higher surface area to heat and light, leading to loss of vitamin C.

Food	Amount	Vitamin C (mg)
Blackcurrants	1 cup	202
Red pepper, raw	1 cup, sliced	174
Guavas	1 fruit	165
Orange juice, commercial	1 cup	124
Grapefruit juice	1 cup	94
Kohlrabi, boiled	1 cup	89
Papaya	1 cup, cubes	86
Lemons	1 fruit	83
Strawberries	1 cup	82
Green pepper	1 cup. sliced	82
Kiwi fruit, peeled	1 medium	74
Oranges	1 fruit	68
Cantaloupe melon	1 cup, diced	66
Broccoli, boiled	½ cup	58
Mangoes	1 fruit	57
Kale	1 cup	53
Brussels sprouts, boiled	½ cup	48
Grapefruit	½ fruit	47
Honeydew melon	1 cup, diced	42
Raspberries	1 cup	37
Cauliflower, boiled	½ cup	27
Tangerines	1 medium	26

Pineapples, raw	1 cup, diced	24
Cabbage, boiled	½ cup, shredded	15

Recommended dietary allowances

	Men	Women	Pregnancy	Lactation
USA	60 mg	60 mg	70 mg	95 mg
UK	40 mg	40 mg	50 mg	70 mg
Australia	40 mg	30 mg	60 mg	75 mg

In a paper published in 1996, researchers at the National Institutes of Health recommended that the RDA for vitamin C be raised to 200 mg per day.[30]

Supplements

Vitamin C is the most widely taken supplement in developing countries. It is available in pills, powders, effervescent tablets, syrups and pastilles. Ascorbic acid is the most widely used and least expensive form, but it causes stomach upsets in some people and can damage tooth enamel. Calcium ascorbate and sodium ascorbate are also readily available and are less likely to have these effects. Some supplements provide vitamin C in the form of C complex which contains bioflavonoids. These compounds occur naturally with vitamin C and, in high enough doses, increase its activity.

Supplements are particularly beneficial for anyone who smokes, eats an unhealthy diet, is under physical or emotional stress, drinks alcohol, lives in a polluted environment, is exposed to toxic chemicals, suffers from recurrent infections or has an increased risk of cancer. Women who take the contraceptive pill, elderly people, pregnant women and those with absorption difficulties are also likely to benefit.

Dosage

Opinions vary widely as to the optimal dose of vitamin C. Linus Pauling, the Nobel Prize winner who studied the effects of large doses of vitamin C on the common cold, flu and cancer, recommended an optimum intake of between 2 g and 9 g per day. Many experts believe that 500 mg is ideal to meet body needs while others feel that 200 mg is adequate. Vitamin C needs vary with age, weight, activity, energy levels, general metabolism and state of health.

In order to maintain blood levels of vitamin C, it is best to take it in divided doses throughout the day. Taking vitamin C with food minimizes adverse effects on the digestive system.

A study reported in 1997 in the *American Journal of Clinical Nutrition* suggests that doses of vitamin C above 200 mg do not increase blood levels of the vitamin significantly and may be excreted. Researchers at the University of Tucson in Arizona, measured blood levels of vitamin C when the dose given was 200 mg and then again when 2500 mg was administered. They found negligible absorption increases between the lower and higher doses.[31]

Doctors who practise orthomolecular medicine use megadose vitamin C therapy in times of specific illness, especially viral infections. They typically use 20 to 40 g daily, often intravenously. With oral doses, some doctors believe that the amount of vitamin C needed is related to the severity of the disease and increase the dose until 'bowel tolerance' is exceeded and diarrhea results.[32]

Toxic effects of excess intake

Vitamin C is safe in relatively large doses but excessive intakes may cause diarrhea, nausea, stomach cramping, excess urination and skin rashes. There is the possibility of kidney stones in those with kidney disease. These effects may occur when doses above 1 g are taken regularly. Chewable vitamin C may lead to tooth decay.

Large doses of vitamin C taken by pregnant women have caused 'rebound scurvy' in newborn babies whose intake returns to normal. It may be advisable to reduce vitamin C intake slowly after taking large amounts.

Results of a study reported in 1998 in *Nature Medicine* suggest that vitamin C may cause cell damage in doses above 500 mg. The researchers gave daily doses of 500 mg of vitamin C to 30 healthy volunteers and then assessed two indicators of oxidative damage in DNA from their blood cells. One of these indicators showed less oxidation in the volunteers, and the other indicator showed more oxidation than before they began taking the supplements. However, this study directly contradicts other studies and focuses only on a single biological marker that is not necessarily known to be a good indicator of oxidative stress.[33]

Therapeutic uses of supplements

Vitamin C supplements are used to treat and prevent many diseases and conditions. For some of these there is research evidence while for others the evidence is mainly anecdotal. Vitamin C supplement use appears to be associated with a lower risk of death in elderly people and vitamin C seems to enhance the beneficial effects of vitamin E. Researchers involved in a study published in 1996 found that those elderly people who took vitamin C and vitamin E supplements had a lower risk of death from any cause and also from both cancer and heart disease. Those taking vitamin E supplements had a 34 per cent lower risk, and those taking both vitamin C and vitamin E had a 42 per cent reduced risk.[34]

Cardiovascular disease

The evidence from epidemiological studies, animal experiments and some clinical trials suggests that vitamin C supplements may protect against the development of cardiovascular disease. In the same study mentioned in the previous paragraph, those taking vitamin E supplements had a 47 per cent lower risk of death from heart disease and those taking both vitamin C and vitamin E had a 53 per cent reduced risk.[34]

Vitamin C may exert its protective effects by lowering total blood cholesterol and harmful LDL cholesterol and raising beneficial HDL cholesterol. Vitamin C also increases the production of prostacyclin, a prostaglandin which decreases the clumping of blood platelets and dilates blood vessels, therefore reducing the risk of heart disease, atherosclerosis and stroke.

High fat meals cause damage to artery linings, which may contribute to the development of atherosclerosis. Research published in 1997 suggests that taking the antioxidant vitamins C and E before a meal may help to prevent this damage. The study which was carried out at the University of Maryland School of Medicine involved 13 women and seven men with normal blood cholesterol levels. Once a week for three weeks, the subjects ate either a high fat meal, a low fat meal, a high fat meal after taking 1000 mg of vitamin C and 800 IU of vitamin E, or a low fat meal after taking the antioxidants. Before and after the meals, the researchers measured blood fat and cholesterol levels, blood pressure and heart rate in the subjects. They also used ultrasound to measure the dilation of an artery in the arm after release of a tourniquet which had been applied for five minutes. If the artery lining is functioning normally, it releases nitric oxide which causes dilation. The results showed that the high fat meal decreased artery lining function for up to four hours afterwards, whereas the low fat meal did not. This is probably due to oxidative stress caused by an accumulation of triglyceride-rich lipoproteins (blood fats). Vitamins C and E prevented this decrease in artery lining function.[35]

A recent US study looked at the effect of either 2 g of vitamin C or a placebo on patients with coronary artery disease. In such patients the arteries leading to the heart are unable to open when the heart requires increased blood flow. Those patients given the vitamin C experienced expansion in their arteries while those given the placebo experienced no effect.[36] Vitamin C has similar effects in those with high cholesterol[37] and in those with chronic heart failure.[38]

When blood is re-supplied to an organ from which it was previously cut off, oxidative damage can occur. This has been found in many types of surgery, for example in heart bypass operations. Vitamin C has also been shown to protect against this reperfusion injury.[39]

Smoking

Vitamin C needs are higher in smokers and several studies suggest that vitamin C may protect against smoking-related damage. It may help to decrease the smoking-related build-up of atherosclerotic plaque by limiting the amount of white blood cells that stick to artery walls.[40] Vitamin C supplements may be helpful in restoring reduced plasma vitamin C concentrations in smokers.[41] Like those with high cholesterol levels and coronary heart disease, the arteries of smokers have a reduced ability to dilate. Vitamin C supplements may counteract this impairment.[42]

High blood pressure

Vitamin C may also be of benefit in the treatment of mild high blood pressure, another risk factor for heart disease and stroke. Some research suggests that vitamin C may have beneficial effects in lowering high blood pressure.[43] Vitamin C supplements improve abnormal artery lining function in hypertensive people.[44]

Cancer prevention

Vitamin C supplements may have a part to play in cancer prevention. Some research suggests that the risk of cancer is lower in those taking supplements. Vitamin C may exert its anticancer effects by acting as an antioxidant and shielding the genetic mechanism of the cell from damage that can lead to cancerous changes. Vitamin C may also strengthen the ability of the immune system to track down and destroy pre-cancerous cells. Vitamin C may exert its protective effects against some cancers by inhibiting the formation of toxic compounds known as nitrosamines from nitrite food additives. These compounds are also found in cigarette smoke and are linked to an increased risk of stomach and lung cancers.

Stomach cancer

Supplements may be useful in helping to prevent stomach cancer. In a 1996 study, researchers gave 32 patients 500 mg of vitamin C twice daily for two weeks. Levels in gastric juices and gut tissues were increased, raising the possibility of increased protection against free radicals.[45]

A 1997 report in the journal, *Cancer*, suggests that vitamin C may inhibit the growth of *Helicobacter pylori*, a stomach bacterium that increases the risk of ulcers and stomach cancer. High concentrations of vitamin C inhibited the growth of bacteria in culture dishes and also in the stomachs of Mongolian gerbils, according to researchers at the International Medical Center of Japan in Tokyo. Vitamin C-rich diets have been found to decrease the risk of stomach cancer. This has been attributed to the antioxidant ability of vitamin C. However, vitamin E, which is also an antioxidant, does not inhibit the growth of *Helicobacter pylori*. This suggests that vitamin C may exert its protective effects through a biochemical mechanism. This research suggests the possibility of a safe, side effect-free alternative to antibiotics for the treatment of ulcers.[46]

Colon cancer

Vitamin C supplements have also been shown to have beneficial effects against the pre-cancerous changes which occur in colon cancer. In a 1992 study, 20 patients with colorectal cancer were given vitamins A, C, and E for six months and 21 patients with adenomas received placebo. The results showed that supplementation with vitamins A, C, and E was effective in reducing pre-cancerous abnormalities.[47] Vitamin C supplements may also be beneficial in the treatment of prostate cancer.[48]

Cancer treatment

Controversy surrounds the use of vitamin C in the treatment of cancer. The Nobel Prize winner, Linus Pauling and his colleagues have used vitamin C to improve survival times in cancer patients, but these results have not been repeated in other studies. Vitamin C may also benefit cancer patients who are undergoing radiation treatment by enabling them to withstand greater doses of radiation with fewer side effects.[49]

Asthma and allergy

There is some evidence that vitamin C is of benefit in reducing the bronchial constriction and impaired breathing seen in asthma and allergic responses. This effect may be due to the antioxidant effect of vitamin C as oxidizing agents promote inflammation and can increase allergic responses. Vitamin C may also improve lung and white blood cell function and decrease respiratory infections and hypersensitivity reactions by reducing histamine levels. However, some studies do not support a beneficial role in vitamin C in asthma. Most studies have been short term and have assessed immediate effects of vitamin C supplementation. The effect of long-term supplementation with vitamin C is unclear.[50]

According to researchers from the University of Washington, antioxidant vitamin supplements may help relieve the symptoms of asthma. The researchers measured the amount of breath expelled by the lungs in 17 asthma sufferers. The subjects took peak flow lung function tests while running on a treadmill and breathing in high levels of polluted air. In those asthmatics whose diets were supplemented with daily doses of 400 IU of vitamin E and 500 mg of vitamin C, an 18 per cent increase in peak flow capacity was seen.

In a 1997 study, 20 asthma patients underwent lung function tests at rest, before and one hour after receiving 2 g of oral ascorbic acid. They were then randomly assigned in a double-blind manner to receive 2 g of ascorbic acid or a placebo one hour before a 7-minute exercise session on a treadmill. Lung function tests were performed after an 8-minute rest. This procedure was repeated one week later, with each patient receiving the alternative medication. In nine patients, a protective effect on exercise-induced hyperreactive airways was seen.[51]

Immunity

Vitamin C boosts immunity by increasing the production of B and T cells and other white blood cells, including those that destroy foreign micro-organisms. It also increases interferon levels and antibody responses and has antiviral and antibacterial effects. These effects lead to improved resistance against infections.

Vitamin C has been shown to help the immune system recover from exposure to toxic chemicals. In a 1997 study, researchers studied the effect of vitamin C on the function of several immune cells (natural killer, T and B cells) in patients who had been exposed to toxic chemicals. Fifty-five patients were given buffered vitamin C in water at a dosage of 60 mg per kg body weight (around 4g for the average man). Twenty-four hours later, the researchers tested immune cell function. The results showed that natural killer cell activity was enhanced up to ten-fold in 78 per cent of patients. B and T cell function was restored to normal.[52]

HIV/AIDS

Vitamin C supplements are likely to be useful in HIV-positive individuals as they have been shown to boost the immune system and prevent damage to nerves. However, caution should be used with very high doses as they can cause diarrhea. Vitamin C has been shown to inhibit HIV in the laboratory and may also kill HIV-infected cells.[53]

Common cold

Vitamin C may reduce the duration of the common cold and also the severity of symptoms such as sneezing, coughing and sniffling. Its use as a cold treatment is controversial but it seems to have several effects, including reducing blood levels of histamine which can trigger tissue inflammation and a runny nose. It may also protect the immune cells and surrounding tissue from damaging oxidative reactions that occur when cells fight bacteria.[54]

It is possible that the effects of supplementation are greater in those with low dietary vitamin C intake. In general, men have lower vitamin C levels than women. In four studies with British girls and women, vitamin C supplementation had no marked effect on common cold. However, in four studies involving British male schoolchildren and students, a reduction in common cold occurrence was found in groups supplemented with vitamin C.[55]

Research suggests that vitamin C supplementation may be beneficial for people who do heavy exercise and who have problems with frequent upper respiratory tract infections. Three placebo-controlled studies have examined the effect of vitamin C supplementation on common cold occurrence in people under acute physical stress. In one study the subjects were school children at a skiing camp in the Swiss Alps; in another they were military troops training in Northern Canada; and in the third they were participants in a 90 km running race. In each of the three studies, a considerable reduction in common cold incidence in the group supplemented with vitamin C at levels of 600 mg to 1000 mg per day was seen.[56]

Cataracts

Many studies show that vitamin C can protect against cataracts, possibly by reducing oxidative damage caused by ultraviolet light. Vitamin C may act to protect the lens of the eye from this damage and protect enzymes within the lens that remove oxidation damaged proteins.

In a study published in 1992, researchers at Harvard Medical School examined the link between dietary intake of vitamins C and E, carotene, and riboflavin and cataract extraction in over 50 000 women taking part in the Nurses Health Study. The results showed that the risk of cataract was 45 per cent lower among women who used vitamin C supplements for ten or more years.[57]

Further results from this study reported in 1997 in the *American Journal of Clinical Nutrition* also suggests that vitamin C supplements taken for long periods can reduce the development of cataracts. Researchers from the US Department of Agriculture and Harvard School of Public Health examined the link between cataract development and vitamin C supplement use over a ten to 12 year period. The subjects were 247 Boston area nurses aged from 56 to 71. The researchers performed detailed eye examinations to determine the degree of opacity (clouding) of the lenses of the eyes of the subjects. Results showed that use of vitamin C supplements for over ten years was associated with a 77 per cent lower prevalence of early lens opacities and an 83 per cent lower prevalence of moderate lens opacities.[58]

Diabetes

Increasing vitamin C intake may improve blood sugar regulation in diabetics. Vitamin C administration in pharmacological doses for four months in Type II diabetes has been shown to have beneficial effects on glucose and lipid metabolism, blood circulation and capillary fragility.

In a 1995 study the effect of magnesium and vitamin C supplements on metabolic control was assessed in 56 diabetics. The study involved a 90 day run-in period followed by two 90 day treatment periods, during which patients received 600 mg of magnesium and 2 g of vitamin C per day. The results showed that vitamin C supplementation improved glycemic control, fasting blood glucose, cholesterol and triglyceride levels.[59]

High blood sugar levels in diabetes cause a compound known as sorbitol to be manufactured from glucose. This contributes to the progression of diabetic complications. Vitamin C has been shown to reduce levels of sorbitol in diabetics. In a 58 day study carried out in 1994, researchers investigated the effect of two different doses of vitamin C supplements (100 or 600 mg) on young adults with Type I diabetes. The results showed that vitamin C supplementation at either dose normalized sorbitol levels in those with diabetes in 30 days.[60] Vitamin C may also help to reduce capillary fragility, which also contributes to complications. The ability of the arteries to dilate is impaired in diabetics. Vitamin C supplements improve the response.[61]

Skin protection

Vitamins C and E taken together may protect against sunburn. In a study published in 1998, German dermatologists found that people who took these vitamins had a higher threshold for sunburn reaction. The researchers tested ultraviolet sensitivity in two groups of ten Caucasian people by exposing a section of skin to UV light. Subjects in one of the groups then took 2 g of vitamin C and 1000 IU of vitamin E for eight days. The UV test was then re-done. Those taking the vitamins showed increased tolerance, particularly at higher UV doses. However, in comparison with the protection afforded by topical sunscreens, this level of protection is small.[62]

Vitamin C-containing cosmetic skin creams such as Cellex-C have also become extremely popular in the last few years. They are designed to protect against pollutants and to promote healing.

Gallstones

Vitamin C is involved in cholesterol metabolism and deficiency may increase the risk of gallstones. In a 1998 study published in the *Journal of Clinical Epidemiology*, researchers in San Francisco found that vitamin C supplements reduced the prevalence of gall bladder disease by half in 2744 postmenopausal women who regularly drank alcohol. Supplement use was also associated with a 62 per cent decrease in gallstone removal. The supplements had no effect on those who did not drink.[63]

Researchers involved in a 1997 study to test the effect of vitamin C supplements on gallstones analyzed blood fat levels, cholesterol metabolism, bile fat composition and cholesterol saturation in 16 gallstone patients. They then treated the patients with 500 mg of vitamin C four times a day for two weeks before surgery. Their findings indicated that vitamin C supplementation may also influence the conditions for cholesterol gallstone formation.[64]

Exercise

Strenuous exercise appears to increase the levels of free radicals in the body, increasing the risk of disorders in which oxidative damage play a part. As an antioxidant, vitamin C may help to prevent this damage. In a 1997 study researchers examined the effects of supplements on oxidative stress in athletes. They found that exercise-induced oxidative stress was highest when those involved in the study did not supplement with vitamin C.[65]

Other uses

Vitamin C has also been used to treat constipation and to speed wound-healing. Recent research suggests that vitamin C may help to enhance the strength of sperm in smokers.[66]

Interactions with other nutrients

Vitamin C acts together with the other antioxidants, vitamin E and beta carotene in many body processes. High levels of vitamin C appear to increase blood levels of the other antioxidants and therapeutic effects appear to be greater when combinations of antioxidants are used. Vitamin C improves the stability and use of vitamin E. However, it may interfere with selenium absorption and supplements should be taken at different times.

Vitamin C may protect against the harmful effects of beta carotene supplements in smokers. (See page 55 for more information.) Smokers tend to have low levels of vitamin C and this may allow a build-up of a harmful form of beta carotene called the carotene free radical which is formed when beta carotene acts to regenerate vitamin E. Smokers who take beta carotene supplements should also take vitamin C.[67]

Vitamin C aids in the body's absorption of iron by helping convert dietary iron to a soluble form. It helps to reduce the ability of food components such as phytates to form insoluble complexes with, and reduce the absorption of, iron. Vitamin C decreases the absorption of copper. Calcium and manganese supplements may decrease vitamin C excretion and vitamin C supplements may increase manganese absorption. Vitamin C also helps to reduce folic acid excretion and deficiency may lead to increased excretion of vitamin B6. Vitamin C helps to protect against the toxic effects of cadmium, copper, vanadium, cobalt, mercury and selenium.

Interactions with drugs

Large doses of vitamin C may increase estrogen levels when taken at the same time as the contraceptive pill. Oral contraceptives may increase requirements but supplements should be taken at a different time.

Aspirin, alcohol, antibiotics and steroids may increase vitamin C requirements. Vitamin C may be useful for preventing the development of tolerance to nitrate drugs which are often used to treat angina.[68]

Cautions

There is some concern that large doses of vitamin C may cause kidney stones because part of the oxalate in calcium oxalate kidney stones comes from metabolized vitamin C. However, this is unlikely to happen in healthy people. It may be advisable for anyone suffering from recurrent kidney stones, kidney disease or who has a defect in vitamin C metabolism to keep their daily intake of vitamin C to around 100 mg.[69]

Large doses of vitamin C may cause a false positive test result for diabetes and affect hemoglobin tests. Large doses may also affect the action of anticoagulant drugs.

A state of dependency can result from prolonged high dose consumption of vitamin C. If you have been taking large doses and decide to stop, a gradual reduction in dose is advisable.

QUICK GUIDE

Essential for

- the absorption and use of calcium and phosphorus, which are vital for functions such as the development of bones and teeth
- healthy nervous and immune systems
- regulation of some hormones
- normal cell growth and maturation

Absorption and metabolism

Vitamin D requires fat for absorption. It is also made in the skin.

Deficiency

Deficiency in children leads to rickets in which bones lose calcium and become soft and curved. In adults, symptoms include bone pain and tenderness, and muscle weakness. Deficiency may also increase the risk of osteoporosis, arthritis and cancer.

Sources

Good sources include fortified milk, oily fish, liver and eggs.

Daily recommended dietary intakes

Men	200 IU
(over 50)	400 IU
(over 70)	600 IU
Women	200 IU
(over 50)	400 IU
(over 70)	600 IU
Pregnancy	200 IU
Lactation	200 IU

Toxic effects of excess intake

These include symptoms of unusual thirst, sore eyes, itching skin, vomiting, diarrhea, and eventually, calcium deposits in the blood vessels, lungs and kidney.

Interactions

Cholestyramine, anticonvulsants, alcohol and mineral oil interfere with the action of vitamin D.

Therapeutic uses of supplements

Supplements have been used to treat osteoporosis and osteoarthritis in elderly people. Synthetic vitamin D analogues are used to treat psoriasis.

Vitamin D is both a hormone and a vitamin. It was identified in the 1920s after a long search for the cause and cure of rickets, which had been a significant health problem since the industrialization of northern Europe. Vitamin D is obtained from food sources and is also manufactured in the skin through the action of sunlight. There are three forms of vitamin D: vitamin D1 (calciferol), vitamin D2 (ergocalciferol) and vitamin D3 (cholecalciferol). Vitamin D2 is the form most commonly added to foods and nutritional supplements. These forms of vitamin D are converted in the liver and kidneys to the hormone, calcitriol, which is the physiologically active form of vitamin D.

What it does in the body

Bones and teeth

The most important role of vitamin D is to maintain blood calcium levels within an acceptable range. It stimulates intestinal calcium absorption and re-absorption in the kidneys, and regulates the metabolism of calcium and phosphorus, which are vital for many body functions including the normal growth and development of bones and teeth. It enables bones and teeth to harden by increasing the deposition of calcium into these structures and may also assist in the movement of calcium across body cell membranes.

Cell growth

Vitamin D is involved in normal cell growth and maturation and may play a part in cancer prevention. In test tube experiments, calcitriol seems to have anticancer properties, inhibiting the growth of human leukemia, colon cancer, skin cancer and breast cancer cells.

Immune system

Vitamin D is involved in the regulation of the immune system. It has several functions including effects on white blood cells known as monocytes and lymphocytes and seems to suppress function of several parts of the immune system.

Hormones

Vitamin D plays a role in the secretion of insulin by the pancreas, thus aiding in the regulation of blood sugar. Vitamin D suppresses both the action of the parathyroid gland and the action of a hormone from this gland and may play a role in the treatment of an overactive parathyroid.

Nervous system

Careful regulation of calcium levels is vital for normal nerve impulse transmission and muscle contraction. Vitamin D plays a role in the functioning of healthy nerves and muscles by regulating the level of calcium in the blood.

Absorption and metabolism

As with other fat soluble vitamins, fat in the intestine is necessary for vitamin D absorption. Vitamin D from food and supplements is absorbed through the intestinal walls and can be stored in the fat cells of the liver, skin, brain and bones in amounts sufficient for many months' consumption. Exposure to sunlight in spring, summer and autumn usually makes up for any shortfall in dietary vitamin D and even brief exposure to sunlight during these times is adequate. There may, however, be problems in winter months in some climates. The production of vitamin D in the body is blocked by anything which blocks ultraviolet light including skin pigment, smog, fog, sunscreen, windows and hats.

Deficiency

Vitamin D deficiency leads to increased production of parathyroid hormone and the removal of calcium from the bones. In children, this results in rickets, a disorder in which the bones are so soft that they become curved from supporting the weight of the body. The equivalent in adults is osteomalacia which involves a softening of bones and causes bone pain and tenderness and muscle weakness. Other signs of deficiency include severe tooth decay and hearing loss, which is due to a softening of the bones in the inner ear.

Studies show that elderly people, particularly those who are housebound or in institutions, may be at high risk of vitamin D deficiency. A study published in 1998 in the *New England Journal of Medicine* found vitamin D deficiency in 57 per cent of a group of 290 patients who were admitted to hospital. In a subgroup of the patients who had no known risk factors for vitamin D deficiency, the researchers found that 42 per cent were deficient. They concluded that vitamin D deficiency was probably a substantial problem.[1]

There is some concern that the increasing use of sunscreens as skin cancer preventives may increase the risk of vitamin D deficiency. This is unlikely to be a problem in children and young people who do not usually wear sunscreen every time they go outside. However, older people who may be more concerned about sun damage to skin and who may go outside less often are more likely to be at risk.

Vitamin D deficiency is more common in winter in cold climates. This decline may lead to an increased risk of bone loss in elderly men and women according to a 1997 study by researchers at Tufts University in Boston. They examined vitamin D levels in 182 men and 209 women aged over 65. Levels were found to be lower in women. In wintertime levels were lower than in summertime. Travel, vitamin D intake and time spent outdoors increased the vitamin D concentrations.[2]

Other groups at risk of deficiency include alcoholics, those with gastrointestinal malabsorption disorders such as celiac disease, those taking anticonvulsant drugs, those who don't drink milk or get much sunlight, those with absorption problems and darker skinned people living in colder climates. As vitamin D is converted in the liver and kidneys to calcitriol, its active form, sufferers of kidney and liver diseases may also be at risk of vitamin D deficiency.

Osteoporosis

Vitamin D regulates bone mineral density and a deficiency may lead to osteoporosis, a disease in which bones become lighter, less dense and more prone to fractures. (See page 653 for more information.) People with a certain type of vitamin D receptor may be more susceptible to osteoporosis. As the structure of the vitamin D receptor is genetically determined, this may eventually lead to a test to identify women at risk of the disease. Research suggests that women with different types of vitamin D receptor respond differently to vitamin D supplements given to build bone.[3]

Arthritis

Osteoarthrtitis

New research suggests that people with osteoarthritis who have low vitamin D intakes suffer more severe symptoms than those whose intakes are high. In a study done in 1996 researchers at Boston University studied more than 500 elderly people with osteoarthritis of the knee. They found that those with the lowest intakes and blood levels of vitamin D were three times more likely to see their disease progress than people with high intakes and blood levels. Vitamin D may help reduce the cartilage damage seen in osteoarthritis.[4]

Rheumatoid arthritis

Severe rheumatoid arthritis is associated with bone loss. In a 1998 study, German researchers investigated the links between disease activity and serum levels of vitamin D in 96 patients. They found that high disease activity was associated with alterations in vitamin D metabolism and increased bone breakdown. Low levels of vitamin D may also increase the proliferation of white blood cells and may accelerate the arthritic process in rheumatoid arthritis.[5] Vitamin D supplements are likely to be useful in retarding these adverse effects of alterations in metabolism.

Cancer

Low levels of vitamin D have been linked to several cancers including those of the colon, prostate and breast. Laboratory experiments show that vitamin D can inhibit the growth of human prostate cancer[6] and breast cancer cells[7]. Lung cancer and pancreatic cancer[8] cells may also be susceptible to the effects of vitamin D. Sunlight also seems to be protective against several types of cancer, including ovarian[9] and breast cancers, and this effect may be mediated by vitamin D levels.

Colorectal cancer

Several studies have suggested a link between low dietary vitamin D intake and colorectal cancer risk. In a 1996 study, researchers conducted a population-based case-control study to examine this relationship among 352 people with colon cancer, 217 people with rectal cancer, and 512 healthy people in Stockholm, Sweden. The researchers used questionnaires to assess the vitamin D intake for the preceding five years. The results showed that those with the highest vitamin D intakes were around half as likely to get cancers of the colon or rectum than those with the lowest intakes.[10]

Results from the Harvard Nurses Health Study published in 1996 suggest a link between vitamin D and colorectal cancer. The study involved 89 448 female nurses and covered the time period from 1980 to 1992 during which 501 cases of colorectal cancer were documented. The results showed a link between intake of total vitamin D and risk of colorectal cancer.[11]

Prostate cancer

Low vitamin D levels are linked to an increased risk of prostate cancer. In a study published in 1996, researchers at Brigham and Women's Hospital in Boston collected blood plasma samples from 14 916 participants in the Physicians' Health Study and measured vitamin D levels. Their analysis included 232 cases diagnosed up to 1992 and 414 age-matched control participants. The results showed a slightly reduced risk of prostate cancer in those with high vitamin D levels.[12]

The way a man's body utilizes vitamin D could affect his risk of prostate cancer. A 1996 National Institute of Environmental Health Sciences study has found that men with a particular type of vitamin D receptor gene are less likely than others to develop the type of prostate cancer that requires surgery. Researchers looked at the receptor genes in 108 cancer patients and 170 men without cancer. The results showed that 22 per cent of cancer patients had two copies of a particular gene, while only 8 per cent of the cancer-free men did. These findings support the theory that vitamin D plays an important role in prostate cancer.[13]

Multiple sclerosis

There is some suggestion that abnormalities in vitamin D metabolism may be linked to multiple sclerosis. The hormonal form of vitamin D can prevent a disease similar to multiple sclerosis in mice. Multiple sclerosis is more prevalent in areas where there is less exposure to sunlight and some researchers believe that vitamin D protects against the disease.[14]

Diabetes

Vitamin D deficiency impairs glucose metabolism by reducing insulin secretion. This is likely to increase the risk of diabetes mellitus. Vitamin D supplements are likely to be useful in preventing diabetes in areas where vitamin D deficiency is common.[15]

In a 1997 study looking at the links between environmental factors and Type II diabetes, vitamin D levels were assessed in 142 Dutch men aged from 70 to 88 years of age. Thirty-nine per cent were found to have low vitamin D levels and tests showed that low vitamin D levels increased the risk of glucose intolerance.[16]

Heart disease

Low vitamin D levels may also increase the risk of atherosclerosis. Research published in 1997 in the American Heart Association journal *Circulation* suggests that a low level of vitamin D increases the risk of calcium build-up in atherosclerotic plaques and that higher levels reduce the risk of build-up. Researchers at UCLA School of Medicine measured the vitamin D levels in the blood of 173 men and women at risk of heart disease and also measured the build-up of calcium in coronary arteries (a common finding in coronary artery disease). The results suggest that calcium may regulate calcium deposition in the arteries as well as in the bone.[17]

Other effects

Vitamin D deficiency may also play a role in inflammatory bowel disease, tuberculosis, stroke and high blood pressure.

Sources

Fish liver oils, sardines, herring, salmon, tuna, liver, eggs and some dairy products are good dietary sources of vitamin D. Milk is often fortified with vitamin D and is a good source, but dairy products other than milk are not usually fortified with vitamin D.

Food	Amount	Vitamin D (IU)
Medicinal cod liver oil	1 tbsp	2271
Pink salmon, canned	100g	624
Tuna, canned in oil	1 can	404
Whole milk, dried	1 cup	380
Oysters	6 oysters	269
Mackerel, canned in oil	100g	252
Shiitake mushrooms, dried	4 mushrooms	249
Sardines, canned in tomato sauce	1 sardine	182
Fortified milk, evaporated	½ cup	97.9
Whole milk, fortified	1 cup	92.7
Skim milk, fortified	1 cup	92.7
Chocolate milk, fortified	1 cup	92.7
Beef salami	1 slice (23g)	80.3
Low fat milk, dried	¼ cup	79.0
Sardines, canned in oil	2 sardines	65.3
Herring, smoked	1 fillet	48.0
Natural raisin bran	30g	45.6
Shrimp	4 large	42.6
All Bran	30g	42.0

Bran flakes	30g	42.0
Corn flakes	30g	42.0
Special K	30g	42.0
Egg yolk	1 large	24.6
Pork sausages	1 sausage, 10cm long	14.6

Recommended dietary allowances

	Men	*Women*	*Pregnancy*	*Lactation*
USA	200 IU	200 IU	200 IU	200 IU
(over 50)	400 IU	400 IU		
(over 70)	600 IU	600 IU		
UK			400 IU	400 IU
Australia	200 IU	200 IU	400 IU	400 IU

The tolerable upper intake limit has been set at 2000 IU per day.

Supplements

Vitamin D supplements are often available in the form of cod liver oil. Anyone on long-term anticonvulsant drug therapy, older people, and those who follow a strict vegan diet may benefit from supplements.

Toxic effects of excess intake

High daily doses of dietary vitamin D over an extended period of time can produce excessive calcium levels in the blood with symptoms of unusual thirst, metallic taste, bone pain, fatigue, sore eyes, itching skin, vomiting, diarrhea, urinary urgency, abnormal calcium deposits in blood vessel walls, liver, lungs, kidney and stomach. High doses also cause the build-up of calcium in the muscles which impairs their function. Doses of less than 1000 IU daily are unlikely to cause any adverse effects and prolonged exposure to sunlight does not cause toxic effects.

Large doses of vitamin D can irritate the urinary tract. There may be a link between excessive vitamin D intake and heart attacks, atherosclerosis and kidney stones in people who are susceptible.

Very high doses of vitamin D supplements may actually increase the risk of osteoporosis. In an article published in 1997, researchers at the Cedars Sinai Medical Center in Los Angeles reported four cases of osteoporosis linked to excessive use of vitamin D supplements. Each of the four patients had high levels of calcium and vitamin D metabolites in their urine and were taking dietary supplements which contained unidentified amounts of vitamin D. When the patients stopped taking the supplements, bone mineral density increased. Excessive vitamin D supplementation for six months or longer upsets calcium balance and affects bone mineral density.[18]

Therapeutic uses of supplements

Supplements are used to treat vitamin D deficiency and its symptoms.

Osteoporosis

Vitamin D is recommended in the treatment of osteoporosis in postmenopausal women. Several research studies suggest that vitamin D supplements reduce the occurrence of fractures in elderly people.

In a study published in 1997, researchers at Tufts University in Boston assessed the effects of calcium (500 mg per day) and vitamin D (700 IU per day) in 176 men and 213 women aged 65 years or older. When bone density was measured after a three-year period, those taking the supplements had higher bone density at all body sites measured. The fracture rate was also reduced by 50 per cent in those taking the supplements.[19]

Vitamin D supplements may also be useful in preventing bone loss in patients taking corticosteroid drugs. In a study published in 1996, researchers at the University of Virginia found that calcium and vitamin D supplements helped prevent the loss of bone mineral density in those taking the drugs for arthritis, asthma and other chronic diseases.[20]

However, other studies have not shown any reduction in fracture rates in those taking vitamin D supplements. A 1996 study which was carried out in Amsterdam looked at the effects of either vitamin D or a placebo on 2500 healthy men and women over the age of 70 who were living independently. The participants received a placebo or a daily dose of 400 IU of vitamin D for a three-and-a-half-year period. Dietary calcium intake was the same in both groups. Forty-eight fractures were observed in the placebo group and 58 in the vitamin D group.[21]

Other uses

Synthetic vitamin D analogs are used to treat the skin disorder, psoriasis, and are also being investigated for their ability to prevent and treat cancer.

Because of its effects on the immune system, many researchers are investigating the possibility of using vitamin D and related compounds to treat autoimmune disorders and to suppress rejection of transplanted organs.

Interactions with other nutrients

Vitamin D is necessary for calcium and phosphorus absorption and metabolism. Pantothenic acid is necessary for the synthesis of vitamin D.

Interactions with drugs

The cholesterol-lowering drug, cholestyramine, and mineral oil laxatives interfere with the absorption of vitamin D. Alcohol interferes with the conversion of vitamin D to its biologically active form.

People taking certain anticonvulsant drugs, such as phenytoin, may decrease the activity of vitamin D by increasing its metabolism. People taking this drug are likely to be at increased risk of osteoporosis and have high vitamin D requirements

Cautions

Vitamin D supplements should not be given to those with high calcium levels or high phosphorus levels, and should be given with caution to those suffering from cardiac or kidney diseases.

QUICK GUIDE

Essential for

- action as an antioxidant to provide protection for cells against free radical damage which may lead to disorders such as heart disease and cancer. It is particularly important in protecting fats, cell membranes, DNA and enzymes against damage.

Absorption and metabolism

Fats and bile are necessary for absorption.

Deficiency

This is rare. Symptoms in infants include irritability, fluid retention and anemia; and in adults, lethargy, loss of balance and anemia. Marginal deficiencies may increase the risk of heart disease, cancer and premature aging.

Sources

Good sources include wheatgerm, nuts and seeds, whole grain cereals, eggs and leafy greens.

Daily recommended dietary intakes

Men	10 mg alpha TE (15 IU)
Women	8 mg alpha TE (12 IU)
Pregnancy	10 mg alpha TE (15 IU)
Lactation	12 mg alpha TE (18 IU)

Toxic effects of excess intake

These are rare and include diarrhea, fatigue, bleeding and headache.

Interactions

Vitamin E absorption is reduced by mineral oil, alcohol and the drug, cholestyramine.

Therapeutic use of supplements

Supplements have been used to treat and prevent many disorders including heart disease, cancer, cataracts, diabetes, asthma, Alzheimer's disease and infertility. Natural forms of vitamin E may be more beneficial than synthetic forms.

Cautions

Supplements should not be taken with anticoagulant drugs and should be used cautiously by anyone with an overactive thyroid, hypertension or rheumatic heart disease.

Vitamin E was discovered in the 1920s when rats fed a vitamin E-deficient diet became unable to reproduce; but it was not officially considered essential for humans until 1966. It is the name given to a group of fat soluble compounds which are also called tocopherols and tocotrienols. The term "tocopherol" comes from the Greek words meaning "to bear offspring". The most abundant and active form of vitamin E is alpha tocopherol.

What it does in the body

Antioxidant properties

Unlike the other vitamins which take part in metabolic reactions or function as hormones, the main role of vitamin E appears to be to act as an antioxidant. Vitamin E is incorporated into the lipid portion of cell membranes and carrier molecules and protects these structures from toxic compounds, heavy metals, drugs, radiation and free radicals. Vitamin E also protects cholesterol from oxidative damage. Because of its antioxidant effects, a diet high in vitamin E appears to be protective against common health conditions such as heart disease, cancer and strokes (See page 417 for more information.)

Immune system

Vitamin E is essential for the maintenance of a healthy immune system as it protects the thymus gland and circulating white blood cells from damage. Vitamin E is particularly important in protecting the immune system from damage during times of oxidative stress and chronic viral illness.

Eyes

Vitamin E is vital for healthy eyes. It is essential for the development of the retina and protects the eyes against free radical damage associated with cataract formation and macular degeneration. It also protects vitamin A in the eyes from damage.

Aging

As an antioxidant, vitamin E may protect against the effects of aging by destroying free radicals which cause degeneration in tissues such as the skin and blood vessels. Studies in mice have shown that high doses of vitamin E may help prevent aging-related damage to proteins involved in immune and central nervous system function. Vitamin E may also protect against the mental effects of aging, such as memory loss.

Absorption and metabolism

Vitamin E requires the presence of fats and bile in the gut to be absorbed. Approximately 20 to 60 per cent of dietary vitamin E is absorbed and it is stored in the liver, heart, fatty tissues, heart, muscles, testes, uterus, blood, adrenal and pituitary glands. Absorption and transport are likely to be reduced in elderly people.

Deficiency

The symptoms of vitamin E deficiency in infants are irritability, fluid retention, hemolytic anemia (the breaking down of red blood cells) and eye disorders. In adults, vitamin E deficiency can lead to nerve damage and symptoms of lethargy, apathy, inability to concentrate, staggering gait, low thyroid hormone levels, decreased immune response, loss of balance and anemia.

Severe vitamin E deficiency is very rare. Those at risk include people with chronic liver disease and fat malabsorption syndromes, such as celiac disease and cystic fibrosis. Hemodialysis patients, those with inherited red blood cell disorders, premature and low birthweight infants, and elderly people may also be at risk of vitamin E deficiency and are often given supplements.

As vitamin E is stored in the body, it can take some time before deficiency symptoms become apparent in someone consuming a diet low in vitamin E. Marginal vitamin E deficiency may be relatively common and several studies have shown an increased risk of heart disease, cancer and other disorders in those with low vitamin E levels.

Cardiovascular disease

Low dietary intake of vitamin E seems to increase the risk of heart disease. This is illustrated by results from the Iowa Women's Health Study published in 1996 in the *New England Journal of Medicine*. Researchers studied 34 486 postmenopausal women with no cardiovascular disease who in early 1986 completed a questionnaire that assessed, among other factors, their intake of vitamins A, E, and C from food sources and supplements. During seven years of follow-up, 242 women died of coronary heart disease. The results showed that high vitamin E consumption reduced the risk of death from coronary heart disease. This association was particularly striking in the subgroup of 21 809 women who did not consume vitamin supplements.[1]

Similar results have been seen in men. Harvard School of Public Health researchers have assessed the links between diet and heart disease in 39 910 US male health professionals aged between 40 to 75 years of age. Participants responded to a questionnaire in 1986 and were then followed up for four years, during which time there were 667 cases of coronary disease. The results showed a lower risk of disease among men with higher intakes of vitamin E. Men consuming more than 40 mg (60 IU) per day had a 36 per cent lower risk than those consuming less than 5 mg (7.5 IU) per day. Men who took at least 67 mg (100 IU) per day for at least two years had a 37 per cent lower risk than those who did not take supplements.[2]

The results of a 1996 study done in Japan suggest that low vitamin E levels increase the risk of a type of angina caused by coronary artery spasm.[3] Animal studies suggest that brain damage after stroke may be greater in those who are vitamin E-deficient

Cancer

There is some evidence that vitamin E can protect against cancer, although studies have shown conflicting results. Some population studies suggest that low vitamin E levels increase the risk of certain cancers, particularly those of the gastrointestinal tract, cervix and lungs.

Cancers of the gastrointestinal tract

Results from the Iowa Women's Health Study suggest that high intakes of vitamin E reduce the risk of colon cancer. Researchers analyzed the links between vitamin E and colon cancer in 35 215 Iowa women aged 55 to 69 years without a history of cancer. During the follow-up period, there were 212 cases of colon cancer. The results showed that low vitamin E intake increased the risk of colon cancer and those in the high intake group had 30 per cent of the risk of those in the low intake group. The protective factor was stronger in the younger women.[4]

Other results from the Iowa Women's Health Study show that higher intakes of antioxidants, including vitamin E, are linked to lower risks of both oral, pharyngeal, esophageal and gastric cancers.[5]

Breast cancer

Researchers at the University of Southern California investigated the relationship between blood levels of various nutrients, including vitamin E, and the risks of breast cancer and proliferative benign breast disease (BBD) in postmenopausal women in the Boston area. Women whose intake of vitamin E from food sources only was high had around 60 per cent less risk of breast cancer compared to those in the low intake group.[6] However, not all studies have shown protective effects.[7]

Cervical cancer

Utah University researchers investigating the relationship between cervical cancer and dietary intake of antioxidant vitamins and selenium in 266 women with cervical cancer and 408 women without the disorder found that women with high vitamin E intakes had a 40 per cent lower risk of cervical cancer.[8] Blood levels of vitamin E have also been found to be low in women with cervical cancer.[9]

Lung cancer

Several epidemiological studies suggest that low vitamin E intakes increase the risk of lung cancer. In 1974 and 1975, researchers at Johns Hopkins School of Hygiene and Public Health, Baltimore, collected blood samples from 25 802 volunteers. They assessed vitamin E levels in samples from 436 cancer cases and 765 matched control subjects. The results showed that high vitamin E levels protected against lung cancer.[10]

Cataracts

Low vitamin E levels may increase the risk of cataract formation. A 1996 Finnish study of over 400 men found an increased risk of cataracts in those with low vitamin E levels. The researchers evaluated the link between vitamin E levels and progression of eye lens opacities in 410 men with high cholesterol. The results showed that those with low vitamin E levels had almost four times the risk of lens opacities when compared with those in the highest intake group.[11]

Parkinson's disease

The results of several studies suggest that high levels of vitamin E can protect against Parkinson's disease. In a 1997 study, researchers at Erasmus University Medical School in Holland examined the relationship between dietary intake of antioxidants and Parkinson's Disease and found a reduction in risk associated with high vitamin E intake. The study involved over 5300 men and women living independently and without dementia. It included 31 people with Parkinson's Disease.[12]

Other symptoms

Low levels of vitamin E are common in those who are HIV-positive and high levels seem to be linked to slower disease progression. Vitamin E deficiency may also be involved in the development of pre-eclampsia.

Sources

The best natural sources of vitamin E are wheatgerm oil, hazelnut oil, sunflower oil, almond oil, wheatgerm, whole grain cereals and eggs. Peaches, avocados, broccoli and leafy greens are also good sources. Different foods have varying amounts of the different forms of vitamin E. For example, soybean oil is composed of about 10 per cent alpha tocopherol with the rest made up of other tocopherols. The specific benefits of the different forms of vitamin E remain to be discovered.

The results of a 1997 study suggest that the mixed forms of vitamin E found in food may be more beneficial than the alpha tocopherol form which is the main ingredient in supplements. Scientists at the University of California compared the abilities of alpha tocopherol and gamma tocopherol to protect against lipid peroxidation by compounds known as peroxynitrites which are formed in response to cigarette smoke, pollution and inflammation. Results showed that the gamma tocopherol form may be better at inhibiting these damaging reactions. About 75 per cent of the vitamin E found in food is the gamma tocopherol form while supplements may not contain any gamma tocopherol and it is possible that taking very high doses of alpha tocopherol may displace gamma tocopherol.[13]

Cooking and processing reduces the vitamin E content of foods such as flours and oils. Cold-pressed oils therefore have a higher vitamin E content than refined vegetable oils. Exposure to light and oxygen also destroys vitamin E.

Food	Amount	Vitamin E (mg alpha TE)
Wheatgerm oil	1 tbsp	26.2
Wheatgerm cereal	1 cup	19.5
Sunflower seeds	¼ cup	17.2
Hazelnuts	½ cup, whole	15.4
Peanuts	½ cup, whole	6.32
Soy beans, cooked	1 cup	3.19

Safflower oil	1tbsp	4.69
Canola oil	1 tbsp	2.93
Corn oil	1 tbsp	2.87
Avocado	1 avocado	2.69
Soybean oil	1 tbsp	2.50
Spinach, cooked	1 cup	1.63
Tomato sauce, canned	½ cup	1.63
Olive oil	1 tbsp	1.68
Broccoli	½ cup, chopped	1.25
Grapes	1 cup	1.06
Blackberries	1 cup	0.97
Parsnip, cooked	½ cup, slices	0.74
Peaches	1 medium	0.69
Brussels sprouts, cooked	½ cup	0.63
Margarine	1tsp	0.60
Eggs	1 large	0.53
Tomatoes	1 medium	0.47
Beet greens, cooked	1 cup	0.41

Recommended dietary allowances

The amount of vitamin E required depends on the amount of polyunsaturated fats in the diet. The greater the amount of these fats in the diet, the greater the risk that they will be damaged by free radicals and exert harmful effects. As vitamin E prevents this damage, recommended intake is roughly proportional to the amount of polyunsaturated fats in the diet. The US RDA is based on an intake of 0.4 mg per g of polyunsaturated fats. Vitamin E is measured in International Units (IU) and more commonly nowadays, mg alpha TE. 1 IU equals 0.67 mg alpha TE.

	Men	*Women*	*Pregnancy*	*Lactation*
USA	10 mg alpha TE (15 IU)	8 mg alpha TE (12 IU)	10 mg alpha TE (15 IU)	12 mg alpha TE (18 IU)
Australia	10 mg alpha TE (15 IU)	7 mg alpha TE (10.4)	7 mg alpha TE (10.4)	9.5 mg alpha TE (14 IU)

No RNI has been given in the UK. A 1991 Department of Health report concluded that a fixed amount is impossible to recommend as required vitamin E needs depend on the intake of polyunsaturated fats, which varies considerably from person to person.

Supplements

Vitamin E supplements are available in natural and synthetic forms. Natural forms of vitamin E are derived from soybean or wheatgerm oil and are indicated by a 'd' prefix. These include d-alpha-tocopherol, d-alpha-tocopheryl acetate and d-alpha-tocopheryl succinate. The synthetic forms are manufactured from purified petroleum oil and are indicated by a 'dl' prefix. These include dl-alpha-tocopherol, dl-alpha-tocopheryl acetate and dl-alpha-tocopheryl succinate. Natural vitamin E supplements containing mixed tocopherols appear to offer the most beneficial effects. Water soluble vitamin E supplements are also available and, although more expensive, may not necessarily be more beneficial. As they require fat for absorption, vitamin E supplements should be taken with food.

In studies where benefits of vitamin E supplementation have been shown, the doses used have usually well exceeded the RDAs. In many studies, daily doses of up to 536 mg (800 IU) or even 804 mg (1200 IU) have been used. It is not possible to get such large amounts of vitamin E from food without consuming a high fat diet. Therefore many experts believe that supplements are necessary.

Toxic effects of excess intake

Vitamin E is considered safe even in large doses. Doses over 536 mg (800 IU) may lead to an increased risk of bleeding, diarrhea, abdominal pain, fatigue, reduced resistance to bacterial infection and transiently raised blood pressure.

Some research suggests that vitamin E may actually be pro-oxidant at high doses; that is, may actually increase free radical damage. The results of a 1997 study done in Scotland showed that red cells of nonsmokers receiving 1050 mg of vitamin E had an increased susceptibility to peroxidation. Also, prolonged supplementation with vitamin E led to a decline in vitamin C concentrations in the blood.[14]

Therapeutic uses of supplements

Vitamin E supplements are used to treat deficiency and to prevent it in those at risk. Supplements are also used in a wide range of disorders where there is an increased need for immune support and protection against free radical damage.

A study published in 1996 by researchers from the National Institute on Aging examined the effects of vitamin E and vitamin C supplement on mortality risk in 11 178 persons aged from 67 to 105 who were taking part in the Established Populations for Epidemiologic Studies of the Elderly Study. From 1984 through 1993 there were 3490 deaths. The results showed that those using the vitamin E supplements had a 34 per cent lower risk of death when compared to those not using vitamin E supplements, and around half the risk of death from coronary disease.[15]

Cardiovascular disease

Several studies have shown that high vitamin E intake can reduce the risk of developing heart disease and improve the symptoms in those who do have the disease. Results from the Nurses Health Study provide evidence for the protective effects of vitamin E. Results published in 1993 assessed the links between vitamin E and heart disease in 87 245 female nurses aged from 34 to 59 who were free of diagnosed cardiovascular disease and cancer in 1980. During the follow-up period of eight years, there were 552 cases of major coronary disease (437 nonfatal heart attacks and 115 deaths due to coronary disease). The results showed that women with the highest vitamin E intakes had 34 per cent less risk of major coronary disease compared to those with the lowest intakes. Most of the reduction in risk was attributable to vitamin E consumed as supplements, a finding which conflicts with some other studies which only show benefit from high dietary intakes. Women who took vitamin E supplements for short periods had little apparent benefit, but those who took them for more than two years had an even lower risk of disease.[16]

Results from a British study known as the Cambridge Heart Antioxidant Study (CHAOS) which were published in *The Lancet* in 1996 provide further evidence of a link between vitamin E supplements and reduction in heart disease risk. In this double-blind, placebo-controlled study, 2002 patients with coronary atherosclerosis were enrolled and followed up for 510 days. 546 patients were given 536 mg (800 IU) daily; 589 were given 268 mg (400 IU) per day and 967 received identical placebo capsules. The results showed that those who received vitamin E supplements had a 75 per cent reduction in the risk of fatal heart attacks. However, when nonfatal events were included there did not appear to be any benefit from the vitamin E supplements.[17]

As part of the Finnish Alpha-Tocopherol, Beta carotene Cancer (ATBC) Prevention Study, researchers studied the preventive effect of vitamin E and beta carotene supplements on major coronary events. A total of 27 271 Finnish male smokers aged 50 to 69 years with no history of heart attack were randomly assigned to receive 50 mg (75 IU) and a 20 mg dose of beta carotene, both supplements, or placebo daily for five to eight years. During this period there were 1204 nonfatal heart attacks and 907 fatal ones. The results showed that major coronary events decreased 4 per cent among those taking vitamin E. Supplementation with vitamin E also decreased the incidence of fatal coronary heart disease by 8 per cent although did not appear to affect the incidence of nonfatal heart attacks. The dose of vitamin E used in this study is smaller than that commonly used.[18]

Vitamin E may help prevent heart disease in a number of ways. It lowers total blood cholesterol levels, and as it is easily incorporated into the harmful LDL cholesterol molecule, it can protect it from oxidation by free radicals. Oxidized LDL cholesterol is more likely to block arteries and contribute to the atherosclerotic process than unoxidised LDL cholesterol. Vitamin E may be able to prevent the free radical damage that occurs when blood is cut off then re-supplied, for example during surgery or in the case of a blood vessel spasm. Vitamin E also has important direct effects on vascular endothelial and smooth muscle cells and also inhibits the clumping together of platelets which helps to reduce atherosclerotic plaque formation.[19] It also seems to inhibit the attachment of white blood cells to artery linings which is caused by LDL cholesterol.[20]

A study published in 1996 suggests that the minimum dose of supplementary vitamin E which will significantly reduce the susceptibility of LDL to oxidation is 335 mg (500 IU) per day.[21]

Angina

Vitamin E appears to play a part in decreasing the risk of angina. Results of the Finnish ATBC Prevention Study found a slightly reduced risk in those taking vitamin E supplements.[22]

Cancer

Vitamin E supplements, especially when combined with selenium, have shown beneficial effects in the prevention of certain types of cancer, including breast cancer. Results from the US National Institute on Aging study mentioned above showed a 22 per cent decrease in the risk of death from cancer in those taking vitamin E supplements.

Vitamin E may protect against cell membrane and chromosome damage that would otherwise lead to cancerous changes in cells. Vitamin E also inhibits the growth of abnormal cells and plays a role in their conversion back to normal cells. Vitamin E can also prevent the formation of certain carcinogens by combining with substances in the intestine. For example, the formation of cancer-causing nitrosamines from dietary nitrites in the stomach may be inhibited by vitamin E.

Prostate cancer

According to more results from the ATBC study published in 1998 in the *Journal of the National Cancer Institute*, vitamin E reduces the risk of prostate cancer among smokers. Researchers studied the effects of 50 mg (75 IU) in Finnish men and the results showed a 32 per cent decrease in the incidence of prostate cancer and a 41 per cent decrease in prostate cancer deaths among the men taking vitamin E, compared with those who took no vitamin E.[23]

Immunity

High doses of vitamin E boost the immune system in elderly people. In a 1997 study of 88 healthy people, aged 65 or older, those who took 200 mg (300 IU) each day for about four months showed an improvement in immune response. Researchers assessed the effects of either 60 mg (90 IU), 200 mg (300 IU) or 800 mg (1333) on a measure of immune system strength known as delayed hypersensitivity skin response. The results showed that those who took 200 mg a day had a 65 per cent increase in immune function. Those taking 60 mg or 800 mg of vitamin E also showed some improvements in immune function but the ideal response was seen in those taking 200 mg. In other tests, those who took the supplements produced six times more antibodies to hepatitis B after being given the vaccine than those who took placebo. They also produced more antibodies against tetanus infection. The study, which was reported in the *Journal of the American Medical Association* provides more support for vitamin E supplementation in older people.[24]

HIV/AIDS

Vitamin E may also help to slow disease progression in HIV-positive people. The results of a nine year study involving 311 HIV-positive men showed that those patients with the highest vitamin E intakes had a 35 per cent decrease in risk of progression to AIDS when compared to those in the lowest intake group.[25]

Diabetes

Vitamin E may improve insulin action in some diabetics. Those with the disorder are particularly susceptible to oxidative damage and vitamin E may play a role in preventing the long-term complications of diabetes. Studies show that vitamin E can protect diabetics against LDL cholesterol oxidation and other adverse effects of the disease.

In a study published in 1996, Louisiana researchers examined whether 67 mg (100 IU) per day had any effect on blood lipid oxidation products and blood lipid profiles of 35 diabetic patients over a three month period. The results showed that vitamin E supplementation significantly lowered lipid peroxidation products and lipid levels in diabetic patients.[26]

Type I diabetes

The results of a 1997 study done in Italy show that vitamin E can protect against damage to beta cells which produce insulin in Type I diabetes patients. The one year study involved 84 patients between 5 and 35 years of age. One group was treated with vitamin E supplements and the other group received nicotinic acid which has been shown to protect pancreatic beta cell function (See page 80 for more information.) All patients were under intensive insulin therapy with three to four injections a day. The results showed that vitamin E was as effective as nicotinic acid in protecting the beta cells.[27]

Cataract

Vitamin E supplements may help to prevent cataract progression, according to a 1998 study published in the journal *Ophthalmology.* Researchers found that among a group of around 750 elderly people, those who took vitamin E supplements had half the risk that their cataracts would progress over a four-and-a-half-year period. Taking a multivitamin pill lowered the risk by one-third.[28]

Fertility

Animal studies suggest that moderate doses of vitamin E may enhance the ability of sperm to fertilize eggs. Recent studies suggest that vitamin E supplements may be useful in treating male infertility by improving sperm function.[29]

Arthritis

Vitamin E has anti-inflammatory and analgesic activity which may be useful in rheumatoid arthritis patients. In a study published in 1997, UK researchers treated 42 patients with 600 mg (895 IU) twice a day or with placebo for 12 weeks. The patients were already receiving anti-rheumatic drug treatment. Laboratory and clinical measures of inflammation were not influenced by the treatment. However, the pain measures; including pain in the morning, pain in the evening, and pain after chosen activity; were significantly decreased after vitamin E treatment when compared with placebo.[30]

Asthma

Antioxidants may help asthmatics. According to researchers at the University of Washington, antioxidant vitamin supplements may help relieve the symptoms of asthma. The researchers measured the amount of breath expelled by the lungs in 17 asthma sufferers. The subjects took peak flow lung function tests while running on a treadmill and breathing in high levels of polluted air. In those asthmatics whose diets were supplemented with daily doses of 268 mg (400 IU) and 500 mg of vitamin C, an 18 per cent increase in peak flow capacity was seen.

Alzheimer's disease

Vitamin E may slow the progression of Alzheimer's disease. Researchers at Columbia University have found that treatment with vitamin E slows the progression of Alzheimer's disease symptoms. In a study reported in 1997 in the *New England Journal of Medicine*, patients were treated with 1340 mg (2000 IU) daily, 10 mg of selegiline daily, a combination of the two, or a placebo for two years. The patients were monitored every three months by the researchers who looked for signs such as the loss of ability to perform basic activities, institutionalization or severe dementia. Researchers found that all the treatment groups had delayed rate of loss of function when compared with the placebo group.[31]

Liver disorders

Vitamin E levels have been found to be low in patients with liver damage and supplements have been shown to protect against liver damage induced by oxidative stress in animal experiments. In a 1997 German study, researchers treated 23 hepatitis C patients with two 268 mg (400 IU) doses per day for 12 weeks. In 11 of 23 patients, the measurements in clinical tests to assess liver damage showed improvement during vitamin E treatment.[32]

Hot flashes

In a study published in 1998, researchers at the Mayo Clinic in Minnesota looked at the effect of vitamin E on hot flashes in 104 women who had survived breast cancer. The women were experiencing at least two hot flashes per day. The study took nine weeks. In weeks two to five, the women took either vitamin E or a placebo and in weeks six to nine, they took the alternative pill. The results showed that in general, women taking vitamin E experienced approximately one less hot flash per day than women taking the placebo.[33]

Skin protection

Vitamins E may help to protect against sunburn. In a study reported in 1998, dermatologists at Ludwig Maximilians University in Germany found that people who take the antioxidant vitamins C and E have a higher threshold for sunburn reaction. The researchers tested ultraviolet sensitivity in two groups of ten Caucasian people by exposing a section of skin to UV light. Subjects in one of the groups then took 2 g of vitamin C and 670 mg (1000 IU) for 8 days. The UV test was then re-done. Those taking the vitamins showed increased tolerance, particularly at higher UV doses. The researchers speculate that combined intake of both vitamins is necessary for protection. However, the researchers stress that in comparison with the protection afforded by topical sunscreens, this level of protection is small.[34]

Exercise

A growing amount of evidence indicates that free radicals play an important role in causing skeletal muscle damage and inflammation after strenuous exercise. The generation of oxygen-free radicals may be increased during exercise as a result of increases in oxygen metabolism in the energy producing organelles of the cell – the mitochondria. These changes may lead to damage to cholesterol and DNA. Increased antioxidant activity can help to prevent this damage and some research suggests that antioxidant vitamin supplementation can be protective in people who regularly exercise heavily.

In a study published in 1998, Pennsylvania State University researchers investigated the effects of high intensity resistance exercise on free radical production and also whether vitamin E supplementation could affect free radical formation or muscle membrane disruption. They divided 12 weight-trained males into two groups. The supplement group received 804 mg (1200 IU) once a day for a period of two weeks and the other group received a placebo. The results showed that high intensity resistance exercise increased free radical production and that vitamin E supplementation decreased muscle membrane disruption.[35]

Other uses

Vitamin E has been used to bring relief from the fibrocystic breast changes which are usually part of the premenstrual syndrome and are considered a risk factor for breast cancer. Some evidence suggests that vitamin E may also help prevent scarring and decrease wound-healing time. Vitamin E has also been used to treat inflammatory bowel disease, periodontal disease and gout due to its antioxidant and anti-inflammatory properties.

Long-term antipsychotic drug use causes nervous system side effects such as involuntary movements of the face and mouth. Vitamin E has been successfully used to treat these side effects.[36]

Pre-treatment with vitamin E may help to stop the adverse effects of surgery on skeletal muscles. When blood is reperfused into muscle after a period of stoppage, oxidative damage tends to occur; and as an antioxidant, vitamin E is effective in reducing this damage.[37]

Interactions with other nutrients

Vitamin E exerts antioxidant effects in combination with other antioxidants including beta carotene, vitamin C and selenium. Vitamin C can restore oxidized vitamin E to its natural antioxidant form. Megadoses of vitamin C may increase vitamin E requirements. Vitamin E can also protect against some of the effects of excessive vitamin A and regulates levels of that vitamin. Vitamin E is necessary for the action of vitamin A and high intake of vitamin A may decrease vitamin E absorption

Vitamin E may be necessary for the conversion of vitamin B12 to its active form and may reduce some of the symptoms of zinc deficiency. Large doses of vitamin E may interfere with the anticoagulant action of vitamin K and may reduce intestinal absorption of vitamin K. Inorganic iron destroys vitamin E, so the two supplements should not be taken together.

Interactions with drugs

Cholestyramine, mineral oil and alcohol may reduce the absorption of vitamin E from the intestine. Vitamin E can enhance the action of anticoagulant drugs on blood clotting and should not be taken in large doses. However, the results of a 1996 study in which 21 people taking chronic warfarin therapy received either vitamin E or placebo suggest that vitamin E can safely be given to patients who require chronic warfarin therapy.[38]

Anticonvulsants such as phenobarbital, phenytoin and carbamazepine may lower plasma vitamin E levels by altering absorption, distribution and metabolism. Isoniazid also decreases vitamin E absorption. Neomycin impairs utilization of vitamin E.

Cautions

Vitamin E should be used cautiously by anyone with an overactive thyroid or rheumatic heart disease. Vitamin E in large doses may aggravate iron deficiency anemia. Vitamin E supplements can cause a transient rise in blood pressure and should be used with caution by anyone suffering from hypertension.

QUICK GUIDE

Essential for

- blood clotting
- bone metabolism
- kidney function

Absorption and metabolism

Vitamin K requires the presence of fats and bile in the gut in order to be absorbed.

Deficiency

Vitamin K deficiency in adults is rare and is usually limited to those who have liver or food absorption disorders. Symptoms include prolonged clotting time, easy bleeding and bruising. It may contribute to osteoporosis. Deficiency can occur in premature babies.

Sources

Good sources include dark leafy greens, oils from green plants and some dairy products. Vitamin K is also produced by gut bacteria.

Daily recommended dietary intakes

Men	80 mcg
Women	65 mcg
Pregnancy	65 mcg
Lactation	65 mcg

Toxic effects of excess intake

Reports of toxic effects are rare. Some forms of supplements may cause anemia. Some studies suggest links between vitamin K injections and an increased risk of childhood cancer.

Interactions

X-rays, aspirin, mineral oil, cholestyramine and anticonvulsant drugs, such as phenytoin, can raise vitamin K requirements. Long-term use of antibiotics can produce vitamin K deficiency.

Therapeutic uses of supplements

Vitamin K supplements are used to prevent hemorrhages and may also be useful in the treatment of osteoporosis.

Cautions

Vitamin K can interfere with the action of anticoagulant drugs such as warfarin.

Vitamin K was discovered in 1929. It is a group of three fat soluble vitamins: vitamin K1 (phylloquinone) which is made by plants, vitamin K2 (menaquinone) which is made by animals, birds and by bacteria in the intestines, and vitamin K3 (menaphthone or menadione), which is synthetic.

What it does in the body

Blood clotting

Vitamin K is used to make prothrombin and other proteins which are important in blood clotting. Vitamin K also plays a role in the conversion of prothrombin to thrombin, another protein important in blood clot formation.

Bone metabolism

A bone protein known as osteocalcin regulates the function of calcium in bone turnover and mineralization. Vitamin K is necessary for the conversion of osteocalcin to its active form. It is also necessary for the function of a protein known as MGP which is present in bones, teeth and cartilage.

Kidney function

Vitamin K is necessary for the production of a urinary protein involved in kidney function which inhibits the formation of calcium oxalate kidney stones. This may account for the fact that vegetarians, whose diets are often high in vitamin K, have a low incidence of kidney stones.

Absorption and metabolism

Vitamin K requires the presence of fats and bile in the gut in order to be absorbed. It is absorbed from the upper small intestine and transported to the liver.

Deficiency

Vitamin K deficiency is rare and usually only occurs in people who have prolonged diarrhea, obstructive jaundice, liver disease or malabsorption problems such as celiac disease. It can also occur in the elderly and in newborn and premature babies. Signs of deficiency are prolonged clotting time, easy bleeding and bruising, frequent nosebleeds, blood-stained urine and bleeding from the gut.

Osteoporosis

Vitamin K deficiency may contribute to osteoporosis as low levels have been found in sufferers of the disease. In a Japanese study published in 1997, researchers investigated the relationship between bone mineral density, vitamin K levels and other biological parameters of bone metabolism in 71 post-menopausal women and 24 women with menopausal symptoms receiving hormone replacement therapy. The results showed that women with reduced bone mineral density had lower levels of vitamin K1 and K2 than those with normal bone mineral density.[1] Low levels have also been seen in osteoporotic men.[2]

Sources

Vitamin K is present in a wide variety of foods. Good sources of dietary vitamin K include dark leafy greens – spinach, broccoli, brussels sprouts – and olive, canola and soybean oils. Cabbage, carrots, avocados, cucumbers, leeks, tomatoes and dairy products such as yogurt are reasonable sources, and meats and cereals also contain some vitamin K. Freezing foods may destroy vitamin K but it remains stable when heated.

Food	Amount	Vitamin K (mcg)
Broccoli, cooked	½ cup, chopped	200
Spinach, raw	½ cup, chopped	106
Avocado	1 avocado	80.4
Turnip greens, raw	½ cup, chopped	66.8
Lettuce	½ cup, shredded	55.9
Cabbage, raw	½ cup, shredded	48.3
Pistachio nuts, dried	½ cup	42.6
Watercress, raw	½ chopped	40.4
Soybean oil	1 tbsp	26.2
Snap beans, raw	½ cup	24.6
Plums	½ cup, slices	18.8
Canola oil	1 tbsp	19.7
Kiwi fruit	1 medium	19.0

Green peas, cooked	½ cup	17.5
Miso, dry	½ cup	14.4
Carrots, cooked	½ cup, slices	13.3
Sweet peppers	½ cup, chopped	8.08
Potatoes with skin	1 medium	8.10
Tomatoes	1 medium	7.38
Celery, raw	½ cup	6.84
Peanut butter	2 tbsp	7.20
Olive oil	1 tbsp	6.62
Cauliflower, boiled	½ cup	5.89
Cucumbers, raw	1 medium	5.72

Recommended dietary allowances

The RDA for vitamin K is 1 mcg per kg of body weight. It is assumed that half the necessary daily intake comes from intestinal bacteria.

	Men	*Women*	*Pregnancy*	*Lactation*
USA	80 mcg	65 mcg	65 mcg	65 mcg

There are no established recommended nutrient intakes for vitamin K in the UK as it is assumed that manufacture by intestinal bacteria provides enough. In Australia there is no RDI but a daily intake of approximately 75 to 150 mcg is considered adequate for adults.

Supplements

Vitamin K is available in some multivitamin supplements. Alfalfa tablets are high in vitamin K.

Toxic effects of excess intake

Reports of toxic effects from natural vitamin K are rare. Large doses of the synthetic form of vitamin K, menadione may cause hemolytic anemia and liver damage and should not be used therapeutically. Side effects of intravenous vitamin K injection include flushing, sweats, chest pain and constricted breathing. Intramuscular injection may cause pain, swelling and eczema. Some research suggests a link between neonatal vitamin K injections and childhood cancer (See below).

Therapeutic uses of supplements

Prevention of hemorrhage

Vitamin K injections may be given to patients before or after surgery to prevent hemorrhage. The injections may be also be used to reduce the risk of excessive bleeding in those with liver disease, jaundice, malabsorption problems or who are taking aspirin or antibiotics.

Hemorrhagic disease of the newborn

Newborn babies are often given a vitamin K injection soon after birth. Vitamin K is not readily transferred from mother to baby, and as newborn babies do not have the intestinal bacteria necessary to produce vitamin K, they are at increased risk of hemorrhage. Premature babies run an especially high risk of brain hemorrhage during delivery because their blood vessels may be too fragile to withstand the surges in blood pressure that can occur. Vitamin K supplements are often given to women who have a high risk of delivering premature babies.

Mothers who are taking anti-epileptic drugs are also given supplements of vitamin K as their babies are at particular risk of vitamin K deficiency. Vitamin K supplements should only be taken on the recommendation of a doctor.

Childhood cancers

In the early 1990s, researchers reported a possible increase in the risk of childhood cancers in children who were given vitamin K injections after birth. These injections are commonly used to reduce the risk of internal bleeding. However, the results of studies are inconclusive. This link was examined in four studies published in the *British Medical Journal* in 1998. The results of two of the four studies suggest that there is no association between vitamin K injections and cancer, one could not exclude the possibility, and the fourth suggested a possible increase in the risk of leukemia.

In the first study, researchers assessed the risk in over 1000 Scottish children up to 14 years of age.[3] They looked at the links between several types of cancer, including leukemia, and did not find an association. In another study, researchers in Oxford, UK compared the incidence of cancer in groups of children from 94 maternity units with different vitamin K policies.[4] Their results showed that a raised risk was occasionally associated with vitamin K, but the overall results were not significant. The researchers are quoted as saying that "it is unlikely that there is a greatly increased risk of childhood cancer attributable to intramuscular vitamin K given to newborns, if indeed there is any." However, in another study the same researchers drew the conclusion that "the risk..... cannot be large, but the possibility that there is some risk cannot be excluded."[5]

The results of the fourth study by researchers in the north of England indicate that there may be some risk.[6] This study involved 685 children who developed cancer before age 15 and 3442 controls. The results showed a two-fold increase in risk of a type of cancer called acute lymphoblastic leukemia in 1 to 6 year olds who had been given vitamin K injections.

Some research suggests that oral supplements in three doses of 1 to 2 mg, the first given at the first feeding, the second at two to four weeks and the third at eight weeks may be an acceptable alternative to injections.[7]

In general, infants taking formula have a lower risk of hemorrhagic disease than those who are breastfed, as vitamin K levels are higher in formula. Maternal vitamin K supplements can reduce the risk of deficiency in breastfeeding newborn babies. In a study published in 1997, University of Wisconsin researchers showed that maternal vitamin K supplements of 5 mg per day increased the vitamin K content of breast milk to levels comparable with that in infant formula. Plasma vitamin K levels of babies increased compared to the placebo group.[8]

Osteoporosis

Vitamin K supplements may improve bone mineralization in postmenopausal women by boosting blood levels of osteocalcin and also possibly by decreasing calcium excretion through the urine. Research evidence suggests that vitamin K intakes much higher than the current recommendations improve biochemical markers of bone formation as well as bone density. Large supplemental doses of vitamin K have been used to treat osteoporosis.

Other uses

Vitamin K may be useful in the treatment of heavy menstrual bleeding. It has also been used with vitamin C to treat morning sickness.

Interactions with other nutrients

High intake of vitamin E (above 400 mg alpha TE (600 IU)) and vitamin A may antagonize vitamin K action and lead to an increased risk of hemorrhage.

Interactions with drugs

X rays and radiation, aspirin, cholestyramine, the anticonvulsant phenytoin and mineral oil laxatives can raise vitamin K requirements. Some snake venoms act by destroying vitamin K, thus causing uncontrolled bleeding. Vitamin K may be injected to stop the bleeding. Long-term use of antibiotics may produce vitamin K deficiency as these drugs can kill not only harmful bacteria but also the beneficial bacteria which produce vitamin K.

Cautions

Vitamin K supplements can interfere with the action of anticoagulant drugs such as warfarin.

Minerals

QUICK GUIDE

Essential for

- healthy bones and joints

Absorption and metabolism

Boron is efficiently absorbed and excreted in the urine.

Deficiency

Boron deficiency may lead to osteoporosis and arthritis.

Sources

Good sources include fruits and vegetables.

Daily recommended dietary intakes

A safe and adequate intake is estimated to be around 1 to 10 mg per day.

Toxic effects of excess intake

Toxic effects include vomiting, diarrhea, skin rash, coma and convulsions.

Interactions

Boron works with calcium, phosphorus, magnesium and vitamin D in bone metabolism, growth and development.

Therapeutic uses of supplements

Boron supplements have been used to treat osteoporosis and arthritis.

Cautions

The boric acid and borax forms of boron are toxic and should never be consumed.

Boron was shown to be an essential element for plants early this century and there is now evidence that it is also necessary for humans. Boron is distributed throughout the human body with the highest concentration in the bones and dental enamel.

What it does in the body

Boron seems to be essential for healthy bone and joint function, possibly via effects on the balance and absorption of calcium, magnesium and phosphorus.[1] It seems to affect cell membranes and the way signals are transmitted across these membranes.

Boron affects the metabolism of steroid hormones and may also play a role in converting vitamin D to its more active form, thus increasing calcium uptake and deposition into bone. Boron also increases male sex hormone levels.

Absorption and metabolism

Boron is efficiently absorbed and excreted in the urine.

Deficiency

Boron deficiency seems to affect calcium and magnesium metabolism, and affects the composition, structure and strength of bone, leading to changes similar to those seen in osteoporosis.[2] This is likely to be due to decreased absorption and increased excretion of calcium and magnesium. Boron deficiency combined with magnesium deficiency appears especially damaging in cases of osteoporosis.[3] Due to its effects on calcium and magnesium metabolism, boron deficiency may also contribute to the formation of kidney stones. Boron deficiency also seems to decrease mental alertness.[4]

There may also be a link between boron deficiency and osteoarthritis. Epidemiological studies indicate that in countries such as Mauritius and Jamaica, where boron intake is low, the incidence of osteoarthritis is around 50 to 70 per cent. In countries such as the USA, UK and Australia, where boron intake is relatively high, the incidence of osteoarthritis is around 20 per cent. Boron concentrations in bones next to osteoarthritic joints may be lower than in normal joints.[5]

Sources

Plant foods such as fruit, vegetables, soybeans and nuts are rich sources of boron but the level in food depends on the soil in which it is grown. The table below can be used as a guide. Wine, cider and beer also contain significant amounts of boron.[6]

Food	Amount	Boron (mg)
Avocado	100g	2.06
Red kidney beans	130g	1.82
Borlotti beans	130g	1.69
Prunes	50g	0.94
Chickpeas	130g	0.92
Peaches, dried	25g	0.81
Hazel nuts	25g	0.68
Raisins	15g	0.67
Apricots, dried	25g	0.53
Red grapes	100g	0.50
Pear	150g	0.48
Plum	100g	0.45
Almonds	15g	0.42
Dates	35g	0.38
Peanut butter	20g	0.38
Brazil nuts	20g	0.34
Orange	130g	0.33
Apple	100g	0.32
Kiwi	120g	0.31
Apple juice	125g	0.29
Currants	15g	0.26
Sultanas	15g	0.24

Recommended dietary allowances

There is no RDA for boron. A safe and adequate daily intake is estimated to be between 1 and 10 mg.

Supplements

Sodium borate is the most common form of supplement. Boron is increasingly used in calcium and bone-replenishing nutritional formulas. It may be particularly useful in those whose magnesium intake is low. This effect may be useful in the prevention of kidney stones. [7]

Because of its effect on testosterone levels, boron supplements have been marketed to athletes on the basis of their ability to increase muscle mass and strength. A 1994 study of the effects on ten male bodybuilders did not find any increases in those with boron supplements. [8]

Toxic effects of excess intake

Toxic effects appear at intakes of about 100 mg. The World Health Organization has banned boron (in the form of boric acid) as a food additive and preservative. Toxic effects include a red rash with weeping skin, vomiting, diarrhea characterized by a blue green color, depressed blood circulation, coma and convulsions. A fatal dose in adults is 15 to 20 g and in children 3 to 6 g. Repeated intakes of small amounts can cause accumulative toxicity.

Therapeutic uses of supplements

Boron may be beneficial in the treatment of osteoporosis. Supplements of around 3 mg per day have been shown to enhance the effects of estrogen in postmenopausal women. This is likely to contribute to its beneficial effects on bone health.[9]

Studies done in 1994 on athletic college women suggest that boron supplements decrease blood phosphorus concentration and increase magnesium concentration. Both of these changes are beneficial to bone-building.[10] Because of its sex hormone-enhancing effects, boron may help to protect against atherosclerosis.[11]

Osteoarthritis

Boron supplements of 6 to 9 mg per day have been used to treat osteoarthritis with some improvement of symptoms. Boron content in arthritic bones may be lower than that of normal bones and extra boron may increase bone hardness.[12]

Other uses

Boron, in the form of boric acid, has been used as a dusting powder or lotion to treat bacterial and fungal infections. It is also a component of some commercial mouthwashes. In borax solution form, boron has been used to treat mouth ulcers, eye infections and as a nasal douche.

Interactions with other nutrients

Boron works with calcium, magnesium, phosphorus and vitamin D in bone metabolism, growth and development. Animal studies show that a deficiency of vitamin D increases the need for boron.

Cautions

The boric acid and borax forms of boron are toxic and should never be consumed. Boron-containing powders should not be applied to body cavities and mucous membranes as the body absorbs too much and toxic effects can occur.

QUICK GUIDE

Essential for

- healthy bones and teeth
- muscle contraction
- a healthy heart and nervous system
- blood pressure regulation and clotting

Absorption and metabolism

Vitamin D is necessary for absorption, which decreases with age.

Deficiency

Deficiency leads to nerve and bone disorders, osteoporosis, high blood pressure, pre-eclampsia of pregnancy and may contribute to colon cancer.

Sources

These include milk and leafy green vegetables.

Daily recommended dietary intakes

Men	1000 mg
(14-18)	1300 mg
(over 50)	1200 mg
Women	1000 mg
(14-18)	1300 mg
(over 50)	1200 mg
Pregnancy	1000 mg
(14-18)	1300 mg
Lactation	1000 mg
(14-18)	1300 mg

Toxic effects of excess intake

Toxic effects include nausea; vomiting; and kidney, heart and muscle damage.

Interactions

Calcium works with magnesium and phosphorus in many body functions.

Therapeutic uses of supplements

These include osteoporosis, high blood pressure, tooth problems, muscle cramps, pre-eclampsia and heart disease.

Cautions

Calcium supplements should be avoided by people who have impaired kidney function, a history of kidney or bladder stones, constipation or dehydration.

Calcium is the most abundant mineral in the body. An average man contains about one and a half kilograms of calcium and an average woman about one kilogram. Over 99 per cent of the calcium in your body is in bones and teeth. The remaining one per cent is found in the blood, lymph and other body fluids, cell membranes and structures inside cells.

What it does in the body

Bones and teeth

The main function of calcium is in the structural development and maintenance of healthy bones and teeth. Bone is made up of both mineral (mostly hydroxyapatite-like crystals) and nonmineral (mostly protein) components. Calcium in the bone is in two forms, one bound tightly and the other more easily removed. Calcium is removed from the tightly bound part of the bone to maintain blood levels only when dietary intake is inadequate and the more mobile stores are exhausted. Bone undergoes a constant remodeling process with 20 per cent of an adult's bone calcium re-absorbed and replaced every year.

Muscle contraction

Calcium plays a vital role in muscle contraction. It is also necessary for heartbeat regulation through its effects on heart muscle.

Nervous system

Calcium is essential for nerve impulse conduction. It plays a role in the release of neurotransmitters and activates some enzymes which generate neurotransmitters.

Cardiovascular system and blood

Calcium interacts with sodium, potassium and magnesium to regulate blood pressure and water balance. A major class of drugs used to lower high blood pressure blocks the channels which transport calcium across muscle cell membranes. Calcium also plays a role in the activation of prothrombin (which is formed from vitamin K in the liver) which is essential to the blood clotting process.

Other functions

Calcium is essential for cell division, healthy immune function, for enzyme activity and for the production and activity of hormones involved in digestion, energy and fat metabolism, and the production of saliva. It is also involved in the transport of nutrients and other substances across cell membranes.

Absorption and metabolism

On average, adults absorb around 25 to 50 per cent of dietary calcium. Some is absorbed passively while some is transported via a vitamin D-mediated process. Most absorption occurs in the small intestine. The calcium then passes into the exchangeable calcium pool that is in the body fluids. This pool turns over 20 to 30 times a day whereas the calcium in bone turns over every five to six years.

Blood levels of calcium are tightly regulated by the hormones calcitonin, parathyroid hormone and vitamin D. These hormones act together to regulate calcium levels as dietary intake and requirements vary. They control absorption from the gut, excretion in the kidney and the rate of bone formation and breakdown. In the absence of vitamin D, less than 10 per cent of dietary calcium may be absorbed. When intake is inadequate, calcium is removed from storage sites in bone and used to keep blood levels constant. Other hormones which affect calcium levels include estrogens, glucocorticoids, thyroid hormone, insulin and growth hormones.

Absorption is enhanced when calcium intake is low[1] and also by moderate exercise. Lactose, vitamin D and adequate (but not excessive) protein improve calcium absorption. High levels of fat reduce absorption. Compounds known as phytates, which are found in dietary fiber; and oxalates, which are found in leafy greens, reduce absorption. The acid environment of the stomach makes calcium salts more soluble, and therefore easier to absorb; and low stomach acid reduces absorption.

Absorption and retention of calcium become less efficient with age,[2] partly due to lower estrogen and testosterone levels; and a postmenopausal woman may only absorb 7 per cent of her dietary intake. The ability to absorb and retain calcium improves during pregnancy although it seems that some calcium is drawn from bone stores later in pregnancy. A study done in 1996 in Cincinnati showed that breastfeeding stimulates increases in calcium absorption and these increases become apparent after weaning or after menstrual periods restart.[3]

Smoking, high refined sugar intake, caffeine, alcohol and excess salt promote calcium excretion, thereby increasing the risk of deficiency. High protein diets also increase calcium excretion, particularly if the protein comes from meat.[4]

Deficiency

Mild calcium deficiency can cause nerve sensitivity, muscle twitching, brittle nails, irritability, palpitations and insomnia. Signs of severe deficiency include abnormal heartbeat, muscle pains and cramps, numbness, stiffness and tingling of the hands and feet, and depression. Children can suffer from rickets, a disease characterized by excessive sweating of the head; slowness in sitting, crawling and walking; insomnia; bone deformities; and growth retardation. In adults, deficiency can lead to osteomalacia with symptoms of bone pain, muscle weakness and delayed healing of fractures.

Those at risk of calcium deficiency include the elderly, people who don't eat dairy products or other high calcium foods, athletes, those on high protein or high fiber diets, and those who drink a lot of alcohol. High dietary levels of phosphorus cause calcium to be removed from bone and excreted. Phosphorus is found in many common foods such as meat, cheese, processed foods and soda drinks, and people who consume large amount of these foods are at increased risk of calcium deficiency. People on weight-reducing diets are also at risk as they may avoid high calorie foods, which are often good sources of calcium.

Studies have shown that calcium is deficient in the diets of many women. The National Osteoporosis Foundation estimates that the average adult in the US gets only 500 to 700 mg per day. Calcium deficiency is relatively common in many countries.

Osteoporosis

Calcium deficiency contributes to osteoporosis, which literally means "porous bones" and in some cases, can be so severe as to cause the bones to break under the weight of the body. Particularly badly affected bones include the spinal vertebrae, the thigh bone and the radius (shorter arm bone). The symptoms of osteoporosis may be absent until fractures occur, although in some cases there may be back pain.

Osteoporosis is most common in elderly white women with a history of borderline calcium intake. Around 35 per cent of women suffer from osteoporosis after menopause and, although it is less common, the problem occurs in a similar way in men. Most of the bone loss seen in osteoporosis occurs in the first five to six years after menopause due to a decline in circulating estrogens and an age-related reduction in vitamin D production.

Good nutrition plays a role in reducing the incidence of osteoporosis by promoting the development of favorable peak bone mass during the first 30 to 40 years of life. Getting enough calcium in early adolescence and early adulthood is vital for bones to reach their maximum density so that they are strong enough to support the body even when they lose density later in life. Studies suggest that calcium intake in adolescence is often below the recommended levels. Researchers involved in a 1994 USDA study measured calcium intake in 51 girls aged 5 to16 years old. They found calcium intake to be below the recommended dietary allowance for 21 out of 25 girls aged 11 or over. These studies suggest that the current calcium intake of American girls during the puberty is not enough to enable bones to develop maximum strength and that increased intakes may be necessary.[5]

However, it is never too late to slow the bone-loss seen in osteoporosis, and early postmenopausal years are also an important time to ensure optimal intake. A 1997 study done at King's College Hospital in London suggests that high calcium intakes are linked to bone mineral density in elderly women. Researchers assessed calcium intake in 124 women aged from 52 to 62 and also measured bone mineral density at the spine, hip and foot (os calcis). Results showed that women with high calcium intakes had higher bone mineral density.[6]

Results from the Rotterdam Study, which involves 1 856 men and 2 452 women aged 55 years and over also show that high calcium intakes also protect against bone loss in men.[7]

Calcium deficiency is only one factor in osteoporosis. There is likely to be a genetic component and other dietary, behavioral and hormonal factors also play a major part. Adequate intakes of vitamin D, magnesium and boron are also necessary to build healthy bones. Body weight is the factor most linked to bone mineral density and, in women, body fat may be at least as important as muscle in maintaining bone mineral content. Weight-bearing exercise, adequate lifelong calcium intake, and moderate alcohol intake all play important roles in preventing osteoporosis. Estrogen replacement therapy is often used to treat osteoporosis.

Bone loss is found to be up to 11 per cent greater during the night. Calcium levels are also lowest during the night and may be affected by the concentration of the hormone, cortisol. These findings may lead to new hormone treatments for osteoporosis.

Cancer

Calcium deficiency may be linked to an increased risk of colon cancer. Research on animals and some epidemiological studies suggest that people with high calcium intakes are less likely to develop colon cancer. Research findings in humans are inconclusive, with some studies showing protective effects while others have not. The overall results seem to suggest that the protective effect of high calcium intake does exist but that it is not very marked.

The association between calcium intake and deaths from gastrointestinal cancer was assessed in a 28-year follow-up study of 2 591 Dutch civil servants and their spouses, aged 40 to 65 years. The researchers found that men and women who died of colorectal cancer had a lower average calcium intake compared to the rest of the population.[8]

Results from the Iowa Women's Health Study published in 1998 showed that calcium can decrease the risk of rectal cancer. Researchers analyzed information from 34 702 postmenopausal women who responded to a mailed survey in 1986. After nine years of follow-up, 144 rectal cancer cases were identified. The results showed that high total calcium intake reduced the risk of rectal cancer.[9] Other results from this study show a reduced risk of colon cancer in women with high intakes of calcium and vitamin D.

In a 1996 study, Harvard University researchers working on the Health Professionals Study assessed the links between calcium intake and colon cancer in almost 48 000 men aged from 40 to 75. They found that higher intake of calcium from foods and supplements was associated with a lower cancer risk until they adjusted their results to take other factors into account. They concluded that calcium may possibly mildly lower the risk of colon cancer.[10] Data from the Nurses Health Study, which involved over 89 000 nurses, also showed a small reduced risk.[11]

Calcium may exert its protective effects by binding to toxic substances such as bile acids and fats and reduce the chance that these will cause cancerous changes in the gut. Calcium may also normalize the growth of cells in the intestinal wall, thus protecting against cancerous changes. Limited evidence suggests that low calcium intake may also increase the risk of breast, cervical and esophageal cancers.

Taiwanese studies done in 1997 and 1998 showed a protective effect both against gastric and colorectal cancers from high levels of calcium in drinking water.[12,13]

Blood pressure

Calcium metabolism seems to be altered in people with hypertension. Several studies suggest that low dietary intake of calcium is associated with an increased risk of developing hypertension and cardiovascular disease. Some research suggests studies show that restriction of calcium increases, and supplementation with calcium lowers, blood pressure. Data from the US Health and Nutrition Examination Survey (NHANES I) showed that hypertensive people consumed 18 per cent less dietary calcium than those with normal blood pressure.[14]

A review published in 1997 in the *American Journal of Clinical Nutrition* showed that experimental data support the view that when adults meet or exceed the recommended dietary allowances of calcium, potassium, and magnesium, high sodium intakes are not associated with high blood pressure. Thus adequate mineral intake may protect against salt sensitivity. (See page 232 for more information.)[15]

Some evidence suggests that a woman who eats a low calcium diet in pregnancy may also increase the chances of her child suffering from high blood pressure.

Muscle cramps

When blood calcium levels drop below normal, the sensitivity of the nerves can increase, leading to muscle cramps. Pregnant women whose diets are deficient in calcium are at greatest risk of muscle cramps.

Teeth

Severe calcium deficiency can lead to periodontal disease (inflammation and degeneration of the bone and gum structures that support the teeth).

Sources

Good sources of calcium include milk and other dairy products, kale, kelp, tofu, canned fish with bones, peanuts, walnuts, sunflower seeds, broccoli, cauliflower and soybeans. Fortified foods such as fruit juices, breads and cereals are also common sources. Calcium in hard water and some mineral waters may be important dietary sources for some people. [16]

Calcium from milk and milk products is absorbed more easily than that from most vegetables, with the exception of dark green leafy vegetables such as kale, broccoli, turnip and mustard greens. A 1990 study showed that more calcium is absorbed from kale than from milk.[17]

Green leafy vegetables such as spinach contain large amounts of calcium but also contain oxalic acid which binds calcium and prevents it from being absorbed. Insoluble fiber, such as that found in wheat bran, reduces calcium absorption; but soluble fiber, such as that found in psyllium and fruit pectins, does not seem to affect absorption.[18]

While dairy products are good sources of calcium, there is concern that their protein content can increase the loss of calcium from bone. Results from the ongoing Nurses Health Study suggest that drinking lots of milk and other dairy foods high in calcium does not protect older women against bone fractures. Researchers analyzed the diets of over 77 000 participants in the study and looked at the rates of bone fractures. Results showed that women who drank two or more glasses of milk per day had around a 45 per cent increased risk of hip fracture and a 5 per cent increased risk of forearm fracture compared to women who drank one glass or less per week. There was also no drop in risk with intake of calcium from other dairy foods.[19]

In another study done in 1995 at the University of California at Berkeley, researchers assessed the effect of calcium supplementation and drinking milk on pre-eclampsia in over 9000 pregnant women. Results showed that women who drank two glasses of milk per day had the lowest risk. The risk for those drinking one glass of milk per day was similarly low but the risk for those drinking less than one glass of milk per day was substantially higher. Women drinking three or more glasses of milk per day also showed increased risk as did those drinking four or more glasses per day.[20]

A varied diet which includes nondairy sources of calcium is likely to be more beneficial in protecting against osteoporosis and other disorders of calcium deficiency.

Food	Amount	Calcium (mg)
Milk, evaporated	1 cup	658
Salmon, canned	½ can	484
Sardines, canned, tomato sauce	5 sardines	455
Milk, dry, nonfat	¼ cup	377
Fruit yogurt	1 tub	338
Milk, nonfat	1 cup	297
Milk, whole	1 cup	291
Cheddar cheese	1 slice	204

Tofu	½ cup	204
Crab meat, canned	1 cup, drained	136
Figs, dried	5 figs	135
Peanuts	1/2 cup	134
Baked beans, canned	1 cup	127
Brazil nuts	½ cup	123
Kale, cooked	1 cup	94
Walnuts	1 cup, shelled	94
Almonds, blanched	¼ cup	89
Milk chocolate	1 bar	84
Tahini paste	1 tbsp	64
Soybeans	1 cup	55
Broccoli, cooked	½ cup	36
Kelp, raw	2 tbsp	17
Honeydew melon	1 cup, diced	10
Cauliflower	½ cup	10

Recommended dietary allowances

Calcium requirements vary throughout a person's lifetime, with greater needs during periods of rapid growth and later in life. Due to mounting evidence that people are not getting enough calcium to prevent osteoporosis and other bone diseases, in 1997 the US government raised the recommendations for how much calcium people should consume every day.

Recommended intakes for pregnant and breastfeeding women are no longer greater than those for other women. This is partly based on recent studies which suggest that changes in calcium metabolism and absorption during pregnancy and breastfeeding are enough to meet the extra demands placed on a woman's body by her baby. A 1998 British study suggests that bone mineral density changes seen during breastfeeding seems to be unrelated to dietary calcium intake.[21]

Two randomized, placebo-controlled trials of calcium supplementation were done on new mothers in 1997 in Cincinnati, Ohio. Researchers tested the effect of 1000 mg of calcium per day on bone density, measured at enrolment and after three and six months. The results showed no effect of either lactation or calcium supplementation on bone density in the forearm, and also no effect of calcium supplementation on the calcium concentration in breast milk.[22]

In another study published in 1998, researchers studied calcium metabolism in 14 pregnant women from before conception to five months after their periods restarted. When the women were pregnant the increased needs were met by improved absorption, and then during the early breastfeeding period calcium excretion decreased. Some calcium was drawn from bone but this was recovered after menstruation restarted, although not to pre-pregnancy levels.[23]

The women involved in this study were all consuming adequate levels of calcium and it is possible that women whose calcium intake is lower than 1300 mg per day may benefit from extra calcium or supplements.

	Men	*Women*	*Pregnancy*	*Lactation*
USA	1000 mg	1000 mg	1000 mg	1000 mg
(14-18)	1300 mg	1300 mg	1300 mg	1300 mg
(over 50)	1200 mg	1200 mg		
UK	700 mg	700 mg		
Australia	800 mg	800 mg	1100 mg	1300 mg
(postmenopause)		1000 mg		

The tolerable upper intake level for children over the age of one and adults has been set at 2500 mg per day.

Supplements

Several dietary studies suggest that in many population groups, calcium intake is inadequate, particularly in women. As few as 10 per cent of elderly people are getting enough calcium to prevent bone loss and are likely to benefit from supplements. Pregnant and breastfeeding women, adolescent girls, postmenopausal women and vegans may also benefit.

What type to take

Calcium supplements are among those most often prescribed by doctors as calcium deficiency is relatively common. They contain different amounts of calcium and are available in various forms including calcium carbonate (which contains 40 per cent calcium), calcium aspartate, calcium citrate (21 per cent calcium), calcium gluconate (9 per cent calcium) and calcium lactate (13 per cent calcium). While multivitamins do contain some calcium, the amount is not usually sufficient to meet daily requirements and separate calcium supplements are more useful.

Bonemeal, dolomite and oyster shells are common sources of calcium, but they should be avoided as they may be contaminated with lead and cadmium, which can be toxic. Antacids are also good sources of calcium, but those containing aluminum or sodium should be avoided as aluminum inhibits calcium absorption and sodium can raise blood pressure. Calcium citrate, which is an acidified form of calcium supplement, is absorbed better than calcium carbonate.[24] This is particularly important in older people who have low stomach acid. Calcium lactate and calcium aspartate are also well-absorbed. Calcium carbonate may cause side effects such as nausea, gas and constipation; but taking it in divided doses with meals may reduce these side effects and improve absorption.[25]

When to take calcium supplements

Absorption of calcium from supplements is considerably reduced in people who have low stomach acid unless the supplements are taken with food. In general, it seems that calcium supplements are better absorbed if they are taken with a meal, although this depends on the type of food eaten at the meal, for example, less calcium will be absorbed if supplements are taken with foods high in calcium, insoluble fiber and oxalates. A 1989 study showed that a light meal improved calcium absorption from milk, calcium carbonate and calcium-citrate-malate sources.[26] However, calcium may decrease the absorption of other minerals such as zinc. Some calcium supplements can interfere with iron absorption, although this does not seem to be the case with calcium citrate and calcium ascorbate as they are acidic.

Some experts advise taking two-thirds of the daily calcium dose at bedtime and the rest in the morning. Others recommend dividing the dose into four parts; i.e. with meals and at bedtime.[27] As bone loses calcium at night, some experts recommend taking supplements then to maintain blood calcium levels.

Calcium and magnesium

If you take a calcium supplement, you should also take a magnesium supplement. This helps to avoid constipation and to balance the effect of calcium on the electrical impulses in the nerves and muscles. Calcium and magnesium work together as mild neuromuscular relaxants. Some experts recommend taking calcium and magnesium in a 2:1 ratio while others suggest 1:1.

Toxic effects of excess intake

Toxic effects are rare as the body can excrete excess calcium with doses up to 2500 mg per day considered safe. Some people may suffer constipation at these doses. Daily intakes above 2500 mg may cause kidney stones and other problems. At very large doses, such as 25 000 mg, vomiting, nausea and loss of appetite can occur. If taken with high levels of vitamin D for long periods, deposition of calcium in the kidneys, heart and other soft tissues can occur. High levels may also impair vitamin K metabolism, reduce iron and zinc absorption, and affect the activity of neurons in the brain which control mood and emotion.

Calcium forms part of the plaque laid down in the arteries in atherosclerosis, although this problem is likely to be due to abnormalities in calcium metabolism rather than excess dietary calcium.

Results from the Health Professionals Follow-Up study which involved 47 781 men suggest that high calcium intakes from both food and supplements increase the risk of prostate cancer.[28]

Therapeutic uses of supplements

Osteoporosis

Research suggests that taking calcium supplements later in life can slow the bone loss associated with osteoporosis. Treatment which combines calcium and estrogen is likely to be better at building bone than treatment with estrogen alone, according to a review published in 1998 in the *American Journal of Clinical Nutrition*.

Researchers analyzed the results of 31 studies and found that the postmenopausal women who took estrogen alone had an average increase in spinal bone mass of 1.3 per cent per year, while those who took estrogen and calcium supplements had an average increase of 3.3 per cent. Increases in bone mass in the forearm and upper thigh were also greater in women taking supplements. The added benefit from the calcium was seen when the women increased their intake from an average of 563 mg per day to 1200 mg per day.[29]

Another study done in 1997 at Tufts University in Boston showed reduced rates of bone loss and fractures in men and women over 65 who took calcium and vitamin D supplements. Researchers assessed the effects of calcium (500 mg per day) and vitamin D (700 IU per day) on 176 men and 213 women aged 65 years or older. After a three-year period, those taking the supplements had higher bone density at all body sites measured. The fracture rate was also reduced by 50 per cent in those taking the supplements.[30]

Calcium supplements have also been shown to increase bone mass in children, although a 1996 study done in Hong Kong found that when the supplements were stopped, the beneficial effects disappeared.[31]

Protection against the side effects of corticosteroid drugs

One of the side effects of corticosteroid drugs, which are often used to treat arthritis, asthma and other chronic diseases, is a loss of bone mineral density and therefore an increased risk of osteoporosis.

In a study done in 1996 at the Medical College of Virginia, researchers showed that calcium and vitamin D supplements can help prevent this loss. In the two-year study, 96 patients with rheumatoid arthritis, 65 of whom were taking corticosteroid drugs, were given 1000 mg calcium and 500 IU vitamin D per day or placebo. The researchers analyzed the bone mineral density of the lumbar spine and femur for one year. In those patients taking corticosteroid drugs and placebo losses of bone mineral density were seen. In those taking the supplements, gains were seen and in those not taking corticosteroids, the supplements did not appear to affect bone mineral density.[32]

Blood pressure

Some studies have shown that calcium supplements lower blood pressure in mildly hypertensive patients, while others have shown no effect.

In an eight-week randomized, placebo-controlled study done in 1985 in the US, researchers assessed the effect of 1000 mg per day of calcium supplements on the blood pressure of 48 people with hypertension and 32 without. Compared with placebo, calcium significantly lowered both systolic and diastolic blood pressures, but only in those with high blood pressure.[33]

Results from the University of Pittsburgh Trials of Hypertension Prevention (TOHP) showed calcium supplements (100 mg per day) to have little effect on blood pressure. The participants were healthy adult men and women (both white and African American) aged 30 to 54 years with high-normal diastolic blood pressure. However, the supplements did seem to lower blood pressure in white women, who are at particular risk of low calcium intakes.[34] Supplements may be beneficial in cases where calcium intake is insufficient, which may be relatively common. Whether calcium can lower blood pressure in cases where there is no apparent deficiency is not clear. Increasing calcium intake may lower blood pressure by increasing the excretion of sodium and calcium supplements may be most useful in those who are salt sensitive. (See page 232 for more information.)

The results of a study, reported in 1997 in the *British Medical Journal*, suggest that women who take calcium supplements in pregnancy have children with lower blood pressures. Researchers measured the blood pressures of almost 600 children of women who had previously been involved in a double-blind trial of the effects of calcium on blood pressure during pregnancy. The results showed that, overall, systolic blood pressure was lower in the calcium group, particularly among overweight children.[35]

Muscle cramps

Calcium can be used to control the incidence of leg cramps in pregnant women, possibly by decreasing nerve irritability. It has also been used to reduce the incidence of menstrual cramps and symptoms associated with premenstrual syndrome.

Pre-eclampsia

Use of calcium supplements during pregnancy may lower a woman's risk of pre-eclampsia, a disorder which occurs in one in every 20 pregnant women. Symptoms of pre-eclampsia are high blood pressure, headache, protein in the urine, blurred vision and anxiety. It can lead to eclampsia, a seizure disorder which can cause complications with pregnancy and even death. There is some evidence that abnormalities in calcium metabolism are involved in pre-eclampsia. Many pregnant women do not consume enough calcium to ensure optimal blood pressure regulation and the results of several clinical trials have suggested that calcium supplements reduce the incidence of pre-eclampsia.[36]

A 1996 analysis of clinical trials which looked at the effects of calcium intake on pre-eclampsia and pregnancy outcomes in 2500 women found that those who consumed 1500 to 2000 mg of calcium supplements per day were 70 per cent less likely to suffer from high blood pressure in pregnancy.[37]

However, in a study published in 1997 in the *New England Journal of Medicine*, researchers found that calcium supplements did not prevent pre-eclampsia. The study, the largest ever done on the subject, involved 4589 healthy, first-time mothers. Half of the subjects received 2000 mg of calcium per day and the other half received a placebo. The researchers then assessed the incidence of high blood pressure and protein excretion in the urine. No significant differences in the groups were found. Supplements did not reduce other complications associated with childbirth or increase the incidence of kidney stones.[38]

The results of this study still leave open the possibility that calcium supplements may be useful as the women included in the study were already consuming higher than average levels of calcium than is typical even before they took the supplements. Women at high risk of pre-eclampsia were also not included in the investigation.

Other uses

Calcium supplements can be useful in congestive heart failure as they increase the contractility of heart muscle. Calcium salts are used intravenously to treat heart attack associated with high potassium and magnesium levels and low calcium levels. They are also used in cases of calcium antagonist drug overdose.

Calcium supplements have also been used to treat allergy complaints, depression, panic attacks, arthritis, hypoglycemia, muscle and joint pains. Calcium salts are a major component of antacids which are used to treat indigestion and ulcers. Taken with magnesium, they may have neuromuscular relaxing effects and may be useful in insomnia.

Interactions with other nutrients

Calcium and phosphorus work together to form healthy bones and teeth. High phosphorus intakes lead to increased calcium excretion. The intake ratio for calcium to phosphorus should be 1:1.

Calcium competes with zinc, manganese, copper and iron for absorption in the intestine, and a high intake of one mineral can reduce absorption of the others. This is of particular concern in the case of iron. Calcium reduces both heme and nonheme iron absorption.[39] (See page 251 for more information.) The practical implications of the inhibitory effect of calcium mean that addition of milk or cheese to common meals such as pizza or hamburgers can reduce iron absorption by 50-60%. Some experts recommend eating foods that provide most of the daily iron intake at a different time to foods which provide most of the daily calcium intake. Thus it is advisable to reduce the intake of dairy products with the main meals providing most of the dietary iron, especially for children, teenagers and women of childbearing age whose iron requirements are high.[40]

This interaction is also a concern in relation to supplements as calcium and iron are both commonly recommended for women. A study done in 1990 on postmenopausal women showed that calcium supplements decrease iron absorption from supplements and from food sources. Orange juice helped to avoid this reduction in absorption probably because it contains citric and ascorbic acids, both of which are known to enhance iron absorption.[41] However, calcium citrate does not appear to reduce iron absorption.[42]

Lead absorption is blocked by calcium in the intestines. Boron supplementation may reduce the excretion of calcium. Aluminum-containing antacids can inhibit calcium absorption. It is unclear whether magnesium inhibits calcium absorption. A 1994 study found no effect of magnesium supplements on calcium absorption.[43] Calcium supplements have been shown to decrease zinc absorption.[44] High calcium diets are being increasingly recommended to prevent osteoporosis and a 1997 study done in the US showed that high calcium diets decreased zinc absorption by 50 per cent and may raise requirements.[45]

Boron seems to be beneficial to calcium metabolism. Calcium interacts with several vitamins, in particular, vitamin D and vitamin K.

Interactions with drugs

Some diuretics, corticosteroids and antidepressants can lead to calcium deficiency. Calcium supplements may decrease the effectiveness of tetracycline antibiotics; the anticonvulsant, phenytoin; and aspirin; and should not be taken at the same time as any of these drugs.

Cautions

Calcium supplements should not be used in people who have impaired kidney function, cardiac arrhythmias, a history of kidney or bladder stones, constipation or dehydration. The calcium citrate form of supplement is less likely to cause kidney stones than calcium carbonate.

Chromium

QUICK GUIDE

Essential for

- normal sugar and fat metabolism because it is part of a compound known as glucose tolerance factor (GTF)

Absorption and metabolism

Absorption of chromium from food is poor.

Deficiency

Symptoms include high blood fat and cholesterol levels, glucose intolerance and other diabetes-like symptoms. Marginal deficiency may play a role in the development of diabetes and heart disease.

Sources

Good sources include liver, eggs, poultry and whole grain cereals. The chromium content of food varies with the location in which the food is grown. The table on the page 207 can be used as a guide.

Daily recommended dietary intakes

Estimated safe requirements are between 50 and 200 mcg per day.

Toxic effects of excess intake

Little is known about the toxic effects of large doses of the form of chromium found in food and supplements.

Interactions

Antacids may decrease chromium absorption.

Therapeutic uses of supplements

Chromium supplements are available in various forms, including brewer's yeast which may contain the most biologically active and absorbable form. Supplements have been used to treat high cholesterol, diabetes, hypoglycemia, heart disease and acne. Supplements are also used as part of weight loss programs.

Cautions

Chromium supplements may decrease insulin requirements in diabetics.

Chromium is an essential trace mineral. It occurs naturally in three different forms with one particular form (chromium III) making up the majority of dietary chromium. The average adult body contains between 0.4 and 6 mg of chromium and older people usually have lower levels. There is a wide geographical variation in chromium levels and population studies suggest that the incidence of diabetes and heart disease is lower in areas where chromium intakes are relatively high.

What it does in the body

Metabolism

Chromium is essential for normal sugar metabolism. It is a component of a compound called glucose tolerance factor (GTF) which works with insulin to move glucose into cells where it can be used to generate energy. Optimal chromium intake appears to decrease the amount of insulin needed to maintain normal blood sugar.

Insulin also plays a role in fat and protein metabolism, thus chromium is necessary for these processes to occur normally. Adequate chromium intake is essential to maintain healthy cholesterol levels.

Absorption and metabolism

Absorption of chromium from food is poor with only 2 to 10 per cent of dietary intake being absorbed. Organic chromium is absorbed more efficiently than inorganic chromium. Absorbed chromium binds to proteins, including transferrin, which transport it in the bloodstream. Chromium absorption is enhanced by the presence of oxalates and it is also higher in cases of iron deficiency. Absorption may decline with age.

Most absorbed chromium is eliminated through the kidneys. Chromium may be stored in the skin, fat, brain, muscles, spleen, kidneys and testes.

Deficiency

Symptoms of chromium deficiency include high blood fat and cholesterol levels and diabetes-like symptoms of glucose intolerance, weakness, depression, confusion, weight loss, thirst, hunger and frequent urination.

Diets high in refined and processed foods, such as flour and sugar, excessive losses from the body in some diseases, alcoholism, prolonged slimming regimes and pregnancy may lead to chromium deficiency. Infection and physical trauma appear to increase chromium requirements and strenuous exercise appears to increase chromium excretion, increasing the risk of deficiency when intake is marginal.

Tissue levels of chromium tend to decrease with age. British researchers involved in a study published in 1997 analyzed chromium levels in hair, sweat, and serum samples obtained from over 40 000 patients.[1] The results showed highly significant age-related decreases which may play a part in the increased risk of diabetes and atherosclerosis in older people. Marginal chromium deficiency may be relatively common, with as many as 50 per cent of people in the USA consuming less than the recommended 50 mcg per day. Preventing chromium deficiency is very important as this is easier than treating the complications which arise as a result.

Diabetes

Chromium deficiency is relatively common in patients with Type II diabetes and may impair the function of GTF, causing the uptake of glucose into cells to become less efficient. Impaired chromium metabolism may also play a role in diabetes of pregnancy.[2] High insulin levels also seem to increase chromium excretion. Chromium deficiency may also lead to hypoglycemia or low blood sugar.

Heart disease

Chromium deficiency may also play a role in heart disease. Poor dietary intake may be linked to higher blood cholesterol levels and therefore increased risk of atherosclerosis. Patients with advanced heart disease often have low chromium levels in their blood. On a population level, decreased chromium levels correlate with increased heart disease.

Sources

Good sources of chromium include liver, egg yolk, brewer's yeast, certain spices such as black pepper and thyme, beef, poultry, broccoli, whole grain cereals, bran, wheatgerm and oysters. The chromium content of food varies with the location in which the food is grown. The table below can be used as a guide.

Food refining and processing remove most of the chromium from food. Hence a diet high in these foods will not contribute much chromium but will require it for metabolism, thus leading to depletion of the body's chromium stores.

Cooking food in stainless steel pots causes chromium to leach into the food if it is acidic and can be an additional source of dietary chromium. Hard tap water can also be a source.

Food	Amount	Chromium (mcg)
Skim milk powder	100g	34
Brown sugar	100g	27
All Bran	100g	26
Ham	100g	26
Cheddar cheese	100g	24
Corned beef	100g	20
Wheatbran	100g	19
Cod, smoked	100g	18
Split peas, dried	100g	13
Soybean flour	100g	17
Pork sausage	100g	16
Beef sausage	100g	15
Mackerel, canned	100g	14
Oysters, canned	100g	14
Wheatgerm	100g	13
Spinach	100g	13
Brown lentils, dried	100g	13
Lamb chops	100g	13
Beefsteak, mince	100g	9.0
Yeast extract	10g	8.7
Yellow butter beans	100g	8.0
Sweetcorn	100g	7.0
Chicken, dark meat	100g	7.0
Potato	100g	5.0

Recommended dietary allowances

There is no RDA for chromium. Estimated safe requirements are between 50 and 200 mcg per day. It is difficult to test chromium levels accurately as there are no reliable established tests and it is possible that chromium accumulates in the tissues while being quickly cleared from blood serum.

Supplements

Chromium supplements are available in various forms including chromium picolinate, chromium chloride, chromium polynicotinate and chromium-enriched yeast. Biologically active forms of chromium such as chromium picolinate and yeast GTF are better absorbed than chromium chloride. GTF is found in brewer's yeast and is considered the most biologically active and absorbable form of chromium. The supplement doses effective in studies are in the region of 200 to 400 mcg per day. Chromium may be more effective if given with niacin, as the nicotinic acid form of niacin is part of GTF.

Toxic effects of excess intake

Little is known about the toxic effects of large doses of the form of chromium found in food and supplements. There have been reports of adverse effects, including irregular heartbeat, with people taking above the recommended 250 mcg dose.

A 1995 study found that chromium supplements caused severe damage to chromosomes of cells grown in the laboratory.[3] However, no studies have yet been done to confirm these potential carcinogenic effects. As toxic effects were not seen with other forms of chromium; including chromium nicotinate, nicotinic acid, and chromium chloride hexahydrate; the researchers concluded that the toxic effects were due to the picolinate part of the molecule.

Therapeutic uses of supplements

Diabetes

Chromium supplements have been successfully used to treat Type I and Type II diabetes, diabetes in pregnancy, and hypoglycemia. Chromium supplementation has been shown to lower fasting glucose levels, improve glucose tolerance and lower insulin levels in Type II diabetics. This helps to keep blood levels stable, thereby preventing damage to blood vessels and organs caused by high levels of blood sugar. The greatest benefits are seen in those who have severe deficiencies. Chromium acts to increase insulin sensitivity by improving insulin binding, insulin receptor number, insulin internalization, beta cell sensitivity and insulin receptor enzymes.[4]

According to the results of a Chinese study published in 1997, daily chromium supplements may help control blood sugar levels and insulin activity in Type II diabetics. The study, conducted by researchers at the US Department of Agriculture and Beijing Medical University, involved 180 Type II diabetics. Chinese people were chosen because of the likelihood that they had not previously used supplements. The participants were divided into three groups: one group was given 1000 mcg of chromium picolinate, the second was given 200 mcg and the third group was given a placebo. After two months, the researchers assessed blood sugar and cholesterol levels. In the 1000 mcg group, levels were significantly reduced. In the 200 mcg group, it took four months to see a reduction in blood sugar levels and this was not as significant as that seen in the first group.[5]

Chromium supplements have been shown to reduce blood fat levels in Type II diabetics. In a study done in 1994 in San Antonio, Texas researchers found that chromium picolinate supplements taken for a period of two months significantly reduced triglyceride levels in 14 men and 16 women.[6]

Hypoglycemia

Research suggests that chromium supplements may improve the symptoms of hypoglycemia in some people.[7]

Heart disease

Chromium supplements have been shown to improve blood cholesterol and lipid levels in both diabetic and nondiabetic subjects. In those whose body levels of chromium are low, chromium seems to reduce total and harmful LDL cholesterol levels while raising beneficial HDL cholesterol levels.

In a study published in 1996, researchers assessed the effects of daily supplements of 200 mcg of chromium and nicotinic acid on blood glucose and lipids, including total cholesterol, HDL cholesterol, LDL cholesterol, and triglycerides. The patients were 14 healthy adults and five adults with Type II diabetes mellitus. The results showed lowered total and LDL cholesterol, triglycerides, and glucose concentrations in patients with Type II diabetes.[8]

Weight loss

Limited research suggests that moderate increases in chromium, in the form of chromium picolinate, may cause weight loss, reduce fat and increase muscle mass. Because of these reports, chromium picolinate supplements have become very popular.

Researchers involved in a 1997 study done in Austria assessed the effects of chromium yeast and chromium picolinate on lean body mass in 36 obese patients during and after weight reduction with a very low calorie diet. During the 26 week treatment period, subjects received either placebo or 200 mcg chromium yeast or 200 mcg chromium picolinate in a double-blind manner. After 26 weeks, chromium picolinate supplemented patients showed increased lean body mass whereas the other treatment groups still had reduced lean body mass.[9]

In a 1997 study done at the University of Texas at Austin, researchers examined the effects of 400 mcg of chromium and exercise training on young, obese women. The results showed that exercise training combined with chromium nicotinate supplementation resulted in significant weight loss and lowered the insulin response to an oral glucose load.[10]

Other uses

Some animal studies have shown that chromium picolinate supplements can prolong life. Further research is needed but this effect may be due to lowering of blood glucose levels similar to that seen in life-prolonging calorie restriction studies.

Chromium may help to boost the bone-building effects of insulin and may have a role in the maintenance of bone density and prevention of osteoporosis.[11] High chromium yeast has also been used to treat acne with some success.[12]

Interactions

Antacids may decrease chromium absorption and may aggravate an existing deficiency. Sugar increases chromium excretion.

Cautions

Diabetics may benefit from chromium supplementation but as their insulin requirements may change as a result, their use of supplements should be monitored by a doctor.

Cobalt is a component of vitamin B12. The average body content of cobalt is less than 1 mg and it is stored in the muscles, bone, liver and kidneys.

What it does in the body

The only known role of cobalt is as part of the vitamin B12 molecule. Many of the functions of vitamin B12 are mediated through the cobalt portion of the molecule. This includes the synthesis of DNA, production of red blood cells, maintenance of nerve function and detoxification of cyanide.

Absorption and metabolism

Cobalt is absorbed as part of the vitamin B12 molecule.

Deficiency

A deficiency of cobalt is equivalent to a deficiency of vitamin B12 with symptoms of pernicious anemia, nerve disorders and abnormalities in cell formation. However, these symptoms cannot be treated with cobalt alone.

Sources

Green leafy vegetables, some fish, liver, kidney and milk contain cobalt. Some of the cobalt in meat, fish and dairy products is present as vitamin B12 and some in other forms. In vegetables and cereals, it is present in other forms and is therefore of little use to humans.

Recommended dietary allowances

There is no RDA for cobalt. World Health Organization sources have suggested a minimum daily intake of 1 mcg. Most intakes are higher and vary according to the amount of mineral present in the soil. For example, intake is much higher in the USA than in Japan.

Toxic effects of excess intake

In animals, large intakes of cobalt (4 to 10 mg per kg of body weight) have caused anemia, loss of appetite and low body weight. Other toxic effects are goiter, hypothyroidism, overproduction of red blood cells and heart failure. High dietary protein levels may protect against cobalt toxicity.

Therapeutic uses of supplements

There are no uses for cobalt supplements. Radioactive cobalt-60 is used to treat some cancers.

QUICK GUIDE

Essential for

- normal metabolism
- healthy bones, joints, skin, blood vessels
- a healthy nervous system
- a healthy cardiovascular system
- the formation of haemoglobin in red blood cells
- a healthy immune system
- its action as an antioxidant

Absorption and metabolism

Copper is absorbed in the stomach and small intestine.

Deficiency

Copper deficiency leads to anemia, connective tissue defects, immune suppression, nerve problems and heart disease.

Sources

Good sources include seafood, meat and whole grains. Copper is also obtained from water pipes and cookware.

Daily recommended dietary intakes

Safe and adequate daily intake is estimated to range from 1.5 to 3 mg.

Toxic effects of excess intake

Toxic effects include fatigue, irritability, vomiting, diarrhea, liver problems and abnormal mental function. High copper levels, especially when associated with low zinc levels, are implicated in several diseases including mental disorders, joint and muscle problems, premenstrual syndrome and high blood pressure.

Interactions

Zinc and copper interact in many body functions.

Therapeutic uses of supplements

Copper supplements have been used to treat heart disease and arthritis.

Copper is an essential trace element for humans, animals and many plants. The average adult contains between 75 and 150 mg copper and about half of this is contained in the skeleton and the muscles. Copper is most concentrated in the brain and liver.

What it does in the body

Copper is an important component in many enzymes in the body. A copper-containing enzyme plays a vital role in energy production in cells. The activity of this enzyme is highest in the heart, brain, liver and kidney.

Connective tissue formation

An enzyme responsible for the production of the connective tissue proteins, collagen and elastin, requires copper. It is therefore necessary for the development and maintenance of blood vessels, skin, bone and joints.

Iron metabolism and blood

Copper is involved in the release of iron from storage sites and is involved in the formation of bone marrow and the maturation of red blood cells.

Brain and nervous system

Copper is necessary for the synthesis of cell membrane phospholipids, and so helps maintain myelin, the insulating sheath that surrounds nerve cells. It also helps regulate neurotransmitter levels.

Antioxidant

Copper is part of the enzyme copper-zinc superoxide dismutase, an antioxidant vital for protection against free radical damage. Maintaining the correct balance between zinc and copper is important in many body functions involving superoxide dismutase.

Immune system

Copper is important in developing resistance to infection. During inflammation or infection, two copper-containing compounds, superoxide dismutase and ceruloplasmin, are mobilized in the body. Copper is also necessary for T cell function and maturation.

Cardiovascular system

Copper is essential for the contractility of heart muscle. It is also necessary for the healthy function of small blood vessels that control blood flow and nutrient and waste exchange. It is also necessary for the functioning of the muscles of the blood vessels and is involved in the functioning of blood vessel linings and platelets which may play a role in blood clotting.[1]

Other functions

The formation of melanin, a natural coloring pigment found in skin and hair, involves a copper-dependent enzyme. The enzyme histaminase, which metabolizes histamine, requires copper. Copper is involved in fat and cholesterol metabolism and in the normal functioning of insulin which regulates glucose metabolism. It also contributes to the synthesis of prostaglandins, compounds that regulate a variety of functions such as heartbeat, blood pressure and wound-healing.

Absorption and metabolism

Around 30 per cent of dietary intake of copper is absorbed in the stomach and upper intestine. It is transferred across the gut wall and carried to the liver where it combines with proteins including ceruloplasmin. This protein is released into the blood and carries copper to body tissues. Adequate protein improves copper absorption. Excretion is mostly via secretion in bile into the gastrointestinal tract and then elimination in the feces.

Deficiency

Symptoms of copper deficiency in babies include failure to thrive, pale skin, anemia, diarrhea, lack of pigment in hair and skin, and prominent dilated veins. In adults, symptoms include anemia, water retention, weakness of blood vessel walls, irritability, brittle bones, hair depigmentation, poor hair texture and loss of sense of taste.

Children at risk of deficiency include those with Menkes' syndrome, a rare disorder which means they are unable to absorb copper. Malnourished, premature infants and those who have iron deficiency anemia are also at risk. Milk, in general, is low in copper; although absorption from breast milk is more efficient than that from cow's milk and formula.

Those who eat large amounts of phytates which bind copper in the gut, those whose diets are highly refined, those who have prolonged diarrhea or those with high intakes of zinc, cadmium, fluoride or molybdenum may be at risk of deficiency.

Immune system

Copper deficiency can lead to reduced resistance to infection as white blood cell activity and cellular immune responses are reduced. The ratio of zinc to copper may also affect immune system effectiveness. Susceptibility to disease seems to increase when copper intake is high and zinc intake is low.

Nervous system

Copper deficiency can impair the function of the nervous system. This impairment causes poor concentration, numbness and tingling, and a variety of nervous system disorders.

Heart disease

A deficiency of copper may contribute to heart disease. Copper deficiencies have been associated with poor heart muscle, a drop in beneficial HDL cholesterol and an increase in harmful LDL cholesterol. In animals, copper intake has also been associated with weakening of heart connective tissue and rupture of blood vessels. Alterations in blood clotting mechanism and the muscular activity of blood vessels may also occur. The ratio of zinc to copper may be important in the regulation of blood cholesterol.

Collagen defects

Copper deficiency leads to poor collagen formation, the protein component of connective tissue which may result in bone deformities, damaged blood vessels, reduced resiliency of skin and other internal and external linings of the body.

Other problems

Copper intakes may be low in rheumatoid arthritis sufferers and may contribute to the incidence of the disease.[2] Copper deficiency may also be involved in high blood pressure.[3]

Sources

Good food sources include liver, shellfish, brewer's yeast, olives, nuts, whole grains, beans and chocolate. Copper from food processing and storage, pesticides and fungicides in food and copper kettles also contribute to copper in the diet. Up to 70 per cent of the copper content of flour may be lost when it is refined.

Food	Amount	Copper (mg)
Beef liver, fried	85g	3.77
Peanuts	½ cup	1.59
Walnuts	1 cup, chopped	1.58
Sesame seeds	¼ cup	1.40
Almonds	1 cup	1.27
Sardines, canned in tomato sauce	1 can	1.01
Oysters	6 pieces	0.80
Crab, cooked	1 cup	0.72
Soybeans, cooked	1 cup	0.66
Sunflower seeds	¼ cup	0.60
Chickpeas, cooked	1 cup	0.55
Avocado	1 avocado	0.53
Lentils, cooked	1 cup	0.48
Tofu	½ cup	0.47
Wheatgerm	½ cup	0.44
Kidney beans, cooked	1 cup	0.41
Beet greens, cooked	1 cup	0.34
Mushrooms, raw	1 cup, slices	0.32
Spinach, cooked	1 cup	0.29
Wholewheat spaghetti	1 cup	0.22
Cocoa powder	1 tbsp	0.21
Brown rice, cooked	1 cup	0.19
Milk chocolate	1 bar	0.17

Recommended dietary allowances

There is no RDA for copper. Safe and adequate intake is estimated to range from 1.5 to 3 mg per day. The UK RNI is 1.2 mg for adults.

Supplements

Copper supplements are available in various forms including copper amino acid chelate, copper gluconate and copper sulfate. Some experts feel that copper should not be supplemented as there is a fine line between therapeutic and toxic doses.

Toxic effects of excess intake

Toxicity of copper is thought to be fairly rare but high concentrations (daily intakes of 200 mg and over) can cause effects such as nausea, vomiting, abdominal pain, diarrhea, muscle pains, heart problems, immune suppression and abnormal mental states. The lethal dose for copper may be as low as 3.5 g. Imbalance in the copper to zinc ratio may be an important factor in copper toxicity.

Patients with ulcerative colitis may accumulate copper in the tissues and the excess of copper may aggravate the disease. High copper levels may also be a risk factor for heart disease.

A study done in 1998 in Wisconsin suggests that high levels of copper in the water supply may increase the rate of gastrointestinal upsets. The researchers assessed copper levels in several homes with new water distribution systems. Their findings suggested that copper-contaminated drinking water was a common cause of nausea, diarrhea, abdominal cramps, and headaches in areas where water supplies are naturally corrosive.[4]

Wilson's disease

Wilson's disease is a rare genetic disorder affecting one in 30 000 people, in which the liver is unable to remove copper from the body. Excessive amounts of copper accumulate, leading to symptoms of liver disease and loss of mental function. Drugs to remove excess copper, and zinc to promote excretion of copper, are used to treat Wilson's disease.

Therapeutic uses of supplements

Copper is used therapeutically to treat deficiency symptoms and iron deficiency anemia. Copper is present in expectorant cough mixtures, cough suppressant preparations and decongestants.

Heart disease

Copper supplements have been shown to have beneficial effects on the oxidation of blood fats. A 1997 study done over four weeks at Ohio State University found that 2 mg per day of copper increased the time taken for LDL cholesterol to become oxidized.[5] This helps to reduce the damage these fats do to arteries and limits the build-up of atherosclerotic plaque.

Arthritis

The wearing of copper bracelets as a cure for arthritis is an old remedy which may have some scientific support. It is possible that the copper combines with compounds in the skin which are then absorbed and exert anti-inflammatory effects. Copper is part of ceruloplasmin which acts as both an anti-inflammatory agent and as an antioxidant, and plays a role in the body's reaction to inflammatory conditions such as rheumatoid arthritis.

Interactions with other nutrients

Copper to zinc ratio

Zinc and copper compete with each other for absorption. Excess zinc intake for prolonged periods can lead to copper deficiency. Altered copper to zinc ratios may play a role in several disorders including heart disease and some types of cancer including those of the breast, lung and gastrointestinal tract. There is some suggestion that this may be useful as a diagnostic test. Copper zinc ratios also seem to be high in violence-prone males (See page 323 for more information.)

Copper-zinc superoxide dismutase levels seem to be altered in rheumatoid arthritis. Those with the disease have higher serum copper/zinc superoxide dismutase levels than those without.[6]

Other vitamins and minerals

Iron and copper interact in several ways. Copper deficiency alters iron metabolism, causing it to accumulate in the liver. Excess iron can lead to copper deficiency. High molybdenum intakes may increase copper excretion. High

Electrolytes

Potassium, sodium and chloride are known as electrolytes as they conduct electricity when dissolved in water. Potassium and sodium become positive ions as they lose an electron when dissolved and chloride becomes a negative ion as it gains an electron when dissolved. A positive ion is always accompanied by a negative ion, hence the close relationship between sodium, potassium and chloride. The electrolytes are distributed throughout all body fluids including the blood, lymph, and the fluid inside and outside cells.

What they do in the body

Water balance

The electrolytes are vital for maintaining a normal balance of water between body cells and the surrounding fluids, and for moving fluids in and out of cells. Sodium is the main positive ion outside cells and potassium is the main positive ion inside cells.

The blood and other fluids require a narrow range of sodium concentration to function properly. This balance is accomplished by the hormone, aldosterone. When sodium intake is high, the aldosterone level is low, and the kidney excretes more sodium into the urine. When sodium intake is low aldosterone is high and the kidney conserves sodium.

Chloride acts as the main negatively charged ion and neutralizes the positively charged sodium and potassium ions. Chloride ions are most abundant in the fluid outside cells but some are found inside the cells.

Muscle contraction

The electrolytes and calcium are involved in muscle contraction. They regulate heartbeat through their effects on heart muscle.

Acid-alkali balance

Sodium plays a role in preserving the acid-alkali balance of the body in close relationship with bicarbonate, phosphate, protein, potassium, chloride, calcium and magnesium.

Nerve impulse transmission

The flow of sodium into the nerve cell and the opposite flow of potassium out of the cell sets up an electrical impulse that travels down the nerve.

QUICK GUIDE

Essential for

- water balance in the body
- muscle contraction
- acid-alkali balance
- nerve impulse transmission
- energy metabolism
- protein and carbohydrate metabolism
- a healthy heart and blood vessels

Absorption and metabolism

Potassium is well absorbed.

Deficiency

Potassium deficiency may lead to an increased risk of high blood pressure.

Sources

Foods high in potassium include fruits, vegetables and whole grains.

Daily recommended dietary intakes

The estimated minimum requirement for a healthy person is 2000 mg.

Toxic effects of high intake

Toxic effects include muscular weakness, ulcers, low blood pressure and, in high enough doses, coma and death.

Interactions

Potassium interacts with sodium, calcium, magnesium and chloride. High sugar intakes can lead to low potassium levels.

Therapeutic uses of supplements

Potassium has been used to treat cases of depletion, fatigue, high blood pressure, cardiovascular disease and kidney stones.

Cautions

Those with kidney disease or ulcers should not take potassium supplements.

The average body contains about 140 g of potassium.

What it does in the body

Potassium has many functions in addition to those mentioned above. It is essential for protein synthesis and for the conversion of blood sugar into glycogen. It activates a number of enzymes, particularly those concerned with energy production. It stimulates normal movements of the intestinal tract.

Absorption and metabolism

Absorption of potassium from the diet is passive and does not require any specific mechanism. Absorption takes place in the small intestine as long as the concentration in gut contents is higher than that in the blood. If food moves rapidly through the bowel then absorption will not be sufficient.

The kidneys are the main regulators of body potassium, maintaining blood levels by controlling excretion, even as intake varies. Some potassium is excreted in sweat. Digestive juices contain significant amounts of potassium but most of this is re-absorbed in the lower gut.

Deficiency

Symptoms of severe potassium deficiency include fatigue, vomiting, abdominal distention, acute muscular weakness, paralysis, pins and needles, loss of appetite, low blood pressure, intense thirst, drowsiness, confusion and eventually coma. Muscle spasms, tetany, heart arrhythmias and muscle weakness can also be caused by increased nerve excitability associated with inadequate intake of potassium.

Causes of potassium deficiency include high sodium diets, surgical operations involving the bowel, extensive burns and injuries, diabetes, Cushing's syndrome, excessive excretion of aldosterone, chronic diarrhea which limits gut re-absorption of potassium, persistent vomiting, influenza, inflammatory bowel disease, anemia, ulcerative colitis, kidney disease, heart disease, chronic respiratory failure, prolonged fasting, therapeutic starvation, bizarre diets, anorexia nervosa, alcoholism and cystic fibrosis.

Several medications can also cause potassium deficiency. These include thiazide diuretics, long-term therapy with corticosteroids and adrenal hormones, laxatives, excessive intake of licorice and carbenoxolone, high dose sodium penicillin, intravenous infusions of glucose and salt solutions not containing potassium, ion exchange resins used to reduce blood cholesterol, and insulin.

The sudden death that can occur in fasting, anorexia nervosa or starvation is often a result of heart failure caused by potassium deficiency.

High blood pressure

Many population studies have found links between low potassium intakes and an increased risk of high blood pressure and death from stroke. Increasing the amount of potassium-rich foods in the diet can lead to a reduction in high blood pressure. The ratio of sodium to potassium in the diet appears to play an important role in the development of high blood pressure. The typical Western diet is low in potassium relative to sodium.

Potassium depletion causes the body to retain more fluid in response to a large dose of salt, and high levels of potassium may enhance the excretion of sodium, thus decreasing blood volume and blood pressure.

Sources

Good sources of potassium include fresh fruits, vegetables, soybean flour, shellfish, beans, wheat bran, salad, nuts, cereals, meat, milk, coffee and tea. Many food additives such as potassium iodate used in bread baking, also contain potassium. Potassium is easily lost in cooking and processing foods.

Food	Amount	Potassium (mg)
Beet greens, boiled	1 cup	1244
French beans, raw	½ cup	1150
Seeded raisins	1 cup	1136
Snapper, grilled	1 fillet	887
Mackerel, cooked, dry	½ fillet	859
Prunes	½ cup	757
Pistachios	½ cup	665
Avocado	½ avocado	602
Potatoes, fried	regular order	541

Potato chips	30g	523
Potato flesh, baked	1 cup	490
Peanuts	½ cup	488
Ham	100g	510
Orange juice	1 cup	471
Melon	1 cup	470
Halibut, grilled	½ fillet	490
Lima beans, boiled	½ cup	461
Apricots, dried	10 halves	482
Bananas	1 fruit	451
Milk	1 cup	424
Green peas, boiled	1 cup	412
Spinach, boiled	½ cup	398
Barley	½ cup	395
Beef	85g	395

Recommended dietary allowances

No RDA has been set in the USA but the estimated minimum requirement for a healthy person is 2000 mg. The typical adult intake may be between 800 mg and 1500 mg. The RNI in the UK is 3500 mg and the RDA in Australia is 1950 to 5460 mg.

Supplements

Potassium supplements are usually in the form of tablets or solutions, often of potassium chloride. Amino acid chelate and protein complexes are also available and these complexes also replace the protein losses which accompany potassium excretion. Potassium is added to sports drinks to help replace that lost in heavy sweating.

Potassium supplements can be irritating to the stomach and should be taken after meals with a glass of water. Slow release or film-coated tablets have been associated with ulcers of the small intestine. The tablets should not be taken with alcohol as this may worsen stomach irritation.

Toxic effects of excess intake

Intakes of potassium in doses larger than 18 000 mg cause muscular weakness, low blood pressure, mental confusion and eventually heart attack. Potassium injection can be fatal. Lower doses can cause nausea, vomiting, diarrhea and abdominal cramps.

A healthy person cannot obtain toxic levels of potassium from the diet. Causes of potassium excess include insufficient production of adrenal gland hormones, acidosis, major infections, and shock after injury in which potassium leaks out of damaged cells into the blood. In severe kidney disease, potassium is not excreted, and excessive levels build up in the tissue.

Therapeutic uses of supplements

Potassium is one of the most commonly prescribed minerals. It is used in situations where body potassium is decreased, such as during diuretic drugs therapy.

High blood pressure

Many studies have found potassium supplements to have beneficial effects in the treatment of high blood pressure. Doses involved usually range from 2.5 to 5 g. In people with normal blood pressure, those who are salt sensitive or who have a family history of hypertension appear to benefit most from potassium supplementation. The greatest blood pressure-lowering effect of potassium supplements occurs in patients with severe hypertension. This effect is pronounced with prolonged potassium supplementation. Potassium may help to lower blood pressure in several ways, including enhancing sodium excretion, by directly dilating blood vessels, or lowering cardiovascular reactivity to body chemicals which constrict blood vessels.

A 1997 analysis of studies on the effects of potassium supplementation on blood pressure confirms that low intake of the mineral plays an important role in high blood pressure, and increasing intake is beneficial in treatment. Researchers at Johns Hopkins University looked at 33 randomized controlled trials with over 2069 participants in which potassium supplements were used. Positive effects were seen with a decrease in mean systolic pressure of 3.11 mm Hg and in diastolic pressure of 1.97 mm Hg. The effects were enhanced in those exposed to a high intake of sodium.[1]

In a study published in 1998 in the American Heart Association journal, *Hypertension*, researchers at the Harvard School of Public health tested the effects of potassium, calcium and magnesium supplements on 300 women (average age 39 years) whose dietary intakes of those minerals were low. The women had blood pressure in the normal range. The women were divided into five groups: the calcium (1200 mg per day), magnesium (336 mg per day) and potassium (1600 mg per day) groups; a group who received all three supplements; and a placebo group. The result showed that potassium supplements lowered blood pressure whereas calcium and magnesium supplements did not. The results also showed that those in the three supplements group had smaller falls in blood pressure than those in the potassium group. The researchers speculate that calcium and magnesium might in some way interfere with the blood pressure-lowering effect of potassium.[2]

Cardiovascular disease

High rates of potassium intake are associated with protection from cardiovascular disease, including strokc, in pcoplc in both developing and industrialized countries who eat diets high in unrefined whole grains and vegetables. Potassium may protect against cardiovascular diseases in a number of ways: by reducing free radical formation; proliferation of vascular smooth muscle cells; platelet aggregation; and blood clotting.[3] Potassium supplements are used to treat heart arrhythmias.

Kidney stones

Higher potassium intakes may be beneficial in preventing kidney stones formation. Researchers at the Kaiser Permanente Medical Centers in Northern California have found that giving potassium-magnesium citrate to kidney stone sufferers reduces the risk of them developing further stones. The stones were of the calcium oxalate type. In the double-blind study reported in the *Journal of Urology*, 64 patients were given either a placebo or the potassium-magnesium citrate compound for up to three years. New kidney stones occurred in 63.6 per cent of the patients taking placebo, but in only 12.9 per cent of those taking the potassium-magnesium citrate compound.[4]

Other uses

Potassium supplements may be of benefit in early menopause to combat fatigue and mood swings. It can also be used to treat infant colic, allergies and headache. During and after diarrhea, potassium replacement may be necessary.

Interactions with other nutrients

Aside from the interactions with other electrolytes discussed above, potassium may have a role in maintaining normal calcium balance in the body as potassium decreases urinary loss of calcium.

Interactions with drugs

Diuretic drugs, particularly the thiazide variety, act by increasing the output of sodium and water from the kidneys but at the same time, potassium excretion is increased. Antibiotics taken on a long-term basis can deplete potassium. High intakes of alcohol, coffee and sugar may lead to potassium deficiency.

Cautions

Those with dehydration, heat cramps, ulcers, kidney disease or who are taking drugs which cause the kidney to retain potassium should avoid potassium supplements.

Sodium

QUICK GUIDE

Essential for

- water balance in the body
- muscle contraction
- acid-alkali balance
- nerve impulse transmission
- energy production
- stomach acid production

Absorption and metabolism

Sodium is easily absorbed.

Deficiency

Sodium deficiency is rare and toxic effects from high intakes are of greater concern. Deficiency may occur in high temperatures due to hard exercise or manual work.

Sources

Foods high in sodium include processed meats, cheese, margarine and butter.

Daily recommended dietary intakes

Men	920-2300 mg
Women	920-2300 mg
Pregnant women	+0 mg
Lactating women	+0 mg

Toxic effects of excess intake

Toxic effects include high blood pressure, premenstrual syndrome and possibly osteoporosis, asthma and urinary stones.

Interactions

Sodium interacts with potassium, calcium, magnesium and chloride in body functions.

Therapeutic uses

Supplementation is usually unnecessary and is an acquired taste. Sodium bicarbonate may be used to treat metabolic and respiratory acidosis.

Sodium is the major positively charged ion in blood and body fluids. The average adult body contains about 90 g of sodium. More than half of this is in the fluids that bathe the cells, about one-third is in the bones, enmeshed in the crystals of insoluble bone minerals, and some is retained within the cells.

What it does in the body

In addition to its functions as an electrolyte, sodium is also a component of ATPase, an enzyme involved in the production of energy. It is necessary for the transport of amino acids and glucose into body cells.

Absorption and metabolism

Absorption of any soluble form of sodium is passive with excess intakes easily absorbed. Excretion of sodium is mainly via the kidneys with increased sodium intake leading to increased excretion. There is a limit on the extent to which the kidneys can concentrate the urine, so large sodium intakes must be balanced by large intakes of water. The highest excretion of sodium occurs at midday and the lowest at night. Some sodium is excreted in sweat.

Deficiency

A deficiency of sodium is unlikely in any diet, except possibly those that are very low in salt and protein. Deficiency may occur with dehydration in heat exhaustion brought on by high temperatures, hard exercise, manual work and in babies, by diarrhea. Symptoms include mental apathy, loss of appetite and sometimes vomiting and muscle cramps. In severe cases, the blood thickens, veins collapse, blood pressure is reduced and the pulse becomes rapid. Deficiency of sodium can also occur after water intoxication which happens when large amounts of water but no sodium are drunk after heavy sweating.

Other causes of low blood sodium levels include kidney disorders, hormonal imbalance, lung cancers, lung infection, liver cirrhosis, toxemia of pregnancy and high blood glucose levels.

Sources

Foods high in sodium include yeast extract, bacon, smoked fish, salami, sauces, cornflakes, canned or boiled ham, biscuits, cheese, margarine and butter. Foods of animal and fish origin usually contain more sodium than whole grains, fruits and vegetables. Large quantities of sodium chloride, sodium bicarbonate or monosodium glutamate (MSG) are often added to foods during cooking, refining, processing and preservation. Many drugs contain sodium.

In babies, the ideal sodium content of food is that found in human breast milk. Untreated cow's milk is much higher in sodium and should not be fed to babies in the first three months of life as excess salt can cause high blood pressure and even death. Babies fed bottled water may be at risk of sodium deficiency as the water does not contain the levels of sodium comparable to those found in breast milk. It should not be used instead of infant formula.

Food	Amount	Sodium (mg)
Salami, pork	100g	2260
Blue vein cheese	100g	1395
Sausages, cooked	100g	1294
Salami, beef	100g	1176
Corned beef	100g	1134
Feta cheese	100g	1116
Baked beans, canned	1 cup	1008
Soy sauce	1 tbsp	914
Olives	100g	872
Chicken soup, can, prepared	1 cup	849
Anchovies, canned, drained	5 fillets	733
Cheddar cheese	100g	620
Potato chips	100g	594
Tuna, canned	1 can	557
Fish, battered, deep fried	1 fillet	484
Pizza, with cheese	1 slice	336
Gravy powder	1 tbsp	332
Lima beans, canned	½ cup, drained	312

Bacon, cooked	3 slices	303
Corn flakes	1 cup	297
Plain cake	1 piece	233
Cod, cooked	1 fillet	140
French dressing	1 tbsp	128
Butter	1 tbsp	117

Recommended dietary allowances

An amount of about 500 mg a day is considered adequate to maintain the body's salt concentration. Intake should be no more than 2.4 g of sodium per day which is the amount found in around one teaspoon of salt. Those who eat few processed foods are probably getting around 1.2 g of sodium in food, leaving around half a teaspoon to be added to stay within recommended limits. Athletes and those who perspire a great deal may need more. The average daily intake of sodium in the USA is about 3 to 6 g with one-third to one-half of this being made up from table salt.

Pregnant women may need to consume 2 to 3 g of sodium per day. This amount should be available from a varied diet of wholesome, minimally processed foods with no salt added during cooking. In Australia, the recommended intake is 920 to 2300 mg per day.

Supplements

A healthy diet without salt supplementation is sufficient to provide for the body's needs. Salt supplementation is an acquired taste. Salt tablets may be useful in cases where sodium is lost through excessive sweating.

Toxic effects of excess intake

Hypertension

Epidemiological studies show that high sodium intakes are linked with high blood pressure. As a person ages, changes in the hormonal systems which regulate the control of water and sodium balance lead to changes in blood pressure. Many studies, including the Intersalt study, have found that high salt diets accelerate the increase in blood pressure that occurs with age. (See page 624 for more information.)

About one-third of the general population and about one-half of those suffering from high blood pressure are "salt sensitive" and show increases in blood pressure when salt intakes are high. Restriction of dietary salt usually leads to decreases in blood pressure in such cases. Family history also contributes to high sodium levels and may play a role in hypertension.

A new study of almost 1500 British people has found that those who eat the most salt tend to have the highest blood pressure. The study, which involved men and women aged 16 to 64, found that as daily salt intakes rose from 1600 mg to 9200 mg, so did blood pressures. A rise in salt consumption from 2300 mg to 4600 mg led to a 7.1 mmHg rise in systolic blood pressure for women and a 4.9 mmHg rise for men. [5]

In a two-month double-blind, randomized, placebo-controlled crossover study published in 1997 in *The Lancet*, researchers found that modest reduction in salt in the diets of elderly people led to lower blood pressure. The study involved 29 patients with high blood pressure and 18 with normal blood pressure. The average blood pressure fall was 8.2/3.9 mm Hg in the normal subjects and 6.6/2.7 mm Hg in those with high blood pressure.[6] In those with normal blood pressure, cutting salt may have little effect, according to an analysis of 83 studies published in the *Journal of the American Medical Association* in 1998.[7]

High blood pressure appears to be associated with an imbalance of minerals where sodium and possibly chloride are too high; and potassium, calcium and magnesium are too low. When sodium levels are too high, the amount of water retained in the body is increased and water is pulled from cells. The result is high blood pressure and water retention which can lead to puffy eyes and swollen feet or fingers. The ratio of sodium to potassium in the diet may also be important in the regulation of blood pressure. Diuretic drugs, which are often used to treat high blood pressure, act by forcing the kidneys to excrete water and sodium at a faster rate.

Dietary sodium restriction is used to control pregnancy-related high blood pressure. It does not seem to lead to any adverse effects on other minerals or the baby. In fact, increasing evidence suggests that the amount of salt in a baby's diet affects blood pressure later in life. In a study published in 1997, Dutch researchers compared the effects of low salt and normal salt diets in 476 children born in 1980. They measured blood pressures in the first week of life and every four weeks after that for a six month period. Fifteen years later, the study participants had their blood pressures measured again and the results showed that children who had been in the low salt group had lower blood pressures than those in the normal salt group.[8]

Stress and sodium

Stress may affect sodium excretion. In certain people, stress seems to contribute to high blood pressure and this may be mediated via effects on sodium excretion. In a 1995 German study, researchers tested the effects of stress on 27 people with normal blood pressure and 21 with high blood pressure. The participants in the study took part in a 30-minute video game after which their excretion of sodium was measured. Seventy per cent of the people showed increased sodium excretion and 30 per cent showed decreased excretion. Those who excreted more sodium showed less stress-associated increases in blood pressure and greater expression of anger.[9]

Inhibited breathing seems to decrease sodium excretion which could mediate the role of behavioral stress in some forms of hypertension. Sodium excretion patterns under stress may be altered with certain types of antihypertensive medication.

Premenstrual syndrome

Salt and water retention are often seen in women with premenstrual syndrome. High salt diets may exacerbate these symptoms, although research results are conflicting.

Osteoporosis

High salt intakes seem to increase calcium excretion, thus lowering bone mineral density and increasing the risk of osteoporosis. In a study published in 1995, Australian researchers investigated the influence of urinary sodium excretion on bone density in a two-year period in 124 postmenopausal women. The results showed that increased sodium excretion was linked to decreases in bone density.[10]

Asthma

Population studies have found links between consumption of table salt and asthma. Some research reports suggest that high dietary sodium intake is a cause of asthma and airway hyper-reactivity, while others show no effect. A 1993 UK study tested the effects of either a placebo or sodium supplements on asthma sufferers who had previously followed a low sodium diet. The results showed a worsening of symptoms and laboratory measurements of disease severity in those patients on the high sodium diets.[11]

Urinary stones

A high urinary sodium-to-potassium ratio may be linked to the formation of urinary stones. Researchers involved in the Gubbio Population Study in Italy assessed the relationship between urinary sodium-to-potassium ratio and urinary stone disease in 3625 men and women aged 25 to 74. Analysis of the results showed that higher ratios were linked to an increased risk of stone formation.[12]

Therapeutic uses of supplements

Sodium bicarbonate is used intravenously to treat metabolic and respiratory acidosis, in the acute treatment of excessive potassium levels, and to make urine alkaline.

Interactions

In addition to the interactions with other electrolytes described above, sodium increases urinary loss of calcium. The hypertensive effect of sodium is enhanced when calcium intake is low.

Chlorine in the body exists in the form of chloride and is an essential mineral in animals and humans. The average adult body contains about 115 g of chloride.

What it does in the body

In addition to its functions as an electrolyte, chloride combines with hydrogen to make stomach acid (hydrochloric acid).

Absorption and metabolism

Excess chloride is excreted in the urine, sweat and gastrointestinal tract. Excessive losses can be caused by heavy sweating and by diarrhea. Urinary excretion of chloride is increased by high salt diets, rickets and liver cirrhosis. It is decreased in cases of chronic kidney disease, the early stages of pneumonia, cancer and gastritis.

Deficiency

Deficiency of chloride is very rare and is known as alkalosis. It may occur when there are excessive sodium losses, for example in heavy sweating, prolonged vomiting or diarrhea. Symptoms include muscle weakness, loss of appetite and lethargy. Athletes can lose large amounts of chloride during endurance exercise.

Sources

Foods rich in sodium are also rich in chloride. These include salt, yeast extract, processed meats, cheese, kelp, olives and bread.

Recommended dietary allowances

No RDA has been established as most diets are high in salt and therefore high in chloride. The suggested minimum requirement is 750 mg per day and most adults consume 3500 to 7000 mg per day due to high salt diets.

Toxic effects of excess intake

Excessive dietary levels of chloride are likely only with increased salt and potassium chloride intakes. The toxic effects of such diets are attributed to sodium and potassium ions, although it is possible that chloride ions may play a role in the increased incidence of high blood pressure when salt intakes are high. Increased blood plasma chloride levels are seen in kidney disease, anemia, heart disease and pregnancy.

QUICK GUIDE

Fluoride is not classed as an essential nutrient but because of its strengthening effect on bones and teeth, it is officially considered to be a beneficial element in humans. The use of fluoride in water remains controversial.

Absorption and metabolism

Excess fluoride is excreted in the urine.

Deficiency

Fluoride deficiency may lead to tooth decay.

Sources

Sources include water, tea, meat, fish, cereals and fruit. The fluoride content of food varies with the location in which the food is grown. The table on page 239 can be used as a guide.

Daily recommended dietary intakes

Men	3.8 mg
Women	3.1 mg
Children (6 to 12 months)	0.5 mg
Children (4 to 8 years)	1.1 mg
Children (9 to 13 years)	2.0 mg

Toxic effects of excess intake

Toxic effects include mottling of the teeth, dermatitis and bone abnormalities.

Therapeutic uses of supplements

Fluoride supplements have been used to treat tooth decay, osteoporosis and otosclerosis (a loss of hearing due to deposits in the ear). Fluoride supplements may be useful in areas where the water is not fluoridated but, as with water fluoridation, their use is controversial. Sodium fluoride is the least toxic form of fluoride supplement.

Fluoride is not classed as an essential nutrient but because of its strengthening effect on bones and teeth it is officially considered to be a beneficial element in humans. Fluoride is found in the teeth, bones, thyroid gland and skin. The average body contains about 2.6 g of fluoride.

What it does in the body

Teeth

Fluoride helps in the formation of strong teeth. It protects them from decay by forming compounds with calcium and phosphorus that are stronger and less soluble than other calcium salts. These compounds remain in bone as they are not as easily re-absorbed into circulation to supply calcium needs. Children whose mothers have sufficiently high fluoride intake during pregnancy seem to have fewer cavities than children of mothers whose diets are lacking in fluoride. A baby's first teeth start forming in the first few months of pregnancy and adult teeth in the last few months. Fluoride affects the strength and susceptibility to decay of these teeth.

Bones

Bones seem to be more stable and resistant to degeneration when the diet is adequate in fluoride.

Absorption and metabolism

Excretion of fluoride is mainly through the kidneys.

Deficiency

Low fluoride levels increase the risk of dental caries in children and possibly, of osteoporosis in adults. The incidence of dental caries is higher in areas where the water is not fluoridated.

Sources

Natural sources of fluoride include tea, meat, fish, cereals and fruit. The fluoride content of food depends on the fluoride content of the soil in which the food is grown. Drinking water contains appreciable amounts of fluoride. Some fluoride is absorbed from toothpaste and other oral solutions.

Food	Amount	Fluoride (mcg)
Tea	100g	1.41
Oatmeal, cooked	100g	10.6
Rice Krispies	100g	5.9
Cottage cheese	100g	5.0
Coffee	100g	5.0
Noodles	100g	4.6
Potatoes, mashed	100g	4.3
Minestrone soup	100g	4.1
Spinach, cooked	100g	3.7
Rice, cooked	100g	3.5
Spaghetti and sauce	100g	3.3
Cheerios	100g	3.3
Peas, cooked	100g	3.0
Toast	100g	2.7
Sausage	100g	2.5
Potatoes, boiled	100g	2.5
Veal	100g	2.3
Special K	100g	2.1
Pork, roast	100g	2.1
Wholewheat bread	100g	1.7
Ham, baked	100g	1.7
Greens, raw	100g	1.5
Chocolate cake	100g	1.3
Fish, fried	100g	1.0

Recommended dietary allowances

The adequate intake levels for fluoride were set in 1997. The amount necessary to protect against tooth decay without causing fluorosis is used as a basis for calculating these values.

	Men	Women	Children 6 to 12 months	Children 4 to 8 years	Children 9 to 13
USA	3.8 mg	3.1 mg	0.5 mg	1.1 mg	2.0 mg

The daily tolerable upper intake levels for fluoride are:

	Men	Women	Children 6 to 12 months	Children 4 to 8 years	Children 9 to 18
USA	10 mg	10 mg	0.9 mg	2.2 mg	10 mg

In most developed countries, fluoride is added to drinking water at a concentration of one part per million. This supplies between 1 and 2 mg fluoride per day.

Supplements

Fluoride supplements may be useful if drinking water is not fluoridated.

Toxic effects of excess intake

Signs of fluoride toxicity include dermatitis and mottling of the teeth as the enamel becomes infiltrated by yellow-brown staining. This is known as enamel fluorosis. If large quantities (20 to 80 mg per day) are taken for long periods skeletal fluorosis may occur. Appetite is depressed, the joints become stiff and painful, the spine, pelvis and limb bones become denser and calcium can be deposited in the muscles and tendons. Fatal poisoning can occur if fluoride is taken in amounts greater than 2500 times the recommended dose.

There is some evidence linking fluoride in water to various types of cancer, although many studies have not found any connection. A study published in 1996 reported on the relationship between fluoride concentration in drinking water and deaths from uterine cancer in Okinawa, Japan. Fluoride was added to the water supplies in the region in the period from 1945 to 1972. The results showed significant links between the time of water fluoridation and deaths from uterine cancer.[1]

A study published in 1997 in the *Journal of the American Dental Association* suggest that some commercially available infant foods contain high levels of fluoride which may put babies at risk of fluorosis. Some foods, particularly those containing chicken, are processed in ways which lead to high fluoride concentrations. Adding water to dry baby food also increases fluoride content.[2]

Therapeutic uses of supplements

Fluoridation of water

Approximately half of the US water supply is fluoridated in an effort to reduce tooth decay. Studies have shown that one part per million of fluoride in drinking water can substantially reduce tooth decay. This effect is particularly noticeable if treatment is started during early childhood when teeth are still forming. However, water fluoridation is a controversial issue and many experts feel that the practice should be discontinued.

Children living in areas were the water is fluoridated are at increased risk of dental fluorosis, in which teeth become mottled with yellow or brown spots. Bottle fed babies are at particular risk if formula is made with fluoridated tap water. Breast milk and ready-to-feed formula contain safe fluoride levels and experts recommend using low fluoride filtered or distilled water with formula. Fluoridation may also increase the risk of dermatitis in sensitive people.

Tooth decay

Fluoride is used in the treatment of dental caries. It is available in the form of fluoride toothpaste, oral fluoride tablets, fluoride gel and mouth rinses with fluoride solutions. It can help reduce sensitivity to external stimuli in gums which have receded to expose dentine. Fluoride supplements discourage the formation of dental caries in children by reducing the susceptibility to erosion of tooth minerals and by preventing the growth of acid-producing bacteria in the mouth.

Osteoporosis

Sodium fluoride, along with calcium, has also been used to treat osteoporosis as it appears to increase bone mass.[3] Researchers involved in a 1998 study published in the *Annals of Internal Medicine* compared the vertebral fracture rates in 200 women over a four-year period. One group was given 20 mg of fluoride and 1000 mg of calcium daily, and the other group received only calcium. The rate of new fractures in the fluoride group was 2.4 per cent compared to 10 per cent in the calcium only group.[4]

Sustained release fluoride in doses of 23 mg per day appears to be more beneficial than forms which are quickly absorbed from the gut.[5] However, a

1996 study done in Argentina suggests that the increases in bone mineral density are not maintained after sodium fluoride therapy is stopped.[6]

The treatment of osteoporosis with fluoride supplements is controversial as there is the possibility that fluoride bone is not always stronger than normal bone. There may be an increase in the number of hairline fractures in the hips, knees, feet and ankles. In 1983/1984, a study of bone mass and fractures was begun in 827 women aged 20-80 years in three rural Iowa communities selected for the fluoride and calcium content of their community water supplies. Residence in the higher-fluoride community was associated with a significantly lower radial bone mass in premenopausal and postmenopausal women, an increased rate of radial bone mass loss in premenopausal women, and significantly more fractures among postmenopausal women.[7] Fluoride therapy may increase the requirement for calcium as more is needed for bone formation.

Fluoride therapy has also been used to prevent rheumatoid arthritis-induced bone loss.[8]

Other uses

Fluoride may also aid in wound-healing after dental surgery, possibly due to antibacterial action. Fluoride supplements have been used to treat Paget's disease, bone pain, and to stabilize loss of hearing in patients with otosclerosis, a disorder in which deposits in the ear lead to deafness.

Interactions with other nutrients

Fluoride works with calcium, phosphorus, magnesium and vitamin D in the formation of healthy bones and teeth. Magnesium and calcium salts may reduce absorption of fluoride supplements. High calcium intakes may increase fluoride excretion. Caffeine may improve fluoride absorption.

Cautions

Fluoride supplements should be used with caution in patients with joint pain or rheumatic disease. Fluoride supplements may exacerbate gastrointestinal disease and ulcers.

QUICK GUIDE

Essential for

- normal metabolism, growth and development as it is a component of thyroid hormones

Absorption and metabolism

Iodine is efficiently absorbed and excess is excreted in the urine.

Deficiency

Iodine deficiency leads to hypothyroidism, goiter and cretinism; and may play a role in fibrocystic breast disease.

Sources

Good sources include vegetables grown in iodine-rich soil, iodised salt, seafood and milk. The iodine content of food varies with the location in which the food is grown. The table on page 246 can be used as a guide.

Daily recommended dietary intakes

Men	150 mcg
Women	150 mcg
Pregnant women	175 mcg
Lactating women	200 mcg

Toxic effects of excess intake

Toxic effects of iodine include a reduction in thyroid hormone secretion, acne, and inflammation of the salivary glands.

Therapeutic uses of supplements

Iodine supplements are used to treat deficiency disorders and have also been used to treat fibrocystic breast disease. Topical iodine is used as an antiseptic.

Cautions

Potassium iodide supplements should be used with caution in pregnancy and in cases of dehydration, acne, heat cramps, adrenal insufficiency, and cardiac disease.

Iodine is an essential trace element for humans. The average adult body contains between 20 and 50 mg iodine, and more than 60 per cent of this is concentrated in the thyroid gland situated at the base of the neck. The rest is in thyroid hormones in the blood, ovaries and muscles. Worldwide soil distribution of iodine is extremely variable and food grown in areas of low iodine does not contain enough of the mineral to meet requirements. Such areas include a band across the middle of the USA, the Midlands and South West England, and areas of China, Continental Europe, Russia and South America.

What it does in the body

Thyroid gland

Iodine is a component of the thyroid hormones triiodothyronine and thyroxin, which determine the metabolic rate of the body. This affects the body's conversion of food into energy and also the way energy is used.

Thyroid hormones are vital for growth and development of all organs, especially the brain, reproductive organs, nerves, bones, skin, hair, nails and teeth. The thyroid is involved in protein manufacture, cholesterol synthesis, carbohydrate absorption and the conversion of carotene to vitamin A. Thyroxin is an important regulator of body weight.

Absorption and metabolism

Iodine is rapidly absorbed from the gut. Excesses are excreted in the urine.

Deficiency

Iodine deficiency leads to various illnesses which are known as iodine deficiency disorders and include hypothyroidism, goiter and cretinism. Intakes of less than 50 mcg per day induce deficiency.

Hypothyroidism and goiter

When body iodine stores are exhausted, the thyroid gland in the neck is influenced by the pituitary gland to increase its activity and can become enlarged. This swelling is known as a goiter. Other symptoms of hypothyroidism include fatigue, apathy, drowsiness, sensitivity to cold, lethargy, muscle weakness, weight gain and coarse skin. Young men and women in iodine-deficient areas are at the greatest risk of developing goiter.

Deficiency of iodine is an important world health problem but is relatively rare in industrialized countries due to iodine fortification of salt. Those who still suffer from goiter may do so because they eat too many foods which block iodine utilization. These foods are known as goitrogens and include raw cabbage, kale, turnips, peanuts, soybeans and cauliflower. Drugs such as disulfiram, thiouracil, thiourea and sulfonamide can also inhibit the thyroid gland and lead to deficiency.

A reduction of salt in the diet, combined with a growing consumption of manufactured food prepared using low iodine salt, may lead to an increased risk of deficiency in areas where there is little natural iodine.

Cretinism

Severe iodine deficiency in a mother's diet during pregnancy increases the risk of miscarriage and stillbirth. If the baby survives to term, it is likely to suffer irreversible mental retardation. This is known as cretinism and is a major cause of preventable intellectual impairment in low iodine areas. Mildly iodine-deficient children have learning disabilities and poor motivation. The developing fetus, newborn and young children are most susceptible to the effects of an iodine-deficient diet, and treatment before conception or in early pregnancy is essential to prevent irreversible damage. Breast milk contains more iodine than formula milk and premature babies who are formula-fed may be at risk of deficiency.

Breast disorders

Iodine deficiency may play a role in fibrocystic breast disease. (See page 609 for more information.) Hypothyroidism and iodine deficiency may also increase the risk of breast cancer, as a higher incidence of disease has been found in iodine-deficient areas.[1]

Sources

Good sources of iodine include vegetables grown in iodine-rich soil, kelp, onions, milk, milk products, salt water fish and seafood. The iodine content of vegetables varies widely with the iodine content of the soil in which they are grown. The table below can be used as a guide.

Sodium or potassium iodide is added to table salt in many countries including the USA, Switzerland, Australia and New Zealand. Salt used in the processing and refining of foods is not usually iodized. Potassium iodate is used in the baking of some bread.

Food	Amount	Iodine (mcg)
Mackerel	150g	255
Mussels	150g	180
Cod	150g	165
Kipper	150g	107
Whiting	150g	100
Yogurt	150g	95
Milk	560g	86
Cockles	50g	80
Fish fingers	75g	75
Pilchards in tomato sauce	100g	64
Scampi	150g	62
Herring	150g	48
Beer	560g	45
Plaice	150g	42
Prawns	150g	42
Eggs	70g	37
Sardines, canned in oil	150g	35
Trout	150g	24
Kidney	150g	23
Liver	150g	22
Tuna	150g	21
Bacon	150g	18
Cheese	40g	18
Potato chips	265g	13

The average iodine intake in the USA is over 600 mcg per day.

Recommended dietary allowances

	Men	*Women*	*Pregnancy*	*Lactation*
USA	150 mcg	150 mcg	175 mcg	200 mcg
UK	140 mcg	140 mcg		
Australia	150 mcg	120 mcg	150 mcg	200 mcg

Supplements

Iodine supplements come in various forms including ammonium iodide, calcium iodide, potassium iodide and kelp. People who live in low soil iodine areas who restrict the salt in their diet and do not eat fish may benefit from iodine supplements.

Toxic effects of excess intake

Symptoms of acute poisoning from ingestion of iodine (rather than iodide) are mainly due to its corrosive effects on the gastrointestinal tract and include vomiting, abdominal pain and diarrhea. Other symptoms may include metallic taste, sore teeth, gum and mouth, and severe headache. Eventually the kidneys fail to produce urine. A fatal dose is 2 to 3 g of iodine. Treatment is with large volumes of milk and starch solutions with 1 per cent solution of potassium thiosulfate.

Toxic effects from the iodide form of iodine are rare and may include a reduction of thyroid hormone secretion, acne, and inflammation of the salivary glands when doses reach 1500 mcg. Dietary intake of iodine should not exceed 1000 mcg per day for any length of time. Toxic symptoms may result from high intakes which occur as part of medical treatment with iodine as iodides. Patients may become hypersensitive after prolonged oral administration.

Topical application of iodine-containing disinfectants may lead to hypothyroidism in newborn babies.

A disorder known as hyperthyroidism of Graves disease is due to an overactive thyroid. It is not due to over-consumption of iodine, but happens as a result of a disruption in the mechanisms that control thyroid hormone function.

Therapeutic uses of supplements

Supplemental iodine is used to treat iodine deficiency disorders. On a large scale, this is often given in the form of iodized salt or as an iodized oil injection.

Fibrocystic breast disease

Some studies have shown that iodine treatment can relieve the symptoms of fibrocystic breast disease. In 1993, Canadian researchers published a review of trials using iodine replacement therapy to treat fibrocystic breast disease. Preparations used included sodium iodide, protein-bound iodide and molecular iodine. Beneficial effects were seen with all the treatments, but molecular iodine was found to be the most beneficial.[2] Thyroid hormone replacement therapy may also be beneficial.

Other uses

Iodine is an antiseptic and can be used to kill bacteria and fungi. Iodine used topically as a douche is effective against a wide range of organisms including candida and chlamydia. Excessive use should be avoided since some iodine will be absorbed into the system and can cause suppression of thyroid function. Iodine tablets are frequently used to disinfect water.

Iodine can also be used to prevent radioactive damage to the thyroid gland. In nuclear accidents, radioactive iodine is released into the atmosphere and can be taken up by the thyroid, possibly causing cancer. Immediate treatment with iodine prevents this uptake.

Cautions

Potassium iodide supplements should be used with caution in cases of dehydration, acne, heat cramps, adrenal insufficiency, and cardiac disease. Prolonged use during pregnancy is not advisable.

QUICK GUIDE

Essential for

- oxygen transport and storage in the blood and muscles
- fatty acid metabolism
- energy production
- maintenance of a healthy immune system

Absorption and metabolism

Vitamin C improves iron absorption. Iron from animal foods is better absorbed than that from plant foods.

Deficiency

Iron deficiency leads to weakness, fatigue, reduced resistance to infection and eventually to anemia.

Sources

These include meat, whole grains and dark green leafy vegetables.

Daily recommended dietary intakes

Men	10 mg
Women (premenopause)	15 mg
Women (postmenopause)	10 mg
Pregnancy	30 mg

Toxic effects of excess intake

These include deterioration of the gut lining and liver damage. Excess intake may increase the risk of atherosclerosis and heart disease.

Interactions

Iron competes with magnesium, copper, calcium and zinc for absorption. Vitamin E supplements should not be taken at the same time as iron supplements.

Therapeutic uses of supplements

Iron supplements are used to prevent and treat deficiency. 'Ferrous' forms of iron are better absorbed than 'ferric' forms (check supplement labels).

Cautions

Supplements should be avoided by those with ulcers, IBD, arthritis, hemochromatosis, hepatitis, by blood transfusion recipients, and during acute infections.

The therapeutic use of iron dates back thousands of years. The Egyptians prescribed it as a cure for baldness and the Greeks recommended iron in wine as a way to restore male potency. Iron is the most abundant element on earth and is an essential trace mineral for humans. The human body contains about 3.5 to 4.5 g of iron. Two thirds of this is present in blood and the rest is stored in the liver, spleen, bone marrow and muscles.

What it does in the body

Oxygen transport and storage

Red blood cells contain a protein called hemoglobin and each hemoglobin molecule contains four iron atoms. The iron in hemoglobin binds oxygen when it passes through blood vessels in the lungs and releases it in the tissues. After releasing the oxygen, hemoglobin binds carbon dioxide, the waste product of respiration, and carries it back to the lungs to be released. Red blood cells and the iron they contain, are recycled and replaced every 120 days. Another iron-containing molecule, myoglobin, carries and stores oxygen in the cells and is therefore essential for cellular activities in all body tissues.

Metabolism

Enzymes involved in many metabolic functions require iron. It is necessary for cell division and growth through its role in DNA synthesis. It is also essential for protein metabolism.

Energy production

Iron plays a role in oxygen transfer in cytochromes, protein molecules involved in the production of energy in cells.

Other functions

Thyroid hormones, which regulate metabolic processes, require iron for production. Iron is involved in the production of connective tissue and several brain neurotransmitters, and in the maintenance of a healthy immune system.

Absorption and metabolism

Healthy people absorb around 5 to 10 per cent of the iron in their daily diets. Absorption is highest in childhood, and reduces with age. Iron is present in animal foods in organic 'heme' form and in plant foods in inorganic 'nonheme' form. The heme and nonheme forms of iron are absorbed by different mechanisms.[1] About 20 to 30 per cent of heme iron is absorbed compared to only 2 to 5 per cent of nonheme iron. Vitamin C consumed in the same meal as nonheme iron improves absorption by up to 50 per cent. Vitamin A and beta carotene can also improve nonheme iron absorption.[2]

Iron must be in ferrous form to be absorbed and the hydrochloric acid of the stomach converts ferric iron to ferrous iron. Iron absorption is a slow process, taking between two and four hours. Iron levels in the body are regulated by absorption, rather than by excretion and low body iron levels lead to improved absorption. In cases of iron deficiency absorption efficiency increases to around 10 to 20 per cent.

Various food factors affect iron absorption and the overall amount of iron absorbed from a meal will depend on the interactions between these factors. Sugars and amino acids may boost absorption. Calcium supplements, zinc supplements, oxalates in green vegetables such as spinach, and tannins in tea and coffee can reduce absorption. Phytates in unleavened whole grain bread reduce iron absorption although this may be reversed in the presence of meat and vitamin C. Milk proteins, albumin and soy proteins may also reduce absorption.

As it is highly chemically reactive, iron can cause damage to proteins and fats in cell membranes. It is therefore bound to proteins in the body to limit its toxic effects and is not excreted in the urine. A protein known as transferrin, binds to iron and is responsible for its transfer to the bone marrow. Iron is stored in the form of ferritin, mostly in the bone marrow, liver and spleen. Body iron stores depend on the iron absorbed from the diet. They are usually in the range of 300 to 1000 mg for adult women and 300 to 1500 mg for men. The levels vary considerably between people and some healthy adult women have almost no body stores. In the iron overload disorder, hemochromatosis, body iron stores may reach 30 g.

About 24 mg iron is released daily from normal breakdown of red blood cells in the liver and spleen, but most of this is conserved by the body. Iron is lost from the body through bleeding, sloughing of cells, menstrual flow and transfer to a developing fetus. Iron losses during a typical menstrual period are about 15 mg. Losses during breastfeeding are about 0.5 mg daily.

Tests which measure iron levels

There are various blood tests to measure the levels of iron in the body.

Serum ferritin

Serum ferritin is the most useful measure of iron status as it accurately reflects body stores and is the earliest laboratory measure to reflect iron deficiency. It can be used to detect iron deficiency and excess. Normal serum ferritin levels are 40 to 160 mcg per liter, with iron deficiency anemia indicated by a level of 12 mcg per liter.

Serum iron

Serum iron is the concentration of iron in the serum (clear) part of the blood. Normally it is about 100 mcg per 100 ml of blood, although this varies during the day by as much as 30 per cent within a single person. Serum iron is sensitive to the day's dietary intake and is not a reliable predictor of iron status.

TIBC

Total iron-binding capacity (TIBC) is the total amount of iron that can be bound by transferrin. Normally it ranges from 250 to 450 mcg per 100 ml of blood. Transferrin saturation is calculated from serum iron and TIBC. It is an index of iron transport rather than storage. In conditions of deficiency TIBC is increased, serum iron is low and transferrin saturation is reduced (around 15 per cent). In the iron overload disease, hemochromatosis, serum iron is normal, TIBC may be decreased and transferrin saturation may be 100 per cent.

Deficiency

Iron deficiency may be the most common nutritional deficiency in the USA. Results from the third National Health and Nutrition Examination Survey (1988-1994) suggest that iron deficiency and iron deficiency anemia are still relatively common in toddlers, adolescent girls, and women of childbearing age. Nine per cent of toddlers aged 1 to 2 years, and 9 per cent to 11 per cent of adolescent girls and women of childbearing age were iron deficient; of these, iron deficiency anemia was found in 3 per cent and 2 per cent to 5 per cent, respectively. These prevalences correspond to approximately 700,000 toddlers and 7.8 million women with iron deficiency; of these, approximately 240,000 toddlers and 3.3 million women have iron deficiency anemia. Iron deficiency occurred in around 7 per cent of older children or those older than 50 years, and in around 1 per cent of teenage boys and young men.[3]

Infants under two years of age are at risk due to their rapid growth rate, low iron reserves and the low iron content of milk and other foods. Teenagers, particularly girls who menstruate, are at risk due to the large amount of iron needed for rapid growth. Deficiencies are also common in women during childbearing years as menstruation, pregnancy and lactation draw heavily on the body's iron stores. Iron deficiency is also common in the elderly as they have reduced stomach acid and therefore reduced absorption ability. Surgery also leads to anemia and this is related to the extent of the surgery.[4]

Other causes of iron deficiency include heavy menstrual periods, frequent blood donation, and diseases of the stomach or bowel which reduce absorption. Some anti-arthritis drugs, which may cause repeated small bleeds from the stomach, may also lead to deficiency. It is important to carefully investigate the source of iron deficiency as slow blood loss from the gut or the uterus may be the cause.

Symptoms of iron deficiency include anemia, fatigue, rapid heartbeat, breathlessness, inability to concentrate, giddiness, disturbed sleep, severe menstrual pain and bleeding, cracks in the corners of the mouth, eye inflammation, mouth ulcers and hair loss. Low blood plasma levels of iron can cause generalized itching especially in elderly people. Fingernails may become thin, brittle and white.

A pregnant woman with an iron deficiency is more prone to infection after delivery, spontaneous abortion and premature delivery. Iron deficiency also increases the risk of low birthweight babies, stillbirth and infant death. Infants born of anemic mothers may also be at risk of anemia.

A new National Institute of Aging study suggests that low iron levels are linked to an increased likelihood of death in elderly people. Researchers looked at the iron status of nearly 4000 men and women aged 71 and over. Results of the five-year study showed that low iron levels increased the risk of total and coronary heart disease deaths. Those with higher iron levels had decreased risk. Men with the highest iron levels had only 20 per cent of the risk of dying of heart disease of those with the lowest levels. Women with the highest levels were about half as likely to die of heart disease compared to those with the lowest levels. Iron levels tend to be lower in people with chronic disease as the body's needs are higher and normal dietary intake may not be sufficient to meet the body's needs. Other research has linked high iron levels with an increased risk of heart disease. This new study suggests that the picture is not that simple.[5]

Anemia

Anemia is the final stage of iron deficiency. (See page 512 for more information.) Before the red blood cells show anemia, deficiency affects iron- dependent enzymes and immune functions. Symptoms include small pale red blood cells, extreme fatigue, difficulty concentrating, breathlessness and dizziness. Symptoms of anemia can develop gradually and may continue without being recognized for some time. Hemoglobin and hematocrit blood tests may not show evidence of anemia in the early stages and serum ferritin and TIBC tests are the best and most sensitive measures of iron levels. Iron levels may also vary from day to day, and the average value from multiple tests provides the best readings.

Iron deficiency anemia is the most common nutritional deficiency in children. It can lead to depressed growth and impaired mental performance. The baby of a well-nourished mother is born with enough iron to last four months and must also obtain iron from breast milk or formula. Although it is low in iron, breast milk is high in lactose and vitamin C which enhance absorption. Infant formula is fortified with iron and vitamin C. Researchers involved in a 1997 Canadian study assessed iron status and feeding practices at 39 weeks of age in 434 infants in Vancouver. They found iron-deficiency anemia in 7 per cent of infants and low iron stores in about 24 per cent.[6]

Some iron-deficient people develop cravings for ice, clay, soil or other materials, a condition known as pica.

Immune system

Immune response can be impaired in iron-deficient people. Chronic yeast infections and herpes infections are more common in those who have low levels of iron in their diets. Certain types of immune cells rely on iron to generate the oxidative reactions that allow these cells to kill off bacteria and other pathogens. When iron levels are low these cells cannot function properly.

Athletes

Heavy exercise may lead to iron deficiency with distance runners particularly at risk. "Sports anemia" is often used to describe a low hemoglobin condition which impairs exercise tolerance and is relatively common at the beginning of training. Symptoms of iron deficiency in athletes include reduction in exercise time, increased heart rate, decreased oxygen consumption and increased blood lactic acid. The deficiency may result from increased metabolic requirements, increased red blood cell breakdown and increased iron losses in sweat. However, unless a person is iron-deficient, supplements do not appear to improve athletic performance. After adaptation, the anemia seems to subside. It may be due to inadequate dietary intake of iron or the use of protein for tasks other than red blood cell production during the early training stages. Iron intake of athletes needs to be carefully monitored.

Other symptoms

Iron deficiency has also been associated with Plummer-Vinson syndrome where a thin web-like membrane grows across the top of the esophagus, making it difficult to swallow. This disease, once fairly common in Sweden, has been eliminated with the use of iron supplements.

Marginal iron deficiency may also contribute to sleeping difficulties, headaches, rheumatoid arthritis and restless legs syndrome

Low iron levels may increase the risk of menstrual difficulties including behavioral changes and sweating and dizziness, decreased efficiency, poor performance at work and daytime napping. Iron deficiency can also adversely affect the heart. Iron-deficient people have abnormal electrocardiogram readings.

Sources

Good sources include liver, meat, beans, nuts, dried fruits, poultry, fish, whole grains or enriched cereals, soybean flour and most dark green leafy vegetables. Flour is enriched with iron. Cooking in cast iron pots can increase the level of iron in food by as much as 20 times, although this form of iron may not be well-absorbed. Acidic foods such as chili and spaghetti sauce are especially good at leaching out the iron from cooking pots. The longer the food cooks in the pot the more iron is absorbed. The substitution of aluminum, stainless steel or plastic pots has reduced iron intake.

Those who choose not to eat red meat, which is the best source of dietary iron, should include dark green leafy vegetables, dried beans and whole cereal grains in their diet. A vegetarian diet is often high in vitamin C which helps in iron absorption.

Food	Amount	Iron (mg)
Branflakes	1 cup	10.8
Lambs liver, fried	100g	8.2

Spinach, cooked	1 cup	6.4
Apricots, dried	1 cup, halves	6.1
Chickpeas, boiled	1 cup	4.7
All Bran	½ cup	4.5
Oysters, fried	6 oysters	4.4
Salmon, canned	1 can	3.8
Oats	½ cup	3.7
Beef, cooked, lean and fat	¾ cup, diced	2.6
Almonds	½ cup	2.6
Tuna, canned	1 can	2.5
Hamburger patty	1 serve	2.4
Pearl barley, boiled	1 cup	2.1
Cashews, salted	½ cup	2.0
Lamb	100g	2.0
Bulgur, boiled	1 cup	1.7
Raisins	½ cup	1.7
Sausages, grilled	2 thick, 10cm long	1.3
Liverwurst	1 slice	1.2
Bread, wholegrain	1 slice	1.1
Pita bread, wholewheat	1 small	0.8
Paté	1 tbsp	0.7
Baked beans	1 cup	0.7

Recommended dietary allowances

	Men	*Women Premenopause*	*Women Postmenopause*	*Pregnancy*
USA	10 mg	15 mg	10 mg	30 mg
UK(over 19)	8.7 mg	14.8 mg	8.7 mg	
(under 19)	11.3 mg			
Australia	7 mg	12 to 16 mg	5 to 7 mg	+10 to 20 mg

Because the iron from red blood cells is recycled and re-used, recommended requirements are small for healthy men and postmenopausal women. Iron requirements increase in pregnancy due to the increase in the mother's blood volume and the demands of the developing baby. (See table)

Iron intakes in North America and Europe average around 5 to 7 mg per 1000 calories. Thus those on low calorie diets may be at risk of deficiency.

Supplements

Iron supplements come in a variety of preparations including syrups, tablets, capsules and injections. These contain varying forms and amounts of iron. Ferrous salts are absorbed better than ferric salts. Ferrous fumarate and ferrous succinate contain the most iron (31.2 and 32.6 mg per 100 mg respectively). Ferrous succinate and ferrous sulfate (the most common) may be the most easily absorbed forms of iron but ferrous sulfate can cause gut irritation. Ferrous gluconate and ferrous fumarate are also well-absorbed and usually less irritating.

Iron supplements are also available in the form of ferritin, an iron protein complex. The hydrolyzed protein chelate form of iron (most effective with the amino acid cysteine) may cause the least side effects but may not be as well-absorbed as other forms. Supplements are usually best absorbed on an empty stomach and people may vary in their tolerance to different iron salts.

Women of childbearing age, the elderly, adolescents, athletes and alcoholics may benefit from supplements. Women who have heavy menstrual blood loss and who use intra-uterine contraceptive devices may need extra iron. The contraceptive pill reduces menstrual blood flow and may lead to decreased iron requirements.

Vegetarians may also benefit from iron supplements as they avoid easily absorbed iron sources such as meat and seafood. In addition, there are compounds in plant fiber which lead to reduced iron absorption. However, increased vitamin C may compensate.

Toxic effects of excess intake

Large doses of iron can cause deterioration of the gut lining, vomiting and diarrhea, liver damage, abdominal and joint pain, weight loss, fatigue, excess thirst and hunger. Immediate medical attention is necessary. It is important to keep iron supplements out of reach of children as doses as low as 3 g can cause death in children and every year there are a few cases of fatal poisoning.

Constipation is the most common side effect associated with iron supplements, although diarrhea can also occur. Side effects can be reduced if the iron supplements are taken in small divided doses with meals. Doses of 25 to 75 mg per day have been taken without side effects, although those with iron overload or kidney disorders might develop symptoms at lower doses.

In most people iron absorption becomes less efficient as blood levels reach optimum and dietary excesses pass out in feces. Accumulation is possible; however, as excesses are not easily excreted once absorbed. Heme iron absorption may be less affected by the iron status of the individual than nonheme iron absorption, making it easier to overdose on diets high in animal foods.

Hemochromatosis

Hemochromatosis is the term used to refer to iron overload disorders. It may be hereditary, due to excessive intake or due to chronic alcoholism. Hereditary hemochromatosis is an inherited condition of defective iron metabolism in which the body lacks the ability to limit iron absorption from the diet and stores greater than normal amounts. This iron is stored in the liver, heart, pancreas, skin and other organs and can generate free radicals which cause serious damage. In the US, the disorder is known to affect 1.5 million people. Many experts believe hemochromatosis is under-diagnosed and may occur in as many as one in 200 people. The effects are usually seen in men over 50 years of age as the disease can often go undetected until mid-life when iron levels reach five to 50 times normal amounts. The initial symptoms are fatigue, achy joints and weakness. Other symptoms include heart disorders, joint pain, cirrhosis of the liver, diabetes and excessive skin pigmentation.

Researchers involved in the Framingham Heart Study have found high iron intakes to be common in elderly people with around 91 per cent of study participants having intakes above the recommended dietary levels. Only one per cent of the people had iron deficiency anemia.

Iron accumulation can contribute to a variety of disorders such as cancer, heart disease, arthritis, osteoporosis, diabetes and psychiatric illnesses. The liver is particularly susceptible to the toxic effects of iron as it is the major site of iron storage in the body. Treatment for hemochromatosis involves repeated bleeding (phlebotomy) to remove excess iron. Therapy for hemochromatosis may also involve a diet rich in bread and cereals, and fruit and vegetables. The amount of meat and alcohol should be limited. Tea or coffee may be drunk with meals as this will reduce iron absorption. Foods and supplements rich in vitamin C, such as fruit and fruit juice, should be avoided with meals.

Early therapy is very important to prevent complications and increase the chance of normal life expectancy. A test is advisable for those with a family history of hemochromatosis.

Cardiovascular disease

The evidence from many scientific studies suggests that high iron levels (above 200 mcg per liter blood ferritin), may lead to an increase in the risk of cardiovascular disease. The increased risk may be due to oxidative damage to the heart and blood vessels and increased oxidation of LDL cholesterol.

A study published in 1998 in the *American Journal of Epidemiology* suggests that men and women, particularly those over 60, are at increased risk of heart disease if they have high levels of iron in their diets. The study, which was conducted in Greece, involved 329 patients with heart disease and 570 people of similar age who were admitted to hospital with minor conditions believed to be unrelated to diet. Results showed that for every 50 mg increase in iron intake per month, men over 60 were 1.47 times more likely to have heart disease than their peers. In women over 60, the risk was even higher, with a 3.61-fold risk for every 50 mg increase.[7]

In a paper published in 1997, Austrian researchers involved in the Bruneck study investigated the links between serum ferritin concentrations and the five-year progression of carotid atherosclerosis in 826 men and women aged 40 to 79 years old. Serum ferritin was one of the strongest risk predictors of overall progression of atherosclerosis, probably due to increased oxidation of LDL cholesterol. Changes in iron stores during the follow-up period modified atherosclerosis risk, in that a lowering was beneficial and further iron accumulation exerted unfavorable effects. High serum ferritin and LDL cholesterol also increased the risk of death from cardiovascular disease.[8]

Another study published in 1998 in the American Heart Association journal *Circulation* suggests that men with high levels of stored iron in the body have an increased risk of heart attack. The Study, which was done in Finland, involved 99 men who had had at least one heart attack and 99 healthy men matched for background and age. The results showed that those men with the highest iron levels had almost three times the risk of heart attack when compared with those with the lowest levels.[9]

Donating blood may help prevent a heart attack according to a 1998 study reported in the *American Journal of Epidemiology.* The results of a Finnish study showed that middle aged men who gave blood had an 88 per cent lower risk of heart attack than those who had not donated. In a group of 2862 men, less than 1 per cent of the blood donors had heart attacks compared with 12.5 per cent of the non-donors.[10]

Cancer

Some studies have shown that iron can inhibit tumor development while others have shown that it might enhance it. Iron may increase the risk of cancer through its effect on free radical formation. In some population studies, high iron levels have been associated with an increased risk of throat and gastrointestinal cancers while others have not shown links.[11] Results from a study assessing the links between body iron stores and cancer in 3287 men and 5269 women participating in the first National Health and Nutrition Examination Survey (NHANES I) found an increased risk with high iron levels.[12] Some experts believe that the findings of increased risk are due to causes such as defects in iron metabolism, rather than diet alone.

Other disorders

High iron levels may also worsen the joint inflammation associated with rheumatoid arthritis. High iron levels may also lead to an increased risk of infection as iron is necessary for bacterial growth. Vitamin A supplementation may help to control the adverse effects in areas where infections are prevalent.[13]

Therapeutic uses of supplements

Prevention and treatment of deficiency

Iron supplements are used to treat cases of iron deficiency anemia, generalized itching and impaired mental performance in the young. The usual dose for treatment of deficiency is 100 mg per day in adults and 2 mg per kg of body weight per day in children. Doses are low to start with and increased gradually to reduce side effects. It may take one to two months to correct anemia and iron supplements may be needed for a further several months afterwards to replenish iron stores.

Pregnancy

Iron supplements are often recommended for pregnant women due to the high demands of the developing baby and may also be useful after pregnancy. During the last three months of pregnancy, 3 to 4 mg of iron are transferred to the baby each day. The number of red blood cells in the mother's blood increases by 20 to 30 per cent. It is often very difficult to meet these increased needs from diet alone, and many doctors recommend iron supplements. They are particularly important for women with low iron stores. Iron is also very important for women who are breastfeeding, especially if they are recovering from blood loss during delivery or depletion of body stores during pregnancy. Breastfeeding causes needs to increase by around 0.5 to 1 mg per day.

Mental function

Iron supplements may improve verbal learning and memory in those susceptible to iron deficiency even in those who are not anemic. In a study published in *The Lancet* in 1996, researchers at Johns Hopkins University evaluated 78 adolescent girls with non-anemic iron deficiency and measured their cognitive ability, memory and concentration. The girls were then divided into two groups, some were given a placebo and some were given iron supplements. After eight weeks, measurements showed an increase in iron levels in the supplement group while the levels in the placebo group remained low. Tests showed that the girls who took the iron supplements performed better on the verbal learning and memory tests than the girls who took placebo. Both groups scored the same on tests measuring their ability to pay attention and concentrate. There was a direct relationship between how much the blood iron levels went up and the ability to learn.[14]

Interactions with other nutrients

Iron in the ferric form oxidizes vitamin E and reduces its effectiveness. Ferrous forms of iron do not usually interact with vitamin E. Vitamin E may reduce the possible harmful oxidative effects of iron.

Iron competes with magnesium, copper, calcium and zinc for absorption in the intestine, and excess intake of one of these minerals could produce a deficiency of the others. Nicotinic acid seems to enhance iron utilization.[15]

Interactions with drugs

Antacids, anti-arthritis drugs, allopurinol for gout, aspirin, and cholestyramine may decrease iron absorption and should be taken several hours apart from supplements. Iron may decrease absorption of thyroxin, tetracyclines, penicillamine, ciprofloxacin or norfloxacin.

Elevated serum levels of iron may reduce the effectiveness of interferon therapy for the hepatitis C virus.

Cautions

Children should not be given large doses of iron supplements. Iron is an important nutrient for bacteria and supplements should be avoided during acute infections, particularly in the young.

Iron supplements should be avoided in cases of peptic ulcers and inflammatory bowel disease as iron can have a corrosive effect and exacerbate these conditions. Blood transfusion recipients and sufferers of thalassemia, hemochromatosis and hepatitis should also avoid iron supplements. Iron preparations by injection may cause a flare-up of rheumatoid arthritis.

QUICK GUIDE

Essential for

- production and transfer of energy
- a healthy heart, bones, muscles and blood vessels
- protein and carbohydrate metabolism
- transport of substances across cell membranes
- manufacture of genetic material

Absorption and metabolism

About 50 per cent of dietary magnesium is absorbed.

Deficiency

Symptoms include fatigue, mental and heart problems. Marginal deficiency may lead to cardiovascular disease, hypertension, diabetes, osteoporosis, asthma, migraine, PMS and kidney stones.

Sources

These include whole grains, nuts and green vegetables.

Daily recommended dietary intakes

Men (under 30)	400mg		
Men (over 30)	420 mg		
Women (under 30)	310 mg		
Women (over 30)	320 mg		
Pregnancy (14 to 18)	400 mg	Lactation (14 to 18)	360 mg
Pregnancy (19 to 30)	350 mg	Lactation (19 to 30)	310 mg
Pregnancy (over 30)	360 mg	Lactation (over 30)	320 mg

Toxic effects of excess intake

Symptoms include skin flushing, nervous depression and fatigue.

Interactions

Calcium and magnesium act together in many body functions. Alcohol, diuretics, antidepressants, estrogen and heart drugs can increase requirements.

Therapeutic uses of supplements

These include treatment of stress, fatigue, cardiovascular disease, migraine, kidney stones, asthma, premenstrual syndrome, osteoporosis, muscle cramps, pre-eclampsia and diabetes.

Cautions

Magnesium supplements should not be used by those who have impaired kidney function or serious heart disease.

Magnesium is one of the most abundant minerals in soft tissue. The average adult body contains about 20 to 28 g of magnesium with about 60 per cent of this present in the bones, and the rest in the muscle, soft tissue and body fluids. Magnesium is found in high concentrations inside cells, particularly those of the brain and heart. Research into the role of magnesium is increasing in clinical importance as growing evidence suggests that magnesium deficiency may play a role in a number of disorders.

What it does in the body

Metabolism

Magnesium is a co-factor in over 300 enzyme reactions, particularly those involving the metabolism of food components and the formation of new compounds essential for good health. All enzymatic reactions requiring the energy storage molecule, adenosine triphosphate (ATP), require magnesium. It is also needed for protein synthesis, DNA manufacture, fatty acid synthesis, anaerobic breakdown of glucose; and the removal of toxic substances, such as ammonia, from the body.

Bone

Magnesium is vital for healthy bone structure.

Interaction with calcium

Calcium interacts with magnesium in many body processes, such as the regulation of blood vessel tone and contraction of muscles, including heart muscle. Calcium stimulates muscles and contracts blood vessels, while magnesium relaxes muscles and dilates blood vessels. Magnesium can contribute to calcium balance by affecting the hormones which control calcium absorption and metabolism, and also influences calcium at the cellular level by interacting with calcium transport mechanisms.

Ion transport

Magnesium is involved in the maintenance of the membrane electric potential and the transport across membranes of sodium, potassium and calcium. Magnesium is involved in nerve impulse transmission.

Hormone action

Magnesium is necessary for the action of a compound which plays a vital role in transmitting messages from hormones and other stimuli which cause chemical reactions inside cells. Magnesium also enhances insulin secretion, and helps it to move into cells, thus facilitating sugar metabolism.

Absorption and metabolism

Magnesium is mostly absorbed in the small intestine. In a normal person, around 50 per cent of dietary magnesium taken is absorbed. However, this depends on the concentration in the diet, with a lower percentage absorbed from a high magnesium diet. Magnesium absorption requires an acidic stomach environment. Absorption is reduced by laxative abuse, infections and allergies. Foods low in protein or high in phosphorus can reduce magnesium absorption.

Oxalates, which are found in some green vegetables and phytates which are found in some grains, may form insoluble complexes with magnesium and prevent it from being absorbed. However, these foods are often high in magnesium which may compensate for the reduced absorption. Vitamin D promotes magnesium absorption. Some reports have suggested that magnesium and calcium compete for absorption but recent studies suggest that calcium does not affect magnesium absorption.[1]

The kidney is the main regulator of blood concentration and total body content of magnesium. Excretion mainly occurs at night. High protein and high sugar diets may increase magnesium excretion.

Deficiency

Magnesium deficiency affects all body tissues. Symptoms of severe deficiency, which is rare, include irritability, personality changes, anorexia, weakness, tiredness, vertigo, convulsions, nervousness, muscle cramps and tremors, tongue jerks and tremors, involuntary eye movements, unsteady gait, irregular heartbeat, palpitations, low blood sugar and sustained muscle contraction. Loss of hair, swollen gums, and damage to the arteries resembling atherosclerosis are symptoms of advanced deficiency. Magnesium deficiency leads to low blood calcium levels.

Deficiency can occur due to malnutrition, surgery, serious burns, kidney disease, pancreatic inflammation, liver disease, absorption disorders, diabetes, hormonal disorders, cancer, heavy exercise and pregnancy. A high dietary intake of phosphate, calcium, vitamin D and saturated fats may also lead to deficiency. Alcoholics and those taking diuretics are particularly at risk as these drugs both cause large urinary magnesium losses.

Marginal magnesium deficiency is considered to be very common and may affect 15 to 20 per cent of the population. It is common in those who eat diets high in processed foods, alcoholics, and in those with malabsorption problems.

Elderly people

Magnesium deficiency is especially prevalent in elderly people. This is due to low dietary intakes and also to the decreases in absorption and increases in excretion associated with aging.

Cardiovascular disease

Inadequate magnesium intake has been linked to several types of cardiovascular disease, including atherosclerosis, heart attack, angina, ischemic heart disease and cardiac arrhythmias. Epidemiological studies show that death rates from coronary heart disease are higher in areas where the water is low in magnesium. In a 1996 study, Swedish researchers investigated these links in 17 municipalities in the southern part of the country which had differing water magnesium concentrations. The study included 854 men who had died of heart attacks between the ages of 50 and 69, and 989 men of the same age in the same area who had died from cancer during the same time period. The results showed that men living in high magnesium water areas had a 35 per cent lower chance of death from heart attack than those who drank low magnesium water.[2] The results of a 1997 study done in Taiwan suggest that magnesium in drinking water helps to prevent death from cerebrovascular disease.[3]

Results from the Atherosclerosis Risk in Communities (ARIC) Study support the association between low serum and dietary magnesium, and various types of cardiovascular disease including high blood pressure. A total of 15 248 people took part, male and female, black and white, aged 45 to 64 years. The results showed that serum magnesium levels were significantly lower in participants with cardiovascular disease, high blood pressure, and diabetes than in those free of these diseases. Low dietary intake was linked to lower beneficial HDL cholesterol levels and thicker carotid artery walls, both of which increase the risk of cardiovascular disease.[4]

Researchers involved in a 1996 study done in Wales found a trend towards protection from ischemic heart disease in men with high magnesium intakes.

However, when other factors were taken into account, the results did not appear to be significant.[5] Magnesium deficiency is also linked to variant angina, a disorder in which coronary heart vessels go into spasm.[6] A 1996 Japanese study found that men with lower magnesium levels had more frequent and severe angina attacks.[7] Magnesium-deficient heart muscle is more vulnerable to lack of oxygen.

Magnesium deficiency may increase the risk of cardiovascular disease in several ways. Chronic magnesium deficiency in animals has been shown to result in microscopic changes in the heart arteries and the development of atherosclerosis. Deficiency also leads to changes in the heart muscle itself, including cell degeneration, fibrosis, necrosis and calcification. Blood fat levels are also affected by magnesium dietary intake. Cholesterol may be more susceptible to oxidative damage when magnesium levels are low. Some of the harmful effects of magnesium deficiency may be due to the products of increased fat oxidation.

Magnesium deficiency also contributes to cardiac arrhythmias, possibly because magnesium is responsible for maintaining potassium concentrations inside muscle cells. Potassium plays a role in heart muscle contraction. Magnesium deficiency has been implicated in mitral valve prolapse, a disorder in which the mitral valve in the heart fails to properly close off the heart chambers from each other during contraction. As many as 85 per cent of sufferers may have chronic magnesium deficiency.

High blood pressure

Results from the ARIC study mentioned above showed that low dietary intakes of magnesium are linked to higher diastolic and systolic blood pressures, possibly due to a reduction in the relaxing effect on blood vessels and by indirect effects on potassium balance. Studies suggest that around 30 per cent of high blood pressure sufferers consume inadequate amounts of magnesium and high blood pressure is more common in areas where the water is low in magnesium.

The Honolulu Heart Study, which looked at the relationship between dietary magnesium intake and blood pressure, found that those in the high intake group had, on average, systolic blood pressures 6.4 mmHg lower and diastolic pressures 3.1 mmHg lower than those in the low intake group.[8] In another survey of over 58 000 women, researchers found that those with magnesium intakes of less than 200 mg per day had a significantly higher risk of developing high blood pressure than women whose intakes were over 300 mg per day.[9] In another study published in 1992, researchers also found that low dietary intakes of magnesium were linked to an increased risk of high blood pressure in over 30 000 men.[10]

Diabetes

Magnesium deficiency results in impaired insulin secretion and reduces tissue sensitivity to insulin. Sub-clinical magnesium deficiency is common in diabetes and occurs because of insufficient magnesium intakes and increased magnesium losses, particularly in the urine. In Type II, or non-insulin-dependent, diabetes mellitus, magnesium deficiency seems to be associated with insulin resistance. It may also be involved in the development of diabetes complications and may contribute to the increased risk of sudden death associated with diabetes. Some studies suggest that magnesium deficiency may play a role in spontaneous abortion and birth defects in diabetic women.

Results from the ARIC study suggest that serum magnesium levels are low in those suffering from diabetes and that intake is related to insulin levels. Magnesium plays a role in the insulin-mediated uptake of glucose into cells, and deficiency may worsen control of diabetes.[11] Low blood magnesium levels are commonly associated with many complications of diabetes, including heart disease and high blood pressure.

According to research presented at the 1997 annual meeting of the American Diabetes Association, low magnesium levels predict Type II diabetes in whites. Researchers from Johns Hopkins University Medical School examined blood levels of magnesium in over 12 000 nondiabetic, middle-aged African American and white subjects and monitored them for six years. No relationship was found between magnesium levels and diabetes in African Americans, but a relationship was seen in whites.

Osteoporosis

Magnesium is vital for normal bone function and deficiency may contribute to osteoporosis. In a 1995 study, results showed that women whose dietary intakes were less than 187 mg per day had a lower bone mineral density than women whose average intakes were more than 187 mg.[12]

Magnesium is essential for the normal function of the parathyroid glands, metabolism of vitamin D, and adequate sensitivity of bone to parathyroid hormone and vitamin D. Magnesium deficiency may impair vitamin D metabolism which adversely affects bone-building.[13] Magnesium deficiency is also known to cause resistance to parathyroid hormone action which affects calcium balance and may cause abnormal bone formation.[14] However, magnesium excess inhibits parathyroid hormone secretion which means that bone metabolism is impaired under positive as well as under negative magnesium balance.[15] Maintaining normal calcium-to-magnesium balance is very important in the prevention of osteoporosis.

Migraine

Magnesium metabolism appears to be altered in some migraine sufferers and deficiency may contribute to symptoms through effects on neurotransmitters and blood vessels, and muscles in the head and neck.[16]

Premenstrual syndrome

Red blood cell concentrations of magnesium appear to be low in women with premenstrual syndrome. The calcium to magnesium ratio also seems to be affected by hormonal fluctuations which may affect neurotransmitter levels and lead to premenstrual symptoms.[17]

Asthma

Epidemiological evidence suggests that a low intake of magnesium is associated with impaired lung function, bronchial hyperreactivity and wheezing.

Kidney stones

Magnesium deficiency leads to kidney stones in animal studies. Magnesium inhibits the precipitation of calcium phosphate and calcium oxalate, two substances which contribute to the formation of kidney stones.

HIV/AIDS

Magnesium deficiency occurs early in the course of HIV infection. This may be relevant to the HIV-related symptoms of fatigue, lethargy and mental impairment.[18]

Exercise

Lack of magnesium decreases energy efficiency, and research has shown that people who are deficient in magnesium may use more energy during exercise. In a recent study, USDA researchers investigated the amount of oxygen needed by healthy women over 50 to perform a certain amount of low intensity work on an exercise bicycle. When their dietary magnesium was inadequate (150 mg daily) they used 10 to15 per cent more oxygen to perform the work and their heart rates climbed by about 10 beats per minute. The results suggest that magnesium deficiency is associated with increased physiological demands to do the same amount of work as when magnesium is adequate.

In a 1998 study, researchers from the University of Texas examined body magnesium concentrations in 26 marathon runners during an endurance run. They found that levels in the muscles and urine dropped significantly, possibly putting the athletes at risk of decreased performance and muscle cramps.[19]

Other symptoms

Magnesium deficiency may also play a role in pre-eclampsia and eclampsia (toxemia of pregnancy), leg cramps, sleeping problems, candida albicans infection, gastric cancer[20], allergies, chronic fatigue syndrome and anxiety. Low blood levels of magnesium are also sometimes found in bulimia nervosa sufferers and patients with irritable bowel syndrome.

Sources

Good sources of magnesium include whole grains, nuts, soybeans, avocados, beans, corn, lemons and dark green leafy vegetables, as magnesium forms part of the green pigment, chlorophyll. Meat is rich in magnesium but it also contains calcium, phosphate and protein which reduce the amount of available magnesium. Flour refining, rice polishing, sugar extraction from molasses and other methods of food processing remove almost all the magnesium from these foods. Modern food production has reduced the average magnesium intake from 400 mg per day to 300 mg per day over the last 70 years.

Drinking water is an important source of magnesium, especially in hard water areas, and is usually better absorbed than magnesium from food.

Food	Amount	Magnesium (mg)
Almonds	½ cup	200
Buckwheat	½ cup	186
Cashew nuts	½ cup	169
Wheat bran	½ cup	168
Spinach, boiled	1 cup	148
Soybeans, cooked	1 cup	141
Wheatgerm	½ cup	130
Peanuts	½ cup	124
Baked beans	1 cup	105
Beet greens	1 cup	92.2
Halibut, baked	85g	87.0
Black-eyed peas, cooked	1 cup	81.7
Brown rice, cooked	1 cup	79.8
Kidney beans, canned	1 cup	75.1

Chickpeas, cooked	1 cup	74.1
Artichokes, steamed	1 artichoke	72.0
Green peas	1 cup	58.9
Apricots, dried	1 cup	58.0
Oatmeal, cooked	1 cup	53.2
Sweetcorn	1 cup	49.4
Raisins	1 cup	45.6
Wholewheat spaghetti, cooked	1 cup	39.9
Avocado	½ avocado	35.0

Recommended dietary allowances

The RDAs for magnesium have recently been revised.

	Men	*Women*	*Pregnancy*	*Lactation*
USA				
(under 30)	400 mg	310 mg		
(over 30)	420 mg	320 mg		
(14 to 18)			400 mg	360 mg
(19 to 30)			350 mg	310 mg
(Over 31)			360 mg	320 mg
UK	300 mg	270 mg		320 mg
Australia	320 mg	270 mg	300 mg	340 mg

The tolerable upper intake limit is set at 350 mg for adults.

Magnesium requirements are increased during rapid growth in children and adolescents. The RDA for adolescent boys is 410 mg and for girls is 360 mg.

Studies have shown that most people may not get sufficient magnesium in their daily diets. Some research indicates that the RDAs for magnesium may be inadequate and that those who exercise may need up to 500 mg per day. Dr. Mildred Seelig, a well-known magnesium researcher, has recommended a daily intake of 6 to 10 mg per kg of body weight per day for optimal health.

Less than 1 per cent of the total body magnesium is present in blood. Thus, blood serum measurements of magnesium that are routinely made in a clinical setting assess only a small part of the total magnesium stores in the body and magnesium in the blood does not necessarily correlate with the amount of magnesium in other parts of the body. More sophisticated tests are not readily available in a clinical setting and even for these tests, results do not necessarily correlate with intracellular magnesium. Thus, there is no readily available test to determine intracellular/total body magnesium status. At present there is little information about the state of magnesium within body pools and deficiencies are difficult to pinpoint.

Supplements

Magnesium supplements are available in a variety of forms, with varying amounts of magnesium. These include magnesium carbonate, magnesium amino acid chelates, magnesium citrate and dolomite. Organic forms of magnesium, such as citrate, aspartate and fumarate, are better absorbed than inorganic forms such as magnesium oxide and magnesium hydroxide, which is why the last two are often used as laxatives. Enteric-coated magnesium supplements may not be as well-absorbed as magnesium in other types of supplements.[21]

Magnesium supplements should not be taken with meals as they neutralize stomach acid. The suggested ratio of intake of calcium to magnesium is about two-to-one although one-to-one may be better. Magnesium supplements may be best taken at night. Alcoholics, people under stress or who exercise heavily, diabetics, anyone taking diuretic drugs (which deplete magnesium), and women who suffer from PMS or who take the contraceptive pill may benefit from supplements.

Toxic effects of excess intake

Magnesium toxicity is rare as the body excretes excess. Symptoms of toxicity include diarrhea, flushing of the skin, thirst, low blood pressure, loss of reflexes, lethargy, weakness, fluid retention, nausea, vomiting and shallow breathing. The most common cause of excess magnesium is renal failure.

Therapeutic uses of supplements

Cardiovascular disease

Heart attack

Low magnesium levels have been found in the blood and cardiac muscle of heart attack victims, and several small studies have shown that magnesium sulfate injections can reduce death rates in heart attack patients, both in the short term and for longer periods.[22] It may act by improving energy production, inhibiting platelet aggregation, reducing vascular resistance, promoting clot breakdown, dilating blood vessels, and improving the function of heart muscle. It also protects the damaged heart muscle against calcium overload and reduces free radical damage.

However, two recently published studies showed different results, although similar doses of magnesium were used. The LIMIT-2-study was a double-blind, placebo-controlled investigation of over 2300 patients with suspected heart attack. Magnesium infusion reduced 28 day death risk by 24 per cent.[23] The ISIS-4-study on over 50 000 patients with suspected heart attack did not show any positive effect of magnesium on death rate.[24]

However, in the ISIS-4 study, magnesium was given after the end of drug therapy to break down blood clots. In LIMIT-2, magnesium infusion was started as early as possible. It seems that in heart attack patients who have been given clot break-down drugs, magnesium therapy is not useful. These studies also suggest that timing of the magnesium treatment is important, and evidence suggests that the injections should be given early. Magnesium injections also show more beneficial effects in higher risk patients.

Cardiac arrhythmias

Magnesium is reasonably well-established as a therapy for certain types of cardiac arrhythmia. It is usually given intravenously.[25] Post-operative administration can also reduce the incidence of arrhythmias following surgery. Magnesium may also enhance the action of digoxin, a drug often used to treat cardiac arrhythmia.

Angina

Magnesium supplements are often used to treat angina, both that caused by atherosclerosis and variant angina caused by coronary artery spasm. In a 1997 study, UK researchers assessed the effects of a 24-hour infusion of magnesium in patients with unstable angina. Thirty-one patients received magnesium sulfate and 31 placebo. After treatment, there were fewer ischemic episodes in the magnesium group, and duration of ischemia in the placebo group was longer than that in the magnesium group.[26]

Other heart conditions

Magnesium has also been used to treat cardiomyopathy, a weakening of heart muscle which leads to reduced efficiency of blood circulation and congestive heart failure. Sufferers of intermittent claudication, a painful condition caused by reduced blood flow to the legs, often have low magnesium levels and may be helped by supplements. Magnesium supplements have been successfully used to treat mitral valve prolapse.[27] Magnesium supplements have been shown to reduce cholesterol and triglyceride levels.

High blood pressure

Magnesium supplements may be useful in the treatment of high blood pressure, although the results of studies have been mixed. Intravenous magnesium has been shown to reduce blood pressure, possibly by relaxing constricted blood vessels. Those with high sodium and low potassium levels and those taking diuretic drugs may benefit from magnesium supplements.

In a 1997 double-blind, placebo-controlled study carried out in Japan, 33 people received either a four-week treatment with oral magnesium supplementation (411 to 548 mg per day) or a placebo. The results showed that the systolic and diastolic blood pressure values decreased significantly in the magnesium group, but not in the placebo group. Measurements made during the study suggest that magnesium may lower blood pressure through its effects on the secretion of adrenal hormones which cause an increase in sodium excretion.[28]

In a 1994 study, 91 middle-aged and elderly women with mild to moderate hypertension who were not on antihypertensive medication were treated with either magnesium supplements or placebo for six months. At the end of the study, systolic blood pressure had fallen by 2.7 mm Hg and diastolic blood pressure by 3.4 mm Hg more in the magnesium group than in the placebo group.[29]

Kidney stones

Magnesium supplements may be helpful in the treatment of kidney stones. In a 1997 study, researchers examined the use of potassium-magnesium citrate in the prevention of recurrent calcium oxalate kidney stones. Sixty-four patients received either a placebo or potassium-magnesium citrate daily for up to three years. The results showed that those in the supplement group had an 85 per cent lower risk of recurrence of stones.[30] Mineral water containing high levels of calcium and magnesium may also be useful in preventing the formation of calcium oxalate kidney stones.[31]

Pregnancy

Magnesium sulfate is routinely used in the USA to prevent convulsions in pre-eclampsia and to break down toxins in pre-term labor. A 1996 research review of trials of magnesium sulfate in the treatment of eclampsia and pre-eclampsia analyzed data from nine randomized trials involving 1743 women with eclampsia and 2390 with pre-eclampsia. The analysis showed that magnesium sulfate is effective in preventing the recurrence of seizures in eclampsia and in preventing them in pre-eclampsia.[32]

Researchers involved in a 1996 study reported in the *Journal of the American Medical Association* found that administration of magnesium sulfate to women before delivery reduced the risk of cerebral palsy in very low birthweight babies.[33]

A 1995 Swedish study showed that magnesium supplements may help reduce the pain and discomfort of night-time leg cramps that up to one-third of pregnant women suffer. Pregnant women tend to have lower blood magnesium levels than those who are not pregnant.[34]

Diabetes

Diabetics can benefit from magnesium supplements as they have been shown to improve glucose tolerance and insulin response and action. Magnesium may help protect against diabetic complications including heart disease and eye disorders.

In a 1994 study, Italian researchers investigated the effects of magnesium supplementation on glucose uptake and use in nine elderly Type II diabetic patients. Each patient was followed up for a period of three weeks before the study and was then given either a placebo or a magnesium supplement for four weeks. At the end of this time, improvements in insulin sensitivity and glucose oxidation were seen in those taking magnesium.[35] Magnesium supplements have also been shown to lower blood pressure in Type II diabetics.[36]

Asthma

Magnesium can act as a bronchial smooth muscle relaxant, and its use in the treatment of asthma is still in investigational stages. In a 1997 randomized, double-blind, placebo-controlled, cross-over study, 17 asthmatic people were given a low magnesium diet for two periods of three weeks, preceded and separated by a one week run-in/wash-out, in which they took either placebo or 400 mg magnesium per day. Asthma symptom scores were significantly lower during the magnesium treatment period.[37] Intravenous magnesium has been successfully used as an emergency treatment for asthma in children.[38] Magnesium sulfate aerosol has also been used effectively.[39]

Migraine

Magnesium supplements may be beneficial in the treatment and prevention of migraine. In a 1996 study, Belgian researchers assessed the effect of oral magnesium on the prevention of migraine in 81 patients aged from 18 to 65. They were either given a placebo or a daily supplement of 600 mg for 12 weeks. In weeks nine to12, the attack-frequency was reduced by 42 per cent in the magnesium group and by 16 per cent in the placebo group. The number of days with migraine and the drug consumption for symptomatic treatment per patient also decreased significantly in the magnesium group.[40] Supplements may also be useful in the treatment of menstrual migraine.[41]

Premenstrual syndrome

Oral magnesium treatment has been shown to relieve menstrual and premenstrual symptoms including mood changes and breast tenderness. In a 1991 study, Italian researchers investigated the effects of a two-month period of magnesium supplementation on premenstrual symptoms in 32 women. The dose used was 360 mg three times a day, from the 15th day of the menstrual cycle to the onset of menstrual flow. The results showed that supplementation was effective in the treatment of premenstrual symptoms related to mood changes.[42]

Chronic fatigue syndrome

Magnesium sulfate injections have been shown to improve the symptoms of chronic fatigue syndrome.[43] Further research is need to determine if oral supplements can show the same effects.

Osteoporosis

Supplements may help to increase bone mineral density in postmenopausal women, thus reducing the risk of osteoporosis. In a 1990 study, US researchers investigated the effect of a dietary program emphasizing magnesium instead of calcium for the management of postmenopausal osteoporosis. Nineteen women on hormonal replacement therapy (HRT) received 500 mg magnesium and 600 mg calcium, and seven other women on HRT did not receive supplements. The results showed that in one year, those women given the supplements had greater increases in bone mineral density than those who were not. Fifteen of the 19 women had had bone mineral density below the spine fracture threshold before treatment; within one year, only seven of them still had values below that threshold.[44]

In a 1993 study, Israeli researchers assessed the effects of supplemental magnesium in 31 postmenopausal women who received six 125 mg tablets daily for six months and two tablets for another 18 months in a two-year trial. Twenty-three symptom-free postmenopausal women were assessed as controls. The results showed that 22 patients responded with a 1 to 8 per cent rise of bone density. The mean bone density of all treated patients increased significantly after one year and remained unchanged after two years. In control patients, the mean bone density decreased significantly.[45]

Other uses

Supplements have also been used in the treatment of epilepsy, glaucoma, attention deficit hyperactivity disorder (ADHD), hearing loss, thalassemia, irritable bowel disorders and alcoholism. Taken with calcium they may have neuromuscular relaxing effects and may be useful in insomnia. Some antacids contain magnesium bound to an alkali that neutralizes stomach acid. It is also used as a laxative (in milk of magnesia) as it draws fluid into the bowel.

Interactions with other nutrients

High doses of zinc decrease magnesium absorption. Magnesium is necessary for thiamin, vitamin C and pyridoxine metabolism. Calcium, sodium, phosphorus and potassium metabolism are linked to magnesium metabolism in bone formation, muscle contraction and nerve transmission. High calcium intake may lead to magnesium deficiency. Magnesium deficiency may be linked to potassium deficiency and supplementation reduces potassium loss. Excess vitamin D may lead to magnesium deficiency.

Interactions with drugs

Antibiotics, antidepressants, estrogen and heart drugs can all affect magnesium levels. Diuretics are a major cause of magnesium deficiency. Magnesium salts may decrease the absorption of other drugs taken at the same time such as digoxin, tetracycline, iron and phenytoin.

Cautions

People with kidney problems and some heart diseases should not take large doses of magnesium.

Manganese

QUICK GUIDE

Essential for

- energy production
- the action of the antioxidant enzyme, superoxide dismutase
- protein metabolism, bone formation
- a healthy nervous system

Absorption and metabolism

Only 3 to 5 per cent of dietary manganese is absorbed.

Deficiency

Manganese deficiency is rare. Marginal deficiency may play a role in osteoporosis and diabetes.

Sources

Good sources of manganese include nuts, whole grains, dark green leafy vegetables and tea. The manganese content of food varies with the location in which the food is grown. The table on page 280 can be used as a guide.

Daily recommended dietary intakes

A safe and adequate daily intake is estimated to be around 2 to 5 mg.

Toxic effects of excess intake

Toxic effects from oral manganese are rare.

Interactions

High intakes of calcium, phosphorus, magnesium, iron, copper and zinc may inhibit manganese absorption.

Therapeutic uses of supplements

Manganese supplements have been used to treat inflammatory conditions, fatigue, mental disorders, epilepsy and diabetes.

Manganese is an essential trace element for humans. The average adult body contains between 12 and 20 mg with the highest concentrations in the bones, liver, kidneys and heart.

What it does in the body

Manganese appears to be involved in many enzyme systems, although its functions are not well understood. It acts as a co-factor for enzymes necessary for energy production and is involved in glucose metabolism, the stimulation of glycogen storage in the liver, protein digestion and cholesterol and fatty acid synthesis. It is also necessary for the synthesis of DNA and RNA.

Manganese is necessary for growth, maintenance of the nervous system, the development and maintenance of healthy bones and joints, the formation of blood clotting factors, female sex hormone function and thyroid hormone function.

Superoxide dismutase

One form of the antioxidant enzyme, superoxide dismutase, contains manganese. Proper function of this enzyme helps protect against free radical damage. (See page 417 for more information.) Laboratory studies have shown that it can protect brain cells from the type of damage seen in stroke and Alzheimer's disease.[1] It may also help to protect against liver damage. Manganese superoxide dismutase levels are higher in alcoholics and may help to protect against oxidative damage by alcohol.[2]

Absorption and metabolism

Only 3 to 5 per cent of dietary manganese is absorbed. After absorption, manganese is transported to the liver.

Deficiency

The first report of a manganese deficiency occurred as recently as 1972 in a man who lived for four months on a manganese-free diet. Symptoms include dizziness, bone problems, reduced growth of hair and nails, weakness, hearing problems, weight loss, abnormal gait, and skin problems. In children, severe deficiency may lead to convulsions, paralysis or blindness.

Marginal deficiency may arise when processed or refined foods form a large part of the diet. Marginal intake of manganese may increase loss of calcium from bone, increasing the risk of osteoporosis. Diabetics often have low manganese levels which may contribute to abnormal blood sugar regulation and decreased pancreatic cell function. Manganese deficiency appears to lead to abnormal glucose transport and metabolism.[3] Manganese deficiency may also play a role in epilepsy and infertility.

Recent research in rats suggests that manganese deficiency may lead to artery damage as a manganese-dependent enzyme is involved in the formation of arterial connective tissue. Damage to artery wall structure can promote the binding of harmful LDL cholesterol and the formation of atherosclerotic plaque.

Sources

Good sources of manganese include cereals, spinach, wholemeal bread, nuts, pulses, fruit, dark green leafy vegetables, root vegetables, tea and liver. As much as 86 per cent of the manganese content is lost when flour is refined and 89 per cent is lost when sugar is refined.

Food	Amount	Manganese (mg)
Wheat bran	½ cup	3.17
Brown rice, cooked	1 cup	1.68
Chickpeas, cooked	1 cup	1.60
Spinach, boiled	1 cup	1.60
Almonds	½ cup	1.53
Buckwheat	½ cup	1.05
Lentils, cooked	1 cup	0.93
Lima beans	1 cup	0.92
Kidney beans, cooked	1 cup	0.80
Green peas	1 cup	0.80
White rice, cooked	1 cup	0.71
Wholewheat bread	1 slice	0.65
Wheat bran bread	1 slice	0.60
Carrots, cooked	½ cup, slices	0.56
Kale	1 cup, chopped	0.51

Tea	1 cup	0.49
Raisins	1 cup	0.48
Prunes, dried	1 cup	0.36
Snap beans, boiled	1 cup	0.35
Beef liver, fried	85g	0.36
Sweetcorn, boiled	1 cup	0.36
Beets, boiled	½ cup, slices	0.26
Brazil nuts	6-8 nuts	0.22

Recommended dietary allowances

Suggested daily intake ranges from 2 to 5 mg. Such amounts are easily obtained from diets high in whole grains and vegetables.

Supplements

Manganese supplements are available in various forms including amino acid chelates, manganese sulfate and manganese gluconate. Manganese most often occurs in multivitamin and mineral supplements in doses of 1 to 9 mg.

Toxic effects of excess intake

Toxic effects from oral ingestion of manganese are very rare and include lethargy, involuntary movements, changes in muscle tone and posture, and coma. Toxic effects known as 'manganese madness' have been observed in manganese miners. Symptoms include unaccountable laughter, impulsiveness, inability to sleep, violent acts, delusions and hallucinations.

Therapeutic uses of supplements

Inflammation

Manganese supplements have been used to treat inflammation, strains and sprains. Activity levels of the enzyme, superoxide dismutase, have been raised by manganese supplementation which may protect against the oxidative damage seen in inflammatory disorders such as arthritis.[4]

Other uses

Manganese supplements have also been used to treat schizophrenia, epilepsy, osteoporosis, multiple sclerosis and anemia. Manganese may be useful in the treatment of diabetes through effects on glucose metabolism.

Interactions with other nutrients

Manganese may inhibit the absorption of copper, iron and zinc. Calcium, iron, copper, manganese and zinc compete for absorption in the small intestine and high intake of one of the minerals reduces the absorption of the others. Magnesium may substitute for manganese in certain conditions when manganese is deficient. Manganese functions with vitamin K in the formation of blood clotting factors.

Molybdenum

QUICK GUIDE

Essential for

- reactions involving the waste products of protein metabolism
- iron utilisation
- carbohydrate metabolism
- alcohol and sulfite detoxification

Absorption and metabolism

As much as 88 to 93 per cent of dietary intake is absorbed.

Deficiency

Deficiency is rare and has only been seen in people who are on long-term tube or intravenous feeding or who have a rare genetic inability to use molybdenum. Symptoms include rapid heartbeat and breathing, headache, night blindness, anemia, mental disturbance, nausea and vomiting.

Sources

Good sources of molybdenum include milk, beans, bread, liver and cereals. The molybdenum content of food varies with the location in which the food is grown. The table on page 285 can be used as a guide.

Daily recommended dietary intakes

An estimated safe and adequate intake is 75 to 250 mcg per day.

Toxic effects of excess intake

These include weight loss, slow growth, anemia, diarrhea, increased blood levels of uric acid and swelling in the joints.

Interactions

Molybdenum competes with copper at absorption sites.

Therapeutic uses of supplements

Supplements have been used to detoxify copper in cases where levels are too high. They have also been used to prevent cancer in areas where the soil content is low.

Molybdenum has been considered an essential trace mineral since the 1950s. The average adult body contains about 9 mg with the highest concentrations in the liver, kidneys, bone and skin.

What it does in the body

Molybdenum is a component of the enzymes, xanthine oxidase, sulfite oxidase and aldehyde oxidase. These enzymes perform many vital functions including the production of uric acid, a nitrogen waste product of protein metabolism; carbohydrate metabolism; iron utilization; and alcohol and sulfite detoxification. They may also act as antioxidants and may play a role in normal sexual function in men.

Absorption and metabolism

Between 25 and 80 per cent of dietary intake is absorbed and excretion is mainly in the urine. Molybdenum is conserved at low intakes and excess molybdenum is rapidly excreted in the urine when intake is high.[1]

Deficiency

Molybdenum deficiency is extremely rare and has only been seen in people who are on long-term tube or intravenous feeding or who have molybdenum co-factor deficiency, a rare genetic inability to use molybdenum. Symptoms of deficiency include rapid heartbeat and breathing, headache, night blindness, anemia, mental disturbance, nausea and vomiting.[2] There may also be problems with sexual function and dental caries. Low molybdenum levels may be linked to an increased allergic reaction to sulfite food additives.

Marginal molybdenum deficiency has been associated with the development of cancer. In China and Japan, people living in areas where the soil is molybdenum-deficient have been found to have an increased risk of stomach and esophageal cancers.[3] This may be because molybdenum-deficient plants are unable to metabolize carcinogenic compounds known as nitrosamines which are thus present in high levels in food.

Sources

Good sources of molybdenum include milk, beans, bread, liver and cereals. The molybdenum content of plants depends on the soil in which they are grown. The table below can be used as a guide.

Food	Amount	Molybdenum (mcg)
Lima beans	100g	870
Small white beans	100g	450
Yellow split peas	100g	250
Oats	100g	180
Green peas	100g	130
Chili beans	100g	110
Raisin bran	100g	76
String beans	100g	60
Spaghetti	100g	41
Macaroni	100g	38
Rice	100g	29
Bakery sweets	100g	27
Bread	100g	21
Cheese	100g	11
Pineapple	100g	9
Eggs	100g	9
Banana	100g	8
Corn	100g	8
Spinach	100g	7
Potatoes	100g	7
Cabbage	100g	6
Chicken	100g	5
Milk	100g	5
Bean sprouts	100g	5

Recommended dietary allowances

There is no RDA for molybdenum. The estimated safe and adequate intake is 75 to 250 mcg per day. Average daily intake in the USA ranges from 50 to 500 mcg per day.

Supplements

Molybdenum is available commercially as sodium molybdate. The maximum daily dose should not exceed 500 mg per day. If you take molybdenum supplements, it is advisable to take 2 to 3 mg of copper to offset the risk of copper deficiency.

Toxic effects of excess intake

Toxic effects of excess molybdenum intake include weight loss, slow growth, anemia, diarrhea, increased blood levels of uric acid and swelling in the joints. This may occur at intakes of 10 to 15 mg.

Therapeutic uses of supplements

Molybdenum has been used to treat copper toxicity in cases such as Wilson's disease where levels are too high.[4] Molybdenum has been used with fluoride to treat dental decay.

Interactions with other nutrients

The molybdenum-containing enzyme, xanthine oxidase, may help to mobilize iron from liver reserves. Molybdenum competes with copper at absorption sites, and amounts of 500 mcg per day have been found to cause significant losses of copper.

Nickel may be an essential trace mineral but its role in the body is unknown. The average adult body contains about 10 mg of nickel and it is found in many body tissues.

What it does in the body

High concentrations of nickel are found in genetic material and it may be involved in protein structure and function. It may also play a role in hormone function, and may activate certain enzymes related to the breakdown or utilization of glucose.

Absorption and metabolism

Nickel is poorly absorbed from the gut and is carried in the body attached to a carrier protein. Most nickel is eliminated in the feces, some in urine and some in sweat.

Deficiency

Nickel deficiency in animals leads to decreased growth, dermatitis, pigment changes, liver damage and reproductive abnormalities. No deficiency symptoms have been reported in humans. Low blood levels of nickel may be found in those with liver and kidney disease.

Sources

Vegetables usually contain more nickel than other foods. High levels have been found in legumes, spinach, lettuce and nuts. Certain products, such as baking powder and cocoa powder, have been found to contain excessive amounts of nickel, perhaps because of nickel leaching from machinery during the manufacturing process. Soft drinking water and acid beverages may dissolve nickel from pipes and containers.

Recommended dietary intakes

Studies indicate a highly variable dietary intake of nickel, but most averages are about 0.2-0.7 mg per day.

Toxic effects of excess intake

Inhaled nickel is toxic and can cause nausea, vomiting and increase the risk of lung cancer. High levels of nickel in the diet may be associated with an increased risk of thyroid problems, cancer and heart disease.

Nickel in jewelry, dental materials, prosthetic joints or heart valves may cause allergic reactions such as contact dermatitis and eczema. Low nickel diets may bring improvement in some patients who are sensitive to nickel.[1]

Phosphorus

QUICK GUIDE

Essential for

- for healthy bones
- acid base balance in the body
- for metabolism of proteins, carbohydrates, fats and DNA
- energy production and exchange

Absorption and metabolism

Phosphorus is efficiently absorbed.

Deficiency

Symptoms are rare and include weakness, loss of appetite, bone pain, joint stiffness, irritability, numbness, speech disorders, tremor and mental confusion.

Sources

These include meat, wheatgerm, poultry, cheese, milk, canned fish, nuts and cereals.

Daily recommended dietary intakes

Men	700 mg
Women	700 mg
Pregnancy (14 to 18)	1250 mg
Pregnancy (over 18)	700 mg
Lactation (14 to 18)	1250 mg

Toxic effects of excess intake

High levels of phosphorus can produce calcium deficiency. Interactions: The functions of calcium, magnesium and phosphorus are closely related, and disturbances in one mineral may affect the other.

Therapeutic uses of supplements

The use of supplements is rare but they have been used to treat bone problems including osteomalacia, osteoporosis and rickets.

Interactions

Phosphorus interacts with calcium and magnesium in body functions.

Cautions

Phosphorus supplements should be avoided in cases of kidney disease, liver disease, heart failure and high blood pressure.

Phosphorus is second only to calcium as the most abundant mineral in the body. It is usually combined with oxygen to make phosphate compounds and is a constituent of all plant and animal cells. The average adult contains around 500 g of phosphorus, around 85 per cent is in the bones and teeth, 14 per cent in the muscles and the rest in the fluid that surrounds the cells.

What it does in the body

Phosphate is the primary ion in extra and intracellular fluid. It aids absorption of dietary constituents, helps to maintain the blood at a slightly alkaline level, regulates enzyme activity and is involved in the transmission of nerve impulses. Phosphorus is a component of some of the major building blocks in the body, including RNA and DNA and lipids, including those in the blood and cell membranes.

Bones and teeth

Phosphorus combined with calcium, usually in the form of hydroxyapatite, is a major component of the structural part of bones and teeth.

Energy production

Phosphorus takes part in almost every metabolic reaction in the body. It is necessary for the conversion of dietary carbohydrate, fat and protein to energy. It is part of the adenosine triphosphate (ATP) molecule which acts as a reservoir of energy in cells.

Calcium-phosphorus balance

Calcium and phosphorus act together and balance each other in many body functions. An excessive intake of one mineral may cause a deficiency in the other. The intake ratio of calcium to phosphorus should be 1:1.

Absorption and metabolism

Nearly 70 per cent of dietary phosphorus is absorbed from the intestine, although absorption depends on intake levels and life cycle changes such as growth, pregnancy and lactation. In general, more phosphorus is absorbed from plant foods than from animal foods. Vitamin D is necessary for phosphorus absorption from the gut and transfer into bone from the blood. Most phosphorus excretion is via the kidney and this is mainly regulated by parathyroid hormone.

Deficiency

Deficiency symptoms include weakness, loss of appetite, bone pain, joint stiffness, osteomalacia, irritability, numbness, pins and needles, speech disorders, tremor, and mental confusion. Red blood cell life becomes shortened, leading to anemia. White blood cells may also be affected leading to reduced resistance to infection.

Deficiencies are unlikely to occur in healthy adults as phosphorus is widespread in many types of foods. Certain medical conditions such as disorders of vitamin D metabolism, kidney or liver disorders, or alcoholism can induce low blood phosphate levels. Large amounts of aluminum-containing antacids can block phosphorus absorption and may lead to deficiency. Low levels of blood phosphorus are fairly common in hospitalized people and those on formula diets. Premature babies are also at risk of phosphorus deficiency.

Sources

Good sources of phosphorus include meat, yeast, wheatgerm, soybean flour, meat, poultry, cheese, milk, canned fish, nuts and cereals. Soft drinks also contain a lot of phosphorus and may contribute to excessive intake. Food additives may contribute 30 per cent of the dietary intake of phosphorus.

Food	Amount	Phosphorus (mg)
Bran cereal	½ cup	770
Rice bran	½ cup	706
Salmon, cooked, dry	½ fillet	571
Mackerel, cooked, dry	½ fillet	490
Oats	½ cup	388
Beef liver, fried	85g	392
Sunflower seeds	¼ cup	369
Raisin bran	100g	372
Oat bran	½ cup	324
Clam, boiled	20 small	304
Buckwheat	½ cup	279
All Bran	30g	280

Tuna, grilled	85g	277
Peanuts	½ cup	261
Wheatgerm	¼ cup	232
Goat's cheese	30g	219
Bulgur, dry	½ cup	210
Dried walnuts	½ cup pieces	181
Swiss cheese	30g	182
Wholewheat cereal	½ cup	168
Cheshire cheese	30g	139
Sardines, canned in tomato	1 sardine	139
Sardines, canned in oil	2 sardines	118
Shredded wheat	30g	106

Recommended dietary allowances

The RDAs for phosphorus are based on an estimate for the preferable ratio (1:1) for calcium and phosphorus. The average American diet contains twice the RDA for phosphorus and the ratio of calcium to phosphorus is often as low as 1:2. The recommended upper intake limit is set at 4 g per day.

	Men	*Women*	*Pregnancy*	*Lactation*
USA	700 mg	700 mg		
(14 to 18 years)			1250 mg	1250 mg
(Over 18 years)		700 mg	700 mg	
UK	540 mg	540 mg	+425 mg	+425 mg
(under 18)	770 mg	620 mg		
Australia	1000 mg	1000 mg	1200 mg	1200 mg

Supplements

These are available in various forms including bonemeal, sodium phosphate and potassium phosphate. A recent study showed that sweet foods supplemented with phosphorus reduced the loss of minerals from dental enamel which these foods normally cause.[1] Acute ingestion of phosphorus (phosphorus loading) may improve aerobic capacity.

Toxic effects of excess intake

High levels of phosphorus lead to calcium deficiency. (See page 191 for more information.) When the diet is high in phosphorus, calcium may be lost in the urine, increasing the risk of disorders such as kidney stones, osteoporosis and atherosclerosis.[2] Soda drinks which contain large amounts of phosphoric acid may contribute to these harmful effects. Excess intakes can also prevent absorption of iron, magnesium and zinc. High levels of phosphorus also decrease vitamin D levels. This may increase the risk of bone disorders and cancer.[3] A 1997 UK study involving 376 heart disease patients found a relationship between high phosphorus levels and the severity of coronary heart disease.[4]

Therapeutic uses of supplements

Sodium phosphate is used as a laxative as it increases the amount of water in the bowel. Phosphate supplements have been used to treat bone problems including osteomalacia, osteoporosis and rickets. They are sometimes given to premature babies. Low phosphate levels caused by disease are treated with supplements by a doctor who can monitor response.

Interactions with other nutrients

The functions of calcium, magnesium and phosphorus are closely related and disturbances in one mineral may affect the other. Calcium aluminum, magnesium and iron reduce phosphorus absorption while vitamin D enhances it.

Cautions

Phosphorus supplements should be avoided in cases of kidney disease, liver disease, heart failure and high blood pressure. Phosphorus salts should not be given with iron salts, calcium salts, zinc salts or antacids as nonabsorbable complexes may form.

Selenium

QUICK GUIDE

Essential for

- the function of the antioxidant enzyme, glutathione peroxidase, which protects against damage to cells
- healthy immune and cardiovascular systems
- hormone production

Absorption and metabolism

Organic selenium is absorbed more efficiently than inorganic forms.

Deficiency

Selenium deficiency may contribute to cancer, heart disease, arthritis, cataracts, autoimmune diseases and birth defects.

Sources

Good sources include organ meats and seafood. The selenium content of food varies with the location in which the food is grown. The table on page 299 can be used as a guide.

Daily recommended dietary intakes

Men	70 mcg
Women	55 mcg
Pregnancy	65 mcg
Lactation	75 mcg

Toxic effects of excess intake

Toxic effects include fatigue, hair loss, nail problems, bad breath and nervous system problems.

Interactions

Selenium and vitamin E work better together than individually.

Therapeutic uses of supplements

Selenium supplements may be useful in preventing heart disease, cancer and cataracts, and in the treatment of asthma and rheumatoid arthritis.

Selenium was identified as an essential trace mineral for humans in the 1970s. The average adult body contains about 20 mg of selenium and most of this is concentrated in the kidneys, liver, heart, spleen and testes.

What it does in the body

Antioxidant activity

As part of the enzyme glutathione peroxidase, selenium acts as an antioxidant. It is extremely powerful and protects red blood cells and cell membranes from free radical damage. Selenium works closely with vitamin E and may enhance its function. Glutathione peroxidase seems to be able to protect against the damaging effects of ultraviolet light.

Immune system

Selenium is important in maintaining resistance to disease. It may enhance the production and effectiveness of white blood cells and protect them from the free radicals they generate in the process of fighting infection. It also appears to increase antibody production, and strengthen the body's surveillance of abnormal cell growth and cancer.

Hormones

A selenium-dependent enzyme is involved in the metabolism of thyroid hormones. Studies have shown that thyroid hormones in elderly people are influenced by selenium status.[1]

Other functions

Selenium is involved in maintaining normal liver function, protein synthesis and protecting against toxic minerals such as arsenic, cadmium, mercury and lead. It plays a role in promoting male sexual reproductive capacity and maintaining healthy eyes, hair and skin. It may be involved in the metabolism of prostaglandins which control inflammation.

Absorption and metabolism

Organic selenium, such as that found in yeast, is more efficiently absorbed than inorganic salts.

Deficiency

Severe selenium deficiency has only been seen in those living off foods grown in selenium-deficient soil. Levels of selenium in soil vary between countries and between different regions in the same country. There are low levels in Europe, parts of the USA, New Zealand and parts of China. There are high levels in Japan, Thailand, Philippines and Puerto Rico.

Severe selenium deficiency leads to the heart disorder, Keshan disease, a potentially fatal cardiomyopathy that affects children in low selenium areas of rural China. Kashin Beck disease, another deficiency disease seen in rural China, resembles arthritis.

Marginal selenium deficiency can occur in alcoholics and those living on refined and processed foods, and may increase the risk of a variety of diseases. Blood selenium levels may also be low in those who are critically ill, AIDS patients, fibrocystic breast disease sufferers, those with Down syndrome, and liver disease patients.

Cancer

Epidemiological studies have shown that those who live in areas of low selenium soil are more prone to cancer than those living in areas where the soil is high in selenium. Blood samples taken from large groups of people show that they are more likely to develop cancer if they have low blood levels of selenium and glutathione peroxidase. Low serum, dietary and soil selenium levels are particularly associated with lung and gastrointestinal tract cancers.

Colorectal cancer

In a 1997 study of the relationship between selenium and colon cancer, researchers at the University of North Carolina determined selenium levels in patients referred for colonoscopy. The results showed that those with the lowest selenium levels had almost four times the risk of colon cancer when compared to those with the highest levels.[2]

A 1998 German study assessed the selenium and glutathione peroxidase levels in 106 colorectal cancer patients and compared these to a gender-matched and age-matched control group. When average selenium levels in the cancer patients were compared with those in the control group, no significant differences were found. However, a significant reduction of serum glutathione peroxidase activity was seen in cancer patients. Those patients with low selenium levels had lower survival times and rates than the patients with higher selenium levels. The lowest selenium level was found for patients with advanced tumor disease.

It is unclear from the results of this study whether low selenium levels are a cause or effect of cancer.[3]

Lung cancer

In a study that started in 1986 and was published in 1993, Dutch researchers examined the links between longterm selenium status and lung cancer among 120 852 Dutch men and women aged 55-69 years. The results showed that the lung cancer risk in those with the highest intake of selenium was half that of those in the lowest intake group. The protective effect of selenium was concentrated in subjects with a relatively low dietary intake of beta carotene or vitamin C.[4]

Cardiovascular disease

Severe selenium deficiency leads to weakened and damaged heart muscle. People living in low selenium areas have lower plasma selenium levels and an increase in the risk of coronary disease, atherosclerosis, platelet aggregation and levels of compounds such as prostaglandins and leukotrienes which play a role in inflammation and platelet aggregation. (See page 560 for more information.) Selenium seems to be able to affect prostaglandin and leukotriene synthesis.

As part of glutathione peroxidase, selenium takes part in the reduction of hydrogen peroxides and lipid peroxides. The concentration of these peroxides, in turn, affects platelet aggregation. Blood platelets of selenium-deficient people show increased aggregation, which selenium administration inhibits. Thus long-term supplementation with low doses of selenium could have a beneficial effect on the prevention of both thrombosis and coronary heart disease in people who are selenium-deficient.[5]

Dutch researchers studying the association between selenium status and the risk of heart attack, compared plasma, red blood cell, and toenail selenium levels and the activity of red blood cell glutathione peroxidase among 84 heart attack patients and 84 healthy people. They found lower selenium levels in all the heart attack patients. Because the toenail selenium level reflects blood levels up to one year before sampling, the results suggest that low selenium levels were present before the heart attacks and, may have played a role in causing them.[6]

However, results from the Physicians' Health Study published in 1995 do not suggest a link between selenium levels and heart attack risk. Researchers analyzed blood selenium levels in 251 subjects who had heart attacks and an equal number of healthy people, matched by age and smoking status. The results did not show significant differences.[7]

HIV/AIDS

As part of the antioxidant enzyme glutathione peroxidase, selenium is necessary to help prevent oxidative damage and to help the immune system function effectively. Levels of this enzyme have been shown to be low in some HIV-positive patients, particularly in those with more advanced stage of the disease, and low selenium levels appear to be associated with low CD4+ lymphocyte counts and with higher death rates in AIDS patients. Deaths from AIDS are higher in areas where soil selenium is low.

Birth defects

Selenium deficiency in women may result in infertility, miscarriages, neural tube defects and retention of the placenta.[8]

Asthma

As an antioxidant, selenium may be able to protect against the damage to lung tissue and enzymes caused by the free radicals produced by inflammatory cells in asthmatic airways. As a component of the enzyme glutathione peroxidase it helps to stabilize cell membranes.

In a New Zealand study done in 1994, researchers examined 708 children for symptoms of wheezing. They then measured selenium levels in blood samples taken eight years previously from 26 of the children with current wheezing, and compared these with levels in 61 healthy children. The results showed that wheezing was more common in those with low levels of selenium.[9] Another New Zealand study, done in 1990, showed that whole blood selenium concentrations and glutathione peroxidase activity were lower in adults with asthma than in those without.[10]

Rheumatoid arthritis

Free oxygen radicals are involved in the inflammatory process seen in rheumatoid arthritis and are generated mainly by white blood cells. Selenium is important to the functioning of the immune system and to the inflammatory process. Low selenium levels among patients with rheumatoid arthritis have been reported from areas with both high and low natural selenium intake. The reduction seems to be related to the clinical disease activity in arthritis patients, and selenium concentrations have been found to fluctuate during the disease.

Cataracts

Reduced antioxidant defenses seem to play a role in cataract formation and selenium deficiency may play a part in this. Glutathione peroxidase is found in high concentrations in the lens and selenium levels in lenses with cataracts have been found to be lower than in normal lenses.[11]

Anemia

Selenium deficiency may play a role in causing or aggravating anemia as glutathione peroxidase protects red blood cells from free radical damage and destruction.

Other effects

A 1996 study done at the USDA Human Nutrition Research Center in San Francisco suggests that people with low selenium levels might experience depressed moods, supporting the idea that selenium plays a special role in the brain. However, the study did not find improvements with selenium supplementation in people eating a typical American diet.[12]

Sources

Good food sources of selenium include organ meats, fish and shellfish, muscle meats, whole grains, cereals, dairy products and vegetables such as broccoli, mushrooms, cabbage and celery. The selenium content of foods depends on the soil in which they are grown. Food processing techniques can remove selenium.

Food	Amount	Selenium (mcg)
Brazil nuts	6-8 kernels	840
Pork kidney, cooked	1 cup, sliced	271
Beef kidney, cooked	1 cup, sliced	212
Lamb kidney, raw	1 cup, sliced	185
Lamb liver, raw	1 cup, sliced	118
Tuna, canned, drained, in water	1 can	133
Tuna, canned, drained, in oil	1 can	130
Flounder, cooked	1 fillet	73.9
Pink salmon, raw	½ fillet	70.9
Macaroni pasta, dry	1cup	62.0
Oysters, cooked	6 oysters	60.1
Turkey, dark meat	1 cup	54.3

Beef liver, pan-fried	100g	57
Mackerel, baked	1 fillet	46.5
Pork, chops, sirloin	85g	43.9
Wheat flour, wholegrain	½ cup	40.3
Wholewheat pita bread	1 pita	28.2
Ocean perch, raw	1 fillet	27.7
Rolled oats	1 cup	26.2
White bread flour	½ cup	26.0
Wheat bran	½ cup	22.1
Wheatgerm	¼ cup	21.9
Oat bran	½ cup	20.1
Special K	1 cup	19.2

Recommended dietary allowances

	Men	*Women*	*Pregnancy*	*Lactation*
USA	70 mcg	55 mcg	65 mcg	75 mcg
UK	75 mcg	60 mcg	75 mcg	75mcg
Australia	85 mcg	70 mcg	80 mcg	85 mcg

Supplements

There are various forms of selenium supplements including organic selenium rich yeast, selenium in the form of selenomethionine, and inorganic sodium selenite. These different types of selenium may act differently, with selenium yeast raising blood selenium levels and sodium selenite more effective at increasing the activity of glutathione peroxidase. Organic selenium seems to be better absorbed and less toxic than the inorganic forms.

Young adults, vegetarians, the elderly, smokers, pregnant women and nursing mothers may benefit from supplements.

Toxic effects of excess intake

Selenium toxicity can occur at doses of 600 to 750 mcg. Early signs of selenium toxicity include fatigue, irritability and dry hair. Other symptoms of excess intake include dental caries in children, hair loss, skin depigmentation, abnormal nails, vomiting, nervous system problems, and bad breath.

Therapeutic uses of supplements

Cancer

Some studies have shown that selenium supplements protect against some types of cancer such as rectal, ovarian, colon, lung and cervical cancers. However there are also studies, including the Nurses Health Study at Harvard, which do not show a protective role for selenium against cancers at any major site. Laboratory studies have shown that selenium can slow tumor cell growth.

A 1996 study looking at the effect of selenium supplements on cancer has found a 50 per cent reduction in deaths from cancer in those taking supplements. Researchers at the Arizona Cancer Center set out to test the effectiveness of selenium supplements on the prevention of skin cancer in over 1300 patients. Participants received a placebo or 200 mcg selenium per day over a period of 4.5 years and a total follow-up of 6.4 years. While the results did not show any reduction in skin cancer risk, the selenium group had a 37 per cent reduction in cancer incidence and a 50 per cent reduction in cancer mortality. The effects appeared strongest for prostate (63 per cent lower risk), colorectal (58 per cent lower risk) and lung (53 per cent lower risk) cancers.[13]

A recent report in the *Journal of the National Cancer Institute* suggests that selenium compounds may inhibit colon cancer in rats. Researchers at the American Health Foundation gave the synthetic organoselenium compounds to rats with high fat diets and found inhibition of tumor incidence. The effects were more pronounced with a low fat diet. There were no toxic effects with either compound.[14]

Heart disease

Selenium may reduce heart disease by protecting against oxidative damage to blood cholesterol. Selenium supplements have been shown to increase HDL cholesterol levels and decrease LDL cholesterol levels. Selenium can also inhibit platelet aggregation, thus reducing the risk of build-up of atherosclerotic plaques in the arteries.

Finnish researchers evaluated the effect of selenium supplementation on 81 patients with heart attacks. Patients received either selenium-rich yeast (100 mcg per day) or placebo in addition to conventional drug therapy for a six-month period. During the follow-up period there were four cardiac deaths in the placebo group but none in the selenium group. There were two nonfatal heart attacks in the placebo group and one nonfatal attack in the selenium group.[15]

A small 1997 German study indicated improvements that patients who were given selenium supplements after heart attacks showed greater improvements in heart function than patients not given supplements.[16]

Asthma

In 1993 Swedish researchers conducted a study of 24 adults with asthma in which half of the patients received 100 mcg of selenium per day for 14 weeks, while the other half received a placebo. Six patients from the selenium-supplemented group and one from the placebo group noticed significant clinical improvement, although neither group showed improvement in laboratory measures.[17]

Rheumatoid arthritis

Selenium supplements may be beneficial in the treatment of rheumatoid arthritis, especially when combined with vitamin E treatment. In some trials, symptoms have been shown to improve as blood selenium levels increase. However, the results of studies are mixed. Selenium may reduce inflammation through its antioxidant action, and through control of prostaglandins, hormone-like compounds that regulate the inflammation process.

In a three month study done in 1997 in Germany, 70 patients with rheumatoid arthritis were randomly divided into two groups. One group was given 200 mcg per day of sodium selenite while the other group was given a placebo. Selenium concentrations in red blood cells of patients with rheumatoid arthritis were significantly lower than found in an average German population. At the end of the experimental period, the selenium-supplemented group showed less tender or swollen joints, and morning stiffness. Selenium-supplemented patients needed less cortisone and other anti-inflammatory medications than the placebo group. Analysis also showed a decrease in laboratory indicators of inflammation.[18]

Other uses

Selenium supplements have been used in the detoxification of arsenic, cadmium and mercury; to treat angina; high blood pressure in pregnancy; and hair, nail and skin problems. Selenium may also play a role in preventing anemia; cataracts; periodontal disease; and improving mood, anxiety, depression and fatigue in some people. Selenium supplements may benefit those with low immune function, such as the elderly.

Shampoos or prescription solutions containing selenium sulfide are used for the treatment of fungal infections, including tinea capitis.

Interactions with other nutrients

The amino acid, methionine, is essential for the absorption, transport and bioavailability of selenium. Combined selenium and vitamin E seems to have synergistic effects in the treatment of heart disease, tissue damage due to restricted blood flow, and cancer. Vitamin C has also been found to have added effects. Large doses of vitamin C can interfere with the absorption and use of inorganic selenium such as sodium selenite.[19]

Silicon

Silicon, the most abundant mineral in the earth's crust, may be an essential element in humans. It is present in bone, blood vessels, cartilage, tendons, skin and hair.

What it does in the body

Silicon is found in areas of active growth inside bones and may be involved in the growth of bone crystals and calcification. Silicon may also play a role in the formation of cartilage and other connective tissue, giving strength and stability. It may help to maintain the elasticity of arterial cell walls.

Deficiency

Silicon deficiency in animals causes weak and malformed bones of the arms, legs and head. Low silicon levels also lead to atherosclerotic lesions in animals due to its role in artery wall formation. Thus silicon deficiency may play a role in cardiovascular disease.

Sources

Silicon is widely available in food. Good sources include wheat, oats, rice, lettuce, cucumbers, avocados and strawberries. Silicon is easily lost in food processing.

Recommended dietary allowances

Average daily intakes of silicon probably range from about 20 to 50 mg per day with the lower values for animal-based diets and the higher values for plant-based diets.

Supplements

Silicon supplements are available in several different forms, including sodium metasilicate and silicic acid.

Toxic effects of excess intake

Silicon is generally regarded as nontoxic.

Therapeutic uses

Silicon supplements have been used to improve strength in hair, skin and nails. Silicon may have a role in the prevention and treatment of osteoporosis as supplements have been shown to increase bone mineral density.

Sulfur

As a constituent of all proteins, sulfur is an essential element for humans. The sulfur content of the average adult body is approximately 100 mg and most of this occurs in the three amino acids, cysteine, cystine and methionine. The rest is in the form of sulfates attached to other substances in body cells.

What it does in the body

Sulfur is found mainly in tissues that contain high amounts of protein. It is a constituent of collagen, the protein found in connective tissue, bones and teeth; and keratin, the protein found in skin, hair and nails. Sulfur gives these tissues strength, shape and hardness.

Sulfur is involved in the formation of bile acids which are important for fat digestion and absorption. As a component of the B vitamins, thiamin and biotin, sulfur helps in the conversion of proteins, carbohydrates and fats to energy. Sulfur plays a part in the reactions that help cells utilize oxygen. It is necessary for blood clotting and for the function of several enzymes including glutathione and coenzyme A, and for the production of the hormone, insulin.

Absorption and metabolism

Sulfur is absorbed in amino acids in the small intestine. Excess sulfur is excreted in the urine and feces.

Deficiency

There is no known sulfur deficiency disease. Protein is the main dietary source and a diet inadequate in protein would be of greater concern.

Sources

Good sources of sulfur include mustard, egg, seafood, beans, milk, milk products, nuts and meat. Protein supplies most of the sulfur in the diet but some comes in the form of sulfates in water, fruit and vegetables.

Recommended dietary allowances

No RDA has been set for sulfur but a diet sufficient in protein will generally provide enough. About 850 mg per day is thought to be sufficient for the basic turnover of sulfur in the body.

Toxic effects

There are no known toxic effects from organic sulfur.

Therapeutic uses of supplements

Sulfur has been used as a mild laxative; a mild antiseptic in ointment form to treat acne, eczema, dermatitis and psoriasis; a parasiticide in lotion form to treat scabies; and as a depilatory agent. Oral sulfur has been used to treat psoriasis. Bathing in water containing sulfur may benefit arthritis sufferers.

Interactions

The poisonous effects of arsenic are due to its ability to bind to the sulfur portion of amino acids and inactivate them.

Vanadium

Vanadium is a trace mineral which has been considered essential for humans since the 1970s. The average adult body contains about 100 mcg of vanadium and it is found in the blood, organ tissues and bones.

What it does in the body

Vanadium may act as a co-factor for enzymes involved in blood sugar metabolism, lipid and cholesterol metabolism, bone and tooth development, fertility, thyroid function, hormone production and neurotransmitter metabolism.

Absorption and metabolism

Vanadium absorption from food may be as low as 5 to 10 per cent. Most is eliminated in the feces. Vanadium is mainly stored in fat and bone.

Deficiency

Vanadium deficiency has not been described in man. Deficiency in animals causes infertility, reduction in red blood cell production leading to anemia; iron metabolism defects; and poor bone, tooth and cartilage formation. It is possible that deficiency in humans may lead to high cholesterol and triglyceride levels and increase susceptibility to heart disease and cancer.

Sources

Good sources of vanadium include whole grain breads and cereals, vegetable oils, nuts, root vegetables, parsley, fish, radishes, dill, lettuce and strawberries. The vanadium content of food depends on the soil in which it is grown. Airborne vanadium may also be an important source. Processed or refined foods may contain higher levels of vanadium than unprocessed foods, possibly because of contamination from stainless steel processing equipment.

Recommended dietary allowances

There is no RDA for vanadium. A daily intake of 10 to 100 mcg is probably safe and adequate.

Supplements

Vanadyl sulfate is the most common form of nutritional supplement.

Toxic effects of excess intake

Vanadium can easily be toxic if taken in synthetic form. It may cause nerve damage, blood vessel damage, kidney failure, liver damage, stunted growth, loss of appetite and diarrhea. Excess vanadium in humans has been suggested as a factor in bipolar disorder.[1]

Therapeutic uses of supplements

Animal experiments have shown that vanadium can mimic the effects of insulin and reduce blood sugar levels from high to normal. These benefits are seen with low doses and there have been limited clinical trials with vanadium salts in patients with Type II diabetes, indicating that vanadium may have therapeutic potential in the treatment of diabetes.[2]

In a study published in 1996, researchers at the Albert Einstein College of Medicine in New York compared the effects of 100 mg/day of oral vanadyl sulfate in moderately obese diabetic and nondiabetic people. The results showed improvements in both liver and skeletal muscle insulin sensitivity in diabetics. Blood fat levels and oxidation were also reduced. Thus vanadium may also be useful in reducing the risk of atherosclerosis in diabetic people.[3]

Vanadium may be beneficial in treating subnormal thyroid function. Limited animal experiments suggest that vanadium may prevent the occurrence of tumors.[4] Vanadium supplements have been used as performance enhancers by athletes, although there is little research evidence to support their effectiveness.[5]

Interactions with other nutrients

Vitamin C, chromium, iron, protein, chloride and aluminum may reduce vanadium absorption.

Zinc

QUICK GUIDE

Essential for

- energy production
- manufacture of genetic material
- detoxification of chemicals, including alcohol
- healthy immune and reproductive systems
- hormone production
- normal growth and development
- healthy brain, teeth, bones and skin

Absorption and metabolism

This ranges from 20 to 40 per cent of dietary zinc.

Deficiency

Symptoms include skin problems, fetal abnormalities, reproductive defects, cardiovascular disease, immune deficiency, loss of eye function and osteoporosis.

Sources

These include seafood, meat and whole grains.

Daily recommended dietary intakes

Men	15 mg
Women	12 mg
Pregnancy	15 mg
Lactation	19 mg

Toxic effects of excess intake

Toxic effects include vomiting, diarrhea, immune problems and heart disease.

Interactions

Zinc and copper interact in many body functions. Zinc helps the body to use vitamin A.

Therapeutic uses of supplements

Zinc supplements are often given to diabetics and pregnant women. They are also used to treat immune deficiency, the common cold, skin disorders, infertility, arthritis, taste disorders, macular degeneration, digestive diseases, prostate problems and to promote wound-healing.

Cautions

Large amounts of zinc may impair copper absorption.

Zinc has been recognized as an essential trace mineral for plants, animals and humans since the 1930s. The average adult body contains between 1.5 and 3 g of zinc with approximately 60 per cent of this in the muscles, 30 per cent in the bones and 6 per cent in the skin. The highest concentrations of zinc are in the prostate gland and sperm in men, and in red and white blood cells. The retina of the eye, liver and kidneys also have high concentrations and there is some zinc in hair.

What it does in the body

Metabolism

Zinc functions in over 200 enzymatic reactions in the body. It plays a key role in the synthesis and stabilization of genetic material. It is necessary for cell division and the synthesis and degradation of carbohydrates, lipids and proteins, and is therefore essential for the growth and repair of tissue.

Antioxidant function

As part of the enzyme copper-zinc superoxide dismutase, zinc helps to protect cells and other compounds against the effects of free radicals.

Cells and tissues

Zinc is vital for the normal structure and function of cell membranes. It is vital for the formation of connective tissue, teeth, bone, nails, hair and skin. Zinc may play a role in calcium uptake in bone and modulate the effects of growth hormones.

Immunity

Zinc is considered one of the most important nutrients for the immune system as it is necessary for healthy antibody, white blood cell, thymus gland and hormone function. It is therefore vital in maintaining resistance to infection and in wound-healing.

Hormones

Zinc is necessary for the secretion, synthesis and utilization of insulin. It also protects the insulin-producing pancreatic beta cells against destruction. Zinc is also involved in the metabolism of the pituitary, thyroid and adrenal glands, the ovaries and the testes. It is vital for healthy male sex hormone and prostate function.

Skin

Normal skin function requires zinc. It is involved in oil gland function, local hormone activation, vitamin A binding protein formation, wound-healing, inflammation control and tissue regeneration.

Pregnancy

Zinc is essential for normal fetal growth and development, and for milk production during lactation. Maternal zinc levels are linked to proper formation of the palate and lip, brain, eyes, heart, bones, lungs and urogenital system of the baby. Adequate zinc is necessary for normal growth, birth weight and completion of full term pregnancy.

Other functions

Zinc is necessary for the production of brain neurotransmitters. Healthy liver function and release of vitamin A from the liver both require zinc. Zinc is also necessary for maintenance of vision, taste and smell and is the most abundant trace mineral in the eye. It is involved in the production of hydrochloric acid in the stomach and in the conversion of fatty acids to prostaglandins, which regulate body processes such as heart rate and blood pressure. Zinc is necessary for muscle contraction and maintaining acid-alkali balance. It also helps detoxify alcohol.

Absorption and metabolism

On average, absorption of zinc is around 20 to 40 per cent of dietary intake, improving when zinc intake is low. Absorption also depends on the food source. More zinc is available from animal and fish sources as these high protein foods contain amino acids which bind to zinc and make it more soluble. Zinc from vegetables, fruits and cereals is less well absorbed as these foods contain compounds such as phytates and oxalates which binds zinc and reduces the amount available for absorption. Food additives and chemicals such as EDTA, which are used in food processing, can also reduce zinc absorption as can large amounts of textured vegetable protein. Zinc absorption decreases with age. People over 65 may absorb half as much zinc as those between 25 and 30 years old.

Zinc is combined in the intestines with picolinic acid which is secreted by the pancreas. This compound requires vitamin B6 for production. The zinc picolinate complex is transported across the absorptive cells of the intestine, then to the liver where some is stored. Vitamin B6 deficiency or a decrease in pancreatic secretion, which is often seen in elderly people, will therefore affect zinc absorption.

Excretion of zinc is mainly via the feces but some is lost in the urine. Excessive sweating can cause losses of up to 3 mg per day. Zinc is not well stored in the body and a reduction in dietary intake leads to deficiency fairly quickly. Plasma or serum zinc levels may not reflect body levels. Red or white blood cell measures of zinc may be the most accurate way to assess body stores.

Zinc absorption does not seem to increase during pregnancy but, according to a 1997 study, can increase nearly two-fold during lactation, presumably in response to the demand for zinc to synthesize breast milk.[1]

Hormone replacement therapy has been shown to decrease zinc excretion. In a study done in 1996, Israeli researchers assessed the effect of estrogen treatment on the excretion of several minerals, including zinc in 37 postmenopausal women. They found that zinc excretion decreased 35 per cent after three months and 26 per cent after one year of treatment.[2]

Deficiency

Symptoms of zinc deficiency include eczema on the face and hands, hair loss, mental apathy, defects in the reproductive organs, delayed sexual maturation, menstrual irregularities, decreased growth rate and impaired mental development. Deficiency may also lead to postnatal depression, loss of the senses of taste and smell, anemia, poor appetite, impaired conduction and nerve damage, white spots on the nails, mental disorders, susceptibility to infections, delayed wound-healing and impotence in men.

Zinc deficiency was first identified in the Middle East in adolescent male dwarfs with poor development of sexual organs. This was caused by high consumption of unleavened bread, which contains zinc-binding phytates.

Acrodermatitis enteropathica, a rare disease in infancy, is caused by a genetic inability to absorb zinc. Skin rashes appear when a baby is young; and when breastfeeding is stopped, gastrointestinal problems, decreased growth and mental abnormalities are seen. The disorder is treated with zinc supplements.

Alcoholic liver disease, trauma such as burns or surgery, stress, weight loss, chronic infections, viral hepatitis, diabetes and some kidney diseases can increase zinc requirements and increase the risk of deficiency. Athletes often have an increased need for zinc. Diseases of the gastrointestinal system such as inflammatory bowel disease and celiac disease, also reduce zinc absorption and may lead to deficiency symptoms. Zinc levels are low in people suffering from sickle cell disease and fat malabsorption disorders.

Results of the Second National Health and Nutrition Examination Survey, published in 1995, suggest that zinc intakes are declining.[3] This is likely to be due to lower meat and higher cereal consumption, food processing methods which reduce zinc content of food and lower soil concentrations of zinc. Those likely to have low intakes include infants; adolescents; women, particularly those who are pregnant; older adults; and those with lower levels of education and higher poverty levels. Pre-school children and vegetarians may also be at risk.

Pregnancy

Zinc deficiency in early pregnancy increases the risk of congenital birth defects, low birth weight, spontaneous abortion, premature delivery, mental retardation and behavior problems in babies; and may also increase the risk of pregnancy induced high blood pressure. Mothers with low zinc intakes may have babies who are more susceptible to infection.

Elderly people

Zinc intakes in older people tend to be much lower than the RDA. This is likely to be due to reduced intake, reduced absorption, the use of medications which affect zinc, and the presence of disease states which alter zinc usage. Zinc deficiency is likely to contribute to clinical conditions commonly seen in elderly people, including poor appetite, slow wound-healing, loss of taste and reduced immune system function.

Alcoholism

Alcoholism increases the risk of zinc deficiency, particularly in those with liver disease. Zinc deficiency in alcoholism is likely to be linked to altered vitamin A metabolism, suppressed immune function, eye problems and sex organ abnormalities. Zinc deficiency may also play a role in fetal alcohol syndrome, birth defects associated with alcohol use by pregnant women.

Diabetes

Alterations in zinc metabolism are seen in people with both Type I and Type II diabetes. Response to insulin may be decreased and excretion in the urine is increased, thus exacerbating the risk of deficiency, with all the associated risks such as poor immune function and increased risk of birth defects.

Zinc deficiency has shown to increase the risk for diabetes in diabetes-prone experimental animals, and low concentrations of zinc have also been shown in the blood of people recently diagnosed with Type I diabetes. The results of a 1995 Swedish study suggest that a low concentration of zinc in drinking water can increase the risk of childhood onset of the disease.[4]

Cardiovascular disease

Population studies suggest that low blood zinc levels are associated with an increased risk of cardiovascular disease. The results of a recent study done over a period of ten years in Finland, which involved 230 men dying from cardiovascular diseases and 298 controls matched for age, place of residence and smoking, found an increased risk of disease in those with low zinc levels.[5] This may be due to an imbalance in the copper-to-zinc ratio.

There is evidence that zinc can protect the inner lining of blood vessels from damage, thus helping to prevent atherosclerosis. This may be due to its membrane-stabilizing, antioxidant and anti-inflammatory properties.[6]

HIV/AIDS

AIDS patients often suffer from zinc deficiency, which adversely affects the immune system. Studies have shown an increased risk of opportunistic infections in AIDS patients with low zinc levels. In a study done in 1996, researchers at the San Francisco General Hospital found that AIDS patients with zinc deficiency had a higher risk of bacterial infections than patients with normal zinc levels. (See page 616 for more information.)

Eating disorders

Low levels of zinc have been found in sufferers of the eating disorder, anorexia nervosa. And this complex disorder may be exacerbated by zinc deficiency. Initial dieting may lead to deficiency which then reduces the senses of taste and smell, thus exacerbating poor appetite.

Eye problems

Zinc deficiency can lead to loss of eye function as several zinc-dependent enzymes play important roles in eye function. Levels of these enzymes decline with age. Zinc deficiency may contribute to macular degeneration of the central part of the retina. Results from the Beaver Dam Eye Study, published in 1996, suggest a link between low zinc intakes and risk of macular degeneration.[7]

Premenstrual syndrome

The symptoms of premenstrual syndrome may be exacerbated by zinc deficiency. In a study published in 1994, researchers at Baylor College of Medicine, Houston,

Texas assessed copper and zinc levels in ten PMS sufferers and compared these to those in non sufferers. Results showed lower zinc levels in the luteal phase (latter half) of the menstrual cycle in PMS sufferers.[8]

Male sexual function

Zinc levels are usually lower in infertile men, leading to decreased testosterone levels and low sperm counts. Zinc deficiency in adolescence can delay puberty and zinc seems to play an important role in controlling serum testosterone levels in normal men. In a 1996 study, researchers investigated the relationship between cellular zinc concentrations and serum testosterone in 40 normal men, aged from 20 to 80. Dietary zinc restriction in normal young men was associated with a significant decrease in serum testosterone concentrations after 20 weeks of zinc restriction, and zinc supplementation of marginally zinc-deficient normal elderly men for six months resulted in an increase in blood levels of testosterone.[9]

Immune system

Immune function is affected by zinc deficiency, which results in a decrease in the numbers of several types of T cells, natural killer cells and other components of the immune response. This leads to increased susceptibility to infection and wound-healing time.

Bones

Diets low in zinc may slow adolescent bone growth and increase the risk of osteoporosis later in life. In a study published in 1996, researchers at the University of California studied two groups of ten monkeys. Both groups were given nutritionally balanced diets but one group received 50 mcg of zinc per gram of food while the other group only received 2 mcg of zinc per gram of food. Eight of the monkeys were then studied throughout their lives to ages equivalent to that of ages 10 to 16 in human girls. The researchers found that the monkeys on low zinc diets had slower skeletal growth, maturation and less bone mass than the other monkeys, with substantial differences noticed in the lumbar spine. The differences were only apparent during rapid growth phases in the monkeys, especially during pregnancy. [10] Zinc excretion appears to be increased in osteoporosis sufferers, probably as a result of increased bone breakdown.

Other disorders

A 1997 Israeli study found low zinc absorption in patients with low disease activity and high disease activity when compared to people without the disease.[11]

Zinc levels may also be lower in people with asthma. A study done in 1996 in the Slovak Republic found lower zinc levels and high copper-to-zinc ratio in asthmatics.[12] Periodontal disease may also be related to zinc deficiency.

Sources

Good sources of zinc include liver, shellfish, oysters, meat, canned fish, hard cheese, whole grains, nuts, eggs and pulses. Vegetables contain smaller amounts of zinc and also contain compounds such as phytates and oxalates which bind zinc, leaving less available for absorption.

The zinc in grains is found mainly in the germ and bran coverings, so food refining and processing reduce the amount of zinc in food. For example, flour refining causes a 77 per cent loss in zinc, rice refining causes a loss of 83 per cent and processing cereals from whole grains causes an 80 per cent loss.

Food	Amount	Zinc (mg)
Oysters, raw	6 oysters	15.6
Crab meat, canned	1 can	5.0
Beef, cooked, lean and fat	100g	4.4
Lamb, cooked, lean and fat	100g	4.4
Lobster, cooked	1 cup	4.2
Salmon, canned	1 can	4.2
Veal, cooked, lean and fat	100g	4.0
Lamb kidney, simmered	100g	3.8
Cashews, salted	½ cup	3.8
Branflakes	¾ cup	3.8
All Bran	½ cup	3.7
Sunflower seeds	½ cup	3.6
Oats	½ cup	3.1
Mixed nuts	¼ cup	2.6
Sausages, grilled	100g	2.5
Lentils, boiled	1cup	2.5
Chickpeas, cooked	1cup	2.5
Peanuts, salted	½ cup	2.4

Pork, cooked, lean and fat	100g	2.4
Plain hamburger	1 serve	2.0
Scallops, heated	6 pieces	1.8
Brown rice, boiled	1 cup	1.3
Tuna, canned	1 can	1.3
Barley, pearl, boiled	1 cup	1.3
Bulgur, boiled	1 cup	1.0
Milk, whole	1 cup	1.0
Fruit yogurt	1 tub	1.0
Cod, cooked	1 fillet	1.0
Peanut butter	2 tbsp	0.9

Recommended dietary allowances

	Men	*Women*	*Pregnancy*	*Lactation*
USA	15 mg	12 mg	15 mg	19 mg
UK	9.5 mg	7 mg		13 mg
Australia	12 mg	12 mg	16 mg	18 mg

Supplements

Zinc supplements are available in various forms such as zinc gluconate, zinc sulfate, zinc picolinate or chelated zinc. Zinc in the form of zinc picolinate may be the best supplement for use in those who do not secrete sufficient picolinate from the pancreas.

Zinc supplements may be best taken first thing in the morning or two hours after meals to avoid the inhibition of absorption by other food constituents. However, taking the supplements with meals helps to reduce nausea which occurs in some people who take zinc on an empty stomach. Supplements should not be taken at the same time as medications, which reduce zinc absorption.

If you regularly take zinc in doses of 25 mg or above it is wise to take 2 to 3 mg of copper to avoid imbalances in the copper-to-zinc ratio.

Toxic effects of excess intake

Toxic effects of zinc are rare as excessive absorption is usually prevented by the abdominal pain, nausea and vomiting that very high doses (around 200 mg) cause. Other symptoms include dehydration, lethargy, anemia and dizziness.

Long-term use of high doses causes secondary deficiency of copper. This has been seen with intakes of zinc as low as 25 mg per day. Long-term use of doses above 150 mg have been reported to cause the suppression of immune function and decreased levels of HDL cholesterol which can lead to heart disease. Excessive use of supplements during pregnancy may be harmful to the fetus.

Therapeutic uses

Growth

Zinc supplements are used in developing countries to treat deficiency-related growth stunting, particularly in young children. A 1998 study done in Guatemala showed that daily zinc supplements of 10 mg improved growth in babies suffering from decreased growth rates.[13] Zinc seems to exert these beneficial effects via growth hormones.

Immune system

Zinc supplementation improves immune function in those who are deficient. It increases the activity of the thymus gland, improves antibody responses and enhances the functioning of white blood cells. It has been shown to inhibit the growth of bacteria and possibly viruses. Zinc supplements have also been shown to boost levels of interferon, a protein which is formed when cells are exposed to viruses and which helps to fight infection.[14]

Researchers at the University of Medicine and Dentistry of New Jersey, Newark, tested the effects of one year of supplementation with zinc and other micronutrients on cellular immunity in elderly people. The patients, aged 60-89, were either given a placebo, 15 mg of zinc, or 100 mg of zinc daily for 12 months. The results showed improvements in some aspects of immunity.[15]

In another double-blind, randomized, controlled trial published in 1998, researchers tested the effects of vitamin A and zinc (25 mg as zinc sulfate) supplements in 136 residents of a public home for older people in Rome. The results showed that zinc supplementation improved cell-mediated immune response.[16]

Many studies show beneficial effects of zinc in the treatment of diarrhea, a major cause of death in children in developing countries. Researchers involved in a double-blind trial carried out in India involving almost 600 children aged 6-35 months found that zinc supplements reduced diarrhea outbreaks.[17]

Oral supplementation with zinc and zinc sulfate gel may shorten healing time in cases of herpes virus infection.

Common cold

There have been several studies of the effect of zinc lozenges on treating the common cold. Some studies have shown benefit while other have not. The authors of a review of the trials, published in 1998 in the *Annals of Pharmacotherapy* concluded that treatment of the common cold with zinc gluconate lozenges, using adequate doses of elemental zinc, is likely to be effective in reducing duration and severity of cold symptoms. Most benefit is seen if the lozenges are started immediately after the onset of symptoms.[18]

In a 1996 randomized, double-blind, placebo-controlled study carried out in Cleveland, researchers tested the effect of zinc gluconate lozenges on the common cold. The study involved 100 participants, and patients in the zinc group received a lozenge containing 13.3 mg of zinc every two hours. The lozenges reduced the duration of cold symptoms from 7.6 days to 4.4 days. However, some people did not like the taste of the lozenges.[19]

The formulation of the lozenges also appears to be important and the addition of citric acid or tartaric acid which binds to zinc ions seems to reduce the benefit. A 1997 study suggests that zinc acetate lozenges may be more effective in treating colds than zinc gluconate, as more zinc ions are released from zinc acetate under physiological conditions.[20]

The most recent study, published in the *Journal of the American Medical Association* in 1998 did not find zinc lozenges to be effective. The study involved 249 students in grades one through 12, some of whom were given 10 mg zinc lozenges five or six times a day for three weeks and some of whom were given placebo lozenges containing no zinc. The study showed that it took children taking zinc lozenges an average of nine days to get over all their cold symptoms, which was the same amount of time for children who took placebo lozenges. More children who took zinc lozenges reported side effects such as bad taste reactions; nausea; mouth, tongue, or throat irritation; and diarrhea.[21]

Wound-healing

Zinc can also be used to enhance wound-healing and both oral and topical preparations have shown benefit. Taken before and after surgery, zinc supplements may speed recovery time. In a double-blind trial published in 1996,

68 patients were involved in an assessment of the effects of zinc supplementation on recovery after severe head injury. One month after injury, those in the zinc group had lower death rates and showed more improvement than those in the placebo group.[22]

AIDS

Studies are being conducted to see whether zinc supplementation has any benefit in the treatment of AIDS. Some studies have shown improvement in immune function while others have not. In a 1995 Italian study, zinc sulfate supplements (200 mg per day for 30 days) were given to HIV-positive patients receiving the medication azathioprine (AZT). Results showed stabilization in body weight and increases in CD4+ lymphocytes and immune-stimulating hormone levels.[23]

Pregnancy

Zinc supplementation in those who are deficient has been shown to improve birth weight and head circumference. In a 1995 study, researchers at the University of Alabama at Birmingham conducted a randomized double-blind placebo-controlled trial involving 580 African-American pregnant women with low blood plasma zinc levels. The women were either given 25 mg of zinc or a placebo. The results showed that in all the women, infants in the zinc supplement group had a significantly greater birth weight and head circumference than infants in the placebo group.[24]

Skin

Zinc is vital for normal skin function and has been used externally to treat acne, eczema, psoriasis and rosacea. The use of zinc supplements for the treatment of acne is controversial and the conflicting results may be due to the variation in the types of supplements used in different studies. (See page 503 for more information.)

Eating disorders

Studies have shown that zinc may be of benefit as part of the therapy for anorexia nervosa by improving taste perception and sense of smell which occur as the disease progresses. Zinc supplements have been found to increase the weight gain of anorexia patients.

Researchers involved in a 1994 Canadian randomized, double-blind, placebo-controlled trial gave a daily dose of 100 mg of zinc gluconate, or a placebo to 35 female anorexia patients until they achieved a 10 per cent increase in body mass index (BMI). The rate of increase in BMI of the zinc supplemented group was twice that of the placebo group.[25]

Taste disorders

Zinc supplements have been used to improve taste perception in people taking medications which reduce taste sensation, and in cancer patients undergoing radiation therapy.[26] This can be valuable in helping to maintain normal weight and nutrient intake during treatment.

Diabetes

Diabetics often excrete excess zinc in their urine and studies have shown beneficial effects of zinc supplementation. Zinc supplementation in animals improves glucose tolerance, and a study carried out in 1995 in France showed zinc gluconate supplements to improve glucose assimilation in humans.[27]

Prostate problems

Zinc supplements may play a role in the treatment of benign prostatic hyperplasia (BPH), an enlargement of the prostate gland seen in 60 per cent of men between 40 and 59 years of age. Zinc treatment, in the form of zinc picolinate or zinc citrate, may be beneficial in reducing the enlargement of the prostate and to reduce the symptoms. The beneficial effects of zinc may be due to its involvement in hormonal metabolism. Zinc inhibits the conversion of testosterone to a more active form, which causes overproduction of prostate cells.[28] It also inhibits the binding of hormones to receptor cells. Zinc also acts to lower levels of another hormone, prolactin, which controls the uptake of testosterone into the prostate.[29] Increasing zinc levels therefore restricts the actions of the hormones and leads to a reduction in prostate size.

Macular degeneration

Zinc supplements have been used to treat age-related macular degeneration, the leading cause of lack of vision in people aged over 55. In one double-blind study, researchers at Louisiana State University found that patients receiving zinc supplements had significantly less vision-loss than those not taking zinc.[30]

Digestive diseases

Zinc supplementation appears to relieve symptoms of inflammatory bowel disease (IBD) such as reduced appetite, suppressed immunity and impaired taste. IBD patients may not be able to absorb zinc properly, and as oral supplementation does not always appear to improve symptoms, intravenous zinc may be necessary. Zinc supplements have also been used to treat celiac disease.

Other uses

Some studies have shown that zinc supplements can reduce free radical damage to blood fats. In a 1996 Italian study, 25 mg zinc sulfate in 136 elderly people decreased plasma lipid peroxides.[31] This can help to reduce the risk of cardiovascular disease.

Zinc supplements have also been used to treat mild mental complaints and Alzheimer's disease. (See page 510 for more information.) A recent Japanese study found low blood levels of zinc in people suffering from tinnitus (ringing in the ears). Supplements improved the condition.[32]

Topically administered zinc acts as an astringent and a weak antiseptic. It is also used in eye drops to treat eye inflammation and as a mouthwash to inhibit plaque growth and protect against tooth disease and fungal and bacterial infections.

Interactions with other nutrients

Interaction with copper

Zinc and copper have related roles in many body functions and the balance between the two nutrients is important. Copper and zinc function together in the antioxidant enzyme copper-zinc superoxide dismutase. High zinc intakes decrease the absorption of copper, and high blood copper content can depress zinc absorption from the intestine.

The ratio of zinc to copper appears to affect the levels of lipoproteins (fat carrying proteins) in the blood. Optimal zinc intake reduces total and harmful LDL cholesterol and raises beneficial HDL cholesterol levels. However, high levels of zinc (160 mg) have been shown to lower HDL cholesterol levels in blood, raise total and LDL cholesterol, induce platelet aggregation and lead to atherosclerosis in animals. These effects may be due to the lowering of copper levels. An imbalance in zinc and copper may also be involved in high blood pressure.

Some research suggests that elevated serum copper and depressed plasma zinc levels are associated with violent tendencies in young men. Based on interviews with patients and their families and reference to a standard behavior scale, researchers identified 135 young men with a history of assault and 18 men with no history of such behavior. They analyzed blood samples and found a higher copper-to-zinc ration in the young men with a history of violence. The researchers speculate that low levels of zinc in the area of the brain known as the hippocampus may somehow alter nerve activity, thus affecting behavior.[33]

Interaction with iron

High iron intake can reduce zinc levels and high zinc intake can reduce iron absorption and encourage iron depletion from body stores.

Interaction with folic acid

A zinc-dependent enzyme is necessary for the metabolism of folic acid. Folic acid may reduce zinc absorption when the dietary zinc intake is low but not when it is high.

Other nutrients

High calcium intakes may reduce zinc absorption. In a study reported in the *American Journal of Clinical Nutrition*, researchers gave 19 healthy postmenopausal women diets which included 890 mg calcium and for some of the study, supplements containing 468 mg calcium. They found that zinc absorption was reduced by 2 mg during the high calcium periods. In another part of the study, calcium supplements were given to ten men and women with a single meal. Zinc absorption was reduced by 50 per cent.[34]

In another study published in 1997, researchers at Ohio State University assessed the effect of 1000 mg calcium supplements on zinc utilization in adolescent girls. They did not find any adverse effects.[35] Zinc supplements may be useful for postmenopausal women who are taking calcium supplements.

Interactions with drugs

Thiazide diuretics, tetracyclines, penicillamine, anticonvulsants such as sodium valproate, caffeine, and other drugs which bind zinc in the gut may reduce zinc absorption. Alcohol interferes with zinc absorption and increases excretion. Contraceptive pills may lower levels of zinc and raise copper levels in the blood, leading to increased zinc requirements.

Long-term use of the anti-hypertensive drugs, enalapril and captopril may lead to zinc deficiency according to an Israeli study published in 1998 in the *Journal of the American College of Nutrition.*[36]

Cautions

Large amounts of zinc may impair copper absorption and reduce the ability to taste sweet and salt. If continued for long periods, the secondary copper deficiency can lead to heart disease.

Other nutrients

Other nutrients

A nutrient is defined as a substance that either provides nourishment or is necessary for normal body functions or structures. The vitamins and minerals covered in the last section are, in most cases, considered to be essential nutrients. Some of the nutrients covered in this section are also essential and must be obtained in the diet. These include the essential fatty acids, alpha linolenic acid and linoleic acid. The role of fats in health and disease is a controversial one and it is only in recent years that scientists have started to understand the beneficial effects of the essential fatty acids.

Other nutrients included here, such as coenzyme Q10, are both manufactured in the body and obtained in food. Increasing evidence suggests that coenzyme Q10 deficiency can occur and supplements have been used to treat a wide range of cardiovascular diseases. Newer supplement products such as glucosamine, lipoic acid, chitosan and shark cartilage are also included here. While there is often little research evidence to support their use, many people have reported benefits that are currently being investigated.

This section also contains a chapter on flavonoids, plant compounds that are found in foods such as fruit, vegetables, red wine, green tea and soy. Scientists are just beginning to understand the disease-preventing properties of the thousands of different compounds found in these foods, and this research helps emphasize the important principle that supplements cannot substitute for an unhealthy diet.

QUICK GUIDE

Two essential fatty acids are necessary for health. These are the polyunsaturated fats, linoleic and alpha linolenic acid. Linoleic acid is an omega-6 fatty acid and alpha linolenic acid is an omega-3 fatty acid.

Essential for

- energy production
- cell membrane formation
- oxygen transfer from air to blood
- hemoglobin manufacture
- prostaglandin function

Deficiency

Symptoms of essential fatty acid deficiency may include fatigue, dry skin, immune weakness, gastrointestinal disorders, heart and circulatory problems, growth retardation, mental problems and sterility. It is likely that a lack of dietary essential fatty acids plays an important role in the development of many common diseases, including cardiovascular disease, cancer, arthritis and asthma.

Sources

Omega-3 fatty acids are found in fish and oils such as flaxseed oil. Linoleic acid is found in safflower, sunflower and corn oils.

Daily recommended dietary intakes

An optimal amount of linoleic acid is around 9 to 18 g per day, while an optimal amount of alpha linolenic acid is around 2 to 9 g per day.

Toxic effects of excess intake

Toxic effects are unknown.

Interactions

Magnesium, selenium, zinc, niacin, vitamins B6, A, C and E are necessary for the conversion of linoleic acid to other omega-6 fatty acids.

Therapeutic uses of supplements

Supplements are used to treat cardiovascular disease, cancer, high blood pressure, arthritis, skin disorders, menstrual pain,diabetes and inflammatory bowel disease. They may also be beneficial during pregnancy and breastfeeding.

Few topics in nutrition cause as much controversy and concern as fat. For years we have been told to cut down on the amount of fat we eat, but the latest research suggests that it is not so much the amount of fat we eat as the balance of the different types. Fats play a critical role in the function of every cell of the body. The type of dietary fat affects the behavior of each one of these cells, how well they perform their vital functions, and the ability to resist disease. There are many kinds of fat in the diet and different types can exert either beneficial or harmful effects. Two essential fatty acids are necessary for health. These are the polyunsaturated fats, linoleic acid and alpha linolenic acid. Essential fatty acids have beneficial effects while high intakes of saturated and hydrogenated fats are linked to an increased risk of degenerative diseases such as cardiovascular disease, cancer and diabetes.

Types of fat

In contrast to the food supply available to man throughout most of history, the typical modern Western diet contains a large amount of fat. Fats are found in both plant and animal foods and there are several different types:

Saturated fats

These are found in animal foods such as meat, butter and cheese, and plant foods such as coconut oil and palm oil. Trans fats are unsaturated fats, which have undergone a chemical process called hydrogenation to turn them into saturated fats. They are found in packaged foods such as pastries, cookies, crackers and baked goods. High intakes of saturated fats are associated with an increased risk of many diseases. As little dietary fat as possible should come from these fats, with a maximum of 10 per cent.

Monounsaturated fats

These include those found in canola, olive and peanut oils, and may also help to lower cholesterol and decrease platelet aggregation. They are also less susceptible to oxidation.

Polyunsaturated fats

These are found in oils of plant origin such as safflower, sesame, sunflower and corn, and may help to lower cholesterol and decrease platelet aggregation, thus reducing the risk of heart disease. However, polyunsaturated oils are susceptible to oxidative damage and may also lower beneficial HDL cholesterol levels. A high intake of polyunsaturated fats has been linked to an increased risk of cancer. Experts recommend that no more than 10 per cent of dietary fat should come from polyunsaturated fats.

Omega-3 and omega-6 fatty acids

Linoleic acid is an omega-6 fatty acid and alpha linolenic acid is an omega-3 fatty acid. These terms refer to characteristics in the chemical structure of the fatty acids. Other omega-3 fatty acids are manufactured in the body using alpha linolenic acid as a starting point. These include eicosapentaenoic acid (EPA) and docosahexaenoic acid (DHA).

Other omega-6 fatty acids can be manufactured in the body using linoleic acid as a starting point. These include gamma-linoleic acid (GLA), dihomo-gamma-linoleic acid (DHGLA) and arachidonic acid.

What they do in the body

Essential fatty acids are involved in energy production, the transfer of oxygen from the air to the bloodstream, and the manufacture of hemoglobin. They are also involved in growth, cell division and nerve function. Essential fatty acids are found in high concentrations in the brain and are essential for normal nerve impulse transmission and brain function.

Cell membranes

Essential fatty acids are components of cell membranes. They are essential for many body functions; including oxygen use and energy production, control of the substances passing in and out of cells, cell to cell communication, and regulation by hormones.

Cell membranes are partly made up of phospholipids, which contain fatty acids. The type of fatty acids in the diet will determine what type of fatty acids go to make up cell membranes. A phospholipid made from a saturated fat has a different structure and is less fluid than one which incorporates an essential fatty acid. This loss of fluidity makes it difficult for the cell to carry out its normal functions, and increases the cell's susceptibility to injury and death. The relative amounts of omega-3 fatty acids and omega-6 fatty acids in cell membranes also affect their function.

Prostaglandins

Essential fatty acids are also involved in the manufacture of prostaglandins, substances which play a role in a number of body functions; including hormone synthesis, immune function, regulation of the response to pain and inflammation, blood vessel constriction, and other heart and lung functions.

There are various types of prostaglandins and these have different effects. Prostaglandins are divided into three main types; those of the 1 and 3 series are usually considered to have beneficial effects while those of the 2 series are usually considered to have harmful effects. EPA, the omega-3 fatty acid that is formed from alpha linolenic acid, is the precursor of the series 3 prostaglandins. Series 1 and 2 prostaglandins are formed from the omega-6 fatty acid, linoleic acid. It can be converted to DHGLA, the precursor of the series 1 prostaglandins and to arachidonic acid, which is the precursor of the series 2 prostaglandins. The types of oils in the diet, including the balance of omega-6 to omega-3 oils, plays a role in determining whether DHGLA is converted to favorable series 1 prostaglandins or to harmful series 2 prostaglandins.

Series 1 and 3 prostaglandins act to dilate blood vessels, reduce clotting, lower harmful LDL cholesterol levels, raise beneficial HDL cholesterol levels and have anti-inflammatory actions. Series 2 prostaglandins have the opposite actions. The balance of prostaglandins in the body is affected by diet and can determine whether a person is at increased risk of disease.

Deficiency

Symptoms of essential fatty acid deficiency may include fatigue, dry skin, immune weakness, gastrointestinal disorders, heart and circulatory problems, growth retardation, mental problems and sterility. It is likely that a lack of dietary essential fatty acids plays an important role in the development of many common diseases.

Modern food production processes have had a large impact on the types of fat in foods. People now eat smaller amounts of essential fatty acids and more refined and unnatural fats and oils, such as trans fatty acids. The commercial refinement of fats and oils has led to a lower availability of essential fatty acids in the diet, and also transforms essential fatty acids into toxic compounds. Refined fats may also prevent the body from using the essential fatty acids that do remain in the diet.

Cardiovascular disease

There are many population studies demonstrating that people who consume omega-3 fatty acid-rich diets have a reduced risk of heart disease. This was first noticed in countries such as Greenland and Japan where fish consumption is particularly high. Studies in other countries have found similar effects. The evidence suggests that eating fish once a week will help prevent coronary heart disease and people with cardiac disease may benefit from eating two fish-containing meals per week.

In a study reported in the *New England Journal of Medicine*, researchers in Holland investigated the relationship between fish consumption and coronary heart disease in a group of men in the town of Zutphen. Information about the fish consumption of 852 middle-aged men without coronary heart disease was collected in 1960. During 20 years of follow-up, 78 men died from coronary heart disease. The results showed that compared to those who did not eat fish, death from coronary heart disease was more than 50 per cent lower in those who ate at least 30 g of fish per day.[1] However, not all studies have shown a reduced risk in those who regularly eat fish. These include the Health Professionals Follow-Up Study.[2,3]

In a study reported in 1989, researchers examined the effects of dietary changes in the prevention of further heart attacks in 2033 men who had recovered from one attack. Some of the men were given various pieces of dietary advice, one of which was to increase the consumption of fatty fish to around two or three portions per week. Those advised to do this had a 29 per cent reduction in death from all causes and a 33 per cent reduction in death from heart attack compared with those who were not advised to eat fish.[4] These beneficial effects may be due to the anti-arrhythmic effects of omega-3 fatty acids.

Results from the Western Electric Study showed a reduced risk of coronary heart disease mortality and nonsudden cardiac death but not a reduced risk of sudden cardiac death with increasing fish consumption. This study involved around 2000 middle-aged men followed up for around 30 years.[5]

The results of this study differ from those obtained from the US Physicians' Health Study published in 1998 in which researchers investigated the links between fish consumption and the risk of sudden death from heart attack in 20 551 US male physicians aged from 40 to 84. The follow-up period was 11 years, and in that time there were 133 sudden deaths. The results showed that men who ate fish at least once per week had around half the risk of sudden cardiac death when compared with men who consumed fish less than once a month. Neither dietary fish consumption nor omega-3 fatty acid intake was associated with a reduced risk of total heart attack, nonsudden cardiac death, or total cardiovascular mortality. However, fish consumption was associated with a significantly reduced risk of death from all causes.[6] The difference in sudden death definition may explain the different results obtained in the two studies. In this study, the association between fish consumption and sudden cardiac death was stronger than that between omega-3 fatty acid intake and sudden cardiac death. It is therefore possible that other substances present in fish may be exerting protective effects.

However, in a 1995 study, researchers at the University of Washington examined the links between risk of heart attack and the consumption of fatty acids from seafood, and assessed both directly and indirectly through examination of blood samples. The study involved 334 patients with primary cardiac arrest and 493 population-based control cases, matched for age and sex. The results showed that an intake of 5.5 g of omega-3 fatty acids (equivalent to one fish-containing meal a week) reduced the risk of heart attack by 50 per cent. Their results also showed a correlation between higher red blood cell levels of omega-3 fatty acids and reduction in risk of heart attack. Those with the highest levels had a 70 per cent reduction in risk compared to those with the lowest levels.[7]

Research done in Finland suggests that a high intake of fish and omega-3 fatty acids is associated with an increased risk of coronary death. In one study, a high intake of local lean fish was associated with a high intake of mercury which may outweigh the benefits of an increase in omega-3 fatty acid intake.[8] High intakes of omega-3 fatty acids are also associated with a lower risk of stroke.[9]

Cancer

The results from some, but not all, epidemiological studies indicate that the level of dietary fat intake and the types of fatty acids consumed influence cancer risk and disease progression. High intakes of omega-6 fatty acids seem to increase the risk of cancers while high intakes of omega-3 fatty acids may provide protection. The fatty acid composition of fat tissue reflects the dietary consumption of essential fatty acids over a period of years. These observations are supported by results from animal studies, which demonstrate that polyunsaturated omega-6 fatty acids stimulate carcinogenesis and tumor growth and metastasis, whereas long-chain omega-3 fatty acids have inhibitory effects. Reducing total fat intake and increasing the ratio of omega-3 to omega-6 fatty acids in the diet may be particularly useful for groups at a relatively high risk of cancer, and may also be useful after surgery to help prevent disease recurrence.[10]

Prostate cancer

Dietary intake of essential fatty acids may play a role in prostate cancer cell proliferation. Epidemiological studies have demonstrated that men whose dietary intake is high in omega-6 fatty acids have a higher incidence of clinical prostate cancer.[11] Diets high in omega-3 fatty acids may have protective effects.

Breast cancer

In a 1994 study done in France, researchers assessed the links between the levels of various fatty acids in breast fat tissue, and the spread of tumors in 121 patients with cancer. The results showed that a low level of alpha linolenic acid was linked to tumor invasion of other tissues.[12]

Other research suggests that omega-3 fatty acids inhibit breast cancer and that the degree of this inhibition depends on background levels of omega-6 fatty acids. Results from the European Community Multicenter Study on Antioxidants, Myocardial Infarction, and Cancer (EURAMIC) study published in 1998, suggest that an increase in the ratio of omega-3 fatty acids to total omega-6 fatty acids in fat tissue decreases the risk of breast cancer. In this study, total levels of omega-3 or omega-6 fat were not consistently associated with breast cancer.[13]

Colon cancer

Population and laboratory studies suggest that omega-3 fatty acids may help to prevent and inhibit colon cancer. In a study published in 1995, death rates for colorectal cancer in 24 European countries were correlated with current fish and fish oil consumption and with consumption 10 and 23 years previously. In men, there was a reduced risk of death from colorectal cancer and current intake of fish; a weaker link with fish consumption ten years earlier; and none with consumption 23 years earlier. The researchers concluded that fish consumption is associated with protection against the later stages of colorectal cancer, but not with the early initiation stages.[14]

Rheumatoid arthritis

A low intake of omega-3 fatty acids may contribute to the development of rheumatoid arthritis. Omega-3 fatty acids have an anti-inflammatory action, most likely due to effects on prostaglandin metabolism. In a population-based case-control study published in 1996, researchers compared diets in 324 women with rheumatoid arthritis and 1245 women with no disease. The results showed that consumption of broiled or baked fish, but not of other types of fish, was associated with a decreased risk of rheumatoid arthritis. Women who ate between one and two servings per week had a 22 per cent lower risk compared with those who ate fish less than once a week. Women who ate fish more than twice a week had a 43 per cent reduced risk.[15]

Asthma

A low dietary intake of omega-3 fatty acids may contribute to or worsen asthma symptoms, most likely due to increased inflammation. The ratio of omega-3 to omega-6 fatty acids has been shown to be low in asthma sufferers.[16] Supplements may be useful in relieving symptoms in some asthmatics, although not all studies have shown beneficial effects.[17]

Depression

Recent research suggests that omega-3 fatty acid deficiency may also be linked to depression and aggression. In a 1998 UK study, researchers assessed the omega-3 fatty acid levels in the diet and in red blood cell membranes of ten depressed patients and compared these with nondepressed patients. The results showed that the severity of depression was linked to red blood cell membrane levels and to dietary intake of omega-3 fatty acids.[18]

Pre-eclampsia

Omega-3 fatty acid deficiency may be linked to pre-eclampsia. In a 1995 study, women with the lowest levels of omega-3 fatty acids were seven times more likely to have had their pregnancies complicated by pre-eclampsia compared with those women with the highest levels of omega-3 fatty acids. An increase in the ratio of omega-3 to omega-6 fatty acids was associated with a reduction in risk of pre-eclampsia.[19]

Other symptoms

Deficiency may also be linked to attention deficit hyperactivity disorder,[20] anorexia nervosa,[21] premenstrual syndrome, skin disorders, inflammatory bowel disease, multiple sclerosis and immune disorders.

Daily intake

The amount of essential fatty acids needed depends on a person's levels of activity and stress, nutritional state and body weight. Three to 6 g (one teaspoon) per day of linoleic acid prevents signs of deficiency in most healthy adults, while an optimal amount may be 9 to 18 g per day. Two to 9 g (one or two teaspoons) of alpha linolenic acid may be a good daily dose. Some omega-3 and omega-6 fatty acids such as EPA and arachidonic acid can be obtained ready made from food rather than being made from linoleic and alpha linolenic acid.

The ratio of omega-3 oils to omega-6 oils may also be important in the development of disease. The omega-6 to omega-3 ratio in healthy populations consuming traditional diets ranges from 5:2 to 1:6. Modern diets have decreased the consumption of omega-3 oils, and the omega-6 to omega-3 ratio is currently around 20:1. Consuming an oil such as flaxseed oil, which has a high omega-3 to omega-6 ratio, can correct a deficiency; but long-term exclusive use may lead to an omega-6 deficiency.

Recent evidence from a number of studies suggests that as little as two to three 3-ounce servings per week of EPA-rich fish may have beneficial effects in preventing disorders such as heart disease and arthritis. The benefits are more pronounced when the diet is low in fat.

Sources

Omega-3 fatty acids

Omega-3 fatty acids such as EPA are found in cold water fish. Mackerel, herring, halibut and salmon contain the most, with lesser amounts in tuna and shrimp.

Flaxseed oil is good source of essential fatty acids and is particularly high in omega-3 oils. It is difficult for the digestive system to break down raw flaxseeds sufficiently to obtain enough essential fatty acids, so using flaxseed oil or grinding the seeds is preferable. As essential fatty acids deteriorate quickly, flaxseeds are best kept in the refrigerator and ground when you need them.

Omega-6 fatty acids

Linoleic acid is found in safflower, sunflower and corn oils. Evening primrose oil, blackcurrant and borage oils contain varying amounts of the omega-6 fatty acid, gamma-linolenic acid (GLA). As GLA is the precursor of beneficial series 1 prostaglandins, supplements are quite popular. However, some studies show that long-term use of these supplements increases arachidonic acid levels and decreases EPA levels which may increase the risk of heart disease and cancer.[22]

Supplements

There are many types of essential fatty acid supplements available, including flaxseed oil, fish oils, evening primrose oil, blackcurrant oil, and borage oil. These are available in capsule and free oil forms. Some experts advise avoiding fish oil supplements because they may have toxic contaminants. Fish oil supplements should not be taken during pregnancy due to the damaging effects of high doses of vitamin A. (See page 40 for more information.)

All essential fatty acids deteriorate rapidly when exposed to light, heat, air and metals. It is important to be aware of the processing and storage methods used when buying supplements. Oils should be organic, unrefined, extracted at temperatures below 98 degrees F, and stored in light-resistant plastic containers.

Toxic effects

The long-term effects of large doses of essential fatty acids are unclear. They may include an increased risk of stroke, nosebleeds and prolonged blood clotting time.

Therapeutic uses of supplements

Manipulating cell membrane structure and prostaglandin metabolism through dietary fats can be used to prevent or treat cardiovascular disease, cancer, inflammatory conditions such as arthritis, allergies, and several other disorders. It may take several weeks to see changes after adding essential fatty acids to the diet.

Cardiovascular disease

Omega-3 fatty acid supplements have been used to treat and prevent various types of cardiovascular disease. Supplements have been shown to have beneficial effects on cholesterol and triglyceride levels. In a 1994 study, researchers assessed the effects of fish oil supplements on 350 men and women aged from 30 to 54 years who were enrolled in a hypertension prevention trial. Once a day for 6 months the participants received either a placebo or 6 g of purified fish oil, which supplied 3 g of omega-3 fatty acids. The results showed that the fish oil increased HDL cholesterol levels significantly. The effect was more marked in the women.[23]

Supplements have also been shown to affect blood clotting through effects on platelets, and to lead to a reduction in production of prostaglandins and other substances that damage artery walls.[24] Other studies have shown that omega-3 fatty acids reduce the build-up of white blood cells in atherosclerotic plaque. A 1997 Australian study showed that flaxseed oil improved the elasticity of artery walls. This tends to decrease with increasing cardiovascular risk and has also been shown to improve with increasing intake of omega-3 fatty acids from fish.[25]

High blood pressure

Dietary omega-3 fatty acid supplementation has been shown to be effective in treating mild high blood pressure. In a 1996 study of 78 patients with untreated mild hypertension, Norwegian researchers found that overall blood pressure was reduced by about six points in people who took fish oil supplements, compared with those who took a corn oil placebo.[26] In some cases it may also be an effective addition to drug treatment.[27] In a 1996 study, 21 men whose blood pressure was not successfully controlled with anti-hypertensive medications were randomized to receive either fish oil (4.5 g omega-3 fatty acids per day) or a placebo. Blood pressure readings were taken at the start of the study and at four and eight weeks. Both systolic and diastolic blood pressures were significantly reduced in the fish oil group at both week four and at week eight.[28] Supplements have also been useful in preventing high blood pressure in heart transplant patients.[29] However, not all studies have shown beneficial effects.[30]

Cancer

Omega-3 fatty acids

Omega-3 fatty acids seem to exert tumor-suppressive effects.[31] A low fat diet that includes omega-3 fatty acid supplements may help to lower the risk of cancer and may also help to prevent the recurrence of tumors in those who have had cancer. In a study published in 1997, Norwegian researchers studied the relationship between incidence of lung cancer and intake of dietary fats, high-fat foods, fish, and fish products in 25 956 men and 25 496 women aged from 16 to 56. During the follow-up period, 153 cases of lung cancer were identified. The results showed that those who took cod liver oil supplements had around half the risk of those who did not.[32]

Essential fatty acids may also boost immune function. Studies on the immune T cells in cancer patients taking fish oil capsules suggest that omega-3 fatty acids bring about beneficial changes. In a Greek study published in 1998, researchers investigated the effect of dietary omega-3 fatty acids and vitamin E on the immune status and survival in both well-nourished and malnourished cancer patients. The study involved 60 patients with solid tumors who were randomized to receive dietary supplementation with either fish oil (18 g of omega-3 fatty acids) or placebo daily. The authors measured various indicators of immune function. The results showed that omega-3 fatty acids had a significant immune-enhancing effect and seemed to prolong the survival of malnourished patients.[33]

GLA

GLA has been shown to be effective in killing cancer cells and is well-established as a topical treatment for some types of cancer, including bladder cancer.[34] It has also been shown to kill various other types of cancer cells.[35,36]

In a 1994 study, 32 breast cancer patients aged 32 to 81 years and classified 'high risk' due to the spread of their tumors to the lymph nodes in their armpits, were studied for 18 months following an Adjuvant Nutritional Intervention in Cancer (ANICA) protocol. This nutritional protocol was added to the surgical and therapeutic treatment of breast cancer and involved treatment with a combination of nutritional antioxidants, (vitamin C: 2850 mg, vitamin E: 2500 IU, beta carotene 32.5 IU, selenium 387 mcg plus secondary vitamins and minerals) essential fatty acids, (1.2 g gamma-linolenic acid and 3.5g of omega-3 fatty acids) and 90 mg of coenzyme Q10 per day.

The researchers measured various biochemical markers of cancer progression, tumor spread and the clinical condition of the patients. Quality of life and survival were also assessed during the trial. The main observations were that none of the patients died during the study period. (The expected number was four); none of the patients showed signs of further distant metastases; quality of life was improved (no weight loss, reduced use of pain killers); six patients showed apparent partial remission.[37]

Arthritis

Omega-3 fatty acids

Fish oils from dietary sources or capsules have been shown to reduce the pain, swelling and stiffness of arthritis. This may be due to the effects on the immune response and on prostaglandins, cytokines and leukotrienes that mediate the inflammatory processes involved in rheumatoid arthritis. Arthritis sufferers may have reduced medication needs if they take omega-3 fatty acids.

In a 1994 study, Belgian researchers enrolled 90 patients in a 12-month, double-blind, randomized trial comparing daily supplementation with either 2.6 g of omega-3 fatty acids, or 1.3 g of omega-3 fatty acids plus 3 g of olive oil, or 6 g of olive oil. The researchers found significant improvement in both the patient's evaluation and in the physician's assessment of pain in those taking 2.6 g per day of omega-3 fatty acids. The number of patients who were able to reduce their anti-rheumatic medications was significantly greater in the group taking 2.6 g of omega-3 fatty acids.[38]

GLA

Research also suggests that GLA-containing essential fatty acids obtained from evening primrose, blackcurrant and borage seed oils are effective in treating rheumatoid arthritis.

In a 1996 double-blind study done at the University of Massachusetts Medical Center, researchers investigated the clinical efficacy and adverse effects of 2.8 g per day of GLA in the treatment of 56 patients with active rheumatoid arthritis. This was followed by a six-month, single-blind trial during which all patients received GLA. Treatment with GLA for six months resulted in statistically significant and clinically relevant reductions in the signs and symptoms of disease activity. During the second six months, both groups exhibited improvement in disease activity. In the group who had continuously received GLA, 16 of 21 patients showed meaningful improvement at 12 months compared with study entry.[39]

In another randomized, double-blind, placebo-controlled study, US researchers investigated the effects of blackcurrant seed oil on arthritis patients over a period of 24 weeks. Treatment with the supplement resulted in reduction in signs and symptoms of disease activity in patients with RA. In contrast, patients given a placebo showed no change in disease.[40] However, results of studies using GLA have been mixed and this may be due to the ability of GLA to raise tissue levels of arachidonic acid while reducing the level of omega-3 fatty acids. Omega-3 fatty acids from fish oil or flaxseed oil may be more beneficial.

Pregnancy and breastfeeding

The omega-3 fatty acid, DHA, is the major structural and functional essential fatty acid in the central nervous system. It is essential for normal development of eye function and vision in the growing fetus. In premature babies, the levels of DHA are positively related to head circumference, birth weight and birth length. These results suggest that increasing omega-3 fatty acids during pregnancy may be beneficial to both mother and child. Essential fatty acids may also help to prevent premature birth.[41,42]

Skin disorders

Essential fatty acids have been shown to have beneficial effects in the treatment of skin disorders. This is likely to be due to effects on prostaglandin metabolism. In a 1997 Italian study, researchers treated 30 eczema patients with GLA (274 mg twice a day), and 30 with placebo for 12 weeks. During this time, the patients assessed their own symptoms and they were also assessed by a dermatologist every four weeks. The patients who received GLA showed gradual improvements in itching, redness, vesicle formation and oozing, which were statistically significant compared with the control group.[43] Borage seed oil capsules have also shown beneficial effects in the treatment of atopic dermatitis,[44] as have evening primrose oil capsules.[45]

Essential fatty acid supplements may be beneficial in psoriasis sufferers. Analysis of blood and fat tissue has shown that the amount of anti-inflammatory alpha linolenic acid decreases, while the level of arachidonic acid, which has inflammatory effects, increases. These changes may be more pronounced in patients with severe psoriasis than in those with a milder form of the disease.[46]

The results of a 1993 study suggest that eating oily fish may help reduce the symptoms of psoriasis.[47] Some small studies suggest that fish oil supplementation may be beneficial in psoriasis. In a 1998 study, researchers from several European centers treated 83 patients with either an omega-3 fatty acid-based lipid emulsion or a placebo. There were significant improvements in symptoms, as assessed both by the patients and the researchers.[48] Essential fatty acid supplements also help to reduce the toxicity of immune-suppressant and vitamin A-derivative drugs.[49]

Menstrual pain

Omega-3 fatty acids have also been shown to relieve menstrual pain. In a 1996 study, researchers assessed the effects of fish oil supplements on girls aged from 15 to 18 who reported suffering from period pain. Twenty-one girls received fish oil supplements (1080 mg EPA, 720 mg DHA and 1.5 mg vitamin E) and the other 21 received a placebo. After two months, the groups switched treatments for another two months. The amount of painkillers that the girls took during each menstrual period was also compared over the four months. After two months of treatment with fish oil, there were marked reductions in symptoms and painkiller use. Placebo treatment did not ease pain.[50]

Diabetes

Diabetics are at increased risk of cardiovascular disease, so increased intakes of omega-3 oils may be beneficial in helping to reduce this risk. There were some concerns that omega-3 fatty acid supplements would worsen blood sugar control in diabetics but more recent studies suggest that this is not the case. In a 1997 Italian study, researchers evaluated the effect of omega-3 fatty acid supplements on 935 patients with high blood fat levels, both with and without glucose intolerance or diabetes. The results showed improvements in blood fat levels and no worsening of blood sugar control.[51]

Diabetics seem to have a reduced ability to convert linoleic acid to GLA. This may lead to defective nerve function, as metabolites of GLA are known to be important in nerve membrane structure, blood flow, and impulse conduction. In a 1993 double-blind, placebo-controlled study, UK researchers compared the effects of placebo and GLA (480 mg per day)on the course of mild diabetic neuropathy in 111 patients over a one-year period. They used various nerve conduction, sensation and reflex tests, and the results of these showed that the change in response to GLA was more favorable than the change with placebo.[52]

Inflammatory bowel disease

Omega-3 fatty acid supplements have been used to treat Crohn's disease. They may be useful in correcting abnormalities in fatty acid and prostaglandin metabolism and act to reduce inflammation. A 1996 Italian study published in the *New England Journal of Medicine* showed beneficial effects of fish oil in treating Crohn's disease. Researchers involved in the one year, double-blind, placebo-controlled study investigated the effects of an enteric fish oil preparation on the maintenance of remission in 78 patients with Crohn's disease who had a high risk of relapse. Every day, the patients received either nine fish oil capsules containing a total of 2.7 g of omega-3 fatty acids or placebo. The proportion of patients in the treatment group who remained in remission after a year was 59 per cent, compared to only 26 per cent of patients in the placebo group. Enteric-coated capsules may be particularly useful as side effects such as unpleasant taste, bad breath and diarrhea are minimized.[53]

Other uses

Essential fatty acids are likely to be useful in the treatment of inflammation due to their effects on prostaglandin metabolism. This may be beneficial in acne, allergies and autoimmune diseases. Other disorders for which they might be beneficial include AIDS, Alzheimer's disease, breast pain, immune disorders and neurological problems.

GLA and alpha linolenic acid have been used to prevent migraine.[54] Some research suggests that essential fatty acids may be beneficial in reducing the frequency and severity of attacks in multiple sclerosis sufferers. These effects may be related to the role played by essential fatty acids in the formation of myelin, the fatty sheath that coats the nerves.

Interactions

Magnesium, selenium, zinc, niacin, vitamins B6, A, C and E are necessary for the conversion of linoleic acid to other omega-6 fatty acids.

Recent evidence suggests that choline is an essential nutrient in humans. Small quantities are synthesized in the liver with the help of vitamin B12, folic acid and the amino acid, methionine; but the amounts made may not be sufficient to meet daily needs.

What it does in the body

Fat metabolism

Choline is involved in fat metabolism and in the transport of fats from the liver.

Cell membranes

Choline is a component of cell membranes and plays a role in the transmission of signals inside cells. Myelin, the insulating sheath around the nerves, and platelet activating factor contain choline.

Neurotransmitters

Choline accelerates the synthesis and release of the neurotransmitter acetylcholine, which is involved in many nerve and brain functions. Dietary intake of choline seems to affect body levels of acetylcholine.

Absorption

Choline may be absorbed better in the form of lecithin.

Deficiency

Choline deficiency symptoms in humans include fatty liver and liver damage. These symptoms have been demonstrated only recently in humans fed choline-deficient diets.[1] This means that choline fulfills one of the criteria for being an essential nutrient. Patients on long-term parenteral nutrition who are not given choline develop fatty infiltration of the liver and other signs of dysfunction. This condition can be improved, and possibly prevented, with choline supplementation. Choline deficiency in animals also leads to nerve degeneration, senile dementia, high blood cholesterol, and liver cancer – possibly by affecting cell signaling or by generating free radicals and DNA alterations.

Nervous system disorders

Uptake of circulating choline into the brain decreases with age. Choline is important for nerve structure and function; and this change may contribute to the type of dementia in which cholinergic nerves are lost.

Sources

Good sources of choline in the form of lecithin include eggs, organ meats, lean meat, brewer's yeast, legumes such as soybeans, grains, and nuts. It is found in green leafy vegetables as free choline.

Recommended intakes

Adequate intake levels for choline have recently been set in the US. The average daily diet supplies around 1000 mg.

Men	Women	Pregnancy	Lactation
550 mg	425 mg	450 mg	550 mg

The tolerable upper intake limit has been set at 3 g per day.

Choline is actively transported from mother to fetus across the placenta and from mother to infant across the mammary gland. Thus, during pregnancy and lactation, dietary requirements for choline are increased.

Supplements

Alcoholics, diabetics and anyone who has deficiency symptoms may benefit from supplements either of lecithin or of choline. Supplemental choline is often in the form of lecithin. The choline content of supplements varies widely.

Toxic effects

Toxic effects at high doses may include reduced appetite, nausea, gastrointestinal problems and a 'fishy' body odor.

Therapeutic uses of supplements

Dementia

Choline supplements have been used to treat the symptoms of brain diseases such as Alzheimer's disease and Huntington's chorea, in which acetylcholine levels are low due to the reduced activity of the enzyme which synthesizes it. Some studies have detected improvements in mental performance after choline treatment.[2] However, results of studies have been mixed. Choline and lecithin may only be useful in the initial stages of the disease. In a 1994 study, lecithin was given to patients with Alzheimer's disease in daily doses of 1000 mg for one month. Results showed slightly improved mental performance, and enhanced cerebrovascular blood flow.[3]

Cardiovascular disease

Choline helps to lower cholesterol levels, as a choline-containing enzyme helps to remove cholesterol from tissues. In a 1995 study, researchers gave lecithin supplements to 32 patients with high cholesterol and triglyceride levels. The dosage used was 3.5 g three times daily before meals. After 30 days of treatment, total cholesterol and triglycerides levels decreased significantly, and beneficial HDL cholesterol levels rose.[4] Choline has also been used to lower homocysteine concentrations, another risk factor for cardiovascular disease. (See page 560 for more information.)

Other uses

Choline supplements (in the form of lecithin) have been shown to bring some benefits in the treatment of bipolar disorder (manic depression).[5] Choline and lecithin are also used to treat liver damage and hepatitis. Supplements have also been used to treat asthma.[6]

Interactions

Severe folic acid deficiency causes secondary liver choline deficiency, and vice versa, in rats. Choline supplements reduce urinary excretion of carnitine.

Inositol

Inositol functions closely with choline. It is not recognized as a vitamin as the body and intestinal bacteria can make it in limited quantities, and no deficiency states have been reported. Inositol is found in the brain, nerves, muscles, bones, reproductive organs, stomach, kidney, spleen, liver and heart. It is a major component of lecithin.

What it does in the body

Fat metabolism

Inositol, like choline, promotes the export of fat from the liver. It is also involved in the control of blood cholesterol.

Cell membranes

Inositol is a component of cell membranes and the myelin which coats the nerves.

Deficiency

Inositol deficiency in animals leads to fat accumulation in the liver, nerve disorders and intestinal problems. No deficiency symptoms have been reported in humans.

Sources

Inositol is found in a wide variety of foods. In plant sources such as citrus fruits, whole grains and seeds, inositol is present mainly in a fiber component known as phytic acid. Intestinal bacteria may act on this compound to release inositol. In animal foods such as liver and beef heart, inositol occurs as myo-inositol.

Recommended intakes

It is difficult to assess recommended daily intakes for inositol due to its synthesis in the body, but the average daily diet supplies approximately 1000 mg. No deficiency or toxicity has been identified for inositol as it is present in a wide variety of foods.

Supplements

Inositol is available in lecithin and as inositol monophosphate.

Therapeutic uses of supplements

Mood disorders

Inositol is sometimes used to treat mental disorders. Researchers involved in a 1997 double-blind controlled trial assessed the effect of 12 g daily of inositol in 28 depressed patients for four weeks. The results showed significant improvement in symptoms compared to placebo. The same researchers also tested the effectiveness of inositol supplements in panic disorders and obsessive compulsive disorder, and found beneficial effects.[1]

Other uses

Low levels of inositol have been found in the nerves of diabetic patients and supplements may be useful in the treatment of diabetic nerve disorders. Inositol has also been used to treat multiple sclerosis. Recent research suggests that myo-inositol can prevent folate-resistant neural tube defects in mice.[2]

Para-aminobenzoic acid

Para-aminobenzoic acid (PABA) is a member of the B complex and is part of the folic acid molecule. It is synthesized by intestinal bacteria.

What it does in the body

PABA may be important for skin, hair and intestinal health.

Deficiency

No deficiency symptoms have been recorded.

Sources

PABA is found in brewer's yeast, wheatgerm, liver, eggs and molasses.

Toxic effects

High doses of PABA may cause nausea, vomiting and possibly liver damage.

Therapeutic uses of supplements

PABA is used as a sunscreen to protect against ultraviolet rays. It has also been used to turn gray hair back to its natural color, although this has not had wide success. PABA has also been used to treat vitiligo, a skin depigmenting condition.

Cautions

PABA is a necessary nutrient for bacteria and may reduce the effectiveness of sulfa antibiotics if taken at the same time.

Laetrile, which is also known as amygdalin, was isolated in 1952 by biochemist Ernest Krebs who named it vitamin B17 and promoted it as a cancer preventative and cure. Laetrile is found in apricot kernels and contains a cyanide molecule which means it may be toxic in large doses. These concerns have led to laetrile being made illegal as a treatment for cancer in the USA.

Laetrile in cancer treatment

In a clinical trial in cancer patients reported in 1982, laetrile did not appear to cause shrinkage of tumors or alleviate cancer symptoms. Survival time was not increased and there were no improvements in feelings of wellbeing.[1] There have also been several reports of laetrile causing serious, life-threatening toxicity when taken in large doses.[2] Krebs claimed that laetrile preferentially killed cancer cells but laboratory evidence suggests that this is not the case.[3]

Absorption

Laetrile is not digested in the stomach but passes into the small intestine where it is acted on by enzymes that split it into various compounds, which are then absorbed.

Sources

Laetrile is found in apricot kernels and in the kernels of other fruits such as plums, peaches, cherries, peaches and apples. Mung bean sprouts and almonds also contain laetrile.

Toxic effects

Laetrile in large doses may be toxic due to its 6 per cent cyanide content. Treatment amounts are usually limited to 1 g to reduce side effects.

Pangamic acid

Pangamic acid was isolated in 1951 by the biochemist Ernest Krebs, who named it vitamin B15.

What it does in the body

Pangamic acid may play a role in the formation of amino acids, glucose oxidation and cell respiration and may act as an antioxidant. It may also lower blood cholesterol and improve circulation.

Deficiency

No deficiency symptoms have been recorded.

Sources

Sources of pangamic acid include apricot kernels, whole grains such as brown rice, pumpkin, sunflower seeds and brewer's yeast. Pangamic acid supplements are not readily available in the USA.

Toxic effects

There are no known toxic effects from even high doses of pangamic acid.

Therapeutic uses of supplements

Much of the research supporting the importance of pangamic acid has been done in the former Soviet Union where it is regularly used for disorders including alcoholism, drug addiction, heart disease and high blood pressure. Pangamic acid has also been used to reduce the build-up of lactic acid and thereby to lessen muscle fatigue and increase endurance.

QUICK GUIDE

Coenzyme Q10 is also known as ubiqinone.

Essential for

- energy production
- ATP formation
- antioxidant action

Deficiency

Coenzyme Q10 deficiency affects the heart. It has also been linked to other conditions such as cancer, muscular dystrophy, diabetes, obesity, periodontal disease, lowered immune function and neurodegenerative disorders such as Parkinson's disease.

Sources

Coenzyme Q10 is found in all plant and animal foods. Good sources include meat, fish and vegetable oils.

Toxic effects of excess intake

Toxic effects are unknown.

Therapeutic uses of supplements

Supplements are used to treat cardiovascular disease, cancer, high blood pressure, periodontal disease, muscular dystrophy. Coenzyme Q10 may also be useful in preventing the side effects of beta blockers and statin-type cholesterol-lowering drugs.

Coenzyme Q10, which is also known as ubiquinone, is one form of a substance known as coenzyme Q which is found in all plant and animal cells. Coenzyme Q10 is the form used for energy production in humans and it can be made from some of the other forms of coenzyme Q in your diet. Coenzyme Q10, was identified in 1957.

What it does in the body

Energy production

Coenzyme Q10 is involved in energy production in cells. It is necessary for the formation of adenosine triphosphate (ATP), a compound which acts as an energy donor in chemical reactions. Coenzyme Q10 is mobile in cell membranes and functions in the transfer of energy and oxygen between blood and body cells and between cell components.

Antioxidant properties

Coenzyme Q10 is an antioxidant and protects against free radical damage to cell structures and other substances in the body. It works together with vitamin E and may protect vitamin E from damage.

Absorption

Plasma levels of coenzyme Q10 are higher in vegetarians. Coenzyme Q10 levels appear to decline with age.

Deficiency

Although coenzyme Q10 can be made in the body, deficiency states can occur. They may be caused by nutritional deficiencies, a genetic or acquired defect in synthesis or because of increased tissue needs due to a medical condition such as heart disease. Coenzyme Q10 deficiency can worsen or cause many disease conditions. Older people in general may need more coenzyme Q10 as levels of this vital nutrient appear to decline with age.

As the heart is one of the most metabolically active tissues in the body and requires a large amount of ATP to function efficiently, coenzyme Q10 deficiency seriously affects the heart. Deficiency has also been linked to a wide range of other conditions including cancer, muscular dystrophy, diabetes, obesity, periodontal disease, lowered immune function, and neurodegenerative disorders such as Parkinson's disease.

Sources

Coenzyme Q is found in all plant and animal cells. Some coenzyme Q10 is made in the body, particularly in the liver, and some is obtained from food. The production process is a complex one involving around 15 different reactions. It is not clear how much coenzyme Q10 from the diet contributes to body stores, but evidence suggests that dietary coenzyme Q10 is an important source. The average person may consume around 5 mg of coenzyme Q10 per day. The main sources are meat, fish and vegetable oils. Soybean, sesame and canola oils are high in coenzyme Q10. Wheat germ, rice bran and soybeans contain reasonable amounts of coenzyme Q10, but vegetables contain relatively little; although spinach and broccoli may be quite good sources.

Supplements

Coenzyme Q10 is available in tablets and capsules. Oil-based supplements may be the best absorbed form. The amount of coenzyme Q10 available from dietary sources is likely to be insufficient to produce the clinical effects of high dose coenzyme Q10. Coenzyme Q10 may take up to four to eight weeks to build up to peak concentration in the body, and it may take several weeks of daily dosing to see noticeable effects.

Toxic effects

No toxic effects have been reported, even at high doses.

Therapeutic uses of supplements

Cardiovascular disease

Increasing scientific evidence suggests that coenzyme Q10 is a safe and effective therapy for a wide range of cardiovascular diseases such as congestive heart failure, cardiomyopathy, high blood pressure, mitral valve prolapse and angina. It has also been used to treat patients undergoing coronary artery bypass surgery. Coenzyme Q10 appears to exert its beneficial effects both by improving energy production and by acting as an antioxidant.

In a study published in 1994, researchers at the University of Texas looked at the usefulness of long-term coenzyme Q10 therapy in clinical cardiology. Over an eight-year period, they treated 424 patients with various forms of cardiovascular disease by adding coenzyme Q10, in amounts ranging from 75 to 600 mg/day to their treatment programs.

Patients were divided into six diagnostic categories including ischemic cardiomyopathy, dilated cardiomyopathy, primary diastolic dysfunction, hypertension, mitral valve prolapse and valvular heart disease.

The patients were followed for an average of 17.8 months. The researchers evaluated clinical response according to the New York Heart Association (NYHA) functional scale and found significant improvements in all the patients. Out of 424 patients, 58 per cent improved by one NYHA class, 28 per cent by two classes and 1.2 per cent by three classes. Statistically significant improvements in heart muscle function were shown using a variety of laboratory tests. Before treatment with coenzyme Q10, most patients were taking from one to five cardiac medications, and during the study, overall medication requirements dropped considerably with 43 per cent of patients stopping between one and three drugs. Only 6 per cent of the patients required the addition of one drug. No apparent side effects from coenzyme Q10 treatment were noted other than a single case of transient nausea. The researchers concluded that coenzyme Q10 is a safe and effective treatment for a broad range of cardiovascular diseases, often in combination with other medications, as it produces improvements in a variety of symptoms and reduces medication needs.[1]

Heart failure

Biopsy samples from patients undergoing cardiac surgery and blood samples from patients with congestive heart failure suggest that mitochondrial dysfunction and energy starvation caused by coenzyme Q10 deficiency contributes to heart failure. The improved cardiac function in patients with congestive heart failure treated with coenzyme Q10 supports this theory.

Several controlled studies using coenzyme Q10 in patients with heart failure have been published. The main clinical problems in patients with congestive heart failure are the frequent need of hospitalization and the high incidence of life-threatening complications. In an Italian study published in 1994 researchers investigated the safety and clinical effectiveness of coenzyme Q10 in treating congestive heart failure that had been diagnosed at least six months previously and treated with standard therapy including digitalis, diuretics and vasodilators. This study involved 2664 patients in NYHA classes I and II, and most of them received 100 mg per day of coenzyme Q10. After three months of treatment, improvement in at least three symptoms was seen in 54 per cent of patients which the researchers interpreted as indicating an improved quality of life.[2]

Hypertension

Coenzyme Q10 deficiency is often seen in patients with hypertension, and several studies have shown beneficial effects of coenzyme Q10 supplements. In a 1994 study, 109 patients with hypertension were treated with an average dose of 225 mg of coenzyme Q10 per day in addition to their existing anti-hypertensive drugs. Most of these patients had been diagnosed with hypertension for a year or more before the study started. Results showed a definite and gradual improvement in symptoms and a reduced need for medication within the first one to six months. Fifty one per cent of patients came off between one and three anti-hypertensive drugs about four months after starting coenzyme Q10 therapy. After this period, blood pressure and medication needs stabilized. Echocardiograms were performed on 39 per cent of the patients at the beginning of the study and during the treatment. In 9.4 per cent of cases, highly significant improvements were seen.[3]

In another study, 26 patients with essential arterial hypertension were treated with 50 mg of coenzyme Q10, twice daily for ten weeks. Blood plasma levels of coenzyme Q10, blood serum total and beneficial HDL cholesterol, and blood pressure were determined in all patients before and at the end of the ten-week period. At the end of the treatment, average systolic blood pressure decreased from 164.5 to 146.7 mmHg and diastolic blood pressure decreased from 98.1 to 86.1 mmHg.[4]

Serum total cholesterol decreased from 222.9 mg/dl to 213.3 mg/dl and serum HDL cholesterol increased from 41.1 mg/dl to 43.1 mg/dl. The researchers also used a test to measure the resistance to blood flow in peripheral blood vessels which showed significant improvements. The results from this study suggest that coenzyme Q10 lowers cholesterol and decreases blood pressure by opening up blood vessels and reducing the resistance to blood flow.

Cardiomyopathy

Cardiomyopathy is the term used for any disease which affects the structure and function of the heart. Coenzyme Q10 deficiency is often found in blood and heart muscle of cardiomyopathy sufferers, and several studies have shown that therapy with coenzyme Q10 produces improvements in heart function as it improves energy production in the muscle. In a 1997 study, seven patients with hypertrophic cardiomyopathy were treated with an average of 200 mg/day of coenzyme Q10. All patients noted improvement in symptoms of fatigue and shortness of breath.[5]

Atherosclerosis

Coenzyme Q10 may help prevent atherosclerosis as it can protect against oxidative damage to fats. In a 1993 Japanese study, researchers measured levels of coenzyme and also levels of various types of cholesterol and other blood fats in 378 people. These included 249 people with no coronary artery disease, 29 patients with the disease who were receiving pravastatin, (a cholesterol-lowering drug) and 104 patients with the disease who were not receiving pravastatin. In the patient groups, the plasma total cholesterol and LDL cholesterol levels were higher and the plasma coenzyme Q10 level lower than in those with no disease.

The researchers found that coenzyme Q10 levels, either alone or when expressed in relation to LDL levels, were significantly lower in the patient groups compared with those with no disease. They concluded that coenzyme Q10 therapy would be beneficial in patients with atherosclerosis.[6]

Heart surgery

Coenzyme Q10 may help to prevent 'ischemia reperfusion injury', one of the main problems that occurs in coronary artery bypass surgery. This term refers to the oxygen-induced damage caused when the blood supply is returned to the heart and arteries after having been cut off during surgery. The heart muscle and the linings of the arteries suffer, and this greatly increases the risk of subsequent coronary artery disease.

A number of medical studies have shown that giving patients coenzyme Q10 supplements before surgery can reduce the damage caused when blood flow is returned. In a 1996 study, 30 patients due to undergo elective surgery for heart disease were randomly divided into two groups. Patients in group I received 150 mg of coenzyme Q10 for seven days before the operation and those in group II received a placebo. Scientists then assessed the amount of oxidative damage by measuring the levels of certain enzymes and chemicals during the surgery. Results showed that those patients who had taken coenzyme Q10 suffered less damage than those who had not.[7]

Angina

Some small studies have shown that coenzyme Q10 supplements can be beneficial in the treatment of angina. In a 1985 Japanese, double-blind, placebo-controlled, randomized, crossover study, the effects of coenzyme Q10 on exercise performance were studied in 12 patients, average age 56 years, with stable angina pectoris. The study involved multistage treadmill exercise tests. The patients were given three daily doses of 50 mg of coenzyme Q10 for four weeks, and results showed a reduction in frequency of angina attacks from 5.3 to 2.5 attacks for two weeks. Consumption of the angina medication, nitroglycerin, was also reduced.[8]

Cancer

As an antioxidant, coenzyme Q10 may have a role to play in both cancer prevention and cancer treatment. In a 1994 study, 32 breast cancer patients, aged 32 to 81 years and classified 'high risk' due to the spread of their tumors to the lymph nodes in their armpits, were studied for 18 months following an Adjuvant Nutritional Intervention in Cancer (ANICA) protocol. This nutritional protocol was added to the surgical and therapeutic treatment of breast cancer and involved treatment with a combination of nutritional antioxidants, (vitamin C: 2850 mg, vitamin E: 2500 IU, beta carotene 32.5 IU, selenium 387 mcg plus secondary vitamins and minerals) essential fatty acids, (1.2 g gamma-linolenic acid and 3.5g of omega-3 fatty acids) and 90 mg of coenzyme Q10 per day.

The researchers measured various biochemical markers of cancer progression, tumor spread and the clinical condition of the patients. Quality of life and survival were also assessed during the trial. The main observations were that none of the patients died during the study period. (The expected number was four); none of the patients showed signs of further distant metastases; quality of life was improved (no weight loss, reduced use of pain killers); six patients showed apparent partial remission.

In one of these six cases, the dosage of coenzyme Q10 was increased to 390 mg. In one month, the tumor was no longer palpable and in another month, mammography confirmed that the tumor had disappeared. Encouraged by these results, the researchers gave 300 mg a day of coenzyme Q10 to another patient who had been surgically treated but still had evidence of some tumor remaining. After three months, the patient was in excellent clinical condition and there was no residual tumor tissue.[9]

Periodontal disease

The treatment of periodontal disease with coenzyme Q10 is controversial and research has produced mixed results, but there have been positive outcomes in some studies.

Muscular dystrophy

Deficiency of coenzyme Q10 has been found in the mitochondria of the muscle tissue of patients with muscular dystrophy.

Two double-blind trials have been carried out involving patients with muscular dystrophies. The first trial involved 12 patients, ranging from 7 to 69 years of age, with diseases including the Duchenne, Becker, and the limb-girdle dystrophies; myotonic dystrophy; Charcot-Marie-Tooth disease; and the Welander disease. The coenzyme Q10 blood levels in these patients were low at the beginning of the study. The patients were then treated for three months with 100 mg daily of coenzyme Q10 or a matching placebo. The second double-blind trial was similar, and involved 15 patients having the same categories of disease. Since heart disease is known to be associated with these muscle diseases, cardiac function was also monitored. The researchers recorded definite improvements in physical performance in both studies.[10]

Exercise

Due to its role in energy production, coenzyme Q10 has also been used to enhance athletic performance. Because exercise increases the risk of oxidative damage, coenzyme Q10 as an antioxidant may have a role to play in protection from such damage. In a 1997 study done in Finland, the effects of coenzyme Q10 supplements were studied in a double-blind cross-over study of 25 cross-country skiers. The results showed that all measured indexes of physical performance improved significantly. Ninety-four per cent of the athletes felt that the supplements had been beneficial in improving their performance and recovery time, whereas only 33 per cent of those in the placebo group did.[11]

Other uses

Coenzyme Q10 may be beneficial in patients with diabetes and may help improve diabetic control. Coenzyme Q10 levels have also been shown to be low in obese people, and when combined with a low-calorie diet coenzyme Q10 may speed up weight loss. Coenzyme Q10 has also been used to treat the neurological disorder, Huntington's chorea, and to improve sperm function and motility.[12]

Interactions with other nutrients

Coenzyme Q10 synthesis requires vitamins B6, C, B12, folic acid, riboflavin, niacin, and pantothenic acid.

Interactions with drugs

Several different types of medications have side effects that include adverse effects on heart function. Some of these drugs, such as doxorubicin, have effects on the heart that are so severe that the amount of time for which they can be used is strictly limited. Research has shown that the toxic effect of doxorubicin is due to its inhibitory effects on coenzyme Q10-dependent enzyme systems. Coenzyme Q10 reduces the toxic effects of doxorubicin on the heart.

Another class of drugs, known as beta blockers, which are used to treat high blood pressure and some other types of cardiovascular disease, have been shown to interfere with the production and function of coenzyme Q10, and to adversely affect heart function. This may explain why, in some cases, long-term therapy with beta blockers can lead to congestive heart failure. Coenzyme Q10 therapy in combination with beta blockers may be beneficial.

In recent years, the drugs lovastatin, pravastatin, and simvastatin have become widely used to treat high blood cholesterol. These medications work by inhibiting an enzyme known as HMG-CoA reductase, and they are very effective in lowering cholesterol levels. However, this enzyme is also responsible for production of coenzyme Q10. Because of this, the cholesterol-lowering effect of these drugs is accompanied by an equivalent lowering of coenzyme Q10 levels.[13] In patients with existing heart failure, lovastatin has been shown to cause increased heart disease with life-threatening results in some patients. Coenzyme Q10 supplements may help to prevent some of the adverse effects of these widely used drugs.

Others drugs, such as phenothiazine neuroleptics and tricyclic antidepressants, also have effects on heart function which seem to be related to inhibition of coenzyme Q10 function.

Amino acids

Amino acids are divided into three main types: essential, nonessential and semi-essential. The essential amino acids are tryptophan, lysine, methionine, phenylalanine, threonine, valine, leucine and isoleucine. Arginine and histidine are considered semi-essential. The non-essential amino acids are tyrosine, glycine, serine, glutamic acid, aspartic acid, taurine, cystine, proline, and alanine.

Meat, fish, eggs, milk and soybeans contain all the essential amino acids and are known as complete proteins. Those foods which are low in some amino acids are called incomplete proteins. For example, legumes are low in methionine and tryptophan, but high in lysine and isoleucine whereas, grains are high in lysine and isoleucine and low in tryptophan and methionine. Two incomplete protein foods, eaten together, can provide a complete protein, for example, baked beans on toast or lentils and rice.

Supplements

Taking one amino acid for a long period of time is not advisable as this may affect the balance and functions of the others. Some experts recommend that single supplements should be taken for no more than two to three weeks.

Essential amino acids

Branched chain amino acids

The branched-chain amino acids, isoleucine, leucine, and valine have been used as supplements for muscle building. Arginine is also used for this purpose. Leucine has also been used to help heal wounds of the skin and bones.

Lysine

Lysine is used to prevent and treat Herpes simplex virus infections. It seems to be more effective for cold sores (herpes type 1) than for genital herpes (type 2). A typical dosage regime is 500 mg three times per day during an infection and 500 mg per day when there are no symptoms.

Phenylalanine

Phenylalanine is used to treat depression, musculoskeletal disorders and various types of pain including back pain, neck pain, osteoarthritis, rheumatoid arthritis, menstrual pain and headaches.

Tryptophan

Tryptophan supplements have been used to treat insomnia and depression.

Semi-essential amino acids

Histidine

Histidine is used to treat allergies, ulcers, anemia, arthritis and high blood pressure.

Nonessential amino acids

Aspartic acid has been used to treat fatigue and depression. Glutamic acid has been used to treat fatigue and alcoholism. Cysteine can be converted to glutathione, which has antioxidant properties and it may be useful in preventing and treating disorders in which free radical damage plays a part. Tyrosine has also been used to treat depression.

Flavonoids

Flavonoids were discovered by Nobel Prize-winning biochemist Albert Szent-Gyorgi, who labeled them "vitamin P". He discovered that they enhanced the function of vitamin C, improving absorption and protecting it from oxidation. Flavonoids that have been shown to have particularly beneficial properties include proanthocyanidins, green tea polyphenols and soy isoflavones. Quercetin and its derivatives; the citrus bioflavonoids, including quercitrin, rutin and hesperidin; have also been fairly well studied.

What they do in the body

Cardiovascular system

Flavonoids are important for blood vessel health. They regulate capillary permeability, thereby stopping fluid, protein and blood cells from seeping out while still allowing oxygen, carbon dioxide and other nutrients to pass through. Many flavonoids enhance capillary strength, preventing them from being easily bruised. This is partly due to the vitamin C-enhancing action of flavonoids. This may help protect against infection and blood vessel diseases.

Flavonoids can also relax the smooth muscle of the cardiovascular system, thus lowering blood pressure. This also improves circulation to the heart itself. Flavonoids are antioxidant and can also prevent oxidation of harmful LDL cholesterol, thereby preventing the build-up of atherosclerotic plaque. They may also stop blood platelets from clumping together which can help to reduce blood clotting and damage to blood vessels.

Anti-inflammatory effects

Flavonoids have anti-inflammatory properties. This is due to their antioxidant effects and to their ability to act against histamines and other mediators of inflammation, such as prostaglandins and leukotrienes.

Other effects

While flavonoids have many properties in common, specific compounds often have specific properties. Some may have estrogen-like activity while others inhibit tumor growth.

Absorption

Flavonoids are usually easily absorbed from the intestine. Excesses are excreted in the urine.

Sources

Flavonoids are found in the edible pulp of fruits such as citrus fruits, rose hips, apricots, cherries, grapes and blackcurrants. Green pepper, broccoli, onions and tomatoes are good vegetable sources and buckwheat is also a rich source. Green tea and red wine also contain several flavonoids. Many herbs are rich sources of flavonoids and these contribute to the therapeutic effects. These include bilberry, hawthorn, ginkgo, yarrow and milk thistle (See page 384 for more information.)

Deficiency

There are no reports of flavonoid deficiencies as most people seem to get enough in their diet to prevent this. It is possible, however, that many people do not eat enough for optimal health.

Recommended intakes

There are no recommended intakes for flavonoids.

Supplements

Bioflavonoid supplements are available in varying types and doses. Pine bark and grape seed extracts are sources of proanthocyanidins. The mix of these flavonoids, like other nutrients, varies from plant species to species. Both sources can be used interchangeably, but grape seed extract may have an advantage over pine bark. Most grape seed extracts contain 92 to 95 per cent proanthocyanidins, whereas pine bark extracts usually contain from 80 to 85 per cent. Grape seed extract also contains small quantities of a beneficial flavonoid found in green tea.

Toxic effects

There are no known toxic effects of large intakes.

Therapeutic uses of supplements

Enhancement of vitamin C action

Flavonoids, particularly citrus bioflavonoids, are often given with vitamin C; for example in the treatment of colds, bleeding problems, bruising and ulcers. Flavonoids may also have antiviral activity.

Cardiovascular disease

As flavonoids have been shown to have antioxidant properties, they are able to protect against heart disease, which may explain the so-called 'French paradox.' This refers to the fact that the French eat much larger amounts of saturated fat and have higher cholesterol levels and blood pressures than Americans, yet are 2.5 times less likely to die of coronary heart disease.

Red wine is a good source of flavonoids and many people have suggested that the liberal French consumption of red wine protects against coronary heart disease. Several studies have found that a glass or two of wine daily protects against heart disease and it seems likely that red wine is more protective than white wine, suggesting that the benefits might be unrelated to the alcohol.

Researchers involved in the Zutphen elderly study assessed the flavonoid intakes of 805 men aged from 65 to 84 years in 1985. The major sources of flavonoid intake were found to be tea, onions, and apples. The men were then followed up for five years, during which time 43 men died of coronary heart disease. Fatal or nonfatal heart attacks occurred in 38 of 693 men with no history of heart attack at the beginning of the study. The results showed that those with the highest flavonoid intake had less than half the risk of death from heart attack when compared to those in the lowest intake group.[1]

In a 1996 study, Harvard researchers assessed the links between heart disease and flavonoid intake in 34 789 male health professionals aged from 40 to 75. Among the 4814 men who reported that they had previously had coronary heart disease, flavonoids showed a protective effect against death from heart attack.[2]

High flavonoid intakes also seem to protect against stroke. Researchers involved in a 1996 Dutch study assessed the diets of 552 men aged 50 to 69 years in 1970 and followed them up for 15 years. The results showed that those with the highest intakes of dietary flavonoids (mainly quercetin) had around 75 per cent less risk of stroke compared to those with the lowest intakes. Black tea contributed about 70 per cent of the flavonoid intake in the study. Men who drunk more than four cups of tea had around a third of the risk of stroke when compared to those who drunk less than two cups of tea.[3] However, in a 1997 study done in Wales, researchers did not find a reduced risk of heart disease with increasing tea consumption.[4] Black tea seems to be more effective in raising antioxidant levels than tea with milk.

Flavonoids are useful in the treatment of high blood pressure due to their capillary-strengthening and blood vessel-dilating effects. They are also useful in capillary fragility disorders such as easy bruising, bleeding of the gums, and also in circulatory disorders of the retina of the eye. They are particularly useful in the treatment of vein and capillary problems such as varicose veins, venous insufficiency (poor return of blood to the heart from the veins of the legs), and eye problems such as diabetic retinopathy and macular degeneration.

Green tea

Green tea contains several polyphenols, the most active of which appears to be epigallocatechin gallate. These compounds have several beneficial effects, including protection from heart disease.

Green tea has been shown to lower cholesterol. In a 1995 Japanese study researchers investigated green tea consumption of 1371 men aged over 40 years. Analysis of their blood samples showed that increased consumption of green tea was linked to decreased serum concentrations of total cholesterol and triglyceride, and increased levels of beneficial HDL cholesterol together with decreased levels of LDL and VLDL cholesterols. Those who drank ten or more cups per day showed better liver function measurements.[5]

Research from Japan has linked green tea consumption with a reduced risk of stroke. In a four-year study of almost 6000 women, the incidence of stroke and cerebral hemorrhage was at least twice as high in those who drank less green tea (fewer than five cups a day) than in those who drank more (greater than or equal to five cups daily).

Cancer

Flavonoids may also help to protect against cancer. Many laboratory experiments have shown that various flavonoids can inhibit the growth and proliferation of cancer cells. Recent animal experiments looking at tumor onset in mice found beneficial effects when their diets were supplemented with red wine solids (which contain no water or alcohol).

In a study published in 1997, Finnish researchers investigated the links between the intake of flavonoids and subsequent risk of cancer in 9959 Finnish men and women aged from 15 to 99 years and initially cancer-free. During the follow-up period, 997 cancer cases and 151 lung cancer cases were diagnosed. The results showed that a high intake of flavonoids reduced the risk of all types of cancer. An inverse association was observed between the intake of flavonoids and incidence of all sites of cancer combined. Those with the highest flavonoid intakes had almost half the risk of cancer compared to those in the lowest intake groups.[6]

Researchers involved in the Iowa Women's Health Study analyzed the tea drinking habits of over 35 000 postmenopausal women and found that those who drank more than two cups of tea a day were 32 per cent less likely to have cancers of the mouth, esophagus, stomach, colon and rectum. They were also 60 per cent less likely to have urinary tract cancer. In those who drank four or more cups per day, the risk of cancer was lowered by 63 per cent.[7]

Onions are high in flavonoids, which may explain the links between their consumption and reduced cancer risk. Researchers involved in The Netherlands Cohort Study assessed the links between onion consumption and the risk of stomach cancer in 120 852 men and women ranging in age from 55 to 69 years. Those whose onion intakes were high had around half the risk of stomach cancer when compared to those whose intakes were low.[8]

Green tea

Green tea preparations and extracts have been shown to inhibit tumor formation and growth in laboratory experiments. The evidence for the protective effect of green tea is strongest for cancers of the digestive tract.

Most of the research on the health benefits of green tea has been carried out in Japan and China. In a study published in 1997, Japanese researchers investigated the links between green tea and cancer in 8552 people over 40. During a follow-up period of nine years, there were 384 cases of cancer. The results showed a lower risk in those who drank green tea, especially among women drinking more than ten cups a day.[9]

The results of a Chinese study suggest that drinking green tea can reduce the risk of esophageal cancer. The study involved 902 patients, aged 30 to 74, who were diagnosed with cancer of the esophagus from October 1990 through January 1993. A group of 1552 healthy volunteers were used as controls. Histories of cancer in the family, diet, smoking and drinking habits were taken into account. The researchers found that for those who refrained from smoking or drinking alcohol, green tea consumption reduced the risk of esophageal cancer in men by 57 percent, and 60 per cent in women. For those who smoked or drank alcohol, green tea exerted little protection.[10]

Another Chinese study showed that drinking green tea also reduced the risk of stomach cancer. This study involved 711 patients and 711 controls. The results showed that those who drank green tea had 30 per cent less risk of stomach cancer.[11] Other studies have shown reduced risks for colon cancer.[12] Green tea may also protect against the carcinogenic changes caused by cigarette smoke.[13]

In a study published in 1998, Japanese researchers investigated the effects of drinking green tea on the progression of breast cancer. The study involved 472 patients with stage I, II, and III breast cancer. The results showed that increased consumption of green tea was linked to a decrease in the spread of breast cancer in premenopausal women. In a follow-up study, the researchers found that increased consumption of green tea was correlated with decreased recurrence of stage I and II breast cancer.[14]

Allergies and autoimmune disease

In addition to their antioxidant effects, the ability of flavonoids to affect enzymes involved in the production of inflammatory substances means they may be useful in the treatment of asthma, allergies, bursitis, arthritis and inflammatory bowel disease.

Quercetin

Quercetin has been shown to exert anti-inflammatory effects. Inflammation is mediated partly by the release of histamine from mast cells. Quercetin may stabilize the membranes of these cells, thereby reducing histamine release. It may also affect leukotriene synthesis.

Diabetes

Quercetin

Quercetin may inhibit the enzyme that converts glucose to sorbitol, a compound which is linked to diabetic complications, including cataracts (See page 593 for more information.) Quercetin-related compounds have been shown to inhibit cataract formation in diabetic animals. Quercetin may also enhance insulin secretion and protect pancreatic cells from free radical damage.

Soy

Soy contains types of flavonoid compounds known as isoflavones. These are also referred to as phytoestrogens because they have both estrogenic and anti-estrogenic properties. When circulating levels of estrogens are high, such as in premenopausal women, these compounds can bind to estrogen receptors and block action of the hormone. When estrogen levels are low, such as in postmenopausal women, phytoestrogens act estrogenically. Phytoestrogen compounds in soy include genistein and daidzein. Evidence from molecular and cellular biology experiments, animal studies, and human clinical trials suggests that phytoestrogens may help to prevent cardiovascular disease, cancer, osteoporosis, and menopausal symptoms. Epidemiological studies suggest that rates of these disorders are lower among populations that eat plant-based diets, particularly among cultures with diets that are traditionally high in soy products. Soybeans also contain other beneficial compounds including phytosterols, which have been shown to lower blood cholesterol, possibly by competing with cholesterol uptake.

Cardiovascular disease

Several studies have shown that the addition of soy foods or extracts to the diet lowers cholesterol. In a 1997 study, 17 healthy men and 17 healthy women with raised levels of total and LDL cholesterol were given either 2 per cent cows' milk products, soybean products or a combination of skim milk products and soy oil, over period of four weeks. During the soybean period, the subjects' mean level HDL cholesterol increased 9 per cent and their mean LDL/HDL cholesterol ratio decreased 14 per cent.[15] Soy compounds may also reduce the oxidation of LDL cholesterol and inhibit clumping together of platelets, both of which slow the atherosclerotic process. They may also improve arterial function.

Cancer

Eating soy foods may lower the risk of cancers, particularly those that are hormone-dependent, such as breast and prostate cancer. Breast cancer rates are lower in countries with soy-based diets and soy products have been shown in many animal experiments to inhibit tumor growth. Genistein may block the stimulatory effect of estrogen on cancer cells. Other hormone-dependent cancers, such as prostate cancer, may also be affected by genistein, which appears to block enzymes that promote tumor growth. Genistein may also inhibit the growth of new blood vessels into tumors.

Researchers involved in a study published in 1997 examined the links between soy and endometrial cancer in 332 women diagnosed with endometrial cancer from various ethnic groups in Hawaii. Their diets were compared with 511 control subjects. High consumption of soy products and other legumes was associated with a decreased risk of endometrial cancer, with those in the high intake group having around half the risk of those in the low intake group.[16] A 1996 US study showed a decrease in breast cancer risk in Asian American women who increased tofu intake.[17]

Menopause and osteoporosis

Japanese women appear to suffer fewer menopausal symptoms than Western women. One of the reasons may be their high consumption of soy foods. Soy compounds may also be useful in preventing osteoporosis which occurs when a decline in circulating estrogen leads to a reduction in bone mass. Estrogen-like compounds such as genistein can help to build bone.

In a 1998 double-blind, randomized placebo-controlled study Italian researchers investigated the effects of daily dietary supplementation of soy protein isolate powder on hot flashes in 104 postmenopausal women. Fifty-one patients took 60 g of isolated soy protein daily and 53 took 60 g of placebo daily. The study lasted 12 weeks. The results showed that soy was much better than placebo at reducing the average number of hot flashes per 24 hours after four, eight, and 12 weeks of treatment. By the end of the twelfth week, women taking soy had a 45 per cent reduction in their daily hot flashes versus a 30 per cent reduction obtained with the placebo.[18]

Lipoic acid

Lipoic acid, which is also known as thioctic acid, is a fat soluble compound produced in the body. It plays an important role in the breakdown of carbohydrates, fats and protein.

What it does in the body

Lipoic acid acts in a complex with thiamin and niacin in the metabolism of glucose. It is also an antioxidant, effective against both water and fat soluble free radicals. Some experts believe that the body synthesizes sufficient lipoic acid for its metabolic function, but additional intake in the diet is necessary for antioxidant function. Lipoic acid may combine with free iron and copper in the body and protect against the oxidative damage exerted by these free ions.

Deficiency

No deficiency symptoms have been reported. Low lipoic acid levels may play a role in disorders such as diabetes, heart disease, and cirrhosis of the liver.

Absorption

Lipoic acid is easily absorbed.

Sources

Liver and brewer's yeast are good sources of lipoic acid.

Supplements

Lipoic acid is available in tablets and capsules.

Toxic effects

There are no reports of toxic effects.

Therapeutic uses of supplements

Diabetes

Lipoic acid has been used to treat diabetics by improving glucose transport and metabolism.[1] High intakes may increase the absorption of glucose into muscle tissue in Type II diabetes.[2] Lipoic acid may also decrease the damaging effects on proteins of high glucose levels.

Lipoic acid may be beneficial in improving nerve blood flow, reducing oxidative stress, and improving nerve conduction in diabetic neuropathy.[3] The effects of lipoic acid on diabetic neuropathy have been studied in two German randomized, double-blind, placebo-controlled trials. In the first of these, 328 patients with Type II diabetes and symptoms of peripheral neuropathy were treated with either intravenous infusion of lipoic acid or placebo for three weeks. The results showed improvements in symptoms. In another study, patients with Type II diabetes and cardiac autonomic neuropathy were treated with a daily oral dose of 800 mg lipoic acid or placebo for four months. Two out of four symptoms test measurements were significantly improved in those taking the lipoic acid compared with placebo.[4]

Other uses

Because of its antioxidant action, lipoic acid may be effective in treating neurodegenerative disorders and other causes of acute or chronic brain damage or nerve tissue damage. Lipoic acid may also inhibit activation of HIV. Supplements have also been used to boost the antioxidant defense system in AIDS patients. Lipoic acid has been used to treat heavy metal poisoning.[5]

Studies have shown beneficial effects of lipoic acid treatment on cataracts in rats.[6] It may be of therapeutic use in preventing human cataracts and their associated complications. Lipoic acid has also been used to treat glaucoma.

Interactions with other nutrients

Lipoic acid may protect vitamins C and E from oxidative damage.

Carnitine

Carnitine is a vitamin-like compound with a structure similar to an amino acid. It is found in food, particularly in meat and dairy products, and can also be made by the body from the amino acid, lysine.

What it does in the body

Carnitine is essential for fat metabolism as it transports fatty acids into the mitochondria, where they are 'burned' to release energy for body functions. Carnitine thus increases the use of fat as an energy source.

Deficiency

Carnitine deficiency may occur due to genetic defects, reduced absorption, dietary deficiency of precursors, and increased requirements due to stress, medication use or disease.

Supplements

Only the L-carnitine form should be used as the D form of carnitine may cause adverse side effects. L-carnitine is available in several different forms including L-propionylcarnitine and L-acetylcarnitine.

Therapeutic uses of supplements

Supplements are used to treat carnitine deficiency.

Cardiovascular disease

Carnitine can be used to treat several types of cardiovascular disease.

Angina

In a 1994 study, Dutch researchers assessed the effect of L-propionylcarnitine on ischemia in 31 untreated male patients with left coronary artery disease. The patients were studied during two identical pacing stress tests 45 minutes before and 15 minutes after administration of 15 mg/kg of L-propionylcarnitine or placebo. The results showed that the L-propionylcarnitine prevented ischemia-induced heart dysfunction through its enhancement of metabolism.[1]

Recovery from heart attack

Carnitine deprivation occurs in heart muscle during heart attack and some studies suggest that supplementation has a beneficial effect on heart function. In a 1995 study, Italian researchers investigated the effects of L-carnitine on heart function in 472 heart attack patients. The patients received either placebo or L-carnitine within 24 hours of the onset of chest pain. The treatments were given at a dose of 9 g per day intravenously for the first five days, and then 6 g per day orally for the next 12 months. The results showed that heart function was better in the carnitine-treated group than in the placebo group. There was a lower incidence of congestive heart failure and fewer deaths in the carnitine-treated group.[2]

Other types of cardiovascular disease

Carnitine supplements have also been used to treat cardiomyopathy, congestive heart failure, peripheral vascular disease, dyslipidemia, diabetes and arrhythmias. Propionyl-L-carnitine has shown beneficial effects in the treatment of intermittent claudication.[3]

It can also be used to lower blood fat levels, aid in weight loss, and improve muscle strength in some cases of weakness. A 1997 Italian study showed that carnitine supplements improved glucose metabolism in healthy people.[4]

Alzheimer's disease

There are several studies which suggest that acetyl-L-carnitine may delay the progression of Alzheimer's disease.[5] In a small double-blind trial published in 1995, seven patients with probable Alzheimer's disease received 3 g/day of acetyl-L-carnitine for one year, while five similar patients were given a placebo. Patients treated with acetyl-L-carnitine showed significantly less deterioration on mental status tests than did patients receiving the placebo.[6]

Interactions with other nutrients

Vitamin C, niacin and vitamin B6 are required for carnitine synthesis from lysine. Carnitine may work with coenzyme Q10. Choline supplementation seems to reduce urinary excretion of carnitine.[7]

Cautions

Carnitine is not recommended in people with active liver or kidney disease, or with diabetes.

Melatonin

Melatonin is a hormone secreted by the pineal gland, which is located at the base of the brain.

What it does in the body

Melatonin functions as an internal biochemical clock and calendar. It has a wide range of physiological effects including modulation of the sleep-wake cycle; temperature; and cognitive, hormone, cardiovascular and immune systems. Melatonin also has antioxidant effects. The melatonin-generating system is light-sensitive, with highest levels of production occurring at night in darkness. Melatonin production declines with age.

Toxic effects

Some users have reported headache, nightmares, hypotension, sleep disorders and abdominal pain. Melatonin may also worsen the symptoms of depression. There have been no studies on the side effects of long-term use.

Therapeutic uses of supplements

Sleep disorders

Melatonin supplements may be useful in improving sleep duration and quality in those in whom the normal cycle is disrupted, such as in those with jet lag and shift workers. Melatonin levels also decrease with increasing age. Melatonin appears to promote sleep by correcting abnormalities in sleep-wake cycles and by exerting a direct soporific effect, especially when administered during the day. Melatonin supplements should be taken in the evening.

In a 1997 placebo-controlled, double-blind, cross-over study, researchers assessed the effects of melatonin in eight males. Following a 7-hour night-time sleep, the participants were given either a placebo or one of three doses of melatonin (1 mg, 10 mg, and 40 mg) at 10 am. All doses of melatonin significantly shortened the time taken to go to sleep. Melatonin also significantly increased total sleep time and decreased wake after sleep onset.[1]

In another placebo-controlled study, researchers studied the effects of single evening doses of melatonin on sleep in 15 healthy middle-aged volunteers. Compared to placebo, the 1.0 mg dose of melatonin significantly increased sleep time, sleep efficiency, non-REM Sleep and REM sleep latency.[2]

Jet lag

Melatonin use in jet lag appears to decrease jet lag symptoms and hasten the return to normal energy levels. In a double-blind placebo-controlled study published in 1993, New Zealand researchers investigated the efficacy of melatonin in alleviating jet lag in 52 flight crew members after a series of international flights. The optimal time for taking melatonin in this group was also investigated. The participants were randomly assigned to three groups: early melatonin (5 mg started three days prior to arrival until five days after return home); late melatonin (placebo for three days then 5 mg melatonin for five days); and placebo. The results showed that the late melatonin group reported significantly less jet lag and sleep disturbance following the flight, compared to placebo. The late melatonin group also showed a significantly faster recovery of energy and alertness than the early melatonin group, which reported a worse overall recovery than placebo.[3]

Cancer

Melatonin seems to affect the immune response to cancer, possibly via effects on cytokines, which inhibit the growth of tumors. In a 1998 study, researchers assessed the effect of melatonin therapy on 31 patients (19 males and 12 females) with advanced solid tumors who had either failed to respond to chemotherapy and radiotherapy or showed insignificant responses. The results showed that in 12 patients, there was no further growth of either the primary tumor or of secondaries. These patients also experienced an improvement in their general wellbeing.[4]

Glucosamine

What it does in the body

Glucosamine, which is made in the body, is needed to make glycosaminoglycans, proteins that are key structural components of cartilage. Glucosamine also stimulates the cells that produce these structural proteins and helps to normalize cartilage metabolism by inhibiting breakdown and exerting anti-inflammatory effects.[1]

Sources

There are no food sources of glucosamine.

Supplements

Glucosamine sulfate seems to be the most beneficial form of glucosamine. It may be given orally, intravenously, intramuscularly, and intra-articularly (injected into joints).

Toxic effects

Toxic effects are rare.

Therapeutic uses of supplements

Glucosamine is used to help the body to repair damaged or eroded cartilage and has been used to treat osteoarthritis. Short-term human trials suggest that glucosamine sulfate may produce a gradual and progressive reduction in joint pain and tenderness, as well as improved range of motion and walking speed. Results of the trials have also shown that glucosamine has produced consistent benefits in patients with osteoarthritis and that, in some cases, it may be equal or superior to anti-inflammatory drugs in controlling symptoms.[2] It is often combined with chondroitin, a substance which has anti-inflammatory properties and protects the cartilage against breakdown. It has also been used to promote wound-healing[3] and to treat psoriasis.[4]

Chitosan

Chitosan is a natural product derived from chitin, a carbohydrate found in the shells of shellfish. It is chemically similar to the plant fiber, cellulose.

Therapeutic uses of supplements

Preliminary research suggests that chitosan can bind to fat in the digestive system and stop it from being absorbed. Chitosan is used to lower cholesterol levels and some evidence suggests that chitosan may be helpful in weight loss.

Shark cartilage

Shark cartilage is a food supplement made from the powdered cartilage of sharks. It is rich in calcium and phosphorus. It also contains amino acids and compounds that seem to inhibit cellular angiogenesis, the ability to generate new blood vessels. Shark cartilage also contains chondroitin sulfate, which has anti-inflammatory properties.

Therapeutic uses

The ability to inhibit angiogenesis means that shark cartilage may be valuable in inhibiting tumor growth, [1] and treating eye disorders such as diabetic retinopathy and macular degeneration. It has also been used to treat AIDS, arthritis, psoriasis, and bowel inflammation.

Cautions

Shark cartilage should not to be used by anyone who is still growing and needs angiogenesis for blood vessel development. Pregnant women, anyone with cardiovascular problems, or anyone recovering from surgery should also avoid shark cartilage.

Betaine hydrochloride

Betaine hydrochloride is a supplemental form of stomach acid; low production of which is associated with many problems including iron deficiency anemia, osteoporosis, allergies, gallstones, skin problems and an increase in bacteria, yeasts, and parasites growing in the intestines.

Therapeutic uses

Taken before, during or after meals, hydrochloric acid supplements may improve digestion of foods which contain protein and/or fat; though not for foods which are mostly carbohydrate.

Cautions

Use of betaine hydrochloride when a person already has normal or excessive stomach acid production or gastritis may increase the risk of gastric irritation or ulcer development.

Digestive enzymes: bromelain and papain

Bromelain is the name given to a group of protein-digesting enzymes obtained from pineapple. It assists digestion in the stomach and small intestine; acts as an anti-inflammatory enzyme to reduce swelling and pain after injury or surgery; has antibiotic activity; and has been shown in some small studies to have anticancer activity. It may also help to reduce the risk of heart disease by reducing blood clotting and arterial plaque formation. Papain, which is extracted from papaya, also helps in protein digestion.

Therapeutic uses

Bromelain has been used to treat several conditions including rheumatoid arthritis, osteoarthritis, thrombophlebitis, varicose veins, athletic injuries, cancer, and to improve recovery after surgery. It may also be useful in preventing E. coli related diarrhea. Bromelain is generally very safe but allergic reactions may occur in sensitive people.

Cautions

Digestive enzymes should not be used by people suffering from inflammation of the stomach lining.

Probiotics

There are several thousand billion bacteria in your body, most of them living in your digestive system. Although there may be as many as 400 species, the most important are *Lactobacillus acidophilus* and *Bifidobacterium bifidum.*

What they do in the body

These have several functions that are vital for good health. They improve the efficiency of your digestive system; manufacture some vitamins, including biotin and vitamin K; and produce antibacterial substances which kill or deactivate harmful bacteria.

Therapeutic uses of supplements

Probiotics are used to prevent and treat antibiotic-induced diarrhea, yeast infections and urinary tract infections. They may also help to protect against colon cancer and the adverse effects of chemotherapy and radiotherapy. Some evidence suggests that probiotics may help to treat allergies and skin conditions, reduce high cholesterol, and improve immunity. They can also be taken as a preventive against food poisoning when travelling. Probiotics should be taken in between meals to avoid extreme stomach acidity and enteric-coated supplemental forms may be preferable.

Probiotics products vary widely in quality and in the bacteria they contain. Products which have been manufactured by a filtration process and which are in powder form in a dark glass container may be preferable. They should be kept in a refrigerator after opening.

Fructo-oligosaccharides

Fructo-oligosaccharides are carbohydrate molecules which are not digested in the human small intestine but fermented in the colon, where they promote the growth of some species of beneficial bacteria, especially bifidobacteria, and may also reduce the growth of harmful species. Fructo-oligosaccharides are found in plants such as onions, asparagus, garlic and wheat.

Fiber supplements

Dietary fiber is the term given to plant foods that the human digestive system cannot digest. There are many different types of dietary fiber, and including these in your diet is one of the most important ways to help your digestive system to function efficiently.

What it does in the body

Benefits include lower blood cholesterol levels,[1] which reduces the risk of heart disease, and a reduction in the formation of cancer-causing compounds in the gut. Fiber also helps to stabilize blood sugar levels.

Therapeutic uses of supplements

While fiber supplements do not substitute for a high fiber diet, they may be useful in certain circumstances. Fiber supplements are available in several forms, such as psyllium seed, oat bran, rice bran, guar gum and flaxseeds. They are used to treat constipation, high cholesterol, irritable bowel syndrome[2] and obesity.

Algae: spirulina and chlorella

Algae are green, or 'blue-green' freshwater, one-celled organisms that can be grown, dried, and used as nutritional supplements.

What they do in the body

They are high in protein and contain all the amino acids. Spirulina is also a good source of iron, potassium, beta carotene and essential fatty acids. Some research suggests that the human body may not be able to absorb the form of vitamin B12 found in spirulina, and it may even block true vitamin B12 absorption.

Therapeutic uses

As it is high in protein, spirulina may be useful in stabilizing blood sugar levels and increasing energy. It is often used by those who are fasting and may also help in weight loss.

Herbal medicines

Herbs have been used as medicines for thousands of years. In fact, many of the pharmaceutical products sold today are synthetic chemicals based on herbal extracts. Herbal medicines may contain a whole plant, parts of a plant, or extracts of either one or a combination of plants. Many people prefer to use herbal medicines because in many cases, they exert beneficial effects without the side effects caused by many pharmaceutical drugs.

In the western world, in the last 10 to 20 years, there has been a tremendous growth in interest in herbal medicine and more natural and less toxic therapies have become increasingly popular. Scientific researchers have also produced a large amount of information on the use of plants and plant substances as medicinal agents. Much of this information provides scientific validation for the uses of plants which have been known to healers for thousands of years.

While herbs are, in many cases, free of the side effects of pharmaceutical drugs, they must be used appropriately. Many herbs have potent effects and may also interact with other medications you may be taking. It is always wise to consult a herbal practitioner if you plan to take herbal medicines, particularly if you are pregnant or have a serious or chronic medical problem.

Commercial herbal preparations are available in a variety of forms including teas, tinctures, fluid extracts, powders, capsules and tablets. Improvements in extraction and concentration processes in recent years have led to the availability of good quality, effective herbal products. The following are some of the most popular and readily available herbs. The term *herb* refers to any plant used for medicinal purposes.

Alfalfa *(Medicago sativa)*

Alfalfa has a powerful reputation as a healing herb. It is a healthy and nutritious source of chlorophyll, beta carotene, calcium, and the vitamins D, E and K. Alfalfa has laxative, diuretic and antiseptic effects. It also has a reputation as a detoxifier, able to improve liver function and cleanse the blood.

Uses

Alfalfa may be helpful in the treatment of urinary tract infections, and kidney, bladder and prostrate disorders. It is also often recommended for bone and joint disorders, digestive problems, skin disorders and ulcers.

Cautions

Anyone with the disease systemic lupus erythematosus (SLE) should avoid alfalfa products.

Aloe vera *(Aloe vera)*

Aloe vera grows throughout most of the warmer parts of the world. It has been used medicinally for thousands of years and has antiviral, antibacterial, anti-inflammatory, moisturising and wound-healing effects. It also stimulates immunity. Taken internally, it soothes gut irritation, aids healing and is laxative.

Uses

When applied to the skin Aloe vera is used to treat burns, minor skin irritations and wounds. Internally it is used to treat constipation, peptic ulcers, diabetes, asthma and viral infections.

Arnica *(Arnica montana)*

Also known as mountain tobacco, arnica is a well known herbal and homeopathic remedy. It has anti-inflammatory and pain-killing properties when used externally.

Uses

Arnica is used to treat bruises, sprains and swellings.

Cautions

Arnica should not be used internally, unless the medicine is in a commercially prepared form. It should not be used on open wounds.

Ashwagandha *(Withania somnifera)*

Widely used in Ayurvedic (traditional Indian) medicine, ashwagandha is also known as Indian Ginseng. It improves the response to stress, possibly via an action on the adrenal glands, and also has anti-inflammatory and sedative effects.

Uses

Ashwagandha is used to treat nervous exhaustion, insomnia and malnutrition. It may also be useful in cases of impotence or infertility due to nervous exhaustion, in convalescence, and in debility associated with chronic inflammatory conditions such as arthritis and Crohn's disease.

Asthma weed *(Chamaesyce hirta)*

Asthma weed acts on the bronchi of the lungs, causing them to relax and making it easier to breathe.

Uses

As is's name suggests, asthma weed is used to treat asthma. It can also be used to treat hay fever and upper respiratory tract catarrh.

Astragalus *(Astragalus membranaceus)*

One of the best known herbs used in Chinese medicine, astragalus strengthens the digestion and stimulates the immune system. It also aids adrenal gland function, acts as a diuretic and dilates blood vessels.

Uses

Astragalus can be used to boost the immune system in people who frequently suffer from infections such as colds. It can also be used in convalescence and to aid in cancer treatment and recovery from chemotherapy.

Cautions

Astragalus shoudl not be used in cases of acute infections or fevers.

Bilberry *(Vaccinium myrtillus)*

Bilberry has a long history of use, both as food and medicine, but renewed interest was sparked when Second World War pilots noticed that their night vision improved after they ate bilberries. Bilberry strengthens capillaries, stabilises collagen, reduces blood clotting, lowers blood sugar, relaxes smooth muscle and helps to prevent and cure ulcers. It also has antioxidant action.

Uses

Bilberry is used to treat eye conditions such as cataracts and macular degeneration, blood vessel problems such as varicose veins, and ulcers.

Black cohosh *(Cimicifuga racemosa)*

Also known as black snakeroot, black cohosh was originally used by the American Indians. It has anti-inflammatory and anti-spasmodic actions. It also acts as a tonic to the uterus and lowers blood pressure. Black cohosh has an oestrogen-like action.

Uses

Black cohosh is often used to treat menopausal problems such as hot flushes and decreases in bone mineral density. It can also be used to treat painful periods. The other main use for black cohosh is in the treatment of rheumatoid arthritis.

Cautions

Black cohosh should not be used during pregnancy or lactation, although it can be used in the later stages of pregnancy to prepare the uterus for birth.

Black haw *(Viburnum prunifolium)*

Mainly a woman's herb, black haw is often combined with crampbark.

Uses

Black haw is used to treat menstrual pain, to prevent miscarriage and prevnet excessive flow at menopause.

Blue flag *(Iris versicolor)*

Commonly grown as an ornamental garden plant, blue flag has a reputation as a blood purifier and cleanser of toxins.

Uses

Blue flag is used to treat skin complaints such as psoriasis and eczema, possibly via its effects on the liver. It is also useful in the treatment of headache and migraine associated with digestive problems and low blood sugar.

Cautions

The root can cause nausea and vomiting. Small doses should be used.

Buchu *(Barosma betulina)*

Buchu is a small shrub native to South Africa where it is often used both as a flavoring agent and as a medicine. It has antiseptic and diuretic properties, and acts as a kidney tonic.

Uses

Buchu is used to treat blood in the urine, bladder infections and other chronic urinary tract disorders. It is also said to be an effective remedy for kidney stones, prostate disorders, cystitis, and rheumatism.

Cautions

Buchu should be used with cautiously in cases of kidney disease.

Burdock *(Arctium lappa)*

Cultivated as a food in Japan, burdock is valued as a blood purifier and cleanser. It stimulates the secretion of digestive juices, especially bile.

Uses

Burdock is used to treat skin conditions such as psoriasis, boils, acne and eczema. It is also used to treat arthritis.

Calendula *(Calendula officinalis)*

Calendula, which is commonly known as marigold, can be used in salads, in skin creams or in medicines. It has anti-inflammatory, antibacterial, antifungal and wound-healing properties when used externally. It also eases muscle spasm and is a useful digestive remedy.

Uses

Calendula is used both internally and externally to treat many conditions including wounds, inflamed lymph nodes, varicose veins, skin ailments, gastritis and ulcers. It can also be used to treat menstrual problems.

Cat's claw *(Uncaria tomentosa)*

Cat's claw has been used by Peruvian Indians to treat a wide range of health problems. It boosts immune and digestive system function and has antiviral and anti-inflammatory effects.

Uses

Cat's claw is used to treat bowel disorders such as Crohn's disease, and colitis. It may also help to treat arthritis and bursitis, and support chemotherapy patients.

Cautions

Cat's claw should not be used during pregnancy.

Cayenne pepper *(Capsicum annuum)*

An essential ingredient in cooking, cayenne is also known as the chilli or hot pepper. It contains carotene molecules which have powerful antioxidant effects. Cayenne can also help digestion, improve circulation and lower cholesterol and blood fat levels. When applied topically, it acts as a pain reliever.

Uses

Topical cayenne pepper preparations are used to relieve pain in cases of arthritis, headaches and diabetic neuropathy.

Cautions

High doses on an empty stomach can cause gut irritation and eventually ulcers in susceptible people.

Chaste tree *(Vitex agnus castus)*

Once used by monks and nuns to curb sexual desire, chaste tree is now highly valued for its ability to regulate female hormones and increase breast milk production.

Uses

Chaste tree is used to treat menstrual and menopausal disorders.

Cautions

Chaste tree should not be used by postmenopausal women, during pregnancy, or by anyone on the contraceptive pill or hormone replacement therapy.

Celery seed *(Apium graveolens)*

The wild version of the well known vegetable, celery has diuretic and antiseptic effects. It also relieves smooth muscle spasm and may lower blood pressure.

Uses

It is used to treat arthritis and urinary tract infections.

Cautions

Celery should not be used during pregnancy or by anyone with kidney disease.

Chamomile *(Matricaria recutita)*

A popular herbal tea, chamomile has many beneficial effects. It is anti-inflammatory, anti-allergy, aids digestion, relieves muscle spasm, is a relaxant and has wound-healing effects.

Uses

Chamomile is used to treat many conditions including asthma, hay fever, sinusitis, gastrointestinal disturbances, menstrual and menopausal problems, nervous tension, insomnia and tension and digestive headaches. Externally it can be used to treat skin problems and conjunctivitis.

Cautions

In rare cases, there may be an allergic reaction to chamomile.

Chickweed *(Stellaria media)*

A common garden weed, chickweed is a vitamin and mineral- rich herb. It is rich in B complex vitamins, iron, copper, calcium and zinc. It can be used externally to relieve itching, and has wound-healing and emollient properties.

Uses

Chickweed is usually used to treat itchy skin problems such as eczema, psoriasis, boils, wounds and bruises.

Cleavers *(Galium aparine)*

Also known as goosegrass and catchweed because of its sticky leaves, cleavers has long been valued as a tonic for the lymphatic system.

Uses

Cleavers is used to treat skin disorders such as psoriasis, eczema and acne. It is also useful in treating swollen glands and urinary stones.

Comfrey *(Symphytum officinale)*

Also known as knitbone, comfrey has a good reputation as a wound healer. It is soothing, healing and anti-inflammatory.

Uses

Comfrey is used to treat fractures, wounds, sprains, psoriasis and eczema. Internally it has been used to treat gastrointestinal problems.

Cautions

Comfrey contains compounds which have caused liver damage in animals. It is not recommended for internal use.

Crampbark *(Viburnum opulus)*

As its name suggests crampbark is a useful remedy for carmping pains as it relaxes muscle tension and spasm.

Uses

It is most often used to treat painful periods and the cramping pains of pregnancy. It can also be used to treat migraine, asthma, angina and hypertension.

Cranberry *(Vaccinium macrocarpon)*

A popular and delicious juice drink, cranberry also has valuable effects on the urinary system.

Uses

Cranberry is used to treat urinary tract infections and as a long term preventive for kidney stones.

Damiana *(Turnera diffusa)*

Originally used in Mexican folk medicine, damiana is an antidepressant and improves mood. It is also mildly diuretic and may enhance the action of testosterone.

Uses

Damiana is used to treat depression, herpes, impotence and sexual problmes of psychological origin in men and women.

Cautions

Damiana should not be used by anyone suffering from irritable bowel syndrome.

Dandelion *(Taraxacum officinale)*

A well known garden weed, dandelion is much valued as a herbal remedy. It is a rich source of vitamins and minerals, including potassium.The root is used to improve digestion as it stimulates the flow of digestive juices, including bile from the liver and gallbladder. This can have beneficial effects on many conditions. The leaves have a diuretic effect.

Uses

Dandelion root is used to treat liver conditions and improve liver function. Both leaves and root can be used to treat arthritis and skin conditions.

Devil's claw *(Harpagophytum procumbens)*

Native to Africa, Devils' claw takes its name from its large, hooked, claw-like fruit. It has strong anti-inflammatory and analgesic properties.

Uses

Devil's claw is used to treat arthritis, liver and gallbladder complaints.

Cautions

Devil's claw should not be used in pregnancy or by anyone with a stomach ulcer.

Dong quai *(Angelica sinensis)*

Dong quai has a reputation as a very valuable remedy for women as it contains compounds which can regulate female hormone action. Dong quai also lowers blood pressure, increases blood flow to the brain and other parts of the body, and has also been shown to have mild tranquillising and pain- relieving effects.

Uses

Dong quai is usually used to treat premenstrual syndrome, menstrual problems, and menopausal symptoms (including hot flushes). It can also be used for treating arthritis, migraines, anaemia and abdominal pain.

Cautions

Dong quai should not be used during pregnancy or in cases of excessive menstrual blood flow as it stimulates the uterus.

Echinacea *(Echinacea angustifolia, E. purpurea, E. pallida)*

Highly valued by the American Indians, echinacea is now used all over the world. It stimulates the immune system, helps in tissue healing and has anti-inflammatory, antiviral, antibacterial and anti-cancer effects.

Uses

Echinacea has long been used to treat infections such as colds and flu. It is also useful in aiding wound-healing, treating arthritis and alleviating the side effects of chemotherapy.

Elder *(Sambucus nigra)*

Elderflowers have diuretic, anti-inflammatory and anti-catarrhal actions. They raise body temperature, causing sweating which is useful in stimulating the immune system. The bark and berries have laxative, diuretic and anti-inflammatory actions.

Uses

Elder is mainly used to treat colds, flu, dry coughs, sinusitis and catarrh.

Elecampane *(Inula helenium)*

Elecampane's Latin name comes from Helen of Troy as the herb was said to spring from her tears. It has antibacterial, antiviral and antifungal effects. It is a digestive tonic, an expectorant, and also reduces coughing by relaxing the bronchial muscles.

Uses

Elecampane is used to treat chronic coughs, bronchitis and asthma. It can also be used for gastrointestinal problems.

Eyebright *(Euphrasia rostokoviana)*

Known throughout history as a treatment for eye problems, eyebright has anti-catarrhal, anti-inflammatory and astringent actions.

Uses

Eyebright is used to treat colds, conjunctivitis, eye inflammation, hay fever, ear disorders and catarrh.

Fennel *(Foeniculum vulgare)*

While the root is eaten as a vegetable, it is the seeds which are used medicinally.

Fennel has anti-inflammatory and diuretic effects. It also acts as a digestive aid and increases milk flow in breastfeeding women.

Uses

Fennel can be used to treat respiratory infections and digestive problems such as gas and bloating. It can be used externally as a gargle and as an eyewash to treat eye infections.

Fenugreek *(Trigonella foenum-graecum)*

Fenugreek has been used as a culinary herb and as a medicine since ancient times. It has expectorant, demulcent, vulnerary, anti-inflammatory, anti-spasmodic, and blood pressure-lowering actions. It also increases the flow of milk in nursing mothers.

Uses

Fenugreek is used to treat sore throats, bronchitis and to improve digestion. It is also recommended for menopausal women.

Cautions

Fenugreek should not be used during pregnancy.

Feverfew *(Tanacetum parthenium)*

Feverfew, a member of the sunflower family, has been used medicinally for centuries. It inhibits the manufacture of substances which promote inflammation.

Uses

Feverfew is mainly used to treat and prevent migraine attacks. It is also used to treat headaches and rheumatoid arthritis.

Cautions

Feverfew should not be used during pregnancy.

Figwort *(Scrophularia nodosa)*

Figwort is used to cleanse and purify the blood.

Uses

Figwort is used to treat skin diseases such as eczema, acne and psoriasis.

Flax *(Linum usitatissimum)*

Highly valued for its fiber and oil, flax has been cultivated for thousands of years. Flax seeds are a good source of beneficial omega-3 fatty acids (See page 329 for more information.) and also have laxative, pain-relieving, emollient and soothing effects.

Uses

Flax seeds can be used to treat respiratory problems, constipation, and to soothe an irritated gut. Externally, flaxseed poultices can be used to treat burns, boils and pain.

Cautions

Very large doses of the seeds (over 100g) have been known to cause poisoning.

Garlic *(Allium sativum)*

Used medicinally for 5000 years, garlic has many well-researched effects. It is antibacterial, antifungal, antiviral and anti-inflammatory. It boosts immune function, helps digestion and has also been shown to have anti-cancer effects. Garlic also reduces cholesterol, blood pressure, blood clotting, and limits free radical damage to blood fats.

Uses

Aside from culinary uses, garlic is most often used to treat high cholesterol and blood pressure. It is also used to treat infections and digestive and respiratory problems.

Gentian *(Gentiana lutea)*

A well known 'bitter' tonic, gentian has been used for centuries to improve digestion. It stimulates the flow of digestive juices including saliva and bile, and helps stimulate gut movement. Gentian improves appetite.

Uses

Gentian is used to stimulate digestive activity whenever this is necessary. It is also used to treat digestive complaints such as dyspepsia, gastritis, diarrhoea, nausea and heartburn.

Cautions

Gentian should be avoided by those with peptic ulcers.

Ginger *(Zingiber officinale)*

Highly valued as a spice, ginger has been used medicinally for thousands of years by Chinese physicians. Ginger acts as an antioxidant and has has antibacterial, anti-inflammatory, anti-clotting and pain-killing properties. It also improves liver function and lowers cholesterol as well as having beneficial effects on the heart. Ginger has anti-ulcer activity and improves the function of the muscles in the gut while helping to relieve spasm. Ginger is also valued for its warming properties.

Uses

Ginger is used to treat motion sickness, nausea and vomiting; inflammatory conditions such as arthritis; and to improve digestion.

Cautions

Large doses on an empty stomach may cause irritation and with long-term use may lead to ulcers.

Ginkgo *(Ginkgo biloba)*

The ginkgo tree is the only survivor of the world's oldest living tree species. It has many valuable effects including stabilising cell membranes, reducing free radical damage, improving blood circulation and enhancing oxygen and glucose use. Ginkgo is particularly beneficial for brain, nerves and blood vessels.

Uses

Ginkgo is used to treat senile conditions, including Alzheimer's disease; hardening of the arteries; depression, and allergies. It is also used as a treatment for oxygen deprivation.

Cautions

Very large doses may cause diarrhoea and vomiting.

Ginseng *(Panax ginseng and Eleutherococcus senticosus)*

There are several types of ginseng, the best known varieties being Korean or Chinese ginseng (*Panax ginseng*) and Siberian ginseng (*Eleutherococcus senticosus*). Korean ginseng is considered to be more stimulating than Siberian ginseng.

Both types of ginseng have a long history of use in Chinese medicine as tonics. They enhance the body's ability to cope with stress, improve energy metabolism, lower blood sugar, boost immunity, enhance liver function, and regulate cell growth.

Uses

The anti-fatigue and anti-stress properties of both types of ginseng are used to increase physical and mental performance in people who are debilitated and suffering from stress. Korean ginseng is also used to treat diabetes, to lower cholesterol, to enhance reproductive system function, to treat menopausal symptoms, to improve immunity and to prevent cancer. Siberian ginseng is often used to treat chronic fatigue syndrome, to combat the side effects of cancer chemotherapy and radiotherapy, and to treat rheumatic pain in the elderly.

Cautions

Ginseng should be avoided by people who have acute infections, high blood pressure or anxiety. Some people experience side effects with ginseng. These include high blood pressure, nervousness, insomnia, skin problems and diarrhoea.

Golden rod *(Solidago virgaurea)*

Also known as woundwort and Aaron's rod, golden rod has diuretic, anti-inflammatory, anti-micorbial and astrigent actions.

Uses

Golden rod is used to treat kidney and urinary infections and stones. It can also be used to treat respiratory catarrh and arthritis.

Goldenseal *(Hydrastis canadensis)*

Highly valued by American Indians as a medicine, wild goldenseal is becoming increasingly rare. It has anti-microbial activity and is active against many disease-causing organisms. Goldenseal prevents bacteria from attaching to cells, stimulates the immune system, lowers fevers, and has anti-cancer effects.

Uses

Goldenseal is used to treat inflammatory digestive conditions such as gastritis, peptic ulcers and colitis. It can also be used to treat painful menstruation and respiratory infections. It can be used as a mouthwash and to treat skin infections.

Cautions

Goldenseal should not be used in pregnancy or in cases of high blood pressure.

Gotu kola *(Centella asiatica)*

Gotu kola has been used as a medicine for thousands of years and has a reputation as an anti-ageing herb. It has wound-healing and sedative properties, and also improves mental function.

Uses

Gotu kola is used to treat wounds, burns, cellulite, cirrhosis of the liver, varicose veins and other blood vessel problems. It is also used to treat insomnia and stress.

Cautions

Gotu kola is toxic in high doses.

Gravel root *(Eupatorium purpureum)*

Also known as kidneyweed, gravel root has beneficial effects on the kidney and urinary system.

Uses

It is used to treat kidney and urinary infections and stones, prostate inflammation and gout.

Gymnema *(Gymnema sylvestre)*

Long used in traditional Indian medicine as a treatment for diabetes, gymnema has been shown to help in blood sugar control, possibly by improving insulin production.

Uses

Gymnema is used to treat Type I and Type II diabetes.

Cautions

Anyone using herbs to treat diabetes should have their blood sugar closely monitored.

Hawthorn *(Crataegus oxyacantha)*

Native to Europe, hawthorn has a reputation as a heart tonic. Hawthorn acts to strengthen blood capillaries and connective tissue. Hawthorn improves the blood supply to the heart, improves the strength of heart muscle contraction, lowers blood pressure and cholesterol levels, and reduces angina attacks.

Uses

Hawthorn is used to treat atherosclerosis, high blood pressure, congestive heart failure, and cardiac arrhythmias.

Horse chestnut *(Aesculus hippocastanum)*

Horse chestnut is a valuable remedy for strengthening veins. It can be used externally and internally.

Uses

Horse chestnut is used to treat vein problems such as varicose veins, haemorrhoids and thrombophlebitis.

Cautions

Horse chestnut should not be used by those with kidney disease.

Hops *(Humulus lupulus)*

Hops have been used to brew beer since Roman times. Highly valued for their medicinal properties, hops have sedative, soporific, diuretic and antibacterial effects. Hops also relieve muscle spasm and act to improve digestion.

Uses

Hops are used to treat insomnia, restlessness and nervous tension. The herb can also be used to treat irritable bowel syndrome, inflammatory bowel disease and dyspepsia.

Cautions

Hops should not be used in cases of depression.

Horseradish *(Cochlearia armoracia)*

Horseradish root stimulates blood circulation and has antibiotic action. It can be used externally and internally.

Uses

Horseradish is used to treat lung and urinary infections, and rheumatic conditions.

Cautions

If using horseradish externally, take care that it does not blister the skin. Anyone with low thyroid function or who is taking thyroxine should avoid horseradish.

Horsetail *(Equisetum arvense)*

Horsetail is a rush-like plant with hollow jointed stems. It is rich in silica and other minerals and has diuretic and healing properties. It also stops bleeding and tones the bladder. Horsetail may also promote the healing of broken bones and connective tissue.

Uses

Horsetail is mainly used to treat urinary tract and prostate disorders such as cystitis, urethritis, kidney stones, prostatitis and incontinence. It may also be useful in the treatment of arthritis and bone diseases. It can be used externally to stop bleeding and heal wounds.

Kava *(Piper methysticum)*

Kava is used to make a drink used in celebrations and rituals in the Pacific islands. It makes drinkers feel calm, relaxed and sociable. Large doses cause sleep.

Uses

Kava is used to treat nervous anxiety, insomnia, restlessness and depression.

Cautions

High doses taken for long periods may cause side effects and should be avoided.

Lemon balm *(Melissa officinalis)*

This essential oil-rich herb has a long history of use as a remedy for nervousness and depression. It has carminative, nervine, anti-spasmodic, anti-depressive, diaphoretic and anti-microbial effects.

Uses

It is used to treat anxiety, depression, insomnia, flatulence, allergies, migraine and viral infections such as herpes.

Linden *(Tilia europea)*

Also known as lime blossom, linden has a long reputation as a nervous tonic.

Uses

Linden is used to treat nervous tension, insomnia, high blood pressure, atherosclerosis, colds, influenza, catarrhal conditions and migraine.

Liquorice *(Glycyrrhiza glabra)*

One of the most widely used herbs, liquorice has an important place in both Western and Eastern herbal medicine. It has hormonal, anti-inflammatory, anti-allergic, antibacterial and antiviral effects. Liquorice has also been shown to stimulate the immune system.

Uses

Liquorice has been used to treat inflammatory and allergic conditions, colds, viral infections, hepatitis, premenstrual syndrome, Addison's disease, peptic ulcers and skin conditions.

Cautions

Long-term use of liquorice can raise blood pressure. It should not be used during pregnancy or by anyone with high blood pressure, liver disease or kidney failure.

Marshmallow *(Althea officinalis)*

Marshmallow has a reputation has a soothing, healing plant. It has demulcent, emollient, diuretic, anti-inflammatory and expectorant actions.

Uses

Marshmallow is used to treat stomach and duodenal ulcers, catarrh, coughs, colds and urinary tract infections.

Meadowsweet *(Filipendula ulmaria)*

Long a remedy for flu, fever, and arthritis, meadowsweet contains an aspirin-type compound called salicylic acid. It has antiseptic, anti-ulcer, anti-inflammatory and diuretic properties.

Uses

Meadowsweet is used to treat rheumatism, ulcers, diarrhoea, kidney problems and gastric acidity.

Motherwort *(Leonurus cardiaca)*

As it's common name suggests, motherwort is useful for women's disorders and as the Latin name suggests, it is also beneficial in treating heart problems.

Uses

Motherwort is used to treat delayed, absent or painful periods, menopausal changes, in childbirth and for heart palpitations.

Milk thistle *(Silybum marianum)*

Milk thistle, which is native to Europe and some parts of the USA, has powerful liver-protecting properties. It prevents damage and improves function.

Uses

Milk thistle is used to treat liver disease, including cirrhosis and hepatitis. It is also used to treat gallstones and psoriasis.

Mullein *(Verbascum thapsus)*

Highly valued has a respiratory remedy, mullein has expectorant, demulcent, diuretic, anti-inflammatory, nervine, anti-spasmodic and astringent actions.

Uses

Mullein is used to treat respiratory disorders, particularly bronchitis.

Mushrooms

Mushrooms, including shiitake, maitake and reishi, are prized in Chinese herbal medicine, and are believed to increase resistance to stress and extend lifespan. These mushrooms can regulate blood pressure, glucose, insulin, cholesterol and triglycerides. They may boost immune function, kill viruses, and protect against cancer. These mushrooms can be used fresh and extracts are also available in capsule form.

Uses

These mushrooms can be used to treat and prevent a wide variety of disorders, including cancer, diabetes, chronic fatigue syndrome, viral infections, high blood pressure, heart disease and fatigue.

Myrrh *(Commiphora molmol)*

Myrrh has an ancient reputation as a cleansing agent and it has antiseptic, anti-fungal and astringent effects. It is often used in mouthwashes.

Uses

Myrrh is used to treat sore throats and infected gums. It can also be useful in the treatment of thrush (*Candida albicans* infection)

Oatstraw *(Avena sativa)*

As well as the seeds, the leaves of the oat plant are used medicinally. Oats has nervine tonic, anti-depressant, nutritive, demulcent and healing properties.

Uses

Oatstraw is used to treat debility, exhaustion, depression and stress. It is useful remedy in those who are convalescing.

Oregon grape root *(Mahonia aquifolium)*

Also known as mountain grape, this herbs has beneficial effects on the liver and gallbladder and has a good reputation as a blood purifier.

Uses

It is used to treat skin disorders such as eczema, psoriasis and acne. As it has laxative effects it is also used in constipation.

Cautions

Oregon grape root should not be used during pregnancy.

Parsley *(Petroselinum crispum)*

One of the most commonly used culinary herbs, parsley also has medicinal uses due to its diuretic action.

Uses

Parsley is used to treat urinary infections and stones. It is also used to improve digestion and treat flatulence.

Cautions

Parsley should not be used in medicinal doses during pregnancy.

Pau d'arco *(Tabebuia avellanedae or T. ipe)*

The native Indians of Brazil use the bark of this tree for many ailments. It has antibacterial, antiviral, anti-parasitic, anti-inflammatory and anti-cancer effects.

Uses

Pau d'arco is used to treat vaginal and intestinal yeast infections. It is also used to treat cancer.

Pellitory-of-the-wall *(Parietaria officinalis)*

Often found in old ruins and walls, pellitory-of-the-wall has soothing, diuretic and astringent properties.

Uses

It is used to treat cystitis, prostate inflammation and urinary stones.

Peppermint *(Mentha piperita)*

Peppermints have been used medicinally for thousands of years. They contain compounds, such as menthol, which help to eliminate intestinal gas, relieve gut and other smooth muscle spasms, stimulate bile flow, and have pain-killing effects.

Uses

Peppermint oil is used to treat irritable bowel syndrome, gallstones, colds and topically, as a painkiller.

Raspberry *(Rubus idaeus)*

The leaves of the raspberry plant are used medicinally. They have a long tradition of use in pregnancy to strengthen and tone the uterus.

Uses

Raspberry leaf is used to prepare mothers for childbirth. It can also be used to treat diarrhea.

Red clover *(Trifolium pratense)*

Rich in compounds known as phytoestrogens, red clover has been used in the treatment of cancer.

Uses

Red clover is used to treat skin conditions such as psoriasis and eczema. It is also useful in the treatment of whooping cough and bronchitis as it has expectorant and antispasmodic action.

Sage *(Salvia officinalis)*

A commonly used culinary herb, sage also has medicinal uses. It has carminative, anti-spasmodic, anti-microbial, astringent and anti-inflammatory actions.

Uses

Sage is used to treat colds, sore throats, hot flashes, painful periods and indigestion.

Cautions

Sage should not be used during pregnancy.

Senna *(Cassia acutifolia and C. angustifolia)*

Senna is well known for its laxative action.

Uses

Senna is used to treat constipation and haemorrhoids/fissures which require soft stools.

Cautions

Senna should not be used for more than 10 days at a time and should not be used at all during pregnancy; lactation; or by those who have intestinal obstructions, inflammatory bowel disease or abdominal pain due to unknown causes.

St John's wort *(Hypericum perforatum)*

St John's wort has a long history of use and has several actions including antidepressant, antiviral and antibacterial effects.

Uses

St John's wort is becoming increasingly popular as a treatment for mild to moderate depression, including menopausal depression. It can also be used to treat viral infections.

Cautions

High doses may cause photosensitivity and gastrointestinal upset.

Saw palmetto *(Serenoa repens)*

Used by the American Indians as a male tonic, saw palmetto inhibits the conversion of the male hormone testosterone to its more active form and also has anti-oestrogenic effects.

Uses

Saw palmetto is mainly used to treat benign prostatic hypertrophy, a disorder in which the prostate gland becomes enlarged. It can also be used to treat urinary tract infections.

Skullcap *(Scutellaria laterifolia)*

Skullcap is valued for its effects as a nervous system tonic.

Uses

Skullcap is used to treat anxiety, depression, insomnia, headaches and premenstrual syndrome.

Slippery elm *(Ulmus rubra)*

A nutritious convalescent food, the powdered inner bark of the tree is the part used medicinally. Slippery elm powder is soothing to the digestive tract and can also be used externally.

Uses

Slippery elm powder is mainly used to treat ulcers and inflammatory conditions of the digestive tract such as gastritis and oesophagitis. It can also be used externally to draw and soothe boils, abscesses and burns.

Stone root *(Collinsonia canadensis)*

Native to canada, stone root has diuretic and vein-strengthening effects.

Uses

Stone root is used to treat kidney stones, gall stones, varicose veins, hemorrhoids and diarrhea

---

Tea tree *(Melaleuca alternifolia)*

The tea tree, which grows only in north east New South Wales, has a long history of use in Aboriginal medicine and is becoming very popular as an antiseptic.

Uses

Tea tree oil is used to treat skin infections, acne, foot problems, fungal nail infections and vaginal infections.

Thyme *(Thymus vulgaris)*

A culinary herb, thyme also has medicinal uses. It has carminative, anti-microbial, anti-spasmodic, expectorant and astringent effects.

Uses

Thyme is used to treat sore throats, colds and coughs. It is also useful in improving digestion and treating flatulence.

Turmeric *(Curcuma longa)*

A member of the ginger family, turmeric is a commonly used curry spice. It has antioxidant, anti-inflammatory, carminative and cholesterol-lowering effects. It is also beneficial for the digestive system.

Uses

Turmeric is used to treat and prevent cardiovascular disease and cancer. It may also be useful in inflammatory conditions.

Uva ursi *(Arctostaphylos uva ursi)*

Uva ursi, which is also known as bearberry, grows in the northern United States and Europe. It has diuretic, astringent and antiseptic properties.

Uses

Uva ursi is used to treat urinary tract infections. The urine must be alkaline for uva ursi to be effective (do not use with cranberry juice which makes the urine acidic).

Cautions

Uva ursi is toxic in high doses and should not be used in pregnancy or by anyone who has a kidney infection.

Valerian *(Valeriana officinalis)*

Valerian, which has a long tradition of use as a sedative, is native to Europe and North America. It acts as a sedative and tranquilliser, relieves anxiety, lowers blood pressure, enhances the flow of bile and relaxes intestinal and other smooth muscles.

Uses

Valerian is mainly used to treat insomnia. It decreases the time taken to go to sleep and improves sleep quality and length.

Cautions

Valerian may cause morning sleepiness in some people. Rarely, some people may be stimulated by valerian.

Vervain *(Verbena officinalis)*

Highly valued by the druids, vervain has an ancient history of use. It has tonic, sedative, anti-spasmodic, diaphoretic, hypotensive and hepatic actions. It also stimulates the flow of mother's milk.

Uses

Vervain is used to treat nervous exhaustion, depression, liver and gallbladder disorders

Cautions

Vervain should not be used in pregnancy.

Wild cherry *(Prunus serotina)*

The bark of this plant is the part that is used medicinally. Wild cherry has anti-tussive, expectorant, astringent, nervine and anti-spasmodic properties.

Uses

Wild cherry is used to treat irritating, nervous and continuous coughs. It can be of value in the treatment of whooping cough and bronchitis.

Wild yam *(Dioscorea villosa)*

Wild yam is now well known as the source of the chemical from which the female hormone progesterone is produced. It has anti-inflammatory, diuretic, anti-spasmodic effects and also stimulates the release of bile from the gall bladder.

Uses

Wild yam is used to treat pain and spasm, especially rheumatic and menstrual pain. It can also be used to treat urinary tract conditions.

Cautions

Some manufacturers claim that wild yam has a progesterone-like action in the body. This claim has not been supported by research.

Willow *(Salix alba)*

White willow is one of the natural sources of aspirin and like that drug, it has anti-inflammatory and analgesic properties.

Uses

Willow is used to treat fevers, arthritis and aches and pains of all kinds.

Yarrow *(Achillea millefolium)*

Also known as soldier's herb, yarrow has been used medicinally for centuries. It has anti-inflammatory, antiseptic and diuretic effects. Yarrow also promotes sweating, lowers blood pressure, relieves muscle spasm, improves digestion and stops bleeding.

Uses

Yarrow is used to treat gastrointestinal problems, menstrual disorders, fevers, colds and haemorrhoids. It is also used for venous problems such as varicose veins, to lower blood pressure, and to reduce clotting.

Promoting optimum health

Promoting optimum health

Health can be viewed as a continuum that ranges from severe illness to optimum health. While it is not the only factor, good nutrition plays a vital role in helping someone to move towards the healthy end of this continuum. Dietary changes and supplements can help an unhealthy person to look and feel better, while someone who feels healthy may become fitter, more mentally alert and recover more quickly from injury, thereby moving further towards optimum health.

Improving the functioning of the immune and digestive systems plays a key role in promoting optimum health. A well-functioning immune system is essential for good health, and poor digestion plays a role in many common diseases, either by directly contributing to symptoms or by exacerbating those due to other causes. A healthy diet which contains optimum amounts of fat, carbohydrate, protein, fiber, vitamins and minerals can help to support good immune and digestive functions.

While everyone can benefit from a diet which boosts immunity and digestive function, there are certain groups of people who need to pay particular attention to diet and intake of vitamins and minerals. This may be due to lifestyle, environmental or other factors. These include vegetarians, older people and those who take medication for long periods. Optimum nutrition is vital during pregnancy, as having a baby is one of the most nutritionally demanding events in a woman's life.

This section also includes a chapter on antioxidants as a growing amount of research suggests that diets high in antioxidants or antioxidant supplements can help to reduce cancer death rates, cold and flu infections and protect against atherosclerosis, heart disease and cataracts. These nutrients may improve immune system function and may even delay some of the effects of aging.

[illegible]

[illegible]

[illegible]

[illegible]

[illegible]

The antioxidant vitamins are vitamin E, vitamin C, and the beta carotene form of vitamin A. Minerals such as selenium, copper, manganese and zinc also have antioxidant properties when combined with certain enzymes. There are many other antioxidant compounds in food, such as bioflavonoids found in fruit and vegetables; coenzyme Q10 found in fish, nuts and lean meats; and sulfur-containing amino acids.

Antioxidants and disease prevention

There is no research which shows that antioxidants *definitely* protect against, or cure any disease. However, growing evidence strongly *suggests* that they have the power to prevent diseases such as cancer, coronary heart disease and cataracts. Studies show that diets high in antioxidants or antioxidant supplements reduce cancer death rates, cold and flu infections and protect against atherosclerosis, heart disease and cataracts. These vitamins may improve immune system function and may even delay some of the effects of aging. This is probably due to their ability to intercept and extinguish free radicals.

Free radicals

Oxygen, the most critical nutrient for life, is the main source of free radicals, which could be the fundamental cause of many chronic diseases and even of the aging process. Free radicals are highly reactive oxygen fragments which are created by normal chemical processes in the cells. They lack electrons and try to steal them from other molecules to regain balance, a process known as oxidation. Free radicals include the superoxide radical, the hydroxyl radical and hydrogen peroxide.

A certain level of free radicals is essential for good health as they are involved in fighting infection and in the contraction of smooth muscles in the blood vessels. Cells have a number of ways of dealing with excess free radicals including the use of enzyme systems and specific antioxidants.

What antioxidants do

An antioxidant is a substance which gives up electrons easily so it can neutralize oxidants, including free radicals. Unfortunately, these protective systems may not always be adequate when the system becomes overloaded with free radicals.

When the antioxidant systems of the body are overwhelmed, free radicals stabilize themselves by stealing electrons from chemically stable compounds, often causing the generation of more free radicals which react further with other compounds, causing yet more damage. These split second chain reactions spread throughout the body, attacking vulnerable sites in the cells and causing damage that can result in chronic disease.

Free radicals can be produced in dangerous amounts by irritants such as cigarette smoke, pesticides, air pollution, ultraviolet light and radiation which are all too common in the environments in which most of us live. Stress and excessive exercise can also produce large amounts of free radicals.

Vitamins may exert their antioxidant effects by acting as circuit breakers. They insert themselves into the free radical chain reaction and are altered without generating further free radicals. Antioxidants interact to protect each other. Vitamin C can react with a damaged vitamin E molecule and convert it back to its antioxidant form. Vitamin C is then returned to its original form by another antioxidant known as glutathione. This may explain the result of studies which show that vitamin C enhances the protective effects of vitamin E.

Free radical damage

- Free radical attacks on DNA, which is the genetic material of the cells, cause cells to die or mutate and possibly become cancerous. Free radicals may be involved in cancers of the lungs, cervix, skin, stomach, prostate, colon and esophagus.
- Free radicals also attack blood fats which may lead to heart and blood vessel disease. When the LDL type of cholesterol reacts with free radicals it becomes damaged and this may lead to atherosclerosis. Unless LDL cholesterol becomes damaged it does not seem to be harmful. Thus the damaging of LDL cholesterol is a critical link between high blood cholesterol and the build-up of vessel-blocking plaques. Atherosclerosis is the major cause of hardening of the arteries and therefore of heart attacks. Levels of another type of cholesterol, known as HDL cholesterol, which may protect against cardiovascular disease, may be lowered by free radical activity.
- Free radicals can also damage cellular enzymes. The processes which depend on these enzymes slow or stop, leading to cell damage and death. Dormant enzymes can also be activated and this can result in tissue damage.
- Cells contain components called mitochondria which are responsible for respiration and energy production. Free radicals can damage mitochondria, affecting the ability of the cell to produce the energy it needs to function.
- Substances which are toxic to nerves can also be released by free radicals, leading to nerve and brain damage, such as that seen in Parkinson's disease.
- Free radicals may be involved in the loss of transparency of the lenses of

the eye, leading to cataracts and macular degeneration.

- Free radicals may be involved in the inflammatory response seen in rheumatoid arthritis and asthma.
- Free radicals may also damage sperm causing infertility and birth defects. They may also be involved in ulcers and other digestive tract disorders, liver damage and reduced resistance to infection and disease.

Reducing free radical damage

Damage from free radicals can be minimized by avoiding excessive exercise, pollution, pesticides, cigarette smoke and other dangerous environmental factors. Eating a diet of foods rich in antioxidants is also extremely important. There are many powerful antioxidant compounds in foods which can strengthen the body's defense systems.

Individual levels of antioxidants depend on many factors including lifestyle, state of health, diet and heredity. People vary in their ability to absorb and metabolize different antioxidants, just as they do in the case of other nutrients. Some people may be able to obtain all the antioxidants they need from a healthy diet and others may benefit from supplements. However, until accurate tests are readily available it is not always easy to identify those who do have higher needs. With diseases where prevention is most important, it may be too late to reverse the adverse effects of free radical damage once susceptible people are identified. Several tests are being developed to measure oxidant stress. Such tests might establish the doses of antioxidant vitamins necessary to provide protection in individuals.

Antioxidants and the aging process

Aging is the accumulation of various adverse changes in cells and tissues that increase the risk of death. Evidence is growing that free radicals are an underlying cause of aging as the biological markers of the process are the same as those caused by free radical damage.

As the mitochondria are where most of the oxygen reactions in the cell occur, they may be the most susceptible to damage by free radicals. It has been suggested that the rate of damage, and therefore aging, in mitochondria may determine how long a person lives. The ability of antioxidants to reduce this damage explains their possible role in slowing the aging process. Research into chemicals which could slow the damage to mitochondria without decreasing energy production is in the early stages but it is expected to increase.

Due to their effects on mitochondria and other elements such as cell membranes and genetic material, free radicals may aggravate the breakdown and sagging of tissues and deterioration of bodily organs involved in the aging process. Many diseases commonly associated with aging, including cancer, heart disease and psychological disorders, appear to be prevented or improved by increasing intake of antioxidants. High levels of antioxidants also increase the effectiveness of the immune system, making older people less susceptible to life-threatening infections.

Experiments with aging animals show that the effectiveness of the body's antioxidant system decreases with age, possibly because of reduced dietary intake, absorption or increased nutrient needs. A steady supply of antioxidant vitamins and minerals should enhance the body's natural defense mechanisms and improve the quality and length of life.

Antioxidant supplements

For a person whose diet does not provide sufficient amounts of the antioxidant vitamins, it may be worth considering taking extra amounts as supplements. Research shows that the protective effects of antioxidant vitamins occur when they are taken at doses much higher than the RDAs. Studies which look at the anticancer effects of vitamin C often use doses of around 1000 mg. This is the amount in 14 oranges. Studies looking at the heart protective effects of vitamin E have used doses of 800 IU (536 mg alpha TE). This is the amount in around eight cups of sunflower seeds.

Those who regularly eat five to nine large servings of fruit and vegetables every day may be able to get enough vitamin C and beta carotene, but a large amount of high fat vitamin E-rich foods would be necessary to reach the levels that have been used to show protective effects.

Antioxidant vitamins are well-tolerated and free from toxicity, even in high doses except in unusual circumstances. In those who have a history or a family history of disease; are under stress; smoke; or live in a polluted environment; antioxidant supplements may be recommended. Suggested doses are:

Vitamin C	100 to 1000 mg
Beta carotene	10 to 30 mg
Vitamin E	67 to 500 mg alpha TE
Selenium	100 to 200 mcg

Other antioxidants

Aside from antioxidant vitamins and minerals, there are several other types of antioxidants available both in foods and supplements. Many of these belong to a family of plant chemicals called flavonoids. (See page 364 for more information). There are also several herbs which have antioxidant activity. These include cayenne or chilli pepper (*Capsicum annuum*), ginger (*Zingiber officinale*), garlic (*Allium sativum*), turmeric (*Curcuma longa*), ginkgo (*Ginkgo biloba*) and bilberry (*Vaccinium myrtillus*). See page 384 for more information on these herbs and the precautions that may be necessary.

Immunity

A well-functioning immune system is essential for good health, as it plays a vital role in protecting the body from the vast numbers of disease-causing organisms and other substances with which it comes into contact. The job of the immune system is to distinguish between normal body cells and foreign or abnormal cells. As with all body systems, immune balance is the key. Overactivity leads to allergies and autoimmune diseases, and underactivity increases the risk of infections. The immune system is also vital for recognizing and destroying cancer cells.

How the immune system works

The immune system is composed of specialized tissues, organs, cells and chemicals that recognize and destroy foreign invaders. The skin and mucous membranes form a barrier against unwanted organisms and substances. Immune cells include white blood cells such as T lymphocytes, which have many functions including control of other immune cells; and B lymphocytes, which produce antibodies. There are also natural killer cells and scavenger cells known as monocytes and macrophages, which engulf foreign particles. The cells of the immune system also produce substances such as interferon, which has antiviral effects.

The best way to keep the immune system working well is to stay in good general health. It is important not to allow infections to persist as this puts a strain on the immune system. Diet, medications, pollution, toxic chemicals, stress levels and emotional state all affect the workings of the immune system. Overuse of antibiotics is common nowadays and may prevent the immune system from becoming strong enough to deal with infectious agents. Other medications that can adversely affect the immune system include steroids. These drugs are often given for long periods in the treatment of disorders such as arthritis and asthma. Improving lymphatic circulation can help to boost the immune system. Exercise, massage and herbal remedies are helpful for this.

Autoimmunity

An autoimmune disease is one in which the immune system mistakenly attacks the body's own tissues. Some of the most common autoimmune diseases include arthritis, systemic lupus erythematosus (SLE), and possibly inflammatory bowel disease. There may be a genetic component to autoimmune diseases and they may also be caused by infections and injuries. Stress and emotional factors also seem to contribute. Supporting the immune system through diet and lifestyle is vitally important in the treatment of autoimmune diseases.

Allergy

An allergy is an inappropriate response by the immune system to a substance that is usually harmless. There are many causes of allergy, the most common being airborne particles such as mold, dust and pollen, certain foods, chemicals and drugs. Allergic responses play a role in many disorders, including asthma and hayfever. Supporting the immune system can be valuable in the treatment of allergic disorders.

Diet and immune function

The strength of the immune system is an important factor in the response to infection. Nutrition plays a vital role in the functioning of the immune system and a poor diet increases the susceptibility to infection and exacerbates autoimmune diseases. Even single nutrient deficiencies can compromise the immune system. Infections also increase the demand for nutrients to help fight infection and repair the damage to tissues.

As well as being good for general health, a low protein, high carbohydrate diet with plenty of fruits, vegetables, and fiber is beneficial for the immune system. An immune-boosting diet is also low in polyunsaturated vegetable oils and products made from them. These fats readily form free radicals that damage immune cells. High protein diets are damaging to the immune system as residues of protein metabolism can cause irritation, especially in people prone to allergy and autoimmunity. Milk protein is a common irritant of the immune system. Foods of animal origin, which tend to be high in protein, often contain residues of antibiotics and steroid hormones that can weaken immunity.

The effectiveness of the immune system declines with age and older people are often more susceptible to infection than younger people. In addition, the elderly are at greater risk of low intake of several vitamins and minerals known to influence the immune response. Recent studies have shown that supplementing the elderly with single nutrients or mixtures of vitamins and minerals at levels that exceed the RDAs significantly improves certain components of the immune response.

Vitamins, minerals and immunity

Vitamin and mineral supplementation can play an important role in the maintenance of normal immune function in the elderly. In a placebo-controlled

1994 study, researchers compared the effects of a vitamin and mineral supplement or placebo on immune responses of 56 people, aged from 59 to 85. Immune function was assessed by the use of the delayed hypersensitivity skin response test after six months and one year. The results showed that immune function was enhanced in the group receiving the supplements but not in the group receiving the placebo.[1] In another study, improved immune response was associated with decreased frequency of infectious diseases, indicating that nutrient-induced immunological improvement clinically enhances the health of elderly people.[2]

Antioxidants

Antioxidants are vital for maintaining optimal immune function as thcy act to prevent free radical damage to immune cells and to the thymus gland. This gland plays an important role in ensuring optimal immune function, via effects on white blood cells and other parts of the immune system.

Antioxidant vitamin concentrations are often lower in those with infections than in those who are healthy. Optimal amounts of antioxidants are necessary for maintenance of the immune response. This is particularly important in older people as age-associated decline of the immune response, particularly of T cell-mediated function, is well documented. The well-known age-related increase in free radical formation and lipid peroxidation contributes to this decline.

Recent clinical trials have found that antioxidant supplementation can significantly improve certain immune responses, including increasing the activation of cells involved in tumor immunity in the elderly. Supplementation with the antioxidant vitamins also protects immune responses in individuals exposed to certain environmental sources of free radicals.[3]

In a 1991 study, 30 elderly hospital patients were randomly allocated to receive either placebo or dietary supplementation with vitamins A, C and E for 28 days. Nutritional status and cell-mediated immune function were assessed before and after the period of supplementation. The results showed that, in those who had taken the supplements, cell-mediated immune function improved, whereas no significant changes were noted in the immune function of the placebo group.[4]

Vitamin A

Vitamin A is vital for the development of the body's barriers to infection and stimulates and enhances many immune functions, including antibody response and the activity of various white blood cells such as T helper cells and phagocytes. This immune-enhancing function promotes healing of infected tissues and increases resistance to infection. Episodes of acute infection may deplete body stores of vitamin A, possibly by increasing excretion, suggesting that vitamin A requirements may be higher during infection.

Death rates and susceptibility to infection and diarrhea are higher in children with vitamin A deficiency, particularly in developing countries. However, vitamin A deficiency may also contribute to susceptibility to infection in developed countries. A 1992 study involving 20 children with measles in Long Beach, California found that half of them were vitamin A-deficient.[5] Measles may increase the body's utilization of vitamin A, possibly because of the rapid destruction of epithelial surfaces.

Vitamin A deficiency is common in HIV-positive people and this may be due to metabolic changes associated with HIV infection. Vitamin A deficiency is often seen in HIV-positive pregnant women and severe deficiency increases infant mortality and the risk of mother-to-child transmission of HIV.

Vitamin A supplements have been used to enhance resistance to infection and to treat measles and respiratory infections, particularly in areas where vitamin A deficiency is widespread. A recent research review analyzing the results of several studies found that adequate vitamin A intake in children resulted in a 30 per cent decrease in deaths from all causes. Children in developing countries are often at high risk of vitamin A deficiency. In developed countries, ensuring adequate vitamin A intake is particularly important in those with life-threatening infections such as measles, and in those at risk of relative deficiency, such as premature infants.[6]

Beta carotene

Beta carotene has been shown to stimulate and enhance many immune system processes. It increases the numbers of immune cells such as B and T lymphocytes, and may enhance natural killer cell activity. T cells play a very important role in determining immune status and are produced by the thymus gland, which is particularly sensitive to free radical damage. Beta carotene protects macrophages, white blood cells which engulf and destroy foreign substances. It also facilitates communication between immune cells and makes the stimulatory action of interferon on the immune system more powerful.

In a 1997 double-blind, placebo-controlled study done in the UK, researchers tested the effects of daily doses of 15 mg of beta carotene in 25 healthy, adult male nonsmokers. Their findings showed improvement in function in various parts of the immune system, including white blood cells known as monocytes, which are involved in surveillance of tumors.[7]

Vitamin C

Vitamin C is critical to immune function as it is involved in antibody production and white blood cell function and activity. Other functions include the production of interferon, an antiviral and anticancer substance. Vitamin C requirements are raised when the immune system is under stress. In a study published in 1997, French researchers assessed vitamin C levels in 18 elderly patients in hospital. The patients were divided into three groups: those with acute infection, those who were malnourished, and a control group. Those with acute infection had considerably lower vitamin C levels than those in the other groups.[8]

A 1994 study tested vitamin C or placebo supplementation on 57 elderly patients admitted to hospital with acute respiratory infections (bronchitis and bronchopneumonia). The researchers found that patients supplemented with vitamin C showed significantly more improvement than those on placebo. This was particularly the case for those starting the trial most severely ill, many of whom had very low plasma and white cell vitamin C concentrations.[9]

Vitamin C has also been shown to help the immune system recover from exposure to toxic chemicals. In a 1997 study, researchers studied the effect of vitamin C on the function of several immune cells (natural killer, T and B cells) in patients who had been exposed to toxic chemicals. Fifty-five patients were given buffered vitamin C in water at a dosage of 60 mg per kg body weight (around 4g for the average man). Twenty-four hours later, the researchers tested immune cell function. The results showed that natural killer cell activity was enhanced up to ten-fold in 78 per cent of patients. B and T cell function was restored to normal.[10]

Vitamin C may reduce the duration of the common cold and also the severity of symptoms such as sneezing, coughing and sniffling. Its use as a cold treatment is controversial but it seems to have several effects, including reducing blood levels of histamine which can trigger tissue inflammation and a runny nose. It may also protect the immune cells and surrounding tissue from damaging oxidative reactions that occur when cells fight bacteria.[11]

Vitamin E

Vitamin E is essential for the maintenance of a healthy immune system as it protects the thymus gland and circulating white blood cells from damage. Vitamin E is particularly important in protecting the immune system from damage during times of oxidative stress and chronic viral illness.

Several studies have suggested that vitamin E supplements can help to boost immune function. A study reported in the *Journal of the American Medical Association* in 1997 provides more support for this. The study involved 88 healthy people, aged 65 or older. Those who took 200 mg (300 IU) each day for about four months showed an improvement in immune response. Researchers assessed the effects of either 60 mg (90 IU), 200 mg (300 IU) or 800 mg (1333) on a measure of immune system strength known as delayed hypersensitivity skin response. The results showed that those who took 200 mg a day had a 65 per cent increase in immune function. Those taking 60 mg or 800 mg of vitamin E also showed some improvements in immune function, but the ideal response was seen in those taking 200 mg. In other tests, those who took the supplements produced six times more antibodies to hepatitis B after being given the vaccine than those who took placebo. They also produced more antibodies against tetanus infection.[12]

Selenium

Selenium is important in maintaining resistance to disease. As part of the antioxidant enzyme, glutathione peroxidase, it may enhance immune function by protecting white blood cells from free radical damage. It also appears to increase antibody production, and accelerate the production of white blood cells and enhance their effectiveness in attacking and destroying harmful micro-organisms.

B vitamins

B vitamins are also essential for the functioning of a healthy immune system. Vitamin B6 plays a vital role in maintaining a healthy immune system by affecting functions such as cell multiplication and antibody production. Many different aspects of the immune system are affected by vitamin B6 deficiency including the quality and quantity of antibodies and the number of white blood cells.[13] Vitamin B6 supplementation may boost the immune system in older people, thus reducing the risk of infection and possibly cancer.

Vitamin B12 deficiency leads to reduced numbers of white blood cells which causes increased susceptibility to infection. Recent research has shown that elderly patients with low vitamin B12 levels have impaired antibody response to bacterial vaccine, even in those with no clinical signs of deficiency.[14]

Biotin deficiency also affects the functioning of the immune system. A recent animal study showed a decrease in white blood cell function with biotin deficiency.[15] Pantothenic acid is necessary for the synthesis of antibodies. It is also involved in wound-healing. Supplements have been used to boost immunity during viral infections[16] and to speed up wound-healing.

Vitamin D

Vitamin D is involved in the regulation of the immune system. It has several functions, including effects on white blood cells known as monocytes and lymphocytes, and seems to suppress some immune functions. Because of its effects on the immune system, many researchers are investigating the possibility of using vitamin D and related compounds to treat autoimmune disorders and to suppress rejection of transplanted organs.

Copper

Copper is important in developing resistance to infection. Copper deficiency can lead to reduced resistance to infection as white blood cell activity and cellular immune responses are reduced. The ratio of zinc to copper may also affect immune system effectiveness. Susceptibility to disease seems to increase when copper intake is high and zinc intake is low.

Iron

Iron is involved in the maintenance of a healthy immune system and the immune response can be impaired in iron-deficient people. Chronic yeast infections and herpes infections may be more common in people who are iron-deficient. Certain types of immune cells rely on iron to generate the oxidative reactions that allow these cells to kill off bacteria and other pathogens. When iron levels are low, these cells cannot function properly.

However, iron is an important nutrient for bacteria and in conditions where iron levels in the tissues are too high, such as the iron overload disorder hemochromatosis, defense against bacterial infections may be impaired. Excess iron can also generate free radicals which can damage the immune system.

Zinc

Zinc is considered one of the most important nutrients for the immune system as it is necessary for healthy antibody, white blood cell, thymus gland and hormone function. It is therefore vital in maintaining resistance to infection and in wound-healing.

Immune function is affected by zinc deficiency, which results in a decrease in the numbers of several types of T cells, natural killer cells and other components of the immune response. This leads to increased susceptibility to infection and wound-healing time.

Zinc supplementation improves immune function in those who are deficient. It increases the activity of the thymus gland, improves antibody responses and enhances the functioning of white blood cells. It has been shown to inhibit the growth of bacteria and possibly viruses. Zinc supplements have also been shown to boost levels of interferon, a protein which is formed when cells are exposed to viruses and which helps to fight infection.[17]

Researchers at the University of Medicine and Dentistry of New Jersey, Newark tested the effects of one year of supplementation with zinc and other micronutrients on cellular immunity in elderly people. The patients, aged 60-89, were either given a placebo, 15 mg of zinc, or 100 mg of zinc daily for 12 months. The results showed improvements in some aspects of immunity.[18] In another double-blind, randomized, controlled trial, published in 1998, researchers tested the effects of vitamin A and zinc (25 mg as zinc sulfate) supplements in 136 residents of a public home for older people in Rome. The results showed that zinc supplementation improved cell-mediated immune response.[19]

Many studies show beneficial effects of zinc in the treatment of diarrhea, a major cause of death in children in developing countries. Researchers involved in a double-blind trial carried out in India involving almost 600 children aged 6-35 months found that zinc supplements reduced diarrhea outbreaks.[20] However, long-term use of zinc in doses above 150 mg have been reported to cause the suppression of immune function.

Other nutrients

Coenzyme Q10

Coenzyme Q10 supplements have also been shown to improve immune function.[21]

Essential fatty acids

Essential fatty acid deficiency may adversely affect immune function and supplements may be useful in promoting optimum function. Studies on the immune T cells in cancer patients taking fish oil capsules suggest that omega-3 fatty acids bring about beneficial changes. Essential fatty acids are also used to treat autoimmune disorders.(See page 329 for more information.)

Herbal medicine and immunity

There are several herbs which have powerful immune-enhancing effects. These include echinacea (*Echinacea angustifolia and E. purpurea*), astragalus (*Astragalus membranaceus*), goldenseal (*Hydrastis canadensis*), licorice (*Glycyrrhiza glabra*), ginseng (*Panax ginseng* and *Eleutherococcus senticosus*), garlic (*Allium sativum*) and cat's claw (*Pau d'Arco*). Mushrooms such as shiitake, reishi and maitake also help to enhance immune system function. See page 384 for more information on these herbs and the precautions that may be necessary.

Improving digestion

Poor digestion plays a role in many common diseases, either by directly contributing to symptoms or by exacerbating those due to other causes. The digestive system needs to be working well to absorb the nutrients in food and to avoid the absorption of food molecules that are not properly broken down. Natural levels of stomach acid and digestive enzymes decrease with age. Food excesses, chemical use, and stress also contribute to the wear and tear on the digestive system. Improving digestion can help alleviate many disease conditions and promote optimum health.

Digestion

In order to be used by the body, food must be broken down into molecules small enough to cross the cell membranes of the gut. This process is known as digestion. These small molcecules are then absorbed into the blood and lymph.

Digestion takes place in the gastrointestinal tract, a continuous tube that extends from the mouth to the anus. The gastrointestinal tract is made up of the mouth, pharynx, esophagus, stomach, small intestine (divided into the duodenum, jejunum and ileum) and large intestine (divided into the cecum, colon and rectum). The teeth, tongue, salivary glands, liver, gallbladder and pancreas also play a part in digestion.

Muscular contractions in the wall of the gastrointestinal tract help to break down food by churning it and mixing it with the various fluids that are secreted into the gut. Digestive organs and the cells that line the tract secrete enzymes that help to break the food down chemically. Peristaltic or wave-like contractions help to propel food through the gut.

Most digestion and absorption takes place in the small intestine. Carbohydrates are mostly digested by pancreatic enzymes secreted into the small intestine. They are absorbed as single sugars, such as glucose and galactose. Protein digestion starts in the stomach and is continued by pancreatic enzymes. Proteins are absorbed as amino acids. Most fat digestion takes place in the small intestine, although some occurs in the stomach. Bile, which is secreted by the liver, and pancreatic enzymes are necessary for this process. Fats are absorbed as monoglycerides and fatty acids.

Fat soluble vitamins A, D, E and K are absorbed along with fats. Most water soluble vitamins are absorbed by diffusion. Vitamin B12 is the exception, and requires a substance known as intrinsic factor for its absorption. Some vitamins are manufactured by bacteria that live in the large intestine.

Supplements and herbs

Eating food slowly and chewing thoroughly are very important in helping to break down food properly before it enters the stomach. People who feel heavy or bloated after meals may benefit from taking digestive enzymes such as bromelain or papain. These enzymes can help to break down protein and fat in the stomach and small intestine.

Stomach acid production usually decreases with age and many people suffer symptoms such as gas, bloating and discomfort after rich meals. Betaine hydrochloride can be used in cases where stomach acid production is insufficient. (See page 381 for more information.) Drinking a small glass of apple cider vinegar before a meal may also be useful.

Probiotics are bacteria that help to maintain a healthy balance of micro-organisms in the gut. They may be useful in those with antibiotic-induced diarrhea, yeast infections and urinary tract infections. They may also help to protect against colon cancer and the adverse effects of chemotherapy and radiotherapy. Some evidence suggests that probiotics may help to treat allergies and skin conditions, reduce high cholesterol, and improve immunity.

Flatulence is a common digestive problem. It can be a symptom of disease or may be related to an inappropriate diet and it is important to identify the cause. There are several herbal remedies that can help to ease the problem. These include sage (*Salvia officinalis*), peppermint (*Mentha piperita*), chamomile (*Matricaria recutita*), hops (*Humulus lupulus*), fennel (*Foeniculum vulgare*) and valerian (*Valeriana officinalis*).

The liver

The liver is the most important metabolic organ in the body and has fundamental effects on health and vitality. Reducing stress on the liver and helping it to heal promotes health and can help to alleviate the symptoms of many disorders. Eating a very low protein, low fat diet; avoiding alcohol, tobacco, drugs and exposure to chemical fumes; drinking plenty of water; and getting plenty of rest can help to take the load off the liver.

After the skin, the liver is the second largest organ in the body. The average adult liver weighs around 1.3 kg. Functions of the liver include:

Carbohydrate metabolism

The liver is especially important in maintaining a normal blood glucose level. When blood glucose is low, the liver breaks down glycogen to glucose and releases glucose into the bloodstream. The liver can also convert other sugars, amino acids and lactic acid to glucose. When the blood glucose level is high, just after a meal, the liver converts glucose to glycogen and to triglycerides for storage.

Fat metabolism

The liver stores some triglycerides, breaks down fatty acids, and converts the breakdown products into ketone bodies. It makes lipoproteins, which are molecules that transport fatty acids, triglycerides and cholesterol to and from body cells. The liver also makes cholesterol and uses it to make bile salts.

Protein metabolism

The liver plays a role in protein synthesis. It also converts amino acids into fats and carbohydrates and converts the ammonia which results from this process into urea which is excreted in the urine.

Detoxification

The liver detoxifies substances such as alcohol and drugs. It can also alter or excrete some hormones.

Other functions

Other functions include excretion of bilirubin, a compound derived from the haem of worn out blood cells; the synthesis of bile salts; storage of vitamins and minerals; and activation of vitamin D.

Supplements and herbs

There are several supplements and herbal remedies that may be useful in improving liver function. Antioxidants help to protect the liver from free radical damage; and carnitine, choline and inositol may help to prevent the accumulation of fat in the liver. Beneficial herbs include a group of plants known as bitters, which stimulate the flow of digestive juices from the glands of mouth, stomach, pancreas and small intestine. Bitters also stimulate liver activity, increasing both bile production and release from the gallbladder. They may also stimulate insulin secretion by the pancreas, and muscle activity in the gut. They help the gut wall repair damage by stimulating repair mechanisms. Bitter herbs include dandelion (*Taraxacum officinale*), gentian (*Gentiana lutea*), goldenseal (*Hydrastis canadensis*), milk thistle (*Silybum marianum*), chamomile (*Matricaria recutita*) and yarrow (*Achillea millefolium*). See page 384 for more information on these herbs and the precautions that may be necessary.

Having a baby is one of the most nutritionally demanding events in a woman's life. Many things influence the success of a pregnancy and every choice a woman makes, from caffeine consumption to vitamin supplements, directly affects the health of her baby. Optimal nutrition is essential as soon as a woman starts thinking about getting pregnant; and avoiding cigarettes, alcohol and drugs is as important as eating a healthy diet.

Nutrition and pregnancy

Women who avoid known risks and eat well before, during and immediately after pregnancy tend to have larger, healthier babies and experience fewer complications. The quality and quantity of a woman's diet plays a vital role in beginning and maintaining the growth and development of her baby, in successful breastfeeding and in a smooth recovery after birth. Poor nutrition can result in low birth weight babies who may have impaired intelligence and a greater risk of disease both earlier and later in life.

Food requirements during pregnancy are similar to those which can be met by eating a normal well-balanced diet that contains a variety of nutrient-dense foods. However, some individual nutrient needs are higher and a pregnant woman should make sure to include plenty of foods high in these particular vitamins and minerals in her diet. All the vitamins and minerals are essential for development of a healthy baby; but getting adequate intakes of calcium, iron, folic acid, phosphorus, magnesium, vitamin B6 and zinc is particularly important. Many women do not consume adequate amounts of these nutrients in their daily diets.

Some nutrients that a baby needs come from limited stores in bones and tissues stockpiled before conception, but most come directly from the mother's diet. Calorie needs increase by about 15 per cent, but the need for some nutrients may double. Eating nutrient-dense foods is vitally important for a woman to get enough vitamins and minerals without putting on too much weight.

Pregnancy is a time of great change in a woman's body. Changes include the growth of placental tissues; the increase in blood volume; increase in cardiac output; accumulation of body water; changes in levels of estrogen, progesterone and other hormones; preparation of breast tissues for lactation; and changes in lung, kidney, reproductive and urinary systems.

Pregnancy and weight gain

Pregnancy is not the time to try and lose weight. In total, it can take as many as 80 000 calories, in addition to those necessary for daily needs, to ensure the development of a healthy baby. After the first three months, most pregnant women need an additional 300 calories per day over and above their pre-pregnancy needs. If a woman does not consume enough calories, her body will use protein for energy instead of cell building.

The amount of weight a woman gains varies with age, height, weight, plans to breastfeed, and the number of babies she is carrying. For a woman of average height and weight, the suggested weight gain is 25 to 35 pounds (11 to 15 kg) or for a woman with twins 35 to 45 pounds (16 to 20 kg). An underweight woman might gain 28 to 40 pounds (13 to 18 kg) and an overweight woman 15 to 25 pounds (7 to 11 kg).

Aside from the weight increase due to the fetus, placenta and amniotic fluid, enlarged uterine and breast tissue, blood volume increases by about 50 per cent and accounts for 4 pounds (2 kg) of weight gain. Pregnant women also accumulate fluid, protein and fat stores, the amount of which varies between women. In the first three months, most women gain only 2 to 4 pounds (1 to 2 kg). After that, the average weight gain is nearly 1 pound (0.5 kg) per week. Exercise such as swimming or gentle yoga can be beneficial for pregnant women, and extra calories may be needed to offset the calorie expenditure through exercise.

Women who gain too much weight during pregnancy do not necessarily have bigger babies. The excess weight is in the form of fat which a woman may find more difficult to lose after the baby is born. Recent studies have shown that maternal obesity may increase the risk of neural tube defects such as spina bifida. A Body Mass Index of 29 or greater nearly doubles the risk of such birth defects. Seriously overweight women may consider losing some weight before trying to get pregnant. After the baby is born most women lose 12 to 14 pounds (5 to 7 kg). With good nutrition and normal activity, the extra weight can be lost within three months to a year.

Pregnancy and alcohol

Most experts advise pregnant women and those who are trying to get pregnant not to drink alcohol. Alcohol is harmful to the baby and impairs absorption, metabolism and utilization of essential vitamins and minerals. Around half of all women have the occasional drink when they are pregnant. Recent research has confirmed that women who drink alcohol before pregnancy but abstain in early pregnancy have babies no smaller than those who never drink alcohol. Women who do drink alcohol in early pregnancy have babies who weigh on average 6 ounces (150 g) less than babies born to those who don't drink. Chronic alcohol use during pregnancy leads to fetal alcohol syndrome, a disorder in which babies are severely damaged.

Pregnancy and essential nutrients

A pregnant woman's diet should consist of fruit, vegetables, grain products, milk and milk products, and protein foods such as legumes, lean meat and fish. Foods which are high in fat and sugar are not usually high in essential nutrients and should only be eaten in small amounts. Caffeine-containing drinks should be limited to one to two cups a day and artificial sweeteners should be avoided as they can contribute to nutrient deficiencies and may have adverse effects on the baby.

A pregnant woman should aim to eat:

- Three to four servings of dairy products a day, such as low fat milk, cheese, yogurt, cottage cheese, hot chocolate made with milk, cheese-topped pizza.
- Four or five servings of cereal grains, such as bread, bagels, muffins, crackers, cereal, rice, spaghetti or noodles.
- One to two servings of meat or protein foods, such as very lean red meat, poultry, fish and eggs.
- One to two servings of cooked dried beans and peas.
- Four to six servings of fruit and vegetables including at least two servings of dark leafy greens and red, yellow or orange vegetables. Two servings should be of vitaminC-rich foods such as an orange, broccoli, grapefruit and tomatoes.

Drinking six to eight glasses of water a day should provide adequate fluid and help prevent constipation, a common problem in pregnancy. Consuming plenty of fiber-rich foods is also helpful for this.

Pregnancy and protein

Protein is vitally important for the growth and development of the baby's tissues, the placenta, the amniotic fluid and the increase in the mother's blood volume. US recommendations are that pregnant women consume at least 60 g of protein daily, and in Australia experts recommend 51 g. The extra protein requirements of pregnancy can easily be obtained by eating an extra serving of lean meat, fish or legumes and drinking an extra glass of milk. However, some experts believe that intakes of dairy products should not increase dramatically as excessive amounts may cause allergies in the baby. If you do not consume dairy products, make sure you include other good sources of calcium in your diet. These include dark leafy greens and tofu. Making sure calorie intake is high enough ensures that protein is used for tissue synthesis rather than for meeting energy needs.

Experts recommend that a pregnant woman should eat two to four servings a day of protein-rich foods such as lean meat, fish, eggs, beans and tofu. One serving is 3° ounces or 100 g. Most people eating Western diets routinely eat more protein than they need so most pregnant women may not have to consciously increase the amount of protein they eat. Some vegetarians and particularly vegans may be the exception to this, and may need to discuss their needs with a dietitian.

Vitamins, minerals and pregnancy

Optimal intake of all vitamins and minerals is essential for a healthy pregnancy. However, requirements for some of these increase considerably and supplements can be very useful in ensuring optimal intake.

Vitamin A

Adequate vitamin A is essential for a baby to develop normally as it plays a vital role in cell development and differentiation, ensuring that the changes which occur in the cells and tissues during fetal development take place normally. Vitamin A may also be involved in cell to cell communication, and deficiency can lead to birth defects. However, the recommended intake of vitamin A during pregnancy does not increase from pre-pregnancy needs, and women who are pregnant or trying to become pregnant should not take large amounts of vitamin A. Daily intakes above 3000 mcg RE (10 000 IU) increase the risks of birth defects such as malformation of the face, head, heart and nervous system.

In a 1995 study, researchers examined the links between vitamin A from food and supplements in almost 23 000 pregnant women. Women who consumed more than 4500 mcg RE (15 000 IU) of preformed vitamin A per day from food and supplements were over three times more likely to have a baby with a birth defect than women who consumed 1500 mcg RE (5000 IU) or less per day. For vitamin A from supplements alone, women who consumed more than 3000 mcg RE (10 000 IU) per day had almost five times the risk of birth defects than women who consumed less than 1500 mcg RE (5000 IU) per day. The risk may be greatest during the first seven weeks of pregnancy.[1]

However, a 1997 study conducted by researchers at the National Institute of Child Health and Human Development did not find a link between vitamin A consumption and birth defects. Their results showed that even in women consuming doses of vitamin A between 2400 mcg RE (8000 IU) and 7500 mcg RE (25 000 IU) the risk of having a baby with a birth defect was no higher than in women taking low doses.[2]

Many manufacturers have reduced the amount of vitamin A in multivitamin supplements or replaced it with beta carotene, which does not pose the same risks. Doses equal to or less than the RDA are not believed to be harmful, but women should not combine supplements with large amounts of pre-formed vitamin A-rich foods such as liver. Vitamin A acne cream has been known to cause birth deformities and is now available only on prescription.

B vitamins

Requirements for thiamin, riboflavin and niacin increase slightly with the increase in calorie intake. Increasing intakes of folate, vitamin B6 and vitamin B12 is particularly important.

Vitamin B6

Vitamin B6 needs increase in pregnancy, and low levels are associated with reduced growth and development of a baby's nervous system.[3] Deficiency may also contribute to water retention, morning sickness, pre-eclampsia and birthing difficulties. It may also lead to diabetic and blood sugar problems in pregnancy.

Vitamin B6 supplements may be useful in treating nausea and vomiting during pregnancy. In a 72-hour study, researchers at the University of Iowa gave 25 mg of vitamin B6 every eight hours to 31 patients, while 28 patients received placebo. At the completion of therapy, only eight of 31 patients in the vitamin B6 group had any vomiting, compared with 15 of 28 patients in the placebo group.[4]

Folate

Optimal folate intake is essential for the development of a healthy baby. A B group vitamin, folate is essential for the processes of DNA synthesis, increased blood volume, cell division and the development of healthy tissues; all of which occur very rapidly during pregnancy. Adequate folate is essential for normal birth weight and nerve development in newborn babies.

Folate deficiency can lead to defects of the brain and spine which are known as neural tube defects. These include spina bifida (open spine) and anencephaly, in which a major part of the brain and skull fails to develop. Neural tube defects are the second leading cause of death from birth defects in the USA, and even mild folate deficiency increases the risk of low birth weight, poor growth and spontaneous abortion.

Making sure folate levels are adequate is vital for any woman who might become pregnant as the high risk period for birth defects is around one month before conception until around one month after. Many women are unaware that they are pregnant during this time. The risk of neural tube defects in the US is around one per 1000 pregnancies, and around 50 per cent of neural tube defects may be preventable by increasing folate intakes.

It is now recommended that a woman who is pregnant or who is planning to become pregnant should consume at least 600 mcg of folic acid per day, up from an RDA of 400 mcg for a nonpregnant women. This folic acid can be obtained from foods such as leafy green vegetables, asparagus, liver, whole grain foods and eggs, or from supplements. In an effort to boost folate intake and help to reduce the occurrence of neural tube defects, cereal products are now fortified with folic acid. However, most doctors recommend folic acid supplements to women who may become pregnant. In fact, it seems that the levels of folate necessary to prevent neural tube defects are more easily derived from fortified foods or supplements than from natural food sources alone. Many experts recommend folic acid supplements and a diet rich in folates for women who are hoping to become pregnant.

In a 1996 study, Irish researchers compared the effectiveness of supplements, fortified foods and nonfortified foods in raising folic acid levels. Sixty-two women were randomly assigned to one of the following five groups: 400 mcg per day of folic acid as a supplement; an additional 400 mcg per day from folic-acid-fortified foods; an additional 400 mcg per day from nonfortified foods; dietary advice, and a control group. The results showed that red blood cell folate concentrations increased significantly only in the groups taking folic acid supplements or food fortified with folic acid. The researchers concluded that advice to women to consume folate-rich foods as the only way to boost folate levels is misleading.[5]

A trial of the effects of vitamin supplements containing folate on the incidence of neural tube defects involving over 4700 women was carried out in Hungary. In the women who did not receive folic acid, there were six babies born with neural tube defects. In the group receiving the supplements, there were none.[6] In an editorial in the *New England Journal of Medicine,* Godfrey Oakley, MD of the Centers for Disease Control in Atlanta, commented that "anyone who chooses to counsel a woman to consume 400 mcg of food-derived folate rather than 400 mcg of supplemental folic acid will be recommending a strategy that has not been proved to prevent birth defects and that leads to lower blood folate concentrations."

Multiple pregnancies, long-term use of oral contraceptives, and anemia may increase folic acid requirements still further. Any woman who has had a baby with a neural tube defect should consult a doctor before trying to conceive as there may be a need for greater amounts of folic acid. Studies have shown that 4 mg of folic acid may reduce the recurrence of neural tube defects by more than 70 per cent in women who have had one baby with a neural tube defect. This extra amount is usually obtained by taking prescribed pure folic acid.

Some studies have shown that folic acid also protects against the most common form of congenital malformations, cleft lip and cleft palate. A recent US study found that it did not. Folic acid stores may take six months to return to normal levels after the birth of a baby.

Vitamin B12

Vitamin B12 requirements increase slightly in pregnant women as vitamin B12 works with folic acid in cell growth, and is essential to the normal development of the baby. Women who follow strict vegetarian or vegan diets may be at risk of deficiencies and should consult a dietitian. Deficiency may lead to infertility and stillbirth.

Vitamin C

Vitamin C recommended intakes increase in pregnancy from 60 mg to 70 mg per day in the US, and from 30 mg to 60 mg in Australia. Vitamin C has a vital role to play in tissue development, and also helps in the absorption of iron and the utilization of other essential minerals. Vitamin C levels may be low in women suffering from pre-eclampsia,[7] a disorder which occurs in one in every 20 pregnant women. Symptoms include high blood pressure, headache, protein in the urine, blurred vision and anxiety. It can lead to eclampsia, a seizure disorder which can cause complications with pregnancy and even death. As an antioxidant, vitamin C may help to prevent the oxidative damage to fats which may worsen high blood pressure.

Pregnant women are usually advised not to take very high doses of vitamin C during pregnancy as this may lead to rebound scurvy after birth in babies no longer receiving large doses of vitamin C.

Vitamin D

Vitamin D is essential for the developing baby and aids in bone and tooth development via its role in calcium absorption. Although the new US government recommendations for Adequate Intake of vitamin D do not increase during pregnancy, supplements may be useful. The Australian NHMRC recommends that pregnant women receive reasonable exposure to sunlight and obtain 400 IU of vitamin D per day. The level of vitamin D in breast milk directly reflects maternal intake, and a severe vitamin D deficiency may lead to rickets in a developing baby. Deficiency is more of a risk in colder climates where the mother has limited exposure to sunlight or avoids vitamin D-fortified milk and milk products. However, pregnant women should avoid large doses of vitamin D as they can be toxic for the developing infant.

Vitamin E

The daily requirement for vitamin E may increase from 8 mg alpha TE (12 IU) to 10 mg (15 IU) during pregnancy, although there is little research on the effects of marginal intakes. Lower vitamin E levels may contribute to high blood pressure and pre-eclampsia. Vitamin E deficiency causes a build-up of fats damaged by free radicals which can lead to constriction of blood vessels and therefore to high blood pressure.[8] Severe vitamin E deficiency in infants can lead to anemia.

Vitamin K

Vitamin K injections are commonly used to reduce the risk of internal bleeding in newborn babies. In the early 1990s, researchers reported a possible increase in the risk of childhood cancers in children who were given vitamin K injections after birth. Subsequent studies suggest that the risk cannot be totally ruled out, but if it exists it is likely to be small. (See page 177 for more information.)

Because of the possibility of an increased risk of cancer, researchers have investigated alternatives to injection. Some research suggests that oral supplements in three doses of 1 to 2 mg, the first given at the first feeding, the second at two to four weeks and the third at eight weeks may be an acceptable alternative.[9]

Calcium

Adequate calcium intake is vital for a baby to develop healthy bones and teeth. A full term baby accumulates about 30 g of calcium in bone mass. A pregnant woman's diet should include three to four calcium-rich foods per day, including low fat milk and milk products, and dark green leafy vegetables. Many women do not get enough calcium in their diets and a pregnant woman will most likely need to consciously increase her intake. Adequate calcium is especially important for pregnant women aged under 25 as their bones are still increasing in density.

A 1998 Australian study found that the lead which accumulates over a woman's lifetime in her bones leaches out into her blood during pregnancy and may pass to the baby, with potentially harmful effects.[10] This is most often seen in the last six months when the fetus draws calcium from the mother for bone development. High intakes of calcium or calcium supplementation may increase blood calcium levels. This reduces the amount of calcium, and therefore lead, which the baby draws from a mother's bones. It is important to avoid lead-containing calcium supplements such as dolomite.

Pregnant women whose diets are deficient in calcium are also at risk of muscle cramps. When calcium levels drop below normal there is an increase in the sensitivity of the nerves which may cause muscles to go into spasm.

The effects of a mother's high calcium diet during pregnancy may also be passed on to her children who will be less likely to suffer from high blood pressure in the future. The results of a 1997 study suggest that women who take calcium supplements in pregnancy have children with lower blood pressures. Researchers measured the blood pressures of almost 600 children of women who had previously been involved in a double-blind trial of the effects of calcium on blood pressure during pregnancy. The results showed that, overall, systolic blood pressure was lower in the calcium group, particularly among overweight children.[11]

The new US RDAs for pregnant and breastfeeding women are no longer greater than those for nonpregnant women. This is partly based on recent studies which suggest that the ability to absorb and retain calcium improves during pregnancy and these changes are enough to meet the extra demands placed on a woman's body by her baby. In a study published in 1998, researchers studied calcium metabolism in 14 pregnant women from before conception to five months after their periods restarted. When the women were pregnant, the increased calcium needs were met by improved absorption; and then during the early breastfeeding period, calcium excretion decreased. Some calcium was drawn from bone but this was recovered after menstruation restarted, although not to pre-pregnancy levels.[12]

In studies done in 1997, researchers tested the effect of 1000 mg of calcium per day on bone density during pregnancy. They took measurements at enrollment and after three and six months. The results showed no effect of either lactation or calcium supplementation on bone density in the forearm, and also no effect of calcium supplementation on the calcium concentration in breast milk.[13] However, the women involved in this study were all consuming adequate levels of calcium, and it is possible that women whose calcium intake is lower than 1300 mg per day may benefit from extra calcium or supplements.

Pre-eclampsia

Calcium supplements have been used to lower a woman's risk of pre-eclampsia as there is some evidence that abnormalities in calcium metabolism are involved in the disorder. Many pregnant women do not consume enough calcium to ensure optimal blood pressure regulation, and the results of several clinical trials have suggested that calcium supplements reduce the incidence of pre-eclampsia.[14] A 1996 analysis of clinical trials which looked at the effects of calcium intake on pre-eclampsia and pregnancy outcomes in 2500 women found that those who consumed 1500 to 2000 mg of calcium supplements per day were 70 per cent less likely to suffer from high blood pressure in pregnancy.[15]

However, the largest study done to date suggests that supplements do not prevent pre-eclampsia. The study, which was published in 1997 in the *New England Journal of Medicine*, involved 4589 healthy, first-time mothers. Half of the subjects received 2000 mg of calcium per day and the other half received a placebo. The researchers then assessed the incidence of high blood pressure and protein excretion in the urine. No significant differences in the groups were found. Supplements did not reduce other complications associated with childbirth or increase the incidence of kidney stones.[16] The results of this study still leave open the possibility that calcium supplements may be useful as the women included in the study were already consuming higher than average levels of calcium than is typical even before they took the supplements. Women at high risk of pre-eclampsia were also not included in the investigation.

In a 1995 study, researchers assessed the effect of calcium supplementation and drinking milk on pre-eclampsia in over 9000 pregnant women. Results showed that women who drank two glasses of milk per day had the lowest risk. The risk for those drinking one glass of milk per day was similarly low but the risk for those drinking less than one glass of milk per day was substantially higher. Women drinking three or more glasses of milk per day also showed increased risk, as did those drinking four or more glasses per day.[17]

Fluoride

Children whose mothers have diets sufficiently high in fluoride during pregnancy seem to have fewer cavities than children whose diets are lacking in fluoride. A baby's first teeth start forming in the first few months of pregnancy and the adult teeth in the last few months. Fluoride affects the strength and susceptibility to decay of these teeth. Excessive fluoride, however, may produce mottled teeth.

Iron

Iron requirements increase in pregnancy due to the increase in the mother's blood volume and the demands of the developing baby. In pregnancy, the mother transfers 500 to 1000 mg of iron to her growing baby, mostly during the last few months. The number of red blood cells in the mother's blood increases by 20 to 30 per cent. This increased demand can lead to iron deficiency if dietary intake does not increase substantially to meet it. A pregnant woman with an iron deficiency is more prone to infection after delivery, spontaneous abortion and premature delivery. Iron deficiency also increases the risk of low birth weight babies, stillbirth and infant death. Infants born of anemic mothers may also be at risk of anemia.

Recommended iron intakes for pregnant women increase from 15 mg to 30 mg per day in the USA, and from 16 mg to 36 mg in Australia. Most women cannot obtain enough iron from dietary sources alone, and the US National Academy of Sciences recommends that pregnant women take a supplement containing 30 mg of iron daily during the last six months of pregnancy. Supplements are particularly important for women with low iron stores. During the later stages of pregnancy, the ability of the body to absorb iron increases.

Good sources or iron include liver, red meats, dried fruits and leafy green vegetables. Vegetarians and vegans need to pay particular attention to their iron intakes as the iron from plant sources may not be as well-absorbed as that from meat.

Iron supplements can cause constipation or nausea which can be reduced by taking the supplements in several small doses with meals and by drinking plenty of water; at least six to eight glasses daily. Iron supplements may adversely affect zinc status, and pregnant women who are taking iron supplements should include zinc-rich foods in their diets.

Magnesium

Magnesium requirements increase in pregnancy as magnesium is involved in many essential bodily functions. Marginal magnesium deficiency is considered to be very common, (15 to 20 per cent of the population) and as physical and emotional stress also increases requirements, pregnant women may be particularly at risk.

Magnesium sulfate is routinely used in the USA to prevent convulsions in pre-eclampsia and to break down toxins in pre-term labor. A 1996 research review of trials of magnesium sulfate in the treatment of eclampsia and pre-eclampsia analyzed data from nine randomized trials involving 1743 women with eclampsia and 2390 with pre-eclampsia. The analysis showed that magnesium sulfate is effective in preventing the recurrence of seizures in eclampsia and in preventing them in pre-eclampsia.[18]

Researchers involved in a 1996 study reported in the *Journal of the American Medical Association*, found that administration of magnesium sulfate to women before delivery reduced the risk of cerebral palsy in very low birth weight babies.[19]

A recent Swedish study showed that magnesium may help reduce the pain and discomfort of night-time leg cramps suffered by up to one-third of pregnant women. The cramps may be caused by magnesium deficiency, and pregnant women tend to have lower blood magnesium levels than nonpregnant women.[20]

Sodium

Pregnant women may need to consume 2 to 3 g per day of sodium. This amount is best obtained from a varied diet of wholesome, minimally processed foods with no salt added during cooking. Dietary sodium restriction is used to control pregnancy-related high blood pressure. It does not seem to lead to any adverse effects on other minerals or the baby.

Zinc

Recommended zinc intakes increase from 12 mg to 15 mg in the USA and from 12 mg to 16 mg in Australia. Adequate zinc is necessary for normal growth, birth weight and completion of full term pregnancy.

Zinc deficiency in early pregnancy can lead to congenital birth defects, low birth weight, spontaneous abortion, premature delivery, mental retardation and behavior problems. Maternal zinc status may also be associated with ease of pregnancy and delivery. Reduced zinc intake in the mother can also lead to children at greater risk of infection due to suppressed immunity.

Many pregnant women do not consume enough dietary zinc and may need supplementation, but should be aware that excessive use of supplements during pregnancy may be harmful for the fetus. Zinc supplementation has been shown to improve birth weight and head circumference. In a 1995 study, researchers at the University of Alabama at Birmingham conducted a trial involving 580 African-American pregnant women with low blood plasma zinc levels. The women were either given 25 mg of zinc or a placebo. The results showed that in all the women, infants in the zinc supplement group had a significantly greater birth weight and head circumference than infants in the placebo group.[21]

Pregnancy and supplements

The US National Academy of Sciences recommends supplements for those women who are vegetarians, smoke cigarettes, drink alcohol or who are carrying twins. Supplementation should begin in the last six months and should be at the following levels:

Iron	30 mg
Vitamin C	10 mg
Zinc	15 mg
Folic acid	400 mcg
Copper	2 mg
Vitamin B6	2 mg
Calcium	250 mcg
Vitamin D	5 mcg

Morning sickness

Morning sickness is common in the first three months of pregnancy. Eating crackers or dry cereal in bed 10 to 15 minutes before getting up, avoiding high fat or fried foods, and drinking liquids in between meals instead of with them, may be successful in alleviating sickness in some cases. Vitamin B6 may also be helpful, (See page 93 for more information.) and many women report successful results with ginger preparations.

Pregnancy and vegetarians

Vegetarian diets are healthy for pregnant women as long as they contain a variety of foods with enough calories and nutrients to meet the extra needs of pregnancy.

As well as consuming sufficient iron and calcium-rich foods, vegetarians must make sure to obtain adequate vitamin B12 from fortified breakfast cereals, soy milk or a B12 supplement. Vegans may need additional vitamin D supplements (10 mcg per day) and vitamin B12 (2 mcg per day). Vegan women who wish to breastfeed may consider taking calcium supplements if they cannot obtain enough calcium from vegetables and nuts.

Breastfeeding

Under normal circumstances, breastfeeding a baby is an important part of pregnancy. Breast milk contains the correct balance of nutrients and also leads to fewer illnesses in the first year of life. It enhances immune function and also offers protection from allergies; although these may develop when a breastfeeding mother's diet is high in cow's milk. Breastfeeding can also help a woman return to her pre-pregnancy weight; and oxytocin, a hormone released during breastfeeding, can help the uterus back to normal size and health.

Calorie requirements may be even greater while breastfeeding than during pregnancy and the mother's diet can affect the quality and quantity of breast milk. A well-balanced diet during breastfeeding is similar to that advisable during pregnancy. Water is the main constituent of mother's milk so an adequate fluid intake is essential. This should be at least eight glasses of water per day. A breastfeeding woman's diet should be high in milk and milk products, protein, whole grains, fruit and vegetables. Caffeine, cigarettes, alcohol and drugs should be avoided.

Vitamin A

The RDA for vitamin A for women who are breastfeeding increases from 800 mcg RE to 1300 mcg RE. This can be met by increasing the intake of beta carotene-rich foods.

Vitamin K

Babies who are formula-fed tend to have a lower risk of hemorrhage than those who are breastfed, as vitamin K levels are higher in formula. Maternal vitamin K supplements may help to reduce the risk of vitamin K deficiency in breastfeeding newborn babies. In a study published in 1997, researchers gave daily doses of 5 mg vitamin K to mothers. This increased the vitamin K content of breast milk to levels comparable with that in infant formula.[22]

Calcium

Recommended calcium intakes for breastfeeding women are no longer greater than those for women who are not breastfeeding. This is partly based on recent studies which suggest that changes in calcium metabolism and absorption during pregnancy and breastfeeding are enough to meet the extra demands placed on a woman's body by her baby. A 1998 British study suggests that bone mineral density changes seen during breastfeeding seems to be unrelated to dietary calcium intake.[23]

Iron

Iron is also very important for women who are breastfeeding, especially if they are recovering from blood loss during delivery or depletion of body stores during pregnancy. Breastfeeding causes needs to increase by around 0.5 to 1 mg per day.

Other vitamins and minerals

Other vitamins and minerals which are required in higher amounts by breastfeeding women include vitamin C, vitamin E, some B vitamins, magnesium, zinc and selenium.

Vegetarians

Vegetarian diets have increased greatly in popularity in the last 20 years, with a growing number of studies linking eating meat to a greater risk of heart disease and other degenerative disorders. A balanced vegetarian diet supplies all the vitamins and minerals the body requires and is usually higher in fiber and lower in fat, cholesterol, protein and sugar than the typical Western diet.

Vegetarian diet and disease

Many medical studies have shown that a low fat vegetarian diet can lessen the risks of developing cardiovascular disease, diabetes, osteoporosis, kidney stones and other common diseases. Vegetarians usually have lower cholesterol and blood pressure than people who eat meat. Low fat, high fiber diets that include a variety of fruits, vegetables, whole grains and beans also help to prevent cancer.

The results of a 17-year study involving 11 000 vegetarians were published in the *British Medical Journal* in 1996. Researchers investigated the links between dietary habits and disease in vegetarians and health conscious people. The results showed that overall, the mortality rate in this group was around half that of the general population, and that daily consumption of fresh fruit was associated with a lower risk of death from any disease.[1]

The vegetarian diet

Vegetarians choose their diets for reasons of culture, belief or health. There is no single vegetarian eating pattern, and diets differ in the extent to which they avoid animal products. Vegans completely exclude meat, fish, poultry, eggs and dairy products. Lacto-vegetarians avoid meat, fish, poultry and eggs. Lacto-ovo vegetarians avoid meat, fish and poultry.

The more restricted the diet, the more care must be taken to ensure that all nutrient needs are met. A vegetarian diet does exclude rich sources of several nutrients such as iron, zinc and vitamin B12, and it is important to include plenty of alternative plant sources of the vitamins and minerals commonly found in meat, fish and eggs. Milk is a good source of calcium and riboflavin, and may supply as much as half the daily needs. Other sources, such as dark green leafy vegetables, must be eaten in quite large quantities in order to meet these needs.

A balanced diet for a lacto-ovo vegetarian might include all of the following foods in a day:

- two to three servings of low fat milk or milk products.
- three to four servings of protein-rich cooked dried beans and peas, seeds or nuts.
- at least five servings of fruits and vegetables.
- at least six servings of whole grain breads and cereals.

Protein

Proteins are made up of 20 main naturally-occurring amino acids and some other minor ones. Some of these amino acids are essential constituents of the diet as they cannot be made in the body, whereas others are nonessential. Meat, fish, eggs, milk and soybeans contain all the essential amino acids and are known as complete proteins. Grains, beans, peas, nuts and seeds contain some amino acids and not others, and are called incomplete proteins. Two incomplete protein foods, eaten together, can provide a complete protein, for example, baked beans on toast or lentils and rice.

A varied vegetarian diet provides adequate amounts of amino acids and usually meets or exceeds requirements for dietary protein. A typical Western diet is probably too high in protein, and vegetarians often eat less protein than meat eaters. This may partly explain their reduced risk of many degenerative diseases as high protein intakes promote excretion of essential minerals.

Fats

Vegetarians often have a higher intake of omega-6 polyunsaturated fats from nuts, seeds and vegetable oils. A high intake of these fats has been linked to an increased risk of cancer, particularly when the omega-6 to omega-3 fatty acid ratio becomes too high. (See page 329 for more information.) Those who avoid fish may not get adequate amounts of omega-3 oils in their diets and should make sure to include plant sources of omega- 3 oils such as flaxseed oil in the diet. Population studies have shown that, compared to vegetarians, those who eat fish tend to have lower blood pressures and lower blood fat levels.[2]

Vegetarians and vitamins

Riboflavin

Riboflavin may be low in vegan diets as the main sources are milk and milk products. Other sources include fortified breakfast cereals, yeast extract and mushrooms. Someone who eats no milk or meat can meet the RDA for riboflavin by including all of the following in a daily diet: three slices of whole meal bread, a cup of almonds, half an avocado and average servings of spinach, broccoli and mushrooms.

Vitamin B12

Animal foods are the only reliable sources of vitamin B12. Vegetarians who eat dairy products generally obtain adequate vitamin B12 from these sources. Vegans tend to have lower vitamin B12 intakes which may not reach recommended levels, and should make sure they include vitamin B12-fortified foods or supplements in their diets. This is particularly important for women who are, or who plan to become, pregnant.

Sea vegetables and fermented soybean products such as miso also contain forms of vitamin B12, although some research suggests that the human body may not be able to absorb these forms and they may even block true vitamin B12 absorption.[3] Many vegetarian and vegan products are fortified with vitamin B12, including yeast extract, vegetable stock and soya milk. In developing countries, food may contain bacteria and other micro-organisms which are a source of vitamin B12. In Western countries better hygiene and food processing removes these sources of vitamin B12.

Vitamin D

Vitamin D is present in vegetarian diets in dairy products. Vegans tend to have low vitamin D intakes, fortified margarine being the major dietary source. In most countries, sufficient vitamin D can be obtained through manufacture in the skin in response to sunlight. Vegans who do not get enough exposure to sunlight may be advised to take a vitamin D supplement; although pregnant women should not take large amounts as there is an increased risk of fetal deformities.

Vitamin E

Vitamin E needs increase in those whose diets are higher in polyunsaturated fats from nuts, seeds and vegetable oils. As vegetarians often have a higher intake of such fats, they need to make sure their vitamin E intake is adequate to protect against harmful free radical damage to these fats. (See page 417 for more information.)

Vegetarians and minerals

Refining removes most of the vitamin and mineral content from grains. For example, flour refining causes a 77 per cent loss in zinc; rice refining causes a loss of 83 per cent; and processing cereals from whole grains causes an 80 per cent loss. It is particularly important for vegetarians who avoid animal sources of minerals like zinc and iron to ensure their intake of whole grains is adequate.

Iron

Both vegetarians and nonvegetarians often have difficulty in meeting RDA for iron, but this is particularly the case in premenopausal vegetarian women. Iron is present in animal foods in organic 'heme' form and in plant foods in inorganic 'nonheme' form. The heme and nonheme forms of iron are absorbed by different mechanisms.[4] About 20 to 30 per cent of heme iron is absorbed, compared with only around 2 to 5 per cent of nonheme iron. Vitamin C consumed in the same meal as nonheme iron improves absorption by up to 50 per cent as it helps to convert dietary iron to a soluble form and also helps counteract the reduction in absorption that occurs in the presence of phytates. Vitamin A and beta carotene can also improve nonheme iron absorption.[5] Tea reduces the absorbability of iron and should be drunk between meals rather than with them.

A premenopausal woman can meet the RDA for iron by including all the following in a daily diet: ten dried apricots; three slices of whole wheat bread; one cup of lentils; and one cup each of cooked spinach, broccoli and green beans.

Iron levels in the body are controlled by absorption. When intakes in the diet are lowered, absorption ability can improve. Some research suggests that this gradually happens in vegetarians. In cases of iron deficiency absorption efficiency increases from around 5 to 10 per cent to about 10 to 20 per cent.

Zinc

Some vegetarians have lower than recommended zinc intakes as they avoid meat and seafood, which are good sources. Phytates also reduce zinc absorption. Vegetarians need to make sure that they include enough zinc-rich pulses, seeds and whole grains in their diets.

The RDA for zinc can be obtained by including all of the following in a daily diet: three slices of wholemeal bread, one cup of cooked chickpeas, a handful of pumpkin seeds, a serving of muesli, two tablespoons of wheatgerm, half a cup of almonds, a serving of peas and one ounce of peanut butter.

Calcium

Although vegans do not eat dairy products – which are the main sources of calcium – with careful planning, it is possible to get enough calcium from plant foods. Vegans may need slightly less calcium than meat eaters as they appear to have better absorption and lower excretion. However, studies of women who have followed vegan diets for long periods indicate that they may be at higher risk of osteoporosis and may benefit from calcium supplements.[6]

Leafy green vegetables, seaweed and tofu made with calcium sulfate are good vegetarian sources of calcium. The amount of calcium in tofu varies from brand to brand, and it is worth comparing quantities between different brands.

The RDA for calcium can be obtained by including all of the following in the daily diet: four ounces of firm tofu processed with calcium sulfate, a cup of cooked spinach, two oranges, a cup of broccoli, four slices of whole wheat bread and a cup of almonds. It can be difficult for vegan children to get enough calcium in their diets as they have to eat relatively large quantities of bulky food.

Iodine

Milk and milk products are important sources of iodine so vegans must be careful to include other iodine-rich foods in their diets. These include seaweed, cereals and vegetables grown in iodine-rich soil.

Vegetarians and supplements

Vegetarians who are not always able to follow a varied, balanced diet may benefit from supplements. Women who are, or who hope to become, pregnant or who are breastfeeding may be advised to take vitamin B, calcium, iron and zinc supplements.

Iron supplements can be useful for premenopausal vegetarian women who often find it difficult to get enough iron. Zinc supplements are also useful and if taken for long periods, it is also advisable to take a copper supplement of around 2 mg per day.

Vegetarian teenagers

Vegetarian diets can be safe for teenagers; although this presents special challenges as teenagers need sufficient calories, protein, vitamins and minerals for rapid growth. Again the key is to eat a variety of foods; including fresh fruit and vegetables, whole grain products, nuts, seeds, beans and peas, and preferably dairy products and eggs.

Vegetarian children

A vegetarian diet can provide the nutrients needed for a child's growth and development. Research into vegetarian children has shown that they are similar to meat eaters in height, weight and skinfold measurement.[7] They are also less likely to be obese. Vegan children tend to be lighter and leaner and may be shorter. Nutritional deficiencies are generally no more common in vegetarian children than among those who do eat meat, although in some cases iron levels may be lower.[8]

Children who eat vegetarian diets often eat fewer convenience foods and dairy products, and more starchy foods such as pulses, fruit and vegetables. Vegetarian girls may start menstruation at a slightly later age which may be protective against breast and other hormone-dependent cancers later in life. Vegetarian diets in children may be beneficial in protecting against disorders such as bowel problems, obesity, cardiovascular disease and cancer by establishing healthy dietary patterns which may be carried on into adult life.

Vegan diets are not usually recommended for children under 18 years of age due to sporadic eating habits and the relatively large volumes of food needed to meet the recommended intakes for nutrients such as calcium, iron and zinc.

Under fives

A diet that is healthy for an adult may not be appropriate for a very young child and high fiber, low fat diets may not be sufficiently high in certain nutrients. Young children need energy and nutrient-dense foods such as cereals, vegetable oils, bananas and avocados. Large intakes of high fiber or watery foods typically found in vegetarian and vegan diets may not be advisable in very young children.

Older people

By the year 2010, one in five people in the developed world will be aged 65 or over and the needs of an aging population will have a huge impact on society in the next century. Increasing research effort is being directed into ways of helping older people stay healthy, independent and mobile. Lifestyle and environmental factors play a part in some of the most common age-related illnesses including heart disease, osteoporosis, cancer, high blood pressure and chronic infection; which means that people have at least partial control over how well they age. Good nutrition early in life affects longevity and quality of life in later years. Aging changes occur at different rates in different people and it is unclear exactly how these are related to diet and other lifestyle factors. However, there is plenty of scientific evidence to show that good eating habits throughout life can help to promote physical and mental wellbeing in older people.

Diet and aging

The dietary needs of people in their fifties or sixties are different from those who are younger. For most vitamins and minerals, needs are higher; although for some nutrients they actually fall. The needs of people in their seventies and eighties are different again. Mainstream nutrition is beginning to recognize these differences and some of the new RDAs take into account the needs of those who are older.

Energy intakes and energy expenditure vary widely among elderly people, and are very different in those who are healthy, sick or institutionalized. Older people tend to consume fewer calories than younger people, probably due to loss of muscle, reduced activity levels and lower metabolic rates. As total food intake decreases, individual nutrient intakes also decrease, making it more important to eat nutrient-dense foods and leaving less room for sweets and other empty calorie foods.

Deficiencies of many nutrients are common in elderly people. Normal changes associated with aging, some medications for chronic disease, and relatively common disorders such as diabetes, high blood pressure, constipation and diarrhea can result in higher requirements for some nutrients. Many social and physiological factors such as loneliness, limited income, reduced interest in food, decreased sense of smell and taste, difficulty in chewing or swallowing and reduced vision may also lead to changes in an older person's diet.

New research findings are being published all the time but relatively little is known about how the aging process affects the ability of the body to digest, absorb and retain nutrients. The diets of elderly people are often deficient in several nutrients including vitamins A, C, D, E, B12, thiamin, riboflavin, pyridoxine, niacin, folic acid, calcium, iron, magnesium and zinc. These deficiencies may be due to lower dietary intake, decreased absorption, altered metabolism or increased excretion. They often develop slowly and may mimic the normal changes of aging. Elderly people are particularly at risk of marginal vitamin and mineral deficiencies and early recognition of malnutrition is very important in preventing diseases, maintaining a healthy immune system and increasing lifespan.

Digestion

As many as 30 per cent of people aged over 65 develop the inability to produce stomach acid which can lead to reduced absorption of certain vitamins and minerals; including folic acid, calcium, iron and vitamin B12. By the age of 80, as many as 40 per cent of people may be unable to produce stomach acid. Improving digestion can be valuable in improving health in elderly people. (See page 430 for more information.)

Immunity

Aging is generally associated with a decline of the immune response, which may be linked to a cumulative marginal deficiency of trace minerals and vitamins. Vitamin and mineral deficiencies, particularly of zinc, selenium, and vitamin B6, all of which are prevalent in aged populations, adversely affect immune responses. Because aging and malnutrition exert cumulative influences on immune responses, many elderly people have poor cell-mediated immune responses and are therefore at a high risk of infection. Supplementation with high doses of single nutrients may be useful for improving immune responses of self-sufficient elderly people living at home. Treating nutritional deficiencies in elderly people can reduce the risk of infections and possibly slow the aging process.[1]

Vitamins, minerals and older people

Vitamin A

Many older people may consume less than recommended levels of vitamin A, which may lead to poor vision, dry skin, lowered immunity, and may contribute to diseases such as cancer. However, large doses of pre-formed vitamin A could be harmful for elderly people as these may be cleared from the blood and tissues more slowly than in younger people. Vitamin A in the form of beta carotene may be more beneficial.

Creams that contain the vitamin A-derivative, tretinoin, may help to combat premature skin aging. In a 1997 study researchers investigated the activity of enzymes known as metalloproteinases which break down collagen, and found that exposure to ultraviolet light increased the activity of these enzymes. This may lead to premature skin aging. The researchers then found that tretinoin could block the enzyme activity, opening up the possibility that tretinoin may be useful in treating patients with signs of premature skin aging.[2]

B vitamins

Low dietary intake of B vitamins is quite common in elderly people and may lead to reduced mental functioning, skin and hair problems, suppressed immunity, depression and other emotional disorders, general weakness, and gastrointestinal problems. Improved nutrition often reverses the symptoms of deficiency, although in some cases permanent damage may occur.

Thiamin

Thiamin deficiency may be relatively common in older people and supplements are likely to be useful in improving quality of life. In a 1997 study, New Zealand researchers measured red blood cell concentrations of a thiamin-dependent enzyme in 222 people aged over 65 years. This measurement was done twice in three months. Thirty-five people who had low levels at both measurement times were divided into two groups. Half were given either a thiamin supplement of 10 mg per day and half were given a placebo for three months. The researchers then assessed blood pressure, body weight, height, body mass index, hand grip strength and cognitive function in the subjects. The results showed that the supplements decreased blood pressure and weight. Those taking the supplements reported improved quality of life, sleep and energy levels.[3]

Vitamin B6

Vitamin B6 requirements increase considerably in elderly people, possibly due to reduced absorption. Low vitamin B6 levels may also lead to increased risk of several disorders, including heart disease. (See page 87 for more information.) In a study published in 1996 Dutch researchers studied the vitamin B6 intake and blood levels in 546 elderly Europeans, aged from 74 to 76, with no known vitamin B6 supplement use. They also examined links with other dietary and lifestyle factors, including indicators of physical health. The results showed that 27 per cent of the men and 42 per cent of the women had dietary vitamin B6 intakes below the mean minimum requirements. Twenty-two per cent of both men and women had low blood levels.[4] The neurological and immunological effects of deficiency are usually reversible with supplementation.

Folate

Many elderly people do not consume enough folate in their diets. In a 1996 Canadian study, researchers investigated folate and vitamin B12 intakes and body levels in 28 men and 30 women aged over 65 years. The results showed that 57 per cent of men and 67 per cent of women were at risk of deficiency.[5] One of the most common disorders in elderly people is cardiovascular disease. There is increasing evidence that folic acid deficiency plays a role in the development of this disease through an increase in homocysteine levels. Supplements may be useful for their protective effects. (See page 105 for more information.)

Folate deficiency may also cause or worsen the mental difficulties often experienced by older people. In a study done in 1996 in Spain, researchers analyzed the relationship between mental and functional capacities and folate status in a group of 177 elderly people. In this study, almost 50 per cent of the people had folate intakes below recommended values. Those with poor test results had significantly lower folate levels.[6]

Vitamin B12

Inadequate vitamin B12 intake is relatively common in elderly people, with 10 to 20 per cent of elderly people having some level of vitamin B12 deficiency. This can result in reduced mental capacity and other neurological disorders that can resemble Alzheimer's disease. Older people often have a reduced capacity to absorb vitamin B12 due to low stomach acid and lack of intrinsic factor, the compound necessary for absorption. A stomach disorder known as atrophic gastritis may also limit absorption. Some experts believe that the incidence of pernicious anemia resulting from low vitamin B12 levels may be more common than previously thought, with up to 800 000 elderly people in the USA suffering from the disease.

Low vitamin B12 levels in older people may also reduce the effectiveness of the immune response. Recent research has shown that elderly people with low vitamin B12 levels may have impaired antibody responses to vaccination even though their immune systems are apparently functioning adequately.[7]

Supplementation can prevent irreversible neurological damage if started early. Elderly people with vitamin B12 deficiency may show psychiatric or metabolic deficiency symptoms even before anemia is diagnosed. Screening for low vitamin B12 levels is necessary in elderly people with mental impairment, although it has also been found that deficiency states can still exist even when blood levels are higher than the traditional lower reference limit for vitamin B12. Patients who are most at risk of vitamin B12 deficiency include those with gastrointestinal disorders, autoimmune disorders, Type I diabetes mellitus and thyroid disorders, and those receiving long-term therapy with gastric acid inhibitors.[8]

Other B vitamins

Mild riboflavin deficiency may be quite common in elderly people whose diets are low in red meat and dairy products. Niacin deficiency is also relatively common.

Vitamin D

Vitamin D absorption from food may decrease with age. Elderly people often also get less exposure to the sun and have a reduced capacity for skin synthesis, a major source of vitamin D. This may increase the risk or worsen the symptoms of osteoporosis, cancer, diabetes and arthritis.

Studies show that elderly people, particularly those who are housebound or in institutions, may be at high risk of vitamin D deficiency. Older people who frequently use sunscreens may also be more likely to suffer from vitamin D deficiency. A study published in 1998 in the *New England Journal of Medicine* found vitamin D deficiency in 57 per cent of a group of 290 patients who were admitted to hospital. In a subgroup of the patients who had no known risk factors for vitamin D deficiency, the researchers found that 42 per cent were deficient. They concluded that vitamin D deficiency was probably a substantial problem.[9]

In recognition of the increased vitamin D needs of older people, the RDAs have been raised. For adults under 50, the RDA is 200 IU; while for those over 50, it is now 400 IU; and for those over 70, it is 600 IU.

Osteoarthrtitis

Osteoarthritis sufferers who have low vitamin D intakes seem to suffer more severe symptoms than those whose intakes are high. In a study done in 1996, researchers at Boston University studied more than 500 elderly people with osteoarthritis of the knee. They found that those with the lowest intakes and blood levels of vitamin D were three times more likely to see their disease progress than people with high intakes and blood levels. Vitamin D may help reduce the cartilage damage seen in osteoarthritis.[10]

Osteoporosis

Vitamin D deficiency increases the risk of osteoporosis in elderly men and women and supplements may be useful in reducing bone loss and the occurrence of fractures. In a study published in 1997, researchers at Tufts University in Boston assessed the effects of calcium (500 mg per day) and vitamin D (700 IU per day) in 176 men and 213 women aged 65 years or older. When bone density was measured after a three-year period, those taking the supplements had higher bone density at all body sites measured. The fracture rate was also reduced by 50 per cent in those taking the supplements.[11] However, other studies have not shown any reduction in fracture rates in those taking vitamin D supplements.[12] Vitamin D supplements may also be useful in preventing bone loss in patients taking corticosteroid drugs.[13]

Antioxidants

Research suggests that the antioxidants beta carotene, vitamin C, vitamin E and selenium may help to prevent aging-related diseases such as cardiovascular disease, cancer, cataracts, rheumatoid arthritis and Alzheimer's disease.

Growing evidence suggests that free radical damage may be an underlying cause of the aging process, thus leaving open the possibility that antioxidants may be able to slow this process.

Beta carotene

As well as exerting protective effects against various aging-related diseases, beta carotene may protect against memory impairment and other loss of mental function in older people. In a recent Dutch study, researchers studied 5182 people aged 55 to 95 from 1990 to 1993. They found that those with intakes of less than 0.9 milligrams of beta carotene per day were almost twice as likely to have impaired memory, disorientation and problem solving difficulty as those with intakes of 2.1 milligrams of beta carotene.[14]

Researchers involved in a 1997 Swiss study found similar results. The study, which was reported in the *Journal of the American Geriatrics Society*, involved 442 men and women, aged from 65 to 94 in 1993. Antioxidant levels were originally tested in 1971 and then again in 1993, when the participants were also given memory-related tests. Higher vitamin C and beta carotene levels were associated with higher scores on free recall, recognition and vocabulary tests.[15]

Vitamin C

Vitamin C deficiency in elderly people can increase susceptibility to many disorders. Low vitamin C levels are associated with lowered immunity, which increases the risk of infection. In a study published in 1997, French researchers assessed vitamin C levels in 18 elderly patients in hospital. The patients were divided into three groups: those with acute infection, those who were malnourished, and a control group. Those with acute infection had considerably lower vitamin C levels than those in the other groups.[16]

Low vitamin C intakes also increase the risk of cardiovascular disease in elderly people. During a study which was begun in 1981, USDA researchers assessed the health and nutrition status of 747 elderly people aged 60 years and over. Particular attention was paid to the foods the participants usually ate and the levels in their blood of the antioxidant vitamins C, E and beta carotene. The researchers following up the subjects from nine to 12 years later found that among people who ate lots of dark green and orange vegetables, there were fewer deaths from heart disease and other causes. The results showed that a daily intake of more than 400 mg and higher blood levels of vitamin C were linked to reduced risk of death from heart disease.[17]

Vitamin E

High vitamin E intakes are linked to lower risks of several disorders including cardiovascular disease, cancer, Parkinson's disease and cataract. Supplements have also shown beneficial effects in several studies. (See page 165 for more information.)

A study by researchers from the National Institute on Aging, published in 1996, examined the effects of vitamin E and vitamin C supplement on mortality risk in 11 178 persons aged from 67 to 105 who were taking part in the Established Populations for Epidemiologic Studies of the Elderly from 1984 through 1993. During the follow-up period, there were 3490 deaths. The results showed that those using the vitamin E supplements had a 34 per cent lower risk of death when compared to those not using vitamin E supplements, and around half the risk of death from coronary disease. Those taking both vitamin C and vitamin E had a 42 per cent reduced risk.[18]

Vitamin E supplements also improve the effectiveness of the immune system in elderly people. In a 1997 study of 88 healthy people aged 65 or older, those who took 200 mg (300 IU) each day for about four months showed an improvement in immune response. Researchers assessed the effects of either 60 mg (90 IU), 200 mg (300 IU) or 800 mg (1333) on a measure of immune system strength known as delayed hypersensitivity skin response. The results showed that those who took 200 mg a day had a 65 per cent increase in immune function. Those taking 60 mg or 800 mg of vitamin E also showed some improvements in immune function but the ideal response was seen in those taking 200 mg.[19] Vitamin E may also provide relief from some of the symptoms of menopause, particularly hot flashes.[20]

Many studies suggest that vitamin E supplements are beneficial for elderly people, as it can be difficult to get high levels of vitamin E in the diet. Most studies use doses that range from 536 mg (800 IU) or even 804 mg (1200 IU). Such doses far exceed the RDAs, and it is not possible to get such large amounts of vitamin E from food without consuming a high fat diet.

Calcium

High calcium intakes are associated with reduced risk of some types of cancer and high blood pressure. Optimal calcium intake is particularly important in preventing the bone-thinning associated with osteoporosis. Although the problem also occurs in men, women are at particularly high risk of osteoporosis, with as many as 35 per cent of women suffering from the disease after menopause. Most of the bone loss seen in osteoporosis in postmenopausal women occurs in the first five to six years after menopause due to low calcium intake, a decline in female hormones, and an age-related reduction in vitamin D production.

It is never too late to slow the bone loss seen in osteoporosis and early postmenopausal years are an important time to ensure optimal calcium intake. Some research shows that taking calcium supplements later in life may lower vertebral fracture rate and prevent bone density decrease in elderly people. The results of the 1997 study mentioned on page 459 provide support for the use of calcium supplements.

Treatment which combines calcium and estrogen is likely to be better at building bone than treatment with estrogen alone. In a 1998 review, researchers analyzed the results of 31 studies and found that the postmenopausal women who took estrogen alone had an average increase in spinal bone mass of 1.3 per cent per year, while those who took estrogen and calcium supplements had an average increase of 3.3 per cent. Increases in bone mass in the forearm and upper thigh were also greater in women taking supplements. The added benefit from the calcium was seen when the women increased their intake from an average of 563 mg per day to 1200 mg per day.[21]

Iron

Iron deficiency is common in elderly people as they often have reduced stomach acid and therefore reduced absorption ability. Low blood plasma levels of iron can contribute to fatigue, heart disease and deterioration in mental functioning.

Iron requirements are lower in women who have reached menopause as they no longer lose iron in menstrual blood. However, deficiency is still relatively common and all elderly people should ensure they get sufficient iron in their diets. A 1997 National Institute of Aging study suggests that low iron levels are linked to an increased likelihood of death in elderly people. Researchers looked at the iron status of nearly 4000 men and women aged 71 and over. Results showed that low iron levels increased the risk of total and coronary heart disease deaths. Those with higher iron levels had decreased risk. Men with the highest iron levels had only 20 per cent of the risk of dying of heart disease of those with the lowest levels. Women with the highest levels were about half as likely to die of heart disease compared to those with the lowest levels.[22]

The iron overload disorder, hemochromatosis, can result in increased risk of heart disease, liver problems and other disorders. This is one of the most common inherited diseases in certain groups of people, and middle-aged and older men may be particularly badly affected. Iron supplements should be avoided in these cases. (See page 258 for more information.)

Magnesium

Marginal magnesium deficiency is considered to be very common, especially in the elderly. Inadequate intake may contribute to cardiovascular disease, high blood pressure, osteoporosis, diabetes and various other disorders. (See page 265 for more information.) Supplements are likely to be beneficial in older people.

Selenium

Selenium is a vital part of the antioxidant enzyme, glutathione peroxidase, and so may protect against free radical damage and its consequences. It is also necessary for thyroid and immune system function, which may be disrupted in older people. Optimal intake may also help combat psychological disorders like depression, anxiety, fatigue and appetite loss.

Sodium

Sodium restriction may be a useful way to lower blood pressure in elderly people suffering from hypertension. In a two-month double-blind, randomized, placebo-controlled crossover study published in 1997 in *The Lancet*, researchers found that modest reduction in salt in the diets of elderly people led to lower blood pressure. The study involved 29 patients with high blood pressure and 18 with normal blood pressure. The average blood pressure fall was 8.2/3.9 mmHg in the normal subjects and 6.6/2.7 mmHg in those with high blood pressure.[23] In those with normal blood pressure, cutting salt may have little effect, according to an analysis of 83 studies published in the *Journal of the American Medical Association* in 1998.[24]

Zinc

Inadequate consumption of zinc-rich foods can result in reduced sense of taste and possibly lead to reduced appetite or increased consumption of sugary or salty foods that may aggravate malnutrition. Zinc is vital for wound-healing and an effective immune response, and a deficiency can leave elderly people susceptible to infection and prolong recovery from illness. Elderly people often have zinc-poor diets and low blood levels.

Menopause

Menopause is when a woman's menstrual periods stop altogether and a woman is said to have gone through menopause when her menstrual periods have stopped for an entire year. This usually occurs between the ages of 45 and 55, although it can happen as early as 35 or as late as 65 years of age. It can also result from the surgical removal of both ovaries. The physical and emotional signs and symptoms that go with menopause usually last around one to two years or more, and vary from woman to woman. The changes are a result of hormonal changes such as estrogen decline, the aging process itself, and stress.

The physical signs and symptoms associated with menopause may include hot flushes, heart palpitations, irregular periods, vaginal dryness, loss of bladder tone, headaches, dizziness, skin and hair changes, loss of muscle strength and tone, and decreased bone mineral density. Emotional changes associated with menopause may include irritability, mood changes, lack of concentration, difficulty with memory, tension, anxiety, depression and insomnia.

Hormone replacement therapy (HRT) is often used to reduce many of the symptoms of menopause. It also offers significant protection against osteoporosis and heart disease. However, it may increase the risk of certain types of cancer and some women are unable or unwilling to use HRT.

Regular exercise and stress reduction techniques can be helpful in reducing the symptoms of menopause. Dietary measures that may be beneficial include limiting or avoiding drinks that contain caffeine or alcohol, spicy foods, and heavy meals. Soy foods such as tofu, which contain compounds known as phytoestrogens, have been shown to reduce menopausal symptoms in many women. A woman's risk of disorders such as heart disease and osteoporosis increases after menopause, and the various dietary measures and supplements outlined above can be used to prevent these.

Herbal medicines and older people

There are many herbs that can be beneficial for older people. These include tonics such as ginseng (*Panax ginseng* and *Eleutherococcus senticosus*), which can improve vitality and resistance to disease; ginkgo (*Ginkgo biloba*), which can improve mental function; damiana (*Turnera diffusa*), which can boost libido; ginger (*Zingiber officinale*), which can improve circulation; and hawthorn (*Crataegus oxyacantha*), which is a heart tonic. Herbs which may be useful during menopause include chaste tree (*Vitex agnus castus*), St John's wort (*Hypericum perforatum*), motherwort (*Leonurus cardiaca*), dong quai (*Angelica sinensis*), and black cohosh (*Cimicifuga racemosa*). See page 384 for more information on these herbs and the precautions that may be necessary.

Exercise

People who exercise regularly are healthier than those who don't. They are less likely to develop diseases such as high blood pressure, heart disease, diabetes and cancer. They usually live longer, look and feel better and younger throughout life, and maintain their independence for longer.

Regular exercise is a vital part of life for many people. Some people include moderate physical activity such as walking in their daily routines while there are others, such as elite athletes, whose lives revolve around training and competition. From the recreational exerciser to the professional athlete, good nutrition is vital for optimal performance through its effects on the functioning of organs, muscles and other tissues. A poor diet combined with increased requirements can impair performance and general health.

Aerobic and anaerobic exercise

There are two basic different types of exercise, aerobic and anaerobic. Aerobic means 'with oxygen' and is any kind of exercise which forces the heart and lungs to work harder to supply the oxygen to the muscles. Aerobic exercise burns calories, strengthens and conditions the heart and lungs and improves general fitness and stamina, improves mental ability, and significantly lowers disease risk. Aerobic exercise includes activities like running, cycling, swimming, fast walking, aerobics classes and dancing.

Anaerobic means 'without oxygen' and is any exercise that requires short bursts of power, such as sprinting or lifting weights. Someone who is exercising anaerobically is using energy sources stored in the muscle rather than oxygen from the air. Because this energy supply is limited, anaerobic exercise can be sustained only for short periods of time. In reality, most exercise is a combination of aerobic and anaerobic exercise. The amount of each is dependent on how hard and fast the exercise proceeds.

Nutrition and exercise

Regular exercise increase demands for calories and most nutrients. It also improves metabolism and elimination. Good nutrition helps to improve performance, prevent bone and muscle breakdown, prevent injuries and, for competitive athletes, can make the difference between winning and losing.

A daily diet built around high levels of complex carbohydrates, moderately low fat levels and moderate protein intake is the best approach for most athletes. It is also important to obtain vitamins and minerals in amounts at least as high as the RDAs. A diet that consists of a wide variety of wholesome, minimally processed foods, fortified foods and, in some cases, supplements is essential to meet these goals.

Body mass and composition

Some people exercise to lose weight and stay healthy while others work out for weight gain. Most athletes avoid high fat diets and strive for low body fat percentages, as body fat does not contribute to athletic performance. Those who exercise tend to have more muscle and less body fat than those who don't.

Water and electrolyte balance

Dehydration can reduce athletic performance and lead to fatigue, and it is vital for those who are exercising to drink enough water. This is particularly important during long endurance events. A general rule is to drink twice as much water as is necessary to quench thirst. Water is also essential for regulating body temperature. Exercise also increases needs for the electrolytes, sodium, chloride and potassium. Magnesium and calcium needs may also be greater. Supplements may be useful during strenuous exercise although sodium supplements are rarely necessary.

Energy

Several factors influence the amount of energy an athlete needs. These include the type, intensity and frequency of training as well as the size, age, sex and genetic make-up of the person. A middle-aged male marathon runner has different requirements to a young female gymnast. The main sources of energy for an athlete are carbohydrates and fats.

In an athletic event, carbohydrates are the initial fuel source. The energy for short bursts of activity all comes from carbohydrates. For longer events the energy comes from both carbohydrates and fats, with the proportions depending on the intensity of the exercise, pre-event diet and the level of training of the athlete.

Protein

Adequate, good quality protein is necessary to preserve lean body mass and maximize athletic performance. Protein is essential for growth, repair and maintenance of body tissues. A typical Western diet provides more than enough protein for athletes and exercisers. Recommended protein intake for adults is estimated to be 0.8 g protein per kg of body weight per day, although some experts feel that the needs for athletes may be higher, with endurance athletes needing up to 1.2 to 1.4 g per kg per day. Athletes who are involved in very intense strength training or endurance sports may need up to 1.4 to 1.8 g per kg of body weight per day, an amount which can easily be met by diet. Those who wish to gain weight also have slightly higher protein requirements. In such cases it may be better to take amino acid supplements rather than increase intake of flesh foods. Many athletes eat two to three times the amount of protein they need. This can put stress on the kidneys and increase the risk of dehydration.

Carbohydrates

Carbohydrate-rich foods are the best fuel source for athletes. Experts recommend that 55 to 65 per cent of an athlete's calories come from carbohydrates. Most of this carbohydrate should be in the form of complex carbohydrate, which is the type found in foods such as whole grain breads, cereals, cooked dried beans and peas, potatoes and corn. Fruits and vegetables are important sources of simple carbohydrates.

The body stores limited amounts of carbohydrates as glycogen. The amount of carbohydrate in the diet is directly related to glycogen storage and athletic performance. Daily high intensity training and endurance events deplete body stores of glycogen and high glycogen stores mean that an athlete can tolerate repeated training and endurance exercise. Physical training enables athletes to store more glycogen and use its limited supply sparingly. About 1800 to 2000 calories are available from glycogen stores and this is usually enough for about 90 minutes of continuous exercise at maximal aerobic pace.

When an event lasts more than one hour an athlete may benefit from consuming carbohydrates during exercise. Drinks, such as diluted fruit juices or sports drinks, which contain less than 24 g of carbohydrate per cup may be the best form for this. It is important to eat a high carbohydrate snack after an exercise session to replace muscle glycogen stores.

Carbohydrate loading

Adequate carbohydrate is essential for athletes to replace glycogen stores depleted by training and competition. This glycogen depletion has led to the practice of carbohydrate loading, which benefits athletes who are involved in training or competition for more than 90 minutes. There are several forms of carbohydrate loading; a common method involves eating a diet that consists of about 60 to 70 per cent carbohydrate about 72 hours before a competition. If muscles are not damaged, 24 to 36 hours of rest before the event will allow maximum glycogen storage.

Fat

Fats are the body's other major energy source. They are twice as dense in calories as carbohydrates. However, fats cannot be used exclusively as an energy source and a small amount of carbohydrate must always be available. Aerobic training increases the ability of the body to use fat as an energy source. Fat is a major source of fuel for exercising muscles but they only store a small amount. When this is used up, fat is taken from body stores.

Body fat stores are more than adequate to provide extra energy and it is not necessary to get large amounts of fat in the diet. Most athlctes eat moderately low fat diets. Health authorities recommend keeping fat intake below 30 per cent of total calories as this has been shown to be beneficial in protecting against various diseases.

Oxygen metabolism and energy production

Several nutrients are vital for the efficient burning of fuel with oxygen and the production of energy. A good diet provides optimal amounts of these nutrients, which include iron, magnesium and other trace elements.

Bone structure

A high density bone structure is vital for optimal athletic performance and the avoidance of injuries such as shin splints. Nutrients such as calcium and vitamin D are vital for healthy bones.

Vitamins, minerals and exercise

Most nutritional studies indicate that vitamin and mineral requirements of athletes are not greater than those of people who don't exercise. Some types of exercise may lead to losses of certain nutrients but these extra requirements can often be met by the extra food intake that is necessary to meet energy requirements.

Supplements

Athletes tend to take nutritional supplements more often than the general population and some may take very high doses. Many athletes believe that the requirements for sport are too high or that their diet is too poor to meet their vitamin and mineral needs. However, most studies also show that blood levels of vitamins and minerals are similar in athletes and nonathletes, suggesting that exercise does not deplete body stores. There are a few possible exceptions, for example, iron in vegetarian athletes.

Many athletes believe that certain supplements can enhance sports performance. Advertising claims for such supplements are often impressive but the vast majority of such supplements are either untested or have failed to show results in the tests that have been done. Megadoses of vitamins are often used by athletes to enhance performance. There is little evidence that they do, unless there are deficiencies. For many athletes, a balanced supplement which contains vitamins and minerals at the RDA level may be useful as nutritional insurance. Supplements are not a substitute for a healthy diet.

Due to increased losses of minerals in sweat and urine, there is a potential increased need for minerals in athletes. Some studies report that mineral intakes among athletes are inadequate, especially among those who are attempting to lose weight for competition. However, most athletes do seem to eat adequate amounts. It is important to eat minerals in balanced ratios. An excess of one mineral can have adverse effects on others in the body. An athlete who eats fortified cereals, sports bars and mineral supplements may be getting excessive doses of certain minerals.

Antioxidants

High intensity exercise may cause excess free radicals to be produced in the cells. The damage from these increase a person's susceptibility to cancer, heart disease, cataracts, premature aging, decreased immunity and other diseases. (See page 417 for more information.)

Free radical production increases as the body's oxygen consumption increases, particularly in the muscle fibers and in the mitochondria, the energy centers of the cell. During exercise, the blood is diverted away from organs not actively involved in the exercise process and then flows back when the exercise is completed. This reperfusion may also cause the production of free radicals, a process that can also occur in muscles during exhaustive exercise. A growing amount of evidence indicates that free radicals also play an important role in causing skeletal muscle damage and inflammation after strenuous exercise. The antioxidant vitamins, C, E and beta carotene, and minerals such as selenium may protect against this free radical damage, giving protection against disease and, possibly, faster recovery from damaging exercise.

Strenuous exercise also leads to a lowering of immune function, putting endurance athletes at increased risk for upper respiratory tract infections during periods of heavy training and after events.[1] This is likely to be due to oxidative damage and antioxidant supplements may be useful in helping to prevent such damage.

Vitamin C

As an antioxidant vitamin C may help to prevent exercise-induced oxidative damage. In a 1997 study, researchers examined the effects of supplements on oxidative stress in athletes. They found that exercise-induced oxidative stress was highest when those involved in the study did not supplement with vitamin C.[2]

Vitamin C supplements may be beneficial for those who exercise heavily and have problems with frequent upper respiratory tract infections. Three placebo-controlled studies have examined the effect of vitamin C supplementation on common cold occurrence in people under acute physical stress. In one study, the subjects were school children at a skiing camp in the Swiss Alps, in another they were military troops training in Northern Canada, and in the third they were participants in a 90 km running race. In each of the three studies, the results showed a considerable reduction in common cold incidence in the group supplemented with vitamin C at levels of 600 mg to 1000 mg per day.[3]

Vitamin E

There is some evidence that vitamin E may decrease muscle fatigue and improve endurance performance. In a 1998 study, researchers investigated the effects of high intensity resistance exercise on free radical production. They also assessed the effects of vitamin E supplementation on free radical formation or muscle membrane disruption. They divided 12 weight-trained males into two groups. The supplement group received 804 mg (1200 IU) once a day for a period of two weeks and the other group received a placebo. The results showed that high intensity resistance exercise increased free radical production and that vitamin E supplementation decreased muscle membrane disruption.[4]

B vitamins

B vitamins are essential for the conversion of carbohydrates to energy, and as calorie and carbohydrate intakes increase, the requirement for B vitamins also increases. However, this increase will usually be covered by the increased food intake if nutrient-dense foods such as whole grain breads and cereals are eaten. There is little evidence that intake of B vitamin supplements improves athletic performance.

Thiamin

Thiamin supplements may be helpful in preventing or accelerating recovery from exercise-induced fatigue. In a study done in 1996, researchers assessed the effects of 100 mg per day of thiamin in 16 male athletes. The athletes exercised on bicycles and changes in blood, heart and lung functioning were measured. In the thiamin supplement group, changes in blood glucose were suppressed and the athletes felt less fatigued.[5]

Vitamin B6

Exercisers and athletes often have low vitamin B6 levels. Exercise causes pyridoxine blood levels to increase during an exercise session, possibly because pyridoxine-dependent enzymes are released from muscle storage or the vitamin is transferred from the liver to the muscles. There is no evidence that vitamin B6 supplements enhance performance.

Pantothenic acid

Pantothenic acid is essential for normal adrenal gland function and the production of cortisone and other adrenal gland hormones. These hormones play an essential part in the body's reaction to stress. Pantothenic acid has been reported to improve athletic performance by improving aerobic capacity and endurance performance, although results of studies have been mixed.

Calcium

Female athletes often have menstrual irregularities, which are due to a disruption of the normal estrogen cycle. Lack of estrogen can lead to a loss of bone mineral density. If this is combined with a diet low in calcium, there is an increased risk of developing stress fractures such as shin splints, weak bones, poor bone healing and eventually osteoporosis. Calcium supplements in doses of around 1000 to 1500 mg per day may be beneficial for such women. Increased loss of calcium can also occur during periods of inactivity.

Recent research suggests that male athletes who train intensively may also lose enough calcium from their bones to increase their chances of stress fractures. In a 1996 study, researchers at the University of Memphis measured the calcium levels of basketball players and found that after intense exercise the players lost an average of 422 mg of calcium in sweat during each session compared with a loss of 40 to 144 mg per day during mild activity. The researchers also found that over ten months, the players' total body bone mineral content declined by 6 per cent. When the players received 2 g of calcium supplements the next season, their lean body mass increased and average bone mineral content increased by 5 per cent.[6]

Chromium

Strenuous exercise may increase chromium excretion. Limited research suggests that chromium supplements, in the form of chromium picolinate may cause weight loss, reduce fat and increase muscle mass. Because of these reports, chromium picolinate supplements have become very popular, particularly among athletes. Most of the research into performance-enhancing effects has been conducted by manufacturers of supplements and there is very little independent research to corroborate the findings.

Iron

Heavy exercise may lead to iron deficiency. Distance runners are at particular risk as running appears to lead to a decrease in body stores of iron. Symptoms of iron deficiency in athletes include reduction in exercise time, increased heart rate, decreased oxygen consumption and increased blood lactic acid. A deficiency may result from increased metabolic requirements, increased red blood cell breakdown and increased iron losses in sweat. However, unless a person is iron-deficient, supplements do not appear to improve athletic performance.

Athletes at risk of iron deficiency include menstruating females; adolescent males whose iron requirements are high due to growth needs; vegetarians who do not eat red meat (the richest source of easily absorbed heme iron); and endurance athletes who may lose a greater amount than usual through blood losses or sweat.

Sports anemia

Sports anemia is often used to describe a low hemoglobin condition that is relatively common at the beginning of training. After adaptation, the anemia seems to subside. It may be due to inadequate dietary intake of iron or the use of protein for tasks other than red blood cell production during the early training stages. Iron intake of athletes needs to be carefully monitored.

Some experts believe that there is a possibility that exercise may have beneficial effects in reducing the risk of heart disease and cancer by lowering body stores of iron which can cause oxidative damage. (See page 257 for more information.)

Magnesium

Strenuous exercise alters magnesium concentrations in muscle and blood. Endurance exercise is particularly likely to do this as higher levels of hormones such as adrenaline and noradrenaline increase urinary loss of magnesium. Stressful conditions such as intense training and competition may also increase the need for magnesium.

In a 1998 study, researchers from the University of Texas examined body magnesium concentrations in 26 marathon runners during an endurance run. They found that levels in the muscles and urine dropped significantly, possibly putting the athletes at risk of decreased performance and muscle cramps.[7]

Athletes on calorie restricted diets may be at particular risk of magnesium deficiency and amounts higher than the RDA may be necessary for those who exercise intensively, possibly in doses as high as 6 mg per kg of body weight. Supplements may help to increase bone mineral density in women athletes who have menstrual irregularities and are at risk of osteoporosis. They may also improve muscle strength in athletes.

Magnesium deficiency decreases energy efficiency and research has shown that people who are deficient in magnesium may use more energy during exercise. In a recent study, USDA researchers investigated the amount of oxygen needed by healthy women over 50 to perform a certain amount of low intensity work on an exercise bicycle. When their dietary magnesium was inadequate (150 mg daily) they used 10 to15 per cent more oxygen to perform the work and their heart rates climbed by about ten beats per minute. The results suggest that magnesium deficiency is associated with increased physiological demands to do the same amount of work as when magnesium is adequate.

Zinc

Athletes can be deficient in zinc as increased needs and increased sweating and urinary excretion may lead to greater requirements. Zinc deficiency can affect energy production, tissue repair and resistance to infection.

Other nutrients

Coenzyme Q10

Due to its role in energy production, coenzyme Q10 has also been used to enhance athletic performance. Because exercise increases the risk of oxidative damage, coenzyme Q10 as an antioxidant may have a role to play in protection from such damage. In a 1997 study done in Finland, the effects of coenzyme Q10 supplements were studied in a double-blind cross-over study of 25 cross-country skiers. The results showed that all measured indexes of physical performance improved significantly. Ninety-four per cent of the athletes felt that the supplements had been beneficial in improving their performance and recovery time, whereas only 33 per cent of those in the placebo group did.[8]

Weight loss

Despite the availability of low fat foods and increasing awareness of the risks, obesity is still on the increase. However, despite the prevalence of obesity, many people do not consume enough essential nutrients to keep themselves healthy, and overweight and poor nutrition are major risk factors for some of the most common diseases in our society. These include high cholesterol levels, atherosclerosis, hypertension, heart disease, diabetes, some types of cancer, gallstones, gout, stroke, gallbladder disease, liver disease, infertility and arthritis. People who are overweight often meet with disapproval in their daily lives and may suffer psychological and social difficulties.

Hand in hand with the increase in obesity has come a national obsession with weight loss. Many overweight people are drawn to fad diets that promise fast results with minimal effort, only to see the weight go back on just as quickly once they return to their regular diet. Such a pattern of repeated weight loss and gain may contribute to lifelong obesity. The only way to lose weight and keep it off is to develop, and stick to a healthy, nutrient-dense, balanced diet and a regular exercise program.

Obesity

Many people think of obesity as an excess of total body weight whereas in fact, it is excess body weight as fat. Being overweight may also be defined in terms of how someone feels about him or herself, and psychological factors play an important role in obesity and weight loss. Many people, particularly young women, think they are overweight when they may actually be underweight. For many people the optimum weight may not be as low as they would like.

An ideal or optimum weight is difficult to define. A commonly used way to assess body weight is the body mass index (usually abbreviated as BMI). A person's BMI is calculated by dividing their weight in kilograms by the square of their height in meters. A BMI within the range 20 to 25 is considered normal. A value of between 25 and 30 is considered overweight and a value over 30 is defined as obese.

Factors contributing to obesity

Obesity is an enormously complex problem and there are various theories as to the cause. It is likely that there are several factors contributing to the weight problem of a particular person. For years the prevailing scientific view was that in order for weight loss to occur, energy (or calories) in needed to be less than the energy (or calories) out. This usually means either eating less or exercising more, and the best results seem to happen when someone does both. However, new research suggests that weight management is more complicated than this and other factors contributing to obesity mean that a calorie is not the same for everyone. Some people seem to have higher metabolic rates and burn up food more efficiently than others. This may be due to a combination of genetic and psychological factors, gender, hormonal imbalances, poor liver function, food allergies and in some cases, medication use.

A healthy weight loss diet

While different diets suit different people, there are some general guidelines that can help people to make better food choices on a weight loss diet. These guidelines are outlined on page 13. A daily diet built around high levels of complex carbohydrates, low fat levels and moderate protein intake is the best approach for those wishing to lose weight. It is also important to obtain vitamins and minerals in amounts at least as high as the RDAs. A diet that consists of a wide variety of wholesome, minimally processed foods, fortified foods and, in some cases, supplements will play a part in safe, effective weight loss.

Calories

The energy value of food is measured in kilocalories, which is usually shortened to calories. The word 'calorie' comes from the Latin for 'heat' and a calorie is defined as the amount of heat needed to raise the temperature of one gram of water by 33.8 degrees Fahrenheit. The metric measurement is kilojoules. One calorie is equivalent to 4.2 kilojoules (kJ).

Food is usually defined in terms of calories as a way of comparing the relative energy value it holds. Fat, carbohydrate and protein are known as macronutrients because they provide energy. Vitamins and minerals are known as micronutrients as they have no energy value.

1 gram of fat provides 9 calories (38 kJ)

1 gram of protein provides 4 calories (17 kJ)

1 gram of carbohydrate provides 4 calories (17 kJ)

Fat

Fat is the most concentrated food source of calories and many weight loss diets are based around limiting fat. Many people trying to lose weight aim to exclude fat from their diets altogether in the belief that this will bring faster results. However, while excessive intakes of certain fats can contribute to obesity and health problems, it is important to remember that some types of fats are essential nutrients and are necessary for health. (See page 329 for more information.)

Carbohydrate

Carbohydrate foods vary in the rate at which they are absorbed into the bloodstream. Foods high in simple sugars such as glucose and sucrose (table sugar) are quickly absorbed and this leads to a sharp rise in insulin production to move the sugar out of the blood. This is followed by a sharp drop in blood glucose and a craving for more sweet food. This contributes to obesity as these foods are high in calories. Complex carbohydrates are absorbed more slowly into the blood than simple carbohydrates, which leads to a slower insulin response. In this way, blood sugar levels tend to be more consistent, avoiding the sharp rises and falls of a diet high in simple sugars. Sucrose also seems to cause a greater increase in blood fat levels than more complex carbohydrates.

In fat tissue, insulin facilitates the storage of glucose and its conversion to fatty acids, and also slows the breakdown of fatty acids. Sharp rises in insulin may contribute to obesity and it seems that blood insulin levels correspond to body fat stores. The longer and more often insulin levels are high, the more likely sugars are to be converted to and stored as fat. Eating large amounts of foods high in both fat and sugar increases weight gain even more.

Eating too many sugar-rich foods such as cookies, cakes and candy that contain refined carbohydrates increases the risk of nutritional deficiencies as there may not be enough room for nutrient-dense foods. Sugars and refined carbohydrates require vitamins and minerals for metabolism but unlike whole grains, they do not contain enough of these vital nutrients.

Exercise

No weight loss program is complete without an exercise component. When a dieter concentrates solely on food restriction to achieve results there is a loss of both body fat and muscle. This is less than ideal as muscle helps burn fat. The most effective weight loss programs involve both diet and exercise.

Aerobic exercise is the best way to lose fat. It burns extra calories, a few hundred or more per hour of exercise, depending on the type of exercise, a person's weight and how hard they exercise. Over time, exercise builds muscle which raises metabolic rate and improves the ability to burn calories and reduce fat tissue. Exercise has the added advantage of increasing metabolic rate for up to 24 hours after exercise has been completed.

More complete exercise programs also include anaerobic exercise as this is the kind which builds strength and flexibility. Strength training can also help with weight loss and improve body image and self-esteem. Building muscle mass will also increase metabolic rate, which burns more. The best fitness programs involve a balance between aerobic fitness and flexibility and strength training.

Vitamin and minerals

Vitamin and mineral supplements can be helpful during and after weight loss as many people on weight loss diets do not consume adequate amounts of vitamins and minerals. Some common sources of nutrients such as calcium and vitamin E are found in high quantities in high calorie foods which people on weight loss diets tend to avoid.

B vitamins

B vitamins are essential for the metabolism of food and optimal intake is necessary to ensure that this takes place effectively. Biotin and pantothenic acid supplements have been used in weight loss programs.

Minerals

Extra minerals may also be useful in preventing deficiency, especially in people whose fiber intakes are high, as fiber reduces absorption of calcium, iron, zinc, copper, manganese, and molybdenum.

Antioxidants

Since weight loss usually involves a mild process of detoxification, with the body burning fat and sometimes other tissues, antioxidants may be useful. These include beta carotene, vitamin C, vitamin E and selenium.

Chromium

Limited research suggests that moderate increases in chromium, in the form of chromium picolinate, may cause weight loss, reduce fat and increase muscle mass. Because of these reports, chromium picolinate supplements have become very popular.

Researchers involved in a 1997 study assessed the effects of chromium yeast and chromium picolinate on lean body mass in 36 obese patients during and after weight reduction with a very low calorie diet. During the 26-week treatment period, subjects received either placebo or 200 mcg chromium yeast or 200 mcg chromium picolinate in a double-blind manner. After 26 weeks, chromium picolinate-supplemented patients showed increased lean body mass whereas the other treatment groups still had reduced lean body mass.[1]

In a 1997 study done at the University of Texas at Austin, researchers examined the effects of 400 mcg of chromium and exercise training on young, obese women. The results showed that exercise training combined with chromium nicotinate supplementation resulted in significant weight loss and lowered the insulin response to an oral glucose load.[2]

Essential fatty acids

Essential fatty acid supplements may also be useful in improving fatty acid metabolism. This is particularly important if the diet is very low in fat. Cold-pressed flaxseed oil is high in both omega-3 and omega-6 fatty acids, and is a good way to obtain these oils. Usually, three or four teaspoons a day are adequate. As cofactors that help in fatty acid metabolism, zinc, magnesium, vitamins A, C, niacin, pyridoxine, biotin, choline and carnitine may also be useful.

Other nutrients

Other nutrients and supplements that have been used to help in weight loss include coenzyme Q10, acetyl-L-carntitine, spirulina and chitosan.

Herbs

Herbs that have been used to aid in weight loss include brindleberry (*Garcinia cambogia*), chickweed (*Stellaria media*), bladderwrack (*Fucus vesiculosus*) and plantain (*Plantago ovata*). See page 384 for more information on these herbs and the precautions that may be necessary.

Drug interactions

From the occasional glass of wine to powerful medications used to fight cancer, drugs have the ability to affect nutritional status and health in a variety of ways. There are more than 100 000 medications available in America and almost two billion prescription drugs are dispensed every year. Many of these drugs affect the way the body uses vitamins and minerals from food. In most cases, medications deplete nutrients gradually and deficiencies may not be noticed until stores are exhausted. Alcohol also affects nutrient status and while light drinking may have some beneficial effects, heavy use carries a high risk of malnutrition. It is important to understand how drugs affect the body in order to minimize adverse effects, enhance recovery and maintain optimal health.

Drug-induced nutrient deficiencies

In most cases, unless drugs are used on a long-term basis, the effects on individual nutrients are not long lasting. Vitamin and mineral deficiencies are more likely to occur in people who take medications for long periods, particularly if their diets are usually low in essential nutrients. This type of medication use typically occurs in those with gastrointestinal disorders, diabetes, cancer, epilepsy, cardiovascular disease and autoimmune diseases. Alcohol, tobacco and oral contraceptives also fall into this category.

Elderly people tend to take more prescription and non prescription medications than any other group and usually also have increased needs, reduced appetite and absorption. This combination means that they are at high risk of drug-induced deficiencies. Children, pregnant women, those on reduced calorie diets and alcoholics are also susceptible.

Prescription and nonprescription drugs can interact with nutrients in a number of ways.

Alterations in appetite

Many medications can increase or decrease appetite, which can lead to a change in the amounts and types of food a person eats. Some drugs, such as some antihistamines and antidepressants can increase appetite. In some cases this may be desirable, but in others there may be an increased risk of obesity and the complications this causes. Many medications reduce appetite. Some are intended to do so, such as amphetamines for weight loss, and others do so as a side effect. If weight loss occurs in those who are already underweight, malnutrition may occur.

Some drugs affect the gastrointestinal system, causing nausea, vomiting, constipation or diarrhea. Others alter the production of saliva and the ability to taste, reducing a person's ability to enjoy food. Some drugs affect mood and alter the desire to eat. Drugs with these effects contribute to reduced intake and can lead to vitamin and mineral deficiencies.

Alterations in absorption

Some medications alter the absorption of vitamins and minerals so that even if dietary intake is sufficient, the body may not absorb enough for optimum health. Other medications bind vitamins and minerals in the intestine and reduce the ability of the body to absorb them; for example mineral oil laxatives reduce absorption of the fat soluble vitamins A, D, E and K.

Other drugs reduce the amount of time food spends in the intestine which means that the body may not have time to absorb all it needs. Others may block absorption sites or alter them so vitamins and minerals cannot pass through. Some drugs may affect absorption by changing the acidity of the stomach and intestines. In some cases the production of digestive juices essential for breakdown and absorption may be reduced.

Alterations in metabolism

Certain drugs alter the availability, storage and use of nutrients. Some of these chemically resemble vitamins and minerals and can bind to the same active sites on an enzyme. However, these drugs may not have the same beneficial effects as a vitamin and this can lead to deficiency symptoms. Other drugs may alter storage.

Some medications increase excretion of certain nutrients. This means that a particular vitamin or mineral is not retained in the body long enough to have beneficial effects; for example, some diuretic drugs increase potassium excretion.

Alcohol

Heavy alcohol use can lead to nutrient deficiencies. Many of the nutritional problems of heavy drinkers occur because of the direct effects of alcohol, but deficiencies are also partly due to the tendency of alcoholics to replace food with alcohol. Heavy alcohol use reduces vitamin and mineral absorption, damages the intestinal lining and can also interfere with the conversion of some nutrients to their active forms. Alcohol-induced disorders such as inflammation of the pancreas and small intestine and liver cirrhosis can also lead to malnutrition.

Vitamin A

Alcohol irritates the digestive tract and inhibits the absorption of vitamin A. It also depletes the body's tissue stores. Deficiency is common in alcoholics and contributes to some of the disorders of alcoholism such as night blindness, skin problems, cirrhosis of the liver and susceptibility to infections. Vitamin A supplements should not be taken with large amounts of alcohol as liver damage may occur.

B vitamins

Alcoholics are classically deficient in B vitamins, and supplements are sometimes used to treat alcoholics and those recovering from the disease. Deficiency is due to low dietary intake, impaired absorption and storage, and reduced conversion to the active form of the vitamin. Alcoholics and binge drinkers are especially prone to thiamin deficiency, which is associated with some of the symptoms of alcoholism such as mental confusion, visual disturbances and staggering gait. If thiamin deficiency is not corrected, permanent brain damage may result. This condition is known as Wernicke Korsakoff syndrome and is usually seen in people who have been addicted to alcohol for many years. Some experts recommend 100 mg of thiamin per day for those who drink alcohol.

Alcohol may increase niacin needs and nicotinamide has been shown to protect against the damage to liver cells caused by drinking a large quantity of alcohol.[1] Alcohol increases breakdown of the biologically active form of vitamin B6 and long-term use may cause liver damage which interferes with the conversion of vitamin B6 to the active form.

Antioxidants

Studies show that alcoholics have lower tissue levels of the antioxidants, beta carotene, vitamin E, vitamin C and selenium.[2] Increased oxidative damage to tissues also occurs as a result of heavy alcohol consumption. The higher needs and reduced intake put alcoholics at increased risk of diseases such as cancer and cardiovascular disease. Studies have also demonstrated that when those at risk cut their alcohol consumption, levels of antioxidants start to normalize.

Beta carotene

Drinking large amounts of alcohol may lower blood levels of carotenes.[3] There have been several studies of the effects of beta carotene supplements on cancer and cardiovascular disease prevention. Some of these studies, including the Finnish Alpha Tocopherol Beta Carotene Cancer (ATBC) Prevention Study, the US Carotene and Retinol Efficacy Trial (CARET), have involved men who smoked and drank alcohol. The results of these studies suggest that beta carotene supplements increase the risk of cancer and cardiovascular disease in those who smoke and drink alcohol. This may be because beta carotene is susceptible to oxidative damage from alcohol and the gases in cigarette smoke, which may lead to the formation of harmful compounds. This suggests that heavy drinkers should not take beta carotene supplements. (See page 54 for more information.)

Vitamin C

Alcohol appears to increase vitamin C excretion and may lead to deficiency.[4] Vitamin C is very important for alcoholics as it protects against oxidative damage and plays a role in the detoxification of alcohol.

Selenium

Alcoholics may have low levels of selenium, increasing the risk of liver damage. Selenium is part of the enzyme, glutathione peroxidase, which is important in protecting against the free radical damage which alcohol causes in the liver. A 1983 English study of selenium status in 391 healthy people showed that a combination of alcohol and smoking was most likely to lead to selenium deficiency.[5]

Vitamin D

Alcohol interferes with the conversion of vitamin D to its biologically active form. This can lead to abnormalities in vitamin D levels which disturb calcium and phosphate metabolism. This contributes to the high frequency of bone fractures and osteomalacia in alcoholics.

Magnesium

Alcoholics are at particular risk of magnesium deficiency. Alcohol causes an increase in the urinary excretion of magnesium and depletes body stores. Magnesium deficiency may exacerbate the symptoms of alcoholism such as high blood pressure, other cardiovascular diseases and osteoporosis.[6] Supplements have been shown to have therapeutic effects in the prevention and treatment of these symptoms. Magnesium sulfate injections may help to diminish the severity of withdrawal symptoms in patients who have recently abstained from alcohol.[7]

Zinc

The enzymes needed for detoxification of alcohol contain zinc, and alcohol may also decrease dietary absorption and increase excretion of zinc. This leads to increased zinc requirements in those who drink a lot of alcohol. Zinc deficiency in alcoholism is likely to be linked to altered vitamin A metabolism, suppressed immune function, neurological problems, eye problems and sex organ abnormalities. Zinc deficiency may also play a role in fetal alcohol syndrome, birth defects associated with alcohol use by pregnant women.

Other minerals

Alcohol abuse also leads to calcium and potassium deficiencies with resulting harmful effects on the cardiovascular system, bones and other body tissues. Alcohol may exacerbate the liver damage caused by the iron overload disease, hemochromatosis, and sufferers should avoid drinking alcohol.

Tobacco

Smoking adversely affects a person's nutritional status in many ways. Cigarette smoke increases the damage caused by free radicals, which may explain the link between smoking and diseases such as cancer. Lung cancer causes more deaths than any other cancer and is strongly linked to smoking.

Antioxidants

Several studies have shown that levels of antioxidants are lower in smokers. Vitamin C needs, in particular, are increased. The RDA for smokers has been increased to 100 mg but needs may in fact be much higher. Despite this, smokers often eat diets which contain lower levels of vitamin C than those necessary to provide protection.

Vitamin C supplementation may help to protect against smoking-related damage. It may help to decrease the smoking-related build-up of atherosclerotic plaque by limiting the amount of white blood cells which stick to artery walls.[8] In a German study done in 1996, supplements were effective in restoring reduced plasma vitamin C concentractions.[9] Like those with high cholesterol levels and coronary heart disease, the arteries of smokers have a reduced ability to dilate. Vitamin C supplements may counteract this impairment.[10]

There have been several large trials examining the effects of antioxidant supplements in smokers. These include the CARET and ATBC studies, which recently reported that large doses of beta carotene may actually increase the risk of lung cancer in smokers. In the ATBC study, the adverse effects appeared stronger in men who drank alcohol and in those who smoked 20 cigarettes a day than in those who smoked less. This is confirmed by the CARET results which showed greater risk in current smokers than former smokers and also in those who drank alcohol. (See page 54 for more information.)

Tobacco smoke may damage beta carotene in ways which cause it to become harmful to body cells. Laboratory research shows that vitamin C may protect against these harmful effects suggesting that, in smokers, vitamin C supplementation should accompany beta carotene supplementation.[11] Vitamin E may also provide protection against the oxidative damage caused by cigarette smoke.

B vitamins

Cigarette smoke may cause a folic acid deficiency in the cells lining the lungs, making them susceptible to damage, which may lead to cancer. Folic acid may also help to prevent the pre-cancerous changes in lung tissue caused by smoking.[12] Heavy smoking may also inactivate vitamin B12.

Antacids

Antacids are commonly used to neutralize stomach acid in cases where excess causes pain. They are also used to treat a condition known as reflux esophagitis where the stomach acid comes up into the esophagus and causes painful inflammation of the membrane lining. This causes heartburn, indigestion or dyspepsia. Cigarettes, coffee, chocolate and fatty foods aggravate the condition. Most indigestion is related to dietary or alcoholic excess, and antacid use is fairly common.

Antacids contain a metal ion, aluminum, magnesium, calcium or sodium, linked to an alkali. Most antacids are a mixture of different ions which minimizes side effects. Long-term use of antacids that contain aluminum hydroxide may inhibit calcium absorption and increase the risk of calcium deficiency and bone disorders. Sodium-containing antacids interfere with calcium absorption and can increase the risk of high blood pressure. Regular use of calcium-containing antacids can be a good source of calcium in the diet but may lead to magnesium and chromium deficiency with long-term use.

As antacids reduce the acidity of the stomach environment, the activity of digestive enzymes is inhibited and absorption of nutrients which require an acid environment for absorption is reduced. These include iron, calcium, zinc, chromium, niacin, folic acid, vitamin A, thiamin and vitamin B12. This reduction in absorption of vitamins and minerals can be lessened if the antacid is taken on an empty stomach rather than with food.

Antibiotics

Antibiotics are widely used in the treatment of infections. Antibiotic-induced vitamin and mineral deficiencies are unlikely to be a problem if the diet is good and use is short-term.

Vitamins

Patients on long-term therapy with some antibiotics can develop deficiencies in some B vitamins, as intestinal bacteria that produce vital nutrients are killed along with the harmful bacteria. These deficiencies could have potentially serious effects, especially for elderly people, and supplements are helpful in preventing them. Long-term use of antibiotics may produce vitamin K deficiency and blood clotting disorders. Antibiotics can kill not only harmful bacteria but also the beneficial bacteria that produce vitamin K. Antibiotics may reduce vitamin C stores.

The antibiotic, isoniazid, which is often used to treat tuberculosis, can cause nerve damage due to its inhibition of vitamin B6 action. Patients with diabetes, malnutrition, or alcoholism may be at higher risk and supplements may be useful to protect against these problems. Several other antibiotics may adversely affect vitamin functions: neomycin interferes with the absorption of vitamin B12 and vitamin D; some antibiotics may cause niacin flushes to become more severe; trimethoprim can raise folic acid requirements; and chloramphenicol may interfere with the red blood cell functions of vitamin B12. There have been reports of benign intracranial hypertension during concurrent use of vitamin A and tetracycline.

Minerals

Tetracycline antibiotics reduce calcium, zinc, iron and magnesium absorption, and calcium salts and magnesium salts that are present in foods and dairy products can form chelates with tetracyclines and cause impaired absorption. The antibacterial efficacy of tetracyclines may be reduced by concurrent use of zinc salts such as zinc sulfate.

Neomycin affects calcium, iron and potassium absorption. Iron may decrease absorption of tetracyclines, penicillamine, ciprofloxacin or norfloxacin. Antibiotics can deplete potassium if taken long-term.

Anticancer medications

Malnutrition is a major cause of deterioration and death in cancer patients, and the effects of anticancer drugs may contribute to this. Good nutrition during chemotherapy can help people cope better with the side effects from the powerful drugs, fight infection more easily and speed recovery of healthy tissue. It is important that the diet includes enough calories to maintain weight and protein to build and repair tissues. A diet high in vitamins and minerals is also very important. In some cases, vitamin and mineral supplements may be useful. However, they should never be taken without a doctor's approval.

Several types of drugs may be used in combination with other types of therapy such as radiation or surgery. The type of therapy depends on the type of cancer, the location and extent and the patient's general health. Anticancer drugs may be given intravenously, intramuscularly, via catheters, topically or orally. It is important that a doctor is aware of any medications taken before chemotherapy is started or during treatment. This includes vitamin and mineral supplements.

Side effects vary from person to person and from drug to drug. Anticancer drugs are designed to kill fast-growing cancer cells and therefore also affect other body cells which are fast-growing, such as cells in the bone marrow, digestive tract, reproductive system and hair follicles. The most common side effects are hair loss, nausea and vomiting, fatigue, susceptibility to infection, and anemia. Recovery time depends on the type of treatment and general health.

Cancer chemotherapy has many side effects, including some nutritional ones. These powerful drugs often affect the digestive system and reduce the desire to eat. Common side effects include sore or dry mouth, altered taste sensation, nausea and vomiting. Diarrhea, constipation and reduced absorption are also common. Nausea and vomiting can be limited by avoiding big meals, eating and drinking slowly, avoiding fatty and sweet foods, and resting after eating.

Keeping mouth, gums and throat healthy can be helped by brushing gently with a soft, clean toothbrush. Mouth sores which prevent eating can be treated with medication. Eating soft, soothing foods, cold or at room temperature; and avoiding irritating, spicy, salty, acidic foods or rough dry foods can also help ease discomfort. Drinking plenty of water, using artificial saliva and sucking candy can help relieve a dry mouth.

If chemotherapy leads to diarrhea, potassium-rich foods are important. Low fiber foods, drinking plenty of water and avoiding fatty, spiced foods, tea, coffee and alcohol can be beneficial. Constipation can be relieved by drinking plenty of fluids, eating high fiber foods and exercising.

Chemotherapy can affect the bone marrow's ability to make red blood cells, leading to anemia. Getting plenty of rest and eating a diet rich in essential nutrients such as iron, folic acid and vitamin B12 can help lessen these effects.

The anticancer drug, methotrexate, alters folic acid metabolism. It acts by suppressing the multiplication of rapidly dividing cancer cells as these cells rely more heavily on folic acid. However, healthy cells also need folic acid and are affected by methotrexate. Folic acid supplements may be taken when on this drug but this should only be under medical supervision. Recent research suggests that long-term treatment with methotrexate also causes loss of bone mineral density.[13] High doses of riboflavin can reduce the effectiveness of methotrexate.

Vitamin C

Some controversy surrounds the use of vitamin C in the treatment of cancer. The Nobel Prize winner, Linus Pauling and his colleagues have used vitamin C to improve survival times in cancer patients, but these results have not been repeated in other studies. Vitamin C may also benefit cancer patients who are undergoing radiation treatment by enabling them to withstand greater doses of radiation with fewer side effects.[14]

Zinc

Zinc supplements have been used to improve taste perception in people taking medications which reduce taste sensation and in cancer patients undergoing radiation therapy.[15] This can be valuable in helping to maintain normal weight and nutrient intake during treatment.

Anticoagulants

Anticoagulant drugs such as warfarin decrease the clotting ability of the blood and are often used to treat heart problems. They act by interfering with the vitamin K-dependent clotting factors. Large doses of vitamin K may interfere with the action of these drugs and are not usually given to people who are taking them. Those taking anticoagulants should keep their intake of vitamin K foods relatively constant. Large doses of vitamin C may also affect the action of anticoagulants.

Vitamin E can enhance the action of anticoagulant drugs on blood clotting and should not be taken in very large doses. However, the results of a 1996 study in which 21 people taking chronic warfarin therapy received either vitamin E or placebo suggest that vitamin E can safely be given to patients who require chronic warfarin therapy.[16]

Anticonvulsants

Anticonvulsant drugs such as phenytoin, phenobarbital, primidone and carbamazepine are used in the treatment of epilepsy. These drugs can affect the metabolism of several vitamins and minerals.

Vitamin D

Long-term use of anticonvulsants may lead to a loss of calcium from bone due to the adverse effect of the medication on the manufacture of vitamin D. It is often recommended that anyone on long-term anticonvulsant therapy take a vitamin D supplement.

Folic acid

Phenytoin, phenobarbital and primidone interfere with the action of folic acid. This may lead to deficiency which can cause anemia and birth defects. Supplementation may be necessary, particularly in pregnant women, but large doses should be used with caution as they can interfere with the effectiveness of the drug and lead to seizure breakthrough. The increase in red blood cell production stimulated by folic acid may also increase the need for vitamin B12.

Vitamin K

Vitamin K levels may also drop on long-term anticonvulsant therapy and supplements are often recommended, particularly for pregnant women as a deficiency can result in an increased risk of hemorrhage in a newborn baby.

Others

Anticonvulsants may lower plasma vitamin E levels by altering absorption, distribution and metabolism. Copper and zinc levels may also be lowered by long-term anticonvulsant therapy.

Antidepressants

The long-term use of antidepressants can affect nutrient intake as these drugs often reduce appetite via effects on mood and the gastrointestinal system. They may also increase excretion of many nutrients. B vitamins (which are often low in those with depression), vitamin C, calcium and magnesium may be particularly affected and supplements may be beneficial in many people. The activation of riboflavin in the liver may be inhibited by major tranquilizers and some antidepressants. Supplements may be beneficial in those taking these drugs on a long-term basis.

Low folate levels have been linked to poorer response to the antidepressant drug, Prozac. In a study published in 1997, researchers examined the relationships between levels of folate, vitamin B12, and homocysteine in 213 depressed patients taking Prozac. The results showed that people with low folate levels were more likely to have melancholic depression and were significantly less likely to respond to the drug.[17]

Lithium

Lithium therapy can cause low sodium levels by reducing re-absorption by the kidney. Lithium should be used with caution in patients following low salt diets. Lithium may also affect calcium and magnesium metabolism and decrease bone mineral content.

Anti-inflammatory medications

The antigout drug, colchicine, reduces the absorption of vitamin B12, increases tissue loss of calcium and potassium and reduces the absorption of folic acid, iron and vitamin A. Nonsteroidal anti-inflammatory drugs (NSAIDS) may cause kidney damage, leading to high potassium levels.

Sulfasalazine can inhibit the absorption and lower the plasma concentrations of folic acid. Thiamin and riboflavin requirements may also increase. Indomethacin may impair vitamin C and thiamin metabolism.

Beta blockers

Beta blockers, which are used to treat high blood pressure and some other types of cardiovascular disease, have been shown to interfere with the production and function of coenzyme Q10, and to adversely affect heart function. This may explain why, in some cases, long-term therapy with beta blockers can lead to congestive heart failure. Coenzyme Q10 therapy in combination with beta blockers may be beneficial.

Corticosteroids

Corticosteroid drugs are widely used in medical treatment for autoimmune diseases such as arthritis, chronic obstructive lung disease, asthma and allergic conditions. Treatment with high doses of corticosteroids causes osteoporosis, particularly in the type of bone found in the lumbar spine.

Corticosteroid cause osteoporosis by several mechanisms; they decrease levels of sex hormones and also directly affect the cells which build and break down bone. They also decrease the absorption of calcium from the intestine. Corticosteroids may also raise folic acid, vitamin B6 and vitamin C requirements.

Vitamin D and calcium supplements may be useful in preventing bone loss in patients taking corticosteroids. In a 1996 study, researchers showed that calcium and vitamin D supplements can help prevent this loss. In the two-year study, 96 patients with rheumatoid arthritis, 65 of whom were taking corticosteroid drugs, were given 1000 mg calcium and 500 IU vitamin D per day or placebo. The researchers analyzed the bone mineral density of the lumbar spine and femur for one a year. In those patients taking corticosteroid drugs and placebo, losses of bone mineral density were seen. In those taking the supplements, gains were seen; and in those not taking corticosteroids, the supplements did not appear to affect bone mineral density.[18]

Arthritis medications

D penicillamine is used in severe and disabling rheumatoid arthritis. It may affect nutrient intake by causing loss of appetite and gastrointestinal disturbances. It can also reduce absorption of iron and zinc and should not be taken with foods containing these minerals. Experts suggest that at least a two-hour period should elapse between the administration of iron salts and oral penicillamine doses. Vitamin B6 needs may also be increased with long-term use of D penicillamine. Supplements in doses of 25 mg per day may be useful.

Aspirin

Aspirin is used as a painkilling and temperature-reducing drug. Frequent use of aspirin may cause bleeding in the stomach and intestines. This may lead to iron deficiency if aspirin is taken for long periods. Patients with vitamin K deficiency should use aspirin cautiously as increased bleeding may result. Vitamin A may protect against stomach ulcers and bleeding in those taking aspirin.

Aspirin may also lead to deficiencies of folic acid, thiamin, vitamin C, potassium and vitamin B12 if used for a long time. Calcium decreases the absorption of aspirin if taken at the same time. The nicotinamide form of niacin causes flushing when taken in large doses. This is caused by blood vessel dilatation, and pretreatment with aspirin may inhibit this effect, which some people find unpleasant.

Asthma medications

Long-term therapy with theophylline, a drug often given to asthmatic patients, lowers vitamin B6 levels. Vitamin B6 supplements may be useful in preventing the side effects of the drug which include headaches, nausea, sleep disorders and convulsions.[19]

Caffeine

Caffeine may increase calcium and potassium losses and reduce zinc absorption. This may contribute to disorders such as high blood pressure and osteoporosis. Caffeine may also raise thiamin requirements. Most studies suggest that the harmful effects of caffeine occur in those who drink more than two cups of coffee per day.

Cardiovascular disease medications

The effect of the heart stimulant drug, digoxin, can be toxic when magnesium and potassium concentrations are too low and when calcium is too high. However, digoxin may not be effective in patients with low calcium levels and small amounts of supplements may be necessary. It is recommended that serum potassium and calcium be monitored regularly in patients receiving digoxin. Digoxin may also lead to thiamin deficiency.

Cholesterol-lowering drugs

In recent years, the 'statin' drugs, lovastatin, pravastatin, and simvastatin have become widely used to treat high blood cholesterol. These medications work by inhibiting an enzyme known as HMG-CoA reductase, and they are very effective in lowering cholesterol levels. However, this enzyme is also responsible for production of coenzyme Q10. Because of this, the cholesterol-lowering effect of these drugs is accompanied by an equivalent lowering of coenzyme Q10 levels. In patients with existing heart failure, lovastatin has been shown to cause increased heart disease with life-threatening results in some patients. Coenzyme Q10 supplements may help to prevent some of the adverse effects of these widely used drugs.

The cholesterol-lowering drug, cholestyramine, reduces the absorption of fat soluble vitamins A, D, E and K, and may lead to deficiencies. Water soluble supplements of these vitamins may be useful. Folic acid, vitamin B12 and iron levels may also be adversely affected, leading to anemia. Cholestyramine may also increase calcium excretion. Colestipol may also lead to folic acid and fat soluble vitamin deficiencies. Niacin may increase the effectiveness of colestipol.

Diabetes medications

The antidiabetic drug, metformin, can inhibit the absorption of vitamin B12, leading to anemia. Other B vitamin deficiencies are also common in patients taking this drug. Niacin may affect the control of blood sugar in diabetics and should be used with caution in patients taking metformin.

Estrogen therapy

Estrogen-containing drugs include oral contraceptives and the hormones used in hormone replacement therapy (HRT). They are often used for long periods and can affect the absorption and use of several nutrients. Some of these effects are beneficial and others may be harmful.

Antioxidants

It has been suggested that estrogen can increase the risk of certain cancers, including those of the breast and cervix. These links have not been confirmed but some studies suggest that estrogen may increase free radical formation. If this is the case, antioxidant vitamin supplements may be useful in protecting against oxidative damage. Oral contraceptive use may also decrease vitamin C and beta carotene levels.[20] Large doses of vitamin C may cause higher blood levels of estrogen when taken at the same time as the contraceptive pill. It is best to take vitamin C supplements separately.

Calcium

HRT is used to increase bone mineral metabolism in postmenopausal women who are at risk of osteoporosis. Estrogen increases calcium absorption, decreases calcium excretion and increases vitamin D levels, thus improving the deposition of calcium into bone.

Folate

Some research suggests that there is a higher risk of abnormalities in cervical tissue in women using oral contraceptives. Supplements are beneficial in preventing cervical dysplasia in these women.[21] (See page 585 for more information.)

Vitamin B6

As estrogen may affect vitamin B6 metabolism and increase needs,[22] supplements may be beneficial for pregnant women, those on the contraceptive pill or those on hormone replacement therapy (HRT) who suffer from mood swings and depression. Vitamin B6 is sometimes known as the women's vitamin.

Other nutrients

Blood levels of vitamin B12, thiamin, riboflavin, magnesium and zinc may be lowered by the contraceptive pill. Copper and vitamin A levels may be raised. The contraceptive pill may reduce menstrual bleeding which decreases iron loss.

High blood pressure medications

There are various types of high blood pressure medications and these vary in their effects on vitamins and minerals. ACE inhibitors such as enalapril raise potassium levels. They should not be used with potassium supplements as heart problems can occur with excessive levels. People taking potassium sparing diuretics such as spironolactone should also avoid potassium supplements as body levels may become too high. Spironolactone may also reduce the availability of vitamin A. Loop diuretics such as bumetanide may cause excessive potassium loss and supplements may be necessary.

Low potassium levels is one of the most common adverse effects associated with thiazide diuretic therapy and can lead to cardiac arrhythmias. This effect is especially important to consider in patients receiving cardiac glycoside therapy (such as digoxin) because potassium depletion increases the risk of toxicity of this drug. Potassium supplements may be necessary in such cases, although they should be used cautiously in patients receiving digoxin. Thiazide diuretics may also decrease calcium excretion and increase magnesium excretion. Magnesium supplements may be useful in patients on long-term diuretic therapy. Zinc absorption may also be reduced. Hydralazine may increase the demand for vitamin B6 as it enhances excretion. Long-term use of frusemide may lead to thiamin deficiency.

Laxatives

Long-term use or overdosage can cause abdominal pain, nausea/vomiting, loss of weight, muscle weakness, laxative dependence, and low potassium and calcium levels. Mineral oil laxatives bind fat soluble vitamins and reduce absorption.

Osteoporosis medications

Taking oral etidronate with vitamin and mineral supplements that contain calcium salts, iron salts such as ferrous sulfate or magnesium salts may be inadvisable. These salts can interfere with the absorption of etidronate, and should not be taken within two hours of the drug. Even though calcium salts should not be taken at the same time as etidronate, patients need to maintain an adequate intake of calcium and vitamin D to avoid low calcium levels.

Psoriasis medications

The vitamin D-derivative drug, calcipotriene, should not be used with high doses of vitamin D and calcium.

Thyroid medications

Excess intake of iodine/iodide can decrease the efficacy of propylthiouracil.

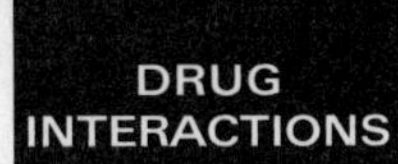

Sedatives and tranquilizers

Barbiturate drugs may enhance excretion and metabolism of vitamin C, and reduce the conversion of vitamin D to its active form.

Vitamin A-derivative drugs

Vitamin A supplements should not be used with the vitamin A-derivative drugs tretinoin, isotretinoin and etretinate. These drugs are used to treat skin disorders such as acne and can be toxic if taken with high levels of dietary vitamin A.

Health problems

Health Problems

The concept of using food to treat ill health is thousands of years old. As far back as 400 BC Hippocrates said "Let food be your medicine and medicine be your food" but it is only in recent years that modern science has enabled us to start to discover and understand the thousands of disease-fighting chemicals in our food. It is now recognized that nutrition has a vital role to play in the prevention and treatment of some of the most prevalent diseases in our society. In the early part of the twentieth century, interest in nutritional science was heightened by the discovery of the first vitamin and its ability to cure a specific disease. Other discoveries followed and common disorders such as scurvy and pellagra were cured by including vitamin rich foods in people's diets.

In the Western world today, severe vitamin and mineral deficiency diseases such as these are rare. In fact, many of the most common diseases in our society are caused by consuming too much of some foods and not enough of others. Diets overloaded with fat, protein, sugar and salt combined with long-term marginal intake of some essential nutrients increase the risk of developing many diseases. Nutrition can also powerfully affect mood, intelligence and mental health.

New scientific discoveries are constantly enhancing our understanding of the role that diet plays in health and disease and there is now good evidence that high intake of certain vitamins and minerals prevents and treats some diseases. However, new findings lead to new questions and it is likely that in the future, nutritional science will expand into areas that can presently only be imagined.

It is important to remember that diet is only one of the factors influencing susceptibility to disease. The information given in this book is not intended to replace appropriate medical investigation and treatment. Foods or supplements should not be substituted for medication without a doctor's approval. This information is not intended as medical advice and individual questions are best answered by a qualified medical practitioner.

Acne

Acne, the most common of all skin problems, is an inflammatory disease of the oil-producing glands in the skin. It usually affects teenagers, although about 20 per cent of cases occur in adults. There are many types of acne, with acne vulgaris being the most common.

Symptoms of acne

Acne is usually divided into two main types, superficial and deep. Superficial acne consists of persistent, recurrent red spots or swellings on the skin. These are known as pimples and they usually occur on the face; but the back, chest, shoulders and neck can also be affected. Spots that bulge under the skin and have no opening are known as whiteheads, while dark pimples with open pores at the center are known as blackheads. Inflamed, fluid-filled lumps known as nodules and cysts can occur occasionally. In deep acne, deep inflamed nodules and pus-filled cysts occur, and these may become abscesses. Scarring becomes more likely as the lesions get deeper.

Causes of acne

There are small glands at the base of hair follicles, known as sebaceous glands, which secrete an oily material called sebum. During puberty, hormonal changes cause these glands to grow larger and produce excess sebum. The cells that line the hair shaft canal are also stimulated to produce more keratin, a fibrous protein which is found in skin and hair.

Acne begins when the openings of these sebaceous glands become plugged with dead skin cells, debris, bacteria and sebum. As the plug grows, it may become visible on the surface of the skin as a whitehead. Contact with air can cause the plug to darken and become a blackhead. When the gland opening is blocked, certain types of bacteria can overgrow and release enzymes which break down sebum and cause inflammation.

Acne is more common in males because they have higher levels of the hormones that stimulate oil and keratin production. Genetic factors may make certain people more susceptible to acne and it is possible that sufferers have higher levels of an enzyme which converts the male hormone testosterone to a more active form. Acne sufferers may also be more susceptible to the increase in sebum production. Acne does not occur because of excessively oily skin or improper cleaning, although these may worsen the symptoms. Another relatively common misconception is that acne is related to sexual activity. This is not the case.

Allergic reactions to certain foods, heat and humidity may make the symptoms of acne worse. In some women who develop acne in their 20s and 30s, aggravation by skin cosmetics may be the cause. Some medications, including anticonvulsants, lithium, anabolic steroids and some types of contraceptive pill, may also exacerbate acne. Acne is usually worse in winter and better in summer due to the beneficial effect of sunlight.

Sudden appearance of acne in adults appears to be on the increase and may be linked to hormonal imbalances. In some women, acne is worse before menstruation, possibly due to increased progesterone secretion. In some cases, acne may become clear or worsen during pregnancy.

While teenage acne almost always heals spontaneously in early adulthood, appropriate treatment can reduce the duration and severity of the disease, and help to avoid complications such as scarring.

Treatment of acne

Acne treatment depends on the severity of the lesions. Washing skin properly with warm water and nonperfumed soap, avoiding oily cosmetics and abrasive scrubs, and regular shampooing of hair to stop it becoming too oily can help to control acne. It is important to minimize the effects of pressure from tight collars or helmets, perspiration and touching, scrubbing and rubbing affected areas. Stress also causes an increase in certain hormones which can affect the severity of acne, and relaxation techniques may be useful in improving symptoms.

Picking and squeezing pimples can result in infection and scarring and should be avoided. There is no instant or permanent cure for acne, although it can be controlled and proper treatment will prevent scarring.

Medications

Mild cases of acne may be treated with various medicated creams and solutions, both prescription and nonprescription. Benzoyl peroxide, which is used on all acne-prone areas of the skin, can prevent as well as treat acne, and is used even when the face is clear. Side effects include burning, excessive drying and redness. Other treatments include clindamycin solution, tretinoin cream and azelaic acid cream.

Oral antibiotics such as tetracycline and minocycline are sometimes prescribed for moderate or severe cases, especially when there is a lot of acne on the back or chest. They reduce the bacteria in the hair follicles. It is usually found that acne symptoms recur after short periods of antibiotic treatment and long-term therapy may be necessary. However there are adverse side effects associated with long term antibiotic use.

Vitamin A-derivative drugs

Synthetic vitamin A-derivative drugs known as retinoids are used to treat cases of severe acne which have not responded to other treatment or which have only shown partial response to antibiotic therapy. There are topical and oral forms of these drugs and they are available on prescription. Visits to a doctor or dermatologist are necessary to monitor the side effects which include dryness and inflammation of the lips, conjunctivitis, photosensitivity, arthritis, bone abnormalities and depression. These drugs can cause birth defects if taken during pregnancy and should also be avoided by breastfeeding women.

Isotretinoin

Isotretinoin (Accutane) is derived from naturally occurring retinoic acid, which is related to vitamin A. It acts to reduce oil production by reducing the size of the sebaceous glands and also exerts anti-inflammatory effects. It is taken by mouth, with food. Care needs to be taken when giving isotretinoin to people with diabetes, alcoholism, inflammatory bowel disease, liver disease and obesity, or those with high blood fat levels.

Tretinoin

Tretinoin is similar to isotretinoin but is more toxic. It prevents the build-up of keratin and increases the turnover of epithelial cells. This prevents the formation of new spots. There are rare reports of nerve damage with topical tretinoin. Symptoms include headaches, depression and memory loss.

Adapalene

Adapalene is a new retinoid which is used on the skin in gel form. Studies have shown that it is as effective as tretinoin gel but is less irritating to the skin.

Hormonal treatment

In women whose acne seems to be particularly related to menstruation, oral contraceptives may relieve symptoms.

Diet and acne

While it does not seem that acne is a food-related problem, oily and sugary foods may exacerbate the symptoms. Foods such as shellfish, iodized salt and milk, which are high in iodine, may also exacerbate acne and should be avoided.[1] Alcohol and tobacco should also be avoided.

Poor nutrition adversely affects the immune system and increases the likelihood of developing infections and inflammatory responses while a healthy low fat, high fiber, nutrient dense diet can boost immunity, reduce inflammation and improve symptoms. While no scientific studies have proven links with any particular food, food allergies may cause acne. Avoiding allergenic foods and improving digestive function may help relieve acne.

Vitamins, minerals and acne

Vitamin A

Dietary vitamin A may reduce sebum production by affecting sebaceous gland activity, but there is no firm evidence that vitamin A can be effective in the treatment of acne at nontoxic doses. Vitamin A supplements should not be taken with vitamin A-derivative acne drugs as this greatly increases the likelihood of toxic side effects.

B vitamins

B vitamins are important for healthy skin function. Vitamin B6 can be useful in treating premenstrual flare up of acne, possibly due to its ability to affect steroid hormone action.[2] Most experts recommend taking it in the second half of the menstrual cycle, that is, one week before and during menstruation. The typical dose is 50 mg per day. Niacin may also be helpful in acne treatment as it improves blood flow to the skin. (See page 79 for more information.)

Nicotinamide (niacin) gel has been used as a topical treatment for acne and was shown in a 1995 study to have comparable effects to the antibiotic, clindamycin. Because clindamycin, like other antibiotics, is associated with the development of resistant bacteria, nicotinamide gel is a useful alternative treatment for acne.[3]

Zinc

Zinc supplements may be useful in the treatment of acne. Serum zinc levels are often low in adolescent boys, who are especially prone to acne.[4] Zinc is involved in many functions which could affect the symptoms of acne. These include hormone activation, regulation of oil-producing gland activity, wound-healing, immune system activity, inflammation and tissue regeneration. High concentrations of zinc decrease the conversion of testosterone to its active form, thus reducing the stimulatory effects on the oil glands.

The results of studies using zinc treatment for acne are mixed. Zinc supplements have been beneficial in reducing the spots and oiliness in some acne sufferers. The inconsistency of the results may be due to the variation in the types of supplements used. Typical doses used to treat acne range from 15 to 30 mg per day.[5,6]

Other vitamin and mineral supplements

Antioxidants such as vitamin E, vitamin C and selenium may help to reduce inflammation and boost the effectiveness of the immune system which can help to reduce infection. It can be difficult to obtain large doses of these vitamins and minerals in the diet and supplements may be useful. Typical doses are 134 to 268 mg alpha TE (200 to 400 IU) for vitamin E, 200 to 500 mg for vitamin C, and 200 mcg for selenium. High chromium yeast has been used to treat acne with some success.[7]

Other supplements and acne

Essential fatty acids

Some research suggests that abnormalities in fatty acid metabolism may contribute to acne.[8] Because of their anti-inflammatory effects, essential fatty acids may be useful in the treatment of acne. Good sources include flaxseed oil and evening primrose oil (See page 329 for more information.)

Herbal medicine and acne

There are several herbal medicines which can be used to alleviate the infectious and inflammatory processes which occur in acne. These include pot marigold *(Calendula officinalis*) which can be used as facial wash, echinacea (*Echinacea angustifolia or E. purpurea*), tea tree oil (*Melaleuca spp*) and goldenseal (*Hydrastis canadensis*).

An important part of a herbal treatment program would also involve blood cleansing and improving elimination of toxins. Herbs that may be useful for this include blue flag (*Iris versicolor*), cleavers (*Galium aparine*), nettles (*Urtica dioica*), burdock root (*Arctium lappa*) and red clover (*Trifolium pratense*). See page 384 for more information on these herbs and the precautions that may be necessary.

Alzheimer's disease is a type of mental deterioration in which sufferers experience a steady and progressive loss of intellectual function due to degenerative changes in the brain. It is the fourth leading cause of death in the USA; and by the age of 80, around one person in three has the disease. Approximately two million people in the USA are currently affected by the disease with women twice as susceptible as men. As the population ages, experts estimate that by 2050 there will be almost 9 million sufferers.

The symptoms of Alzheimer's disease

The most common early symptom of Alzheimer's disease is memory loss. This develops gradually and at first almost imperceptibly, with symptoms that resemble ordinary memory lapses. Other intellectual functions such as comprehension and language skills also deteriorate until the person loses the ability to learn and remember anything new. Familiar places and people become unrecognizable and ordinary activities become increasingly difficult. Sufferers often become irritable, restless and easily agitated. They may become disorientated and wander off and get lost. In the later stages of the disease, they are unable to carry out daily activities and become dependent on others for basic needs such as eating and washing.

When symptoms occur before age 65, the disease is referred to as presenile dementia of the Alzheimer's type; and after 65 as senile dementia of the Alzheimer's type. The average time a person survives with the disease is seven years, although some patients may live for up to 20 years.

Diagnosis of Alzheimer's disease

The only way to definitely confirm the presence of Alzheimer's disease is to perform a brain biopsy which is obviously not possible when the person is alive. Because of this, a physician diagnoses the disease based on physical, neurological and psychiatric signs. However, diagnosis is difficult as the symptoms of the disease are similar to those seen in other disorders; such as other types of dementia, anemia, depression, drug side effects and nutritional deficiencies. Alzheimer's disease is often diagnosed when these other causes have been ruled out. Research has shown that Alzheimer's disease is often unrecognized.[1] Advances in technology such as brain imaging and testing may make it easier to diagnose the disease.

Changes in the brain in Alzheimer's disease

In Alzheimer's disease, there is general destruction of nerve cells in several key areas of the brain devoted to mental functions. Nerve fibers grow tangled and protein deposits known as plaques build-up in the nerve cells. These plaques are usually made up of compounds known as beta amyloid peptides, which are toxic to nerve cells. There is also a reduction in brain neurotransmitters, including acetylcholine.

Causes of Alzheimer's disease

Although people are more likely to develop Alzheimer's disease as they grow older, it is not a natural result of the aging process. There is currently an enormous amount of research being carried out into possible causes, identification and treatment of Alzheimer's disease. It seems likely that several factors are involved in the development of the disease.

Genetic factors

Family history and twin studies suggest that there is likely to be a genetic component to Alzheimer's disease. It seems that several gene mutations are linked to the disease. Recent research in this area has centered around a blood protein known as APO-E which acts as a natural antioxidant and protects nerve cells against free radical damage. It occurs in several different forms and, as with all proteins, these forms are determined by genes. People with one particular form of the gene, known as APO-E4 seem to be at higher risk of Alzheimer's disease. Patients with the gene are also likely to get the disease at an earlier than average age. Scientists are also discovering other genetic factors which appear to increase the risk of Alzheimer's disease. These discoveries may lead to a test which could identify those at risk of the disease in its early stages, thus enabling treatment to be started before damage to brain cells progresses too far.

Oxidative damage and inflammation

Research suggests that abnormalities in oxidative metabolism may play an important role in Alzheimer's disease. Free radicals may be involved in the formation of the plaques of beta amyloid protein seen in the brains of Alzheimer's patients. People with Down Syndrome are more susceptible to Alzheimer's disease and there is evidence that the neuronal degeneration seen in Down Syndrome may be due to oxidative damage.

Inflammation may also be an important part of the Alzheimer's disease process. Anti-inflammatory drugs such as ibuprofen appear to reduce the risk of developing the disease.[2]

Environmental toxins

Some experts believe that environmental toxins contribute to Alzheimer's disease. Research indicates that Alzheimer's disease is more prevalent in certain cultural environments. Results from the Honolulu-Asia Aging Study showed that Japanese men who live and grow old in Hawaii are twice as likely to develop Alzheimer's disease as Japanese men who live and grow old in Japan.[3] The reasons for this are unknown, although environmental and dietary factors may play a part.

Some experts believe that aluminum may play a role in the development of Alzheimer's disease. The plaques and tangles in the brains of people with Alzheimer's disease often contain aluminum compounds. Foods made with baking powder as well as some antiperspirants and antacids contain aluminum compounds, which can also be absorbed from pots and pans used to cook acidic foods. But aluminum is one of the most common substances on earth, and very little of it is absorbed by healthy bodies. Neither people with peptic ulcers who use large amounts of antacids nor metal workers constantly exposed to aluminum have an especially high rate of Alzheimer's disease. It seems likely that the accumulation of aluminum in plaques and tangles is probably a result rather than a cause of the brain damage that produces dementia.

Researchers have found that children of young fathers are more susceptible to the disease. Studies suggest that the rate of Alzheimer's disease declines steadily with increase in the father's age: the child of a 15-year-old is at four times higher risk than the child of a 65-year-old.

Treatment of Alzheimer's disease

There is currently no known cure for Alzheimer's disease and it has not been possible to stop or reverse the brain damage that occurs. Most available drugs only have a temporary effect on the progression of the disease. Those that have been used include hydergine, piracetam, acetyl-L-carnitine, selegiline, tacrine and donezepil. Other drugs now being investigated include anti-inflammatory drugs, hormone replacement therapy and nerve growth factors.

Other types of drugs have been used to treat the common symptoms of the disease such as anxiety, depression and disturbed sleeping patterns.

As it is likely that Alzheimer's disease involves several steps, it is possible that therapy may one day involve the combined use of several types of drugs with small effects on individual steps.

There are several studies which suggest that estrogen therapy can reduce the risk of Alzheimer's disease in postmenopausal women, possibly due to its action as an antioxidant or its effect on nerve growth factors.

Diet and Alzheimer's disease

Poor nutrition is related to Alzheimer's disease, although whether this is a cause or a result of the disease is not clear. A diet which is lacking in essential vitamins and minerals may increase the risk of Alzheimer's disease. Loss of interest in food and inability to prepare and eat nutritious food in the later stages of the disease may also contribute to deterioration of a patient's condition.

The results of a recent study suggest that a high fat diet may be linked to the development of Alzheimer's disease.[4] Researchers found that in countries where people eat diets high in fat, there is a higher prevalence of Alzheimer's disease. However, it is likely that other factors also play a part.

In another study, researchers at Case Western Reserve University are investigating lifestyle histories of 104 Alzheimer's disease patients and 223 people who do not have the disease. Preliminary results after five years are showing that those people without the disease are consuming significantly greater amounts of antioxidant nutrients: alpha carotene, beta carotene, lutein, lycopene and vitamin C; and significantly more servings of fruits and vegetables.[5]

Other types of dementia

The second most common cause of dementia is multi-infarct dementia. This is also irreversible and results from a series of small strokes that damage arteries supplying blood to the brain. Diet may play a role in preventing and controlling this form of dementia through effects on blood pressure and other risk factors.

The third most common cause of dementia appears to be excessive alcohol intake, due to the direct effects of alcohol on nerves and also to the effects of alcohol on nutritional status. Alcoholic dementia may be at least partially reversible with abstinence and good nutrition. Other causes are vitamin B12 and folic acid deficiencies; these are reversible dementias. In all types of dementia, adequate nutrition may improve physical wellbeing and improve the quality of life.

Vitamins, minerals and Alzheimer's disease

Antioxidants

As there is evidence that oxidative damage plays a role in the tissue injury seen in Alzheimer's disease,[6] antioxidants may have a role to play in preventing the brain from free radical damage. Studies have shown that certain parts of the brains of Alzheimer's disease sufferers may be more susceptible to free radical damage than those without the disease. Antioxidant supplements may reduce this susceptibility.[7]

Patients with Alzheimer's disease have been shown to have lower levels of vitamins A, C, E and zinc. In one study, serum concentrations of vitamins A and E and major carotenes were determined in patients with Alzheimer's disease, multi-infarct dementia and control subjects. The results showed that both Alzheimer's and multi-infarct dementia patients had significantly lower levels of vitamin E and beta carotene than controls.[8]

Vitamin E

As an antioxidant, vitamin E may have a role to play in preventing the oxidative damage seen in Alzheimer's disease. In a 1997 study done in the US, researchers looked at the effects of vitamin E and the drug, selegiline, on the clinical deterioration seen in Alzheimer's disease. The study involved 341 patients who were divided into four groups. One group received selegiline, another received 1000 IU (670 mg) of vitamin E, another group received both, and the last group received a placebo. The patients were followed to see when they reached one of the following endpoints: death, institutionalization, inability to do certain basic activities of daily living, or severe dementia. The results showed that treatment with either selegiline or vitamin E slowed progression of the disease.[9]

Vitamin B12

Vitamin B12 deficiency can produce symptoms which include confusion, memory changes, delirium and depression. Alzheimer's disease sufferers may be prone to vitamin B12 deficiency[10] and some studies have shown a relationship between vitamin B12 levels and the severity of mental impairment in Alzheimer's disease.[11]

In another study, intravenous vitamin B12 was shown to improve intellectual functions such as memory, emotional functions and communication in patients with Alzheimer's disease. Improvements in cognitive functions were relatively constant when the vitamin B12 levels in the cerebro-spinal fluid were high.

Improvements in communication functions were seen when a certain level of vitamin B12 was maintained for a longer period.[12]

Thiamin

Some studies have found lower levels of thiamin in the brains of Alzheimer's disease patients, which has an impact on mental function.[13] Clinical data suggest that high dose thiamin may have a mild beneficial effect in some patients with Alzheimer's disease but it does not appear to halt the progress of the disease.[14] Thiamin appears to increase the effect of the neurotransmitter, acetylcholine, in the brain.

Zinc

The metabolism of zinc may be altered in Alzheimer's disease.[15] Results from the Nun Study, a study of aging and Alzheimer's disease, showed that low zinc levels in the blood were associated with more senile plaques in the brains of those who died from the disease.[16] In another study zinc supplements (27 mg per day) led to improvements in memory, understanding and communication in eight out of ten patients who took them.[17]

Choline

Levels of acetylcholine are lower in Alzheimer's disease sufferers due to the reduced activity of the enzyme which synthesizes it. Choline, which is part of the vitamin B complex, is involved in the synthesis of acetylcholine and some studies have detected improvements in mental performance after treatment with it.[18,19] However, results of studies have been mixed. Choline and lecithin (which contains choline) may only be useful in the initial stages of the disease.

Acetyl-L-carnitine

Acetyl-L-carnitine is a compound which is involved in energy metabolism in the cell. It also acts as an antioxidant and may enhance or mimic the function of acetylcholine. There are several studies which suggest that it may delay the progression of Alzheimer's disease.[20] In a small double-blind trial published in 1995, seven patients with probable Alzheimer's disease received 3 g/day of acetyl-L-carnitine for one year, while five similar patients were given a placebo. Patients treated with acetyl-L-carnitine showed significantly less deterioration on mental status tests than did patients receiving the placebo.[21]

Herbal medicines and Alzheimer's disease

Several studies have suggested that the herb, *Ginkgo biloba* is beneficial in the treatment of Alzheimer's disease. In a study reported in the *Journal of the American Medical Association* in 1997, US researchers conducted a 52-week, randomized double-blind, placebo-controlled trial involving mildly to severely demented outpatients with Alzheimer disease or multi-infarct dementia. They used tests to assess the cognitive functioning of the patients and also included assessments by the caregivers of the patients as part of the outcome measurement. The results showed that the ginkgo extract stabilized and, in a substantial number of cases, improved the cognitive performance and the social functioning of demented patients for six months to one year.[22] See page 397 for more information on Ginkgo and the precautions that may be necessary.

Anemia

Anemia is a relatively common condition which has a variety of causes. It is a group of signs and symptoms which occur when there is a low level of red blood cells or the amount of hemoglobin they contain, a low blood volume, or abnormally formed red blood cells. There are over 400 types of anemia, many of them very rare. This chapter focuses on nutritional deficiency anemias.

Symptoms of anemia

In order for red blood cells to carry oxygen to the tissues, they must contain sufficient amounts of hemoglobin, an iron-containing protein molecule. If red blood cell and/or hemoglobin concentrations are low in the blood, less oxygen is transported to the tissues. This results in symptoms such as a tendency to tire easily, shortness of breath, palpitations, poor concentration, weakness, susceptibility to infections and pale skin. Left untreated, anemia can be life-threatening.

Types of anemia

There are several different types of anemia. The most common include anemia due to excessive blood loss, anemia due to excessive red blood cell destruction, and anemia due to deficient red blood cell production.

Causes of anemia

Causes of anemia include genetic defects, disease, inflammation, infection, medication side effects and, most commonly, nutritional deficiencies. Identifying the cause is extremely important in order to rule out serious illness and to ensure that treatment is successful.

Anemia can result from slow or rapid blood loss. While causes of rapid blood loss are usually clear, causes of slow blood loss may be less obvious and include bleeding from the gastrointestinal tract, hemorrhoids and menstrual difficulties.

Old and abnormal red blood cells are removed from the circulation and destroyed, mainly by the spleen. The most common cause of excessive destruction of red blood cells is abnormal shape, which is often a result of a vitamin or mineral deficiency.

Anemia due to lowered red blood cell production is the most widespread type. Lack of a number of vitamins and minerals can lead to deficient red blood cell production; most commonly, iron, vitamin B12 and folic acid. When identifying the cause of anemia it is important to remember that it may be due to a deficiency of more than one nutrient. Vitamin B12 and folic acid deficiency anemias may occur together, as may iron and vitamin B12 deficiency anemias.[1]

Laboratory evaluation of anemia

Laboratory tests which are used to diagnose anemia include measurements of hematocrit (the volume of packed red blood cells) and hemoglobin levels.

Normal hematocrit is 47 per cent (± 5) for men and 42 per cent (± 5) for women. Anemia is diagnosed when this level falls below 42 per cent for men and 37 per cent for women. Normal hemoglobin levels are 16 (± 2) g/dL for men and 14 (± 2) g/dL for women. Anemia is diagnosed when this level falls below 14 (± 2) g/dL for men and 12 (± 2) g/dL for women.

Iron deficiency anemia

Iron plays a vital role in red blood cell production, and deficiency is the most common cause of anemia. As many as 20 per cent of women in general and 80 per cent of those who exercise may be iron-deficient. Severe deficiency leads to anemia as hemoglobin concentration falls below the normal range and red blood cells become small and pale. The prevalence of iron deficiency anemia in the USA is about 2 to 5 per cent and it is also a major problem in developing countries.

As well as the symptoms of anemia described above, someone suffering from severe iron deficiency anemia may crave dirt or paint; a condition known as pica.

Causes of iron deficiency anemia

Iron deficiency anemia can be due to increased iron losses and/or inadequate intake. As iron is poorly absorbed, many people find it difficult to meet their daily needs. For those whose needs are higher or whose absorption is poor, the risk of iron deficiency anemia increases. This is particularly the case in infants under 2 years old, pregnant women, teenage girls, and elderly people. Women are more likely to suffer from iron deficiency as they store less iron than men and lose iron monthly in menstrual blood. Iron deficiency anemia is relatively common in elderly people, particularly those who are in hospital.

There are many other factors which put someone at risk of iron deficiency, with multiple risk factors increasing the likelihood. These include an increased rate of body growth, excessive menstrual blood loss, regular blood donation, intensive exercise, a vegetarian diet, chronic aspirin use, low iron intake, low vitamin C intake, excess tea and coffee, fad diets, poverty, alcohol abuse, depression and gastrointestinal disease such as celiac disease. If several of these factors are present, the risk is obviously greater. In the absence of these risk factors, a careful search for gastrointestinal blood loss is necessary.[2]

Anemia is the final stage of iron deficiency. Before the red blood cells are affected, iron stores are reduced but there are no clinical effects. The next stage is biochemical deficiency without symptoms; and as depletion continues, iron-dependent enzymes are affected, and immune functions requiring iron may be affected. Symptoms of anemia can develop gradually and may continue without being recognized for some time.

Iron deficiency anemia in pregnancy

When a woman becomes pregnant, her iron requirements increase from around 15 mg per day to 30 mg, due to the needs of the developing fetus. This increase can be difficult to obtain in the diet and most anemia during pregnancy is due to dietary iron deficiency. Women whose iron stores are never built up are at particular risk. Women who become iron deficient during pregnancy may find it difficult to rebuild iron stores. Even women with normal hemoglobin levels are advised to take iron supplements during pregnancy to prevent depletion of iron stores and reduce the risk of anemia due to abnormal bleeding or a subsequent pregnancy. Research shows that women who take iron supplements during pregnancy do not suffer the same postnatal reduction in hemoglobin and ferritin as those who don't take supplements. A 1996 Italian study examined the effectiveness of different types of iron supplements in pregnant women. The results showed that oral ferrous gluconate in liquid form was more effective and better tolerated than other solid or liquid preparations containing elementary iron.[3]

Iron deficiency anemia in children

Iron deficiency anemia is the most common nutritional deficiency in children. If a mother has had adequate iron in her diet, a baby is born with enough iron to last four to six months. The main source of iron for babies is breast milk which, although it is low in iron, is high in lactose and contains vitamin C so the iron is well-absorbed. Infant formula is fortified with iron and vitamin C.

Iron deficiency anemia has been implicated in emotional, social and learning difficulties in children and adults. Iron deficient babies are often irritable and have no interest in their surroundings, and adults lacking iron can be affected in job performance, mood and memory, and have trouble concentrating. Children who were anemic as infants do not perform as well in intelligence tests as those who were adequately nourished. Recent research suggests that iron supplements do not improve mental ability in anemic infants, and prevention of iron deficiency in children is therefore very important.[4]

Laboratory evaluation of iron deficiency anemia

In addition to the laboratory measures described above, there are specific tests which can help to diagnose iron deficiency anemia. These tests, which include serum ferritin and TIBC (total iron-binding capacity) measures are more sensitive predictors of iron deficiency. Iron levels may fluctuate throughout the menstrual cycle in women and the average values from multiple tests may provide the best readings.

Serum ferritin measurement accurately reflects body stores and this is usually the earliest laboratory measure to reflect iron deficiency. It is a sensitive test and is not affected by day-to-day fluctuations in intake. Normal serum ferritin levels are 40 to 160 mcg per liter, with iron deficiency anemia indicated by a level of 12 mcg per liter. However, a normal serum ferritin does not rule out iron deficiency as certain conditions such as infection, inflammation, liver disease, some cancers and recent strenuous exercise can raise serum ferritin levels.

Treatment of iron deficiency anemia

The first step in the treatment of iron deficiency anemia is the identification and elimination of any source of excess blood loss, wherever possible.

If iron stores are mildly lowered (serum ferritin less than 20 mcg per liter) or depleted, (less than 15 mcg per liter) increasing the levels of iron and vitamin C in the diet, and avoiding excess tea, coffee and compounds in whole grains which can reduce iron absorption will help to boost iron levels. If these lifestyle measures are difficult, it is advisable to take iron supplements.

In cases of iron deficiency anemia (serum ferritin less than 10 to 12 mcg per liter) supplements are necessary and should correct anemia within two months. However, they may need to be taken for at least six months until iron stores are replenished. (See page 257 for more information.) Hemoglobin levels need to be monitored continuously, and if improvements are not seen, it is important to check for continued hemorrhage, underlying infection or malignancy, insufficient iron intake or, very rarely, inadequate absorption of oral iron.

Vitamin B12 deficiency anemia

Severe vitamin B12 deficiency causes macrocytic anemia in which the red blood cells fail to mature properly and are fewer in number, larger in size and contain less oxygen-carrying hemoglobin than normal. Symptoms are similar to those of iron deficiency and include tiredness, pallor, lightheadedness, breathlessness, headache and irritability.

Causes of vitamin B12 deficiency anemia

Pernicious anemia

One of the most common causes of vitamin B12 deficiency anemia is the lack of a protein known as intrinsic factor, which is produced by the stomach and is necessary for vitamin B12 absorption. In this case, it is known as pernicious anemia. Lack of intrinsic factor tends to be an inherited tendency and is commonly seen in those over 60 years old. Researchers involved in a study done in California in 1996 used their results to estimate that as many as 800 000 elderly people in the United States have undiagnosed and untreated pernicious anemia.[5]

Other causes

Vitamin B12 deficiency can occur in those whose dietary intakes of vitamin B12 are inadequate. It is also seen in babies who are breastfed by vegan mothers. Deficiency may also be due to malabsorption disorders, some types of gastritis, hyperthyroidism, kidney and liver diseases.

Diagnosis and treatment of vitamin B12 deficiency anemia

Because vitamin B12 is used very slowly and is stored in the body, deficiency symptoms may take a long time to appear. Body stores may be sufficient to last for three to five years in the absence of intrinsic factor or sufficient dietary intake.

The Schilling test is used to measure the ability of a person to absorb vitamin B12. (See page 111 for more information.) If vitamin B12 deficiency is due to inadequate dietary intake, it may be treated with dietary supplements. If it is due to lack of intrinsic factor, it is usually treated with vitamin B12 injections.

Vitamin B12 deficiency anemia and folic acid supplements

A high intake of folic acid can mask vitamin B12 deficiency as it can prevent the red blood cell changes but not the other symptoms of vitamin B12 deficiency. These include potentially irreversible nerve damage. Some experts are concerned that fortifying foods with folic acid may lead to vitamin B12 deficiency in susceptible people, such as the elderly and those on vegan diets. The US Food and Drug Administration recommends keeping total folic acid intake below 1 mg per day, unless under medical supervision.

Folic acid deficiency anemia

Folic acid deficiency also causes macrocytic anemia and the symptoms are similar to those of iron and vitamin B12 deficiency.

Causes of folic acid deficiency anemia

The most common causes of folic acid deficiency are inadequate intake and reduced absorption due to malabsorption disorders or prolonged use of certain medications. Folic acid requirements are raised in liver disease, chronic hemolytic anemias, psoriasis, and with long-term dialysis which can also increase the risk of deficiency. Folic acid stores in the body are limited and a deficiency can develop within a few months.

Folic acid deficiency anemia due to inadequate intake

Poor dietary intake of folic acid-rich foods such as green vegetables is common. Folic acid in food is destroyed by light and heat. Alcohol interferes with folic acid metabolism and alcoholics are at particular risk of folic acid deficiency as they also usually have poor diets.

Folic acid deficiency anemia due to medication use

Folic acid deficiency may occur because of long-term use of certain medications. These include anticonvulsants, barbiturates and oral contraceptives which reduce absorption; the anticancer drug, methotrexate; and some antimicrobial drugs such as trimethoprim and pyrimethamine, which alter the metabolism of folic acid.

Folic acid deficiency anemia in pregnancy

During pregnancy, daily folic acid requirements increase from 180 mcg to 400 mcg. Requirements are also increased during breastfeeding. The raised requirements put women at risk of folic acid deficiency anemia. Folic acid supplements are recommended during pregnancy as they help to reduce this risk and also the risk of neural tube defects.

Diagnosis and treatment of folic acid deficiency anemia

A diagnosis of folic acid deficiency can be confirmed by a laboratory test which measures red blood cell levels of folic acid. Folic acid deficiency anemia is treated with supplements. The usual dose given to replenish tissue stores is 1 mg per day. As previously mentioned , it is important to rule out the possibility of vitamin B12 deficiency anemia before folic acid supplements are given.

Other B vitamin deficiencies and anemia

Vitamin B6 deficiency can also cause anemia, as hemoglobin and red blood cells are not formed normally. Supplements can improve the symptoms within a few weeks. Riboflavin may enhance the effectiveness of iron supplementation treatment of anemia, as it appears that iron utilization is impaired in riboflavin deficiency.[6]

Vitamin E deficiency anemia

Although it is very rare, one of the symptoms of vitamin E deficiency is hemolytic anemia (where the red blood cells are broken down faster than the bone marrow can replace them). This may be related to the ability of vitamin E to protect cell membranes from free radical damage. This type of anemia is sometimes seen in babies born prematurely, and vitamin E supplements may be useful in prevention of symptoms[7], although there is some controversy over this.[8]

Other vitamins and minerals and anemia

Vitamin C

Vitamin C plays an important role in iron absorption, and vitamin C deficiency may lead to anemia due to reduced iron absorption. Vitamin C is also involved in folic acid metabolism which may affect red blood cell formation.

Copper

In adults, symptoms of copper deficiency include anemia as red blood cell development is inhibited. Copper plays a role in iron absorption and mobilization and can stimulate hemoglobin synthesis. Copper deficiency anemia may occur if large doses of zinc are taken for long periods, as zinc competes with copper for absorption.[9] Iron deficiency anemia may improve more quickly if both copper and iron supplements are given.

Cobalt

A deficiency of cobalt is equivalent to a deficiency of vitamin B12 with symptoms of pernicious anemia, nerve disorders and abnormalities in cell formation. However, the anemia cannot be treated with cobalt alone.

Selenium

Selenium is a component of the enzyme, glutathione peroxidase, which protects red blood cells from free radical damage and destruction. Selenium deficiency may play a role in, or aggravate anemia, and it has been found that increasing selenium intake in animals sometimes corrects anemia.[10]

Zinc

Prolonged high intakes of zinc may lead to copper deficiency anemia. Zinc deficiency occurs in sickle cell anemia and sufferers may benefit from supplements.[11]

Arthritis

Arthritis is the name given to problems that cause swelling, pain and stiffness in joints. It can mean anything from slight tightness to severe pain and disability. There are over 100 types of arthritis, including osteoarthritis, rheumatoid arthritis and gout. As many as one in seven Americans may suffer from arthritis, with women more commonly affected than men. Arthritis is the number one cause of disability in America, limiting everyday activities for about seven million people. As the population becomes older, this number is expected to increase.

Osteoarthritis

Symptoms of osteoarthritis

Osteoarthritis is the most common joint disease. Initially, the onset is subtle and gradual, and usually involves one or only a few joints. Pain is the earliest symptom, usually made worse by exercise. Morning stiffness follows inactivity but this only lasts around 15 to 30 minutes and improves with exercise.

Osteoarthritis occurs when degenerative changes take place in the cartilage in the joints, causing a roughening or loss of surface. There is increased bone formation in the area under the cartilage. This bone becomes stiffer and tiny fractures occur. Joints may lose their proper shape and become enlarged, or develop bony bumps that can limit movement. More women than men suffer from osteoarthritis and symptoms usually start to show in middle age. As many as 75 per cent of those aged over 70 show some evidence of the disease, with knees and hands being the most commonly affected sites. The cervical and lumbar spine is also commonly affected.

Causes of osteoarthritis

There are many causes of osteoarthritis; including changes in bone and cartilage with aging, and wear and tear on the joints from abnormal physical stresses such as obesity, injury, inflammatory processes and hormonal effects. There seems to be an imbalance in the processes that repair and maintain the joints. Genetic factors seem to play a role and long periods of weight-bearing exercise may increase the risk.[1] Low estrogen levels seem to increase the risk of osteoarthritis and hormone replacement therapy appears to reduce it.[2]

Diagnosis of osteoarthritis

In addition to symptom analysis, X-rays may be used to diagnose osteoarthritis as they show shrunken joints and bone abnormalities. Blood studies may also be used to rule out other disorders.

Treatment of osteoarthritis

There is currently no way of stopping or reversing the changes which occur in osteoarthritis. Exercise is very important, as it maintains healthy cartilage and range of motion and develops the stress-absorbing tendons and muscles. Daily stretching exercises are particularly important as are periods of rest. Drugs such as aspirin are sometimes used to treat inflammation and for pain relief. Muscle relaxants may also be used. Knee and hip replacement surgery may be necessary in severe cases.

Vitamins, minerals and osteoarthritis

Vitamin D

Recent research suggests that older people whose knees are affected by osteoarthritis may run the risk of worsening their symptoms if they do not get enough vitamin D. Results from the Framingham Osteoarthritis Cohort Study published in 1996 showed that men and women with low dietary intakes and blood levels of vitamin D had three times the risk of their symptoms becoming worse than men and women with high intakes. However, they did not find a link between low vitamin D levels and the risk of developing osteoarthritis in a previously normal knee.[3]

Anti-arthritis drugs, including corticosteroids, and reduced activity and exposure to sunlight in those with the disease may contribute to low vitamin D levels. Vitamin D supplements may be beneficial in those already suffering from osteoarthritis who have low intakes. However, very high doses of vitamin D should be avoided as they may cause calcium to be deposited in the tissues causing irreversible damage.

Antioxidants

Other results from the Framingham Osteoarthritis Cohort Study suggest that high intakes of antioxidant nutrients may reduce the risk of cartilage loss and disease progression in people with osteoarthritis. A three-fold reduction in risk of progression was found for those with high vitamin C intakes. Those with high vitamin C intake also had a reduced risk of developing knee pain. A reduction in risk of disease progression was seen for beta carotene and vitamin E intake but was less consistent. Antioxidant nutrients did not seem to affect the initial appearance of the disease.[4]

B vitamins

A controlled, double-blinded, crossover study done in 1994 found that patients taking vitamin B12 and folic acid supplements had less pain and stiffness than others not taking the supplements. The study involved 26 people diagnosed for an average of 5.7 years with osteoarthritis of the hands who had been medicated by prescribed NSAIDs. They were randomly given either 6400 mcg folate or 6400 mcg folate plus 20 mcg vitamin B12 or lactose placebo each for two months. The results showed that right and left hand grip values were higher and the number of tender hand joints was less in the supplements group. There were no side effects in the vitamin group.[5]

Other nutrients

Epidemiological studies suggest that there may be a link between boron deficiency and osteoarthritis. In countries such as Mauritius and Jamaica, where boron intake is low, the incidence of osteoarthritis is around 50 to 70 per cent. In countries such as the USA, UK and Australia, where boron intake is relatively high, the incidence of osteoarthritis is around 20 per cent. Boron concentrations in bones next to osteoarthritic joints may be lower than in normal joints and supplements of 6 to 9 mg per day have been used to treat osteoarthritis with some improvement of symptoms. This may be because boron increases bone hardness.[6]

Glucosamine

Short-term studies in sufferers of osteoarthritis suggest that glucosamine sulfate may produce a gradual and progressive reduction in joint pain and tenderness, as well as improved range of motion and walking speed. Results of the trials have also shown that glucosamine has produced consistent benefits in patients with osteoarthritis and that, in some cases, it may be equal or superior to anti-inflammatory drugs in controlling symptoms.[7]

Rheumatoid arthritis

Symptoms of rheumatoid arthritis

Rheumatoid arthritis occurs when the membrane linings around the joints become inflamed and the joint surfaces and tendons become distorted or even broken. The effects of rheumatoid arthritis differ from person to person and include fatigue, soreness, stiffness and aching. The hand and wrist joints on both sides of the body are often affected, and become warm, painful, swollen and tender, leading to difficulty with movement. Stiffness lasting at least 30 minutes after getting up in the morning or after prolonged inactivity is common; and early afternoon fatigue and malaise also occur. Deformities may develop rapidly. Osteoarthrtitis often develops in joints affected by rheumatoid arthritis, causing further destruction.

Rheumatoid arthritis occurs in around 1 per cent of people and female sufferers outnumber males by three to one. The disease usually starts around age 25 to 50, but it can occur at any age. When the disorder occurs in children under 16 years old, it is known as juvenile rheumatoid arthritis. The onset of rheumatoid arthritis is usually gradual, but in some cases it can be sudden. Stress may worsen the disease symptoms.

Causes of rheumatoid arthritis

Rheumatoid arthritis is an autoimmune disease, occurring when the immune system attacks joint tissue, releasing antibodies and other chemicals that cause pain, swelling and damage. The cause of the disease is unknown but genetic factors may play a role. However, not all patients with a high genetic susceptibility to the disease actually develop it. Researchers believe that even in patients who are genetically predisposed to rheumatoid arthritis, the disease must be initiated by an environmental agent. Possible triggers include viral infections, smoking, obesity, blood transfusions, food allergies and intolerances, and diets high in refined foods.

Diagnosis of rheumatoid arthritis

In addition to symptom analysis, blood tests are often used to confirm the presence of the disease. Most sufferers have antibodies known as rheumatoid factor in their blood.

Treatment of rheumatoid arthritis

As there is presently no cure for rheumatoid arthritis, treatment aims to relieve pain, reduce inflammation and slow joint damage. The disease may vary from person to person, and developing an individual treatment plan is important. Clinical evidence suggests that early diagnosis of arthritis and prompt treatment can alter the disease process, improve quality of life and extend longevity. Once the disease becomes more aggressive, it is more difficult to manage and treat.

Medications

Drugs which can be used to treat the symptoms of rheumatoid arthritis include aspirin and other nonsteroidal anti-inflammatory drugs (NSAIDs) which cut down inflammation. Penicillamine, hydroxychloroquine, sulfasalazine, methotrexate and azathioprine may also be used. Gold is sometimes used to treat rheumatoid arthritis and recent research suggests that long-term wearing of gold rings slows progression of the disease in the joints near the rings.[8] In severe cases, powerful corticosteroids may be given. These drugs are related to cortisone, a natural hormone produced by the human body. Unfortunately, their effectiveness declines over time and they have several undesirable side effects if they are used for long periods, including immune suppression and osteoporosis. (See pages 487 and 490 for more information.) New genetically engineered drugs which affect the inflammatory immune response may soon become available.

Lifestyle measures

A balanced mixture of rest and exercise is important in the treatment of rheumatoid arthritis; rest being important during periods when the disease flares up and exercise when it is not so severe. Stretching and heat treatments can make exercises easier. In a study reported at the 1996 American College Of Rheumatology meeting, moderate exercise performed for a total of three hours over a six-week period substantially reduced joint stiffness in adults with rheumatoid arthritis. Obesity aggravates the symptoms of arthritis and weight loss can often bring improvement.

There are various devices such as joint splints, gloves and orthopedic shoes which can help to relieve symptoms and help patients to perform activities necessary for daily life. Stress relief and pain management techniques may also be valuable in the treatment of rheumatoid arthritis. A 1995 study involving 141 rheumatoid arthritis patients showed that those who underwent special stress management counselling had better coping skills, felt less helpless, reported less pain and had greater mobility several months later than patients who either attended an education program or had no counselling at all.[9]

Rheumatoid arthritis and diet

There is some evidence that a connection exists between diet and rheumatoid arthritis. However, no dietary therapy is widely accepted. Some experts believe that diets high in refined foods and food intolerances and allergies may lead to the development of the disease. Many sufferers find that eating meat and dairy products worsens symptoms while some people have benefited from avoiding foods of the nightshade family which contain a substance called solanine. These include potatoes, tomatoes, peppers, eggplant and tobacco. Avoiding caffeine, alcohol and food additives may also be helpful. Vegetable juices containing carrot, celery, beetroot and cucumber may also be beneficial in some patients.

Certain foods, such as oily fish, which contain anti-inflammatory omega-3 fatty acids may help reduce the pain of tender joints and morning stiffness of rheumatoid arthritis. In a 1996 population-based case-control study, researchers compared 324 women with rheumatoid arthritis cases and 1245 women without the disease. They used a food frequency questionnaire to ascertain diet during a one-year period five years before the women first visited their physicians because of joint symptoms. The results showed that women who ate broiled or baked fish more than twice a week had almost half the risk of rheumatoid arthritis.[10]

Recent research also suggests that a vegetarian diet may lessen the symptoms of arthritis in some people. It is unclear whether benefits come from eating more of certain foods or less of others. Fasting is also an effective treatment for rheumatoid arthritis, but most patients relapse when they start eating again. In a Norwegian randomized, single-blind controlled trial done in 1991, researchers assessed the effect on 27 patients of fasting followed by one year of a vegetarian diet. After a seven to ten day fast, patients were put on individually adjusted gluten-free vegan diets for three and a half months. They were then allowed to eat a lactovegetarian diet for the remainder of the study. A control group of 26 ate an ordinary diet throughout the whole study period. After four weeks, the diet group showed a significant improvement in both symptoms and laboratory measures of disease severity. In the control group, only pain score improved score. The benefits in the diet group were still present after one year.[11] Follow-up studies done a year later found that those patients who had benefited from the vegetarian diet continued to show improvement in symptoms.[12]

Rheumatoid arthritis sufferers are often poorly nourished. Many people lose their appetite and tend to lose weight during the active phase of the disease. Drug treatment and the intestinal changes which can occur in the course of the disease may worsen malnutrition. Deficiencies of folic acid, vitamin C, vitamin D, vitamin B6, vitamin B12, iron, magnesium, selenium and zinc are often found in patients with rheumatoid arthritis but it is unclear whether nutrient deficiencies are a cause or a result of the disease.

Vitamins, minerals and rheumatoid arthritis

Antioxidants

Research suggests that rheumatoid arthritis sufferers have low levels of antioxidant vitamins and minerals which may contribute to inflammation. Sufferers of the disease appear to have higher levels of free radicals in their blood and joint fluid.[13] This may be due to increased activity of white blood cells known as macrophages. If these free radicals are not neutralized by antioxidants, they can cause inflammation and damage to tissues.

In a study published in 1997, researchers from the Training Center for Public Health Research in Maryland examined thousands of blood samples donated in 1974. They then specifically tested those from 21 people who were diagnosed with rheumatoid arthritis two to 15 years after donating their blood. The results showed that those with rheumatoid arthritis had 29 per cent lower beta carotene in their blood before they were diagnosed, 5 per cent less vitamin E and 7 per cent less vitamin A.[14] Other studies have found low levels of vitamin C in rheumatoid arthritis sufferers.[15]

It is unclear from this study whether these lower levels of antioxidants are a cause or an effect of the disease. It is possible that the antioxidants in the blood are being used to combat free radical damage caused by the disease, or alternatively, that decreased intake, absorption or transport increases the risk of oxidative damage. Increasing intake of antioxidant nutrients is beneficial in reducing some of the inflammation caused by free radical damage to joint linings in rheumatoid arthritis sufferers.

In a study published in 1997, UK researchers investigated whether there was any additional anti-inflammatory or analgesic effects of vitamin E in rheumatoid arthritis patients who were already receiving anti-rheumatic drugs. The study involved 42 patients who were given 600 mg alpha TE (895 IU) twice a day or placebo for 12 weeks. The results showed that although laboratory measures of disease activity were unchanged, the patients reported less pain.[16]

B vitamins

Folic acid levels are low in arthritis sufferers taking the anti-inflammatory drug, methotrexate, which interferes with the conversion of folic acid to its active form. Methotrexate reduces inflammation but can also have toxic side effects. Studies have shown that folic acid supplements do not interfere with the beneficial action of the drug but may be useful in protecting against the side effects.[17]

Riboflavin levels may be low in rheumatoid arthritis sufferers. In a 1996 study, UK researchers investigated this link in patients and in those without the disease. The results showed that biochemical riboflavin deficiency was more frequent in patients with active disease. Riboflavin is necessary for the action of an enzyme which has anti-inflammatory activity, and deficiency could reduce the activity and beneficial effect of that enzyme.[18] Niacin, vitamin B6 and pantothenic acid have also been used to treat arthritis.

Vitamin D

Vitamin D may be useful in preventing the bone loss that occurs with severe rheumatoid arthritis. Researchers involved in a 1998 study investigated the links between disease activity and blood levels of vitamin D in 96 patients. They found that high disease activity was associated with alterations in vitamin D metabolism and increased bone breakdown. Low levels of vitamin D may also increase the proliferation of white blood cells, and may accelerate the arthritic process in rheumatoid arthritis.[19]

Calcium

Blood calcium levels are often lower than normal in those with rheumatoid arthritis. Corticosteroids used in the treatment of rheumatoid arthritis can cause bone loss, which may increase the risk of osteoporosis. Supplementation with calcium and vitamin D can help prevent this loss. In a recent two-year study, 96 patients with rheumatoid arthritis, 65 of whom were taking corticosteroid drugs, were given 1000 mg calcium and 500 IU vitamin D per day or placebo. The researchers analyzed the bone mineral density of the lumbar spine and femur once a year. In those patients taking corticosteroid drugs and placebo losses of bone mineral density were seen. In those taking the supplements gains were seen and in those not taking corticosteroids, the supplements did not appear to affect bone mineral density.[20]

Copper and zinc

Copper and zinc metabolism may be altered in rheumatoid arthritis patients. They may have higher than normal urinary copper excretion rates, and serum copper and ceruloplasmin (copper protein complex) levels are also raised in arthritis sufferers while zinc levels are usually lower. Zinc and copper function in the antioxidant enzyme, superoxide dismutase; levels of which may be altered in arthritis sufferers.[21] Some studies have shown beneficial effects of zinc and/or copper supplements in arthritis while others have not.

Iron

Some experts believe that high iron intake may aggravate joint inflammation in rheumatoid arthritis, possibly by increasing free radical damage. Some studies have found that the iron antidote, deferoxamine is useful in the treatment of rheumatoid arthritis. It may act by lowering iron levels in joint tissue and reducing the inflammation. Iron absorption, however, is decreased in rheumatoid arthritis and anemia is a relatively common complication of the disease.[22]

Manganese

Manganese supplements have been shown to have beneficial effects in the treatment of rheumatoid arthritis. Manganese is a component of the enzyme superoxide dismutase, which acts as an antioxidant and reduces inflammation. Manganese needs may be increased in rheumatoid arthritis sufferers.[23]

Selenium

Several studies indicate that selenium levels are low among patients with rheumatoid arthritis. Selenium is part of the enzyme glutathione peroxidase, which acts as an antioxidant and has anti-inflammatory effects. It acts by inhibiting certain hormone-like substances known as prostaglandins and leukotrienes which cause inflammation. Clinical studies have not clearly shown that selenium supplements bring improvements in the condition of rheumatoid arthritis sufferers. Vitamin E and selenium together may have beneficial effects.

In a 1997 German study, 70 patients with rheumatoid arthritis were randomly divided into two groups. One group was given 200 mcg per day of sodium selenite while the other group was given a placebo. Selenium concentrations in red blood cells of patients with rheumatoid arthritis were significantly lower than found in an average German population. At the end of the three-month experimental period, the selenium-supplemented group showed less tender or swollen joints, and morning stiffness. Selenium-supplemented patients needed less cortisone and other anti-inflammatory medications than the placebo group. Analysis also showed a decrease in laboratory indicators of inflammation.[24]

Other nutrients and rheumatoid arthritis

Omega-3 fatty acids

Several research studies suggest that taking omega-3 fatty acids either in food or supplement form reduces the stiffness and pain of rheumatoid arthritis and may also reduce the need for anti-inflammatory medication.This may be due to effects on several parts of the inflammatory process.

Dietary fats are involved in the manufacture of hormone-like compounds known as prostaglandins, which can exert harmful or beneficial effects. Fats in vegetable oils lead to production of harmful inflammatory prostaglandins while fish oils contain fats such as omega-3 fatty acids which lead to the production of anti-inflammatory prostaglandins. Omega-3 fatty acids also seem to affect levels of other chemicals known as cytokines and leukotrienes which are produced by white blood cells and mediate the inflammatory processes involved in rheumatoid arthritis. Omega-3 fatty acids are found in fish oils and plant oils such as flaxseed oil.

In a study done in 1994 in Belgium, 90 patients were enrolled in a 12-month, double-blind, randomized study comparing daily supplementation with either 2.6 g of omega-3 fatty acids, or 1.3 g of omega-3 fatty acids plus 3 g of olive oil, or 6 g of olive oil. The researchers found significant improvement in both the patient's evaluation and in the physician's assessment of pain in those taking 2.6 g per day of omega 3 fatty acids. The number of patients who were able to reduce their anti-rheumatic medications was significantly greater in the group taking 2.6 g of omega 3 fatty acids.[25]

The omega-6 fatty acid, gamma-linoleic acid is found in evening primrose, blackcurrant, and borage seed oils. These supplements may also be effective in treating rheumatoid arthritis.[26]

Herbal medicine and arthritis

Herbal medicines that may be useful in the treatment of arthritis include Devil's claw (*Harpagophytum procumbens*), celery (*Apium graveolens*), ginger (*Zingiber officinale*), parsley (*Petroselinum crispum*), willow (*Salix alba*), cayenne (*Capsicum annuum*), dandelion (*Taraxacum officinale*), cranberry (*Vaccinium macrocarpon*), black cohosh (*Cimicifuga racemosa*), wild yam (*Dioscorea villosa*) and feverfew (*Tanacetum parthenium*). See page 384 for more information on these herbs and the precautions that may be necessary.

Asthma

Asthma is a chronic lung condition that affects around 16 million people in the US. It is most common in children aged under 10, although people of all ages can be affected. Although asthma is seldom fatal, it is quite serious and is the leading cause of school absenteeism and pediatric hospital admission.

Symptoms of asthma

Asthma is a lung disease characterized by airways obstruction that is reversible (but not completely in some patients), either spontaneously or with treatment; airways inflammation; and increased airways responsiveness to a variety of environmental and emotional stimuli.

Symptoms of asthma include a tightening of the chest, cough, wheezing, shortness of breath and mucus production. However, these symptoms are not always present. They come in episodes set off by various triggers. Some people with asthma experience only mild and infrequent attacks while, for others, these can be frequent and serious, requiring emergency medical treatment.

There are several mechanisms which contribute to the airway narrowing which occurs during an asthma attack. The smooth muscles which surround the airways constrict or spasm, making the airways narrower. Fluid also leaks from the blood vessels, filling the cells that line the airways and causing swelling. If the attack is prolonged, inflammatory cells from the bloodstream also leak out with the fluid. The airways are lined with hair-like projections known as cilia, and a thin layer of mucus. In an asthma attack, too much mucus is produced and the cilia cannot move it. Sometimes air becomes trapped in the mucus which blocks parts of the airway.

Causes of asthma

The tendency to have extra irritable airways may have an inherited component, or may be acquired. The early onset of asthma is sometimes triggered by a child not being breastfed. Allergies are a common trigger of asthma, including those to pollen, mold, house dust, animal dander, certain foods and medicines. However, allergies alone will not cause asthma as not all allergic people have asthma and not all asthmatics are allergic. Respiratory infections also aggravate asthma, as can exercise, stress, cigarette smoke, odors, pollution, perfumes and cleaning solutions.

Treatment of asthma

Asthma is a serious disease and can be fatal if left untreated. Most asthma symptoms are controlled with the proper use of various medications, regular medical care and self-monitoring of air flow and symptoms. Even a well controlled asthmatic who is usually symptom-free may experience occasional attacks, often as a result of viral respiratory tract infections.

Corticosteroids are often used to treat chronic asthma. These drugs, which can be inhaled or taken orally, work by decreasing the swelling and inflammation of the airways. Inhaled steroids are more commonly used whereas oral steroids are usually used to treat more severe cases. Side effects of corticosteroid drugs include thinning of bones, ulcers, thin skin, easy bruising and suppression of normal adrenal gland response to stress. In a study published in 1996, researchers at the University of Virginia found that calcium and vitamin D supplements helped prevent the loss of bone mineral density in those taking corticosteroid drugs.[1]

Bronchodilators, in either oral or inhaled form, are used to treat occasional symptoms of asthma. These drugs work to open up the airways, easing breathing. Oral bronchodilators are rarely used because they can cause side effects such as restlessness, insomnia, headache, loss of appetite, increased heart rate, dizziness, nausea, and vomiting. Long-term use of theophylline may also be associated with behavioral problems and learning disabilities. The drug seems to lower vitamin B6 levels and supplements may be useful in preventing some of the side effects.[2]

Asthma which is triggered by allergies to pollen may be treated by immunotherapy. Yoga, relaxation, deep breathing techniques and chest massage are useful for people with asthma, including children. Regular exercise to improve lung function can also be valuable.

Diet and asthma

Food allergies sometimes cause asthma and it is useful to identify trigger foods and avoid them. Common ones include eggs, wheat, even gluten (found in wheat, oats, barley and rye), dairy products, nuts, citrus fruits, seafood, and foods containing additives or food dyes. Wine, beer and preserved fruit, which often contain sulfur dioxide, may also cause allergic reactions. Many asthmatics react to as little as five parts of sulfur dioxide per million. Such preservatives are also used by some restaurants to keep fruits and vegetables at salad bars looking fresh and attractive. Monosodium glutamate (MSG) can also cause problems for some asthmatics and should be avoided. Hidden sources of MSG are often included on food labels as 'hydrolyzed protein', 'autolyzed yeast', 'sodium caseinate', and 'calcium caseinate'. Very cold food and drink and sometimes overeating may also trigger an attack.

Anyone who suffers from asthma should eat a healthy, whole-foods diet based on lean proteins, grains, fruits, and vegetables. Large amounts of saturated and animal fats should be avoided as should dairy products which tend to increase the production of mucus. Recent research suggests that Western diets may be linked to asthmatic and allergic reactions in children.[3] Vegan and vegetarian diets have been tried as therapy for asthma and have shown benefit in some people, possibly due to the elimination of allergens and/or altered fatty acid metabolism.

Vitamins, minerals and asthma

Antioxidants

There is a lot of evidence to suggest that oxidative stress results in inflammation and tissue damage in the respiratory system, and later in immune damage. Those with low levels of antioxidants in their cells may be at increased risk of developing asthma. Dietary selenium deficiency lowers red blood cell glutathione peroxidase activity and is associated with an increased risk for asthma; and low dietary intakes of vitamins C and E also appear to increase asthma risk. High body iron stores increase free radical production and may elevate asthma risk. Higher intakes of antioxidants may significantly reduce oxidative stress and prevent or minimize the development of asthmatic symptoms.

According to researchers from the University of Washington, antioxidant vitamin supplements may help relieve the symptoms of asthma. The researchers measured the amount of breath expelled by the lungs in 17 asthma sufferers. The subjects took peak flow lung function tests while running on a treadmill and breathing in high levels of polluted air. In those asthmatics whose diets were supplemented with daily doses of 400 IU of vitamin E and 500 mg of vitamin C, an 18 per cent increase in peak flow capacity was seen.

Vitamin E

Some research suggests that vitamin E may have a protective effect against asthma. In a study reported in 1995, researchers evaluated the links between diet and asthma over a ten-year period in 77 866 women aged from 34 to 68.

Women with the highest vitamin E intakes had around half the risk of asthma compared to those with the lowest intakes.[4]

In a 1995 study, vitamin E supplements were added to the treatment regime of asthmatics, and increases in levels and activity of white blood cells was seen, suggesting improvements in the effectiveness of the immune system.[5]

Vitamin C

Low vitamin C intake may be linked to the incidence of asthma. Epidemiological studies show associations between oxidant exposure, respiratory infections, and asthma in children of smokers. There is also evidence that oxidants produced in the body by overactive inflammatory cells contribute to ongoing asthma. Vitamin C is the major antioxidant substance present in the airway surface liquid of the lung, where it could be important in protecting against both damage from toxic chemicals and free radicals which may worsen the symptoms of asthma.[6] Low vitamin C levels are associated with increased bronchial reactivity.[7]

Symptoms of asthma in adults appear to be increased by exposure to environmental oxidants and may be decreased by vitamin C supplementation; although not all studies show positive results. Vitamin C has been shown to improve lung function, white blood cell function and motility, and to decrease respiratory infections and hypersensitivity reactions by reducing histamine levels. Most of the studies conducted so far have been short term and have assessed the immediate effects of vitamin C supplementation. The effect of long-term supplementation with vitamin C is unclear.[8]

In a 1997 double blind study, 20 asthma patients underwent lung function tests at rest, before, and one hour after receiving 2 g of oral vitamin C. The study involved a seven-minute exercise session on a treadmill and lung function tests were performed after an eight-minute rest. This procedure was repeated one week later, with each patient receiving the alternative medication. In nine patients, a protective effect on exercise-induced hyper-reactive airways was seen.[9]

B vitamins

Increased intake of vitamin B6 may reduce the symptoms of asthma in some sufferers, particularly children. A study done in the 1970s looked at the effect of five months of pyridoxine therapy (200 mg daily) in asthmatic children and found significant improvement in symptoms and decreased need for anti-asthma medications such as bronchodilators and cortisone.[10] Researchers involved in a 1985 study found a dramatic decrease in frequency and severity of wheezing or asthmatic attacks in those taking vitamin B6 supplements.[11] However, not all studies have found beneficial effects.[12]

Vitamin B12 therapy may also be of value in childhood asthma. Some studies have shown benefits with vitamin B12 injections, particularly in those who are sensitive to sulfites.

Magnesium

Magnesium appears to play an important role in lung function as it relaxes bronchial smooth muscle. This dilates airways and reduces the effects of inflammation. It may also affect the function of immune cells which release inflammatory chemicals. Intravenous infusion of magnesium sulfate has been used to treat asthma attacks and produces a rapid widening of the airways,[13] and magnesium sulfate aerosols have also been used effectively.[14] Magnesium sulfate administration has also been used to enhance the effect of bronchodilator drugs. Many drugs used in the treatment of asthma cause a loss of magnesium.

As well as being used to treat acute asthma, magnesium may be useful in the prevention of the disease as some research has shown that low dietary magnesium intake is linked with impaired lung function and asthma. In a 1994 study of 2633 adults aged from 18 to 70, UK researchers found that high dietary magnesium intake was associated with a significantly better lung function and a reduction in lung hyper-reactivity.[15]

In a 1997 double-blind, placebo-controlled study, 17 asthmatics were fed a low magnesium diet for two periods of three weeks, preceded and separated by a one week run-in/wash-out, in which they took either placebo or 400 mg magnesium per day. Asthma symptom scores were significantly lower during the magnesium treatment period.[16] Intravenous magnesium has been successfully used as an emergency treatment for asthma in children

Selenium

As an antioxidant, selenium acts to protect cells against oxidative stress. It is an essential component of the enzyme glutathione peroxidase, which reduces hydrogen peroxide and other organic peroxides to harmless substances. By detoxifying peroxides, glutathione peroxidase helps to stabilize cell membranes. Inflammatory cells in asthmatic airways produce oxygen-derived free radicals and peroxides which damage lung tissue and enzymes. Selenium may be able to protect against this damage.

In a study done in 1994 in New Zealand, researchers surveyed 708 children and found symptoms of wheezing in just over 20 per cent. For 26 of the children with current wheezing and for 61 healthy children, researchers measured selenium levels in blood samples which had been taken eight years earlier. The results showed that wheezing was more common in those with low levels of selenium, suggesting a possible link. However, current serum levels were not measured.[17] Other studies have shown reduced selenium concentrations in adults. Researchers involved in another New Zealand study done in 1990, found that whole blood selenium concentrations and glutathione peroxidase activity were lower in adults with asthma than in those without.[18]

In a 1993 study, Swedish researchers conducted a study of 24 adults with asthma in which half of the patients received 100 mcg of selenium per day for 14 weeks, while the other half received a placebo. Six patients from the selenium-supplemented group and one from the placebo group noticed significant clinical improvement, although neither group showed improvement in laboratory measures.[19]

Sodium

Some research reports suggest that high dietary sodium intake contributes to asthma and airway hyper-reactivity. A 1993 UK study tested the effects of either a placebo or sodium supplements on asthma sufferers who had previously followed a low sodium diet. The results showed a worsening of symptoms and laboratory measurements of disease severity in those patients on the high sodium diets.[20]

Other nutrients

Essential fatty acids

Low intakes of omega-3 fatty acids may contribute to the occurrence of asthma. The ratio of omega-3 to omega-6 fatty acids has been shown to be low in asthma sufferers.[21] Supplements may be useful in relieving symptoms in some asthmatics, although not all studies have shown beneficial effects.[22]

Herbal medicine and asthma

Herbal treatment of asthma involves the use of anti-catarrhal and expectorant remedies to ensure that there is the minimum build-up of sputum in the lungs. Other herbs can be used to soothe and support the use of expectorants. Anti-spasmodic plants ease the spasm response in the muscles of the lungs and anti-microbials are useful in preventing secondary infections. Herbs which calm the nervous system are useful to alleviate the stress-related aspects of asthma.

Herbs which have been used to treat asthma include elecampane (*Inula helenium*), mullein (*Verbascum thapsus*), astragalus (*Astragalus membranaceus*), licorice (*Glycyrrhiza glabra*), asthma weed (*Chamaesyce hirta*) and wild cherry (*Prunus serotina*). See page 384 for more information on these herbs and the precautions that may be necessary.

Cancer is a group of over 100 diseases in which abnormal cells grow and spread in an uncontrolled way. It is one of the leading causes of death in developed countries, with lung cancer responsible for more deaths than any other type of cancer. Many factors play a role in the development of cancer, and these may vary between the different types of disease. They include nutritional, environmental, genetic, social, emotional, psychological and spiritual factors. It is only in the last 20 years that diet has been accepted as playing a vital part in the prevention of cancer.

The cancer process

Normally, cells divide to produce more cells only when the body needs them. If cells divide when new ones are not needed, they form a mass of excess tissue, called a tumor. Tumors can be benign (not cancer) or malignant (cancer). The cells in malignant tumors can invade and destroy nearby tissues and organs. Cancer cells can also break away from a malignant tumor and travel through the body to form new tumors in other places. The spread of cancer is called metastasis.

Cancer develops in two stages, an initiation stage and a promotion stage. During the initiation stage, the genetic code of a healthy cell is altered by a substance known as a carcinogen. This is followed by the promotion stage in which the abnormal cell is encouraged to multiply. The initiation stage happens frequently and quickly while the promotion stage is more lengthy. In some cases it may take as long as 30 years for cancer to become apparent.

Symptoms of cancer

As cancer occurs in many forms, the symptoms of one type of cancer may be quite different to those of another. However, there are certain warning signs that often occur. These include:

- Change in bowel or bladder habits
- A sore that does not heal
- Unusual bleeding or discharge
- Thickening or lump in the breast or any other part of the body
- Indigestion or difficulty swallowing
- Obvious change in a wart or mole on the skin
- Nagging cough or hoarseness.

However, these symptoms are not always warning signs of cancer as they can also be caused by less serious conditions. A person who has any of these symptoms should see a doctor who can determine what the problem is. There are several tests which can help to determine if cancer is the cause of a particular medical problem. These include a biopsy, in which a sample of tissue is removed and checked under a microscope for cancer cells.

Causes of cancer

Many factors contribute to the development of cancer. Some of the most common include smoking, chemical pollutants, excess sun exposure, radiation, some pharmaceutical drugs, alcohol, viruses and psychological influences. Nutritional factors include food chemicals, obesity, diets high in saturated and polyunsaturated fats and protein, and nutrient deficiencies.

Cancer treatment

Cancer is treated with surgery, radiation, chemotherapy, hormones, or biological therapy. Treatment may involve just one method or a combination of methods. The choice of therapies depends on many factors including the type and location of the cancer, whether the disease has spread, a patient's age and general health.

Cancer prevention

While it is impossible to avoid all cancer-causing substances, it is possible to lower the risk of developing the disease by avoiding risks where feasible, and increasing consumption of nutrients that act to prevent development of cancer. It is important to avoid exposure to the risk factors mentioned above. Other lifestyle factors, including effective relaxation and stress management techniques can play a large part in reducing the risk of developing cancer. Regular checkups and self-examinations can also be useful in preventing death from cancer as they may reveal the disease at an early stage, when treatment is likely to be effective.

Diet and cancer prevention

Between 20 and 60 per cent of deaths from cancer may be diet-related, making diet second only to tobacco as the most influential factor in the development of cancer. Cancers particularly influenced by diet include those in the colon, prostate, ovary, uterus, breast, skin, vulva, kidneys, cervix, stomach, esophagus, mouth and liver. The body has many mechanisms to thwart the progress of cancer; such as detoxification of carcinogens, preventing and correcting damage to DNA, immune stimulation, and sealing off an abnormal cell growth. All these mechanisms rely on good nutrition.

A good diet can prevent cancer and a bad one can increase the risk, but it is not always clear exactly what is good and what is bad. It is known that nutrients play a role in contributing to or preventing cancer, but the exact relationship between dietary ingredients and cancer is elusive. There are many different types of cancers and some of these can take years to develop, thus making it difficult to pinpoint cause and effect. Food contains many chemicals, known and unknown, and the effects of many of these have not yet been investigated.

The dietary guidelines from the American Cancer Society are:

- Choose most of the foods you eat from plant sources.
- Limit your intake of high fat foods, particularly from animal sources.
- Be physically active: achieve and maintain a healthy weight.
- Limit consumption of alcoholic beverages, if you drink at all.

Foods to avoid

Food contains many substances which can cause cell mutations or promote cancer. High intakes of saturated fat, sugar, alcohol, artificial sweeteners and food additives may cause cancer. Alcohol may promote the growth of abnormal cells, and food additives known as nitrites which are found in processed meats can be converted in the body to carcinogenic nitrosamines. Frying, smoking, barbecuing and broiling fatty meat and fish may produce cancer-causing chemicals, and these foods should be avoided as much as possible.

Foods to include

There are many substances in food which prevent the development or progression of cancer. No specific diet is guaranteed to prevent cancer but a diet which is low in fat and high in fruit and vegetables will help reduce the risks. Fruit and vegetables are rich in vitamins, minerals, fiber and other cancer-preventing compounds. A person whose diet is high in fruit and vegetables also tends to eat less fatty and high calorie foods. Studies from many different countries consistently show that diets high in fruit and vegetables reduce the risk of cancer.

Most experts recommend eating at least two fruits and three vegetables, especially dark orange and green ones, every day. Eating a variety of foods is also very important as no single food provides all the nutrients a person needs, and different nutrients protect against different types of cancer. Cruciferous vegetables such as broccoli, cabbage and cauliflower may have particularly beneficial effects as they contain high levels of vitamins and minerals and other phytochemicals.

Fiber

Fruit and vegetables are also high in fiber. A high fiber diet may reduce the risk of several cancers, including colon and rectal cancer, by binding to potentially toxic bile acids, moving food more quickly through the intestines and exerting beneficial effects on gut bacteria. Fiber has also been shown to protect against other cancers such as those of the breast and prostate.

Fat

Maintaining a healthy weight is very important as obesity increases the risk of developing cancer, and many studies have shown that low fat diets protect against cancer. High fat diets are associated with an increased risk of many types of cancers. This is particularly true for diets high in saturated fats such as those from animal sources. High levels of certain polyunsaturated fats also appear to increase the risk of some cancers while monounsaturated fats do not. (See page 7 for more information).

Vitamins, minerals and cancer

Dietary antioxidants

There is a lot of evidence to suggest that insufficient amounts of antioxidants can increase the risk of cancer. In groups of people who have low levels of these nutrients, the cancer rates are higher. Vitamin C is the body's most powerful water soluble antioxidant while vitamin E and carotenes are lipid soluble. Antioxidants neutralize metabolic products, including free radicals; prevent carcinogens from attacking DNA and cell membranes; inhibit chromosome aberrations; restrain replication of transformed cells; suppress actions of cancer promoters; and induce regression of pre-cancerous lesions. Antioxidants can also boost immunity and counter the immune-suppressive effects of oxidized cholesterol and other substances, and may also slow or halt the growth of tumors by enhancing communication between cells, and stimulating the activity of the immune system.

Vitamin A

Many studies suggest that high blood levels of vitamin A can help prevent certain forms of cancer, particularly cancers of epithelial tissues, such as the lung, mouth, stomach, colon, cervix and uterus. Vitamin A plays an important role in the growth and differentiation of cells, strengthening the immune system and suppressing cell transformation into cancerous cells. Vitamin A deficiency-related changes resemble cancer in these cells.

Breast cancer

Breast tissue may be particularly sensitive to the tumor-suppressive action of vitamin A. In a study published in 1997, researchers at Harvard School of Public Health compared the concentrations of various forms of vitamin A in the breast fat tissue from 46 cancer patients and 63 women with benign breast lumps. They found an increased risk of disease in those with low levels of vitamin A.[1]

Results of a 1997 study suggest that the development of lung cancer may be due to a decreased ability of cells to respond to vitamin A-related compounds known as retinoids. When researchers at the University of Texas looked at the lung tissue from 79 patients with lung cancer and 17 without lung cancer they found that all the healthy cells carried receptors that bound retinoids. However, only 42 to 76 per cent of the cancerous cells had this ability. Of the six different types of retinoid receptors, three were found at lower levels in cancer cells.[2] This study raises the possibility that increasing dietary intake of vitamin A or taking supplements can be used to reduce the risk of lung cancer.

Carotenes

Many population studies have suggested that diets high in carotenes can protect against several types of cancer including those of the cervix, ovaries, uterus, mouth, gastrointestinal tract, lung, prostate and breast. Other types of studies have shown that cancer victims often have lower carotenoid levels than healthy individuals.

In a study published in 1991, researchers investigated the links between beta carotene and cancer in New Zealand families. The study involved 389 people diagnosed with cancer and 391 hospital patients without cancer. They also assessed the family members of the study participants to compensate for the fact that changes in beta carotene levels may have occurred after the cancer developed. Low levels of beta carotene were found in people with a number of cancers, including those of the lung, stomach, esophagus, small intestine, cervix, and uterus. Low levels of beta carotene were also found in the relatives of these cancer patients. The strongest findings were those for lung cancer. In this study patients with cancers of the breast, colon, prostate, and skin did not have lower levels of beta carotene and neither did their families. The results of this study suggest that the cancer sites associated with low levels of beta carotene are, in general, sites for which smoking is a strong risk factor.[3]

Lung cancer

Several population studies have investigated the links between lower levels of carotenes and lung cancer. In a study published in 1998, researchers at Johns Hopkins University measured nutrient levels in blood samples from 258 patients with lung cancer and compared these with those in samples from 515 people free of cancer. Blood concentrations of cryptoxanthin, beta carotene, lutein and zeaxanthin were significantly lower among the cancer patients. Small differences were noticed for alpha carotene and lycopene.[4]

In a 1994 study, researchers compared the diets of 413 non-smokers suffering from lung cancer with those of 413 people without cancer. The results showed that high dietary intake of fruit and vegetables and beta carotene was linked to a decreased risk of lung cancer in both men and women.[5]

Breast cancer

In a study published in 1998, researchers in Missouri examined blood levels of various nutrients in women who developed breast cancer after donating blood to a bank over a ten year period. They then compared these levels to women who were free of cancer. They found lower levels of the carotenes beta cryptoxanthin, lycopene, lutein and zeaxanthin in patients who developed breast cancer.[6] In a study published in 1996, Italian researchers investigated the relationship between selected nutrients and breast cancer risk in 2569 women with the disease and 2588 women with no history of cancer. The results showed significantly less risk in women with high beta carotene intakes.[7]

In a 1994 study published in the *British Journal of Cancer*, West Australian researchers investigated the effect of increased intake of beta carotene on survival in breast cancer patients. Over a six-year period, only one death occurred in the group with the highest consumption of beta carotene, while there were eight and 12 deaths in the intermediate and lowest groups of consumption respectively.[8]

In a study published in the *Journal of the National Cancer Institute* in 1996, researchers examined the links between dietary intake of carotenes(including nonfood supplements), and premenopausal breast cancer risk. The study involved 297 premenopausal women 40 years of age or older who were diagnosed with breast cancer from November 1986 to April 1991. These were compared with 311 women without cancer. The results showed a reduction in risk associated with high intake of several nutrients including beta carotene, lutein and zeaxanthin.[9]

Prostate cancer

High beta carotene intakes may improve survival in those with prostate cancer, according to results from the Chicago Western Electric Study published in 1996. The study involved 1899 middle-aged men who were followed for a total of 30 years. During that time, 132 men developed prostate cancer and survival was found to be less likely in those with low beta carotene intakes.[10]

Lycopene-rich tomatoes seem to be linked with a lower risk of prostate cancer. In a study published in 1995, researchers at Harvard Medical School assessed the links between diet during a one-year period, and prostate cancer in almost 48 000 men in the Health Professionals Follow-up Study. They found that men who ate more foods such as tomatoes, pizza and tomato sauce which are high in lycopene were less likely to be at risk of prostate cancer.[11]

Colon cancer

In a 1997 study done in Italy, researchers assessed carotenoid levels in four healthy patients, seven patients with pre-cancerous lesions and seven patients with colon cancer. They found significantly lower carotenoid levels in the cancer patients.[12]

Cervical cancer

Population studies suggest that low carotenoid levels, including beta carotene may increase the risk of cervical cancer. In a 1993 study, researchers examined the relationship between cervical cancer and carotenoid levels in 15 161 women who donated blood in 1974. Over the next 16 years, 50 women developed cancer. The blood samples of these women were compared with those from 50 women free of cancer and the results showed that the levels of total carotenes, alpha carotene, beta carotene, cryptoxanthin, and lycopene were significantly lower among cancer cases than they were among controls.[13] Laboratory studies show that beta carotene can slow the growth of cervical cancer cells.[14] Increasing intake of beta carotene may help to overcome this tissue-specific deficiency.[15]

Vitamin C

People with high vitamin C intakes seem to have a reduced risk of almost all forms of cancer. The protective effect seems to be strongest for cancers of the esophagus, larynx, mouth and pancreas. Vitamin C also seems to provide some protection against cancers of the cervix, liver, stomach, rectum, breast and lungs.[16] However, in many of these studies it is not possible to tell whether the protective effect is due to vitamin C, vitamin E, or carotene, to a combined effect of these nutrients, or even due to additional substances found in food. Results from the Western Electric Study published in 1995 suggest a link between low vitamin C levels and death from cancer. The researchers obtained information on diet and other factors from 1556 employed, middle-aged men. During the follow-up period, 231 men died from cancer. The results showed that those with the highest vitamin C and beta carotene intakes were 40 per cent less likely to die of cancer than those with the lowest intakes.[17]

Prostate cancer

Vitamin C seems to improve survival in those with prostate cancer. Researchers involved in the Western Electric Study examined the links between dietary beta carotene and vitamin C and the risk of prostate cancer in 1899 middle-aged men over a 30-year period. During this time, prostate cancer developed in 132 men. The results showed that associations between vitamin C intake and risk of prostate cancer differed depending on whether the cancer was diagnosed during the first 19 years of follow-up or the next 11 years of follow-up. Overall, higher intakes of vitamin C and beta carotene were linked to improved survival.[18]

Lung cancer

Vitamin C may also help to protect against lung cancer. Researchers involved in a 1997 study obtained dietary information from 561 men from the Dutch town of Zutphen, in 1960, 1965, and 1970. During the period from 1971 to 1990, 54 new cases of lung cancer were identified and analysis of the diets of the men showed an increased risk of lung cancer in those with lower fruit and vegetable and vitamin C intakes.[19]

Stomach cancer

Results from a study published in 1995 suggest that low vitamin C intake is linked to an increased risk of stomach cancer. In the 1960s, researchers collected detailed dietary information and in 1987, they assessed average food intakes. They then examined the links between this information and death from stomach cancer. The results showed that the average intake of vitamin C was strongly related to the risk of stomach cancer. However, vitamin C intake was not related to the risk of lung and colorectal cancer in this study.[20] Other studies have shown similar results.[21]

Colon cancer

In a study published in 1992, researchers investigated the links between fruits and vegetables and vitamin C intake in 11 580 residents of a retirement community who entered the study free from cancer. During the period from 1981 to 1989 a total of 1335 cases of cancer were diagnosed. The results showed a decreased risk of colon cancer in women with higher vitamin C intakes. Supplemental use of vitamins A and C also showed a protective effect on colon cancer risk in women.[22]

In a 1994 study, Italian researchers investigated the relationship between estimated intake of certain nutrients, including vitamin C, and the risk of disease in 828 patients with colon cancer, 498 with rectal cancer and 2024 people without cancer. Those in the highest intake group for vitamin C had a 60 per cent lower risk of cancer than those in the low intake group.[23]

Breast cancer

The results of a 1994 study suggest that women with high vitamin C intakes have a lower chance of dying of breast cancer than those with the low intakes.[24] The study involved 678 women who were diagnosed with the disease from January 1982 through June 1992. However, results from the Nurses Health Study did not show a protective effect against the disease.[25]

Vitamin E

Several population studies show that low levels of vitamin E are linked to the development of certain cancers, including those of the mouth, liver, lung, colon, rectum, cervix and breast.

Cancers of the gastrointestinal tract

Results from the Iowa Women's Health Study show that high intakes of antioxidants including vitamin E are linked to lower risks of colon, oral, pharyngeal, esophageal and gastric cancers.[26] As part of the study, the results of which were published in 1993, researchers analyzed the links between vitamin E and colon cancer in 35 215 women aged 55 to 69 years without a history of cancer. During the follow-up period, there were 212 cases of colon cancer. The results showed that low vitamin E intake increased the risk of colon cancer, with those in the high intake group having 30 per cent of the risk of those in the low intake group. The protective factor was stronger in the younger women.[27]

Breast cancer

Some studies suggest that low vitamin E levels increase the risk of breast cancer. In a study published in 1992, researchers investigated the relationship between blood levels of various nutrients including vitamin E, and the risks of breast cancer and proliferative benign breast disease (BBD) in postmenopausal women. Women who had a high intake of vitamin E from food sources only, had around 60 per cent less risk of breast cancer compared to those in the low intake group.[28] However, not all studies have shown protective effects.[29]

Cervical cancer

In a 1990 study, Utah University researchers investigating the relationship between cervical cancer and dietary intake of antioxidant vitamins and selenium in 266 women with cervical cancer and 408 women without the disorder found that women with high vitamin E intakes had a 40 per cent lower risk of cervical cancer.[30] Blood levels of vitamin E have also been found to be low in women with cervical cancer.[31]

Lung cancer

High vitamin E intakes may decrease the risk of lung cancer. In 1974 and 1975, researchers at Johns Hopkins School of Hygiene and Public Health, Baltimore, collected blood samples from 25 802 volunteers. They assessed vitamin E levels in samples from 436 cancer cases and 765 matched control subjects. The results showed that high vitamin E levels protected against lung cancer.[32]

Selenium

Epidemiological studies suggest that the risk of cancer is reduced in areas where the soil is high in selenium. Blood samples taken from large groups of people also show that they are more likely to develop cancer if they have low blood levels of selenium and the antioxidant selenium-containing enzyme, glutathione peroxidase. Low serum, dietary and soil selenium levels are particularly associated with lung, gastrointestinal tract and prostate cancers. Selenium may be most effective when combined with vitamin E.

Colorectal cancer

In a 1997 study of the relationship between selenium and colon cancer, researchers at the University of North Carolina determined selenium levels in patients referred for colonoscopy. The results showed that those with the lowest selenium levels had almost four times the risk of colon cancer when compared to those with the highest levels.[33]

In a German study published in 1998, researchers investigated the selenium and glutathione peroxidase levels in 106 colorectal cancer patients and compared these to those in people without cancer. When average selenium levels in the cancer patients were compared with those in the control group, no significant differences were found. However, a significant reduction of serum glutathione peroxidase activity was seen in cancer patients. Those patients with low selenium levels had lower survival times and rates than the patients with higher selenium levels. The lowest selenium level was found for patients with advanced tumor disease. It is unclear from the results of this study whether low selenium levels are a cause or effect of cancer.[34]

Lung cancer

In a study published in 1993, Dutch researchers examined the links between long-term selenium status and lung cancer among 120 852 Dutch men and women aged 55-69 years. The results showed that the lung cancer risk in those with the highest intake of selenium was half that of those in the lowest intake group. The protective effect of selenium was concentrated in subjects with a relatively low dietary intake of beta carotene or vitamin C.[35]

Antioxidant supplements

The supplements most widely used to protect against cancer are the antioxidants. There have been several studies showing that high doses of antioxidants are beneficial, particularly in those who are deficient. A five-year study of almost 30 000 adults in Linxian, China found a 13 per cent reduction in cancer death rates in those given vitamin E, selenium and beta carotene supplements.[36] Several studies suggest that the most beneficial effects are seen when antioxidants are given in combination rather than alone. Antioxidants protect each other from damage and interact in many body functions.

Vitamin A

Lung cancer

Vitamin A supplements have been used to prevent cancer recurrence in smokers who had undergone surgery for lung cancer. In a 1993 study, researchers gave daily doses of 90 000 mcg RE (300 000 IU) to 307 patients took for one year. After a follow-up period of 46 months, the number of patients with either recurrence or new tumors was 56 (37 per cent) in the vitamin A group and 75 (48 per cent) in the control group. Eighteen patients in the treated group developed a second primary tumor, and 29 patients in the control group developed 33 second primary tumors.[37]

Other studies support the use of vitamin A as a cancer preventive in those at high risk of disease. In a 1998 study done in Western Australia, 1024 blue asbestos workers known to be at high risk of diseases such as mesothelioma and lung cancer, were enrolled in a cancer prevention program using vitamin A.

Half the subjects given 30 mg per day of beta carotene and the other half 7500 mcg RE (25,000 IU). The workers were followed up for a five-year period. Four cases of lung cancer and three cases of mesothelioma were observed in those in the vitamin A group, and six cases of lung cancer and 12 cases of mesothelioma in the beta carotene group. In the retinol group, there was also a significantly lower rate of death from all causes.[38] When the researchers compared these results with those workers who had not taken part in the study, they found that those taking part in the study had significantly lower death rates than non-participants.[39]

Leukoplakia

Vitamin A has also been shown to exert protective effects against leukoplakia, a pre-cancerous change in mucous membranes. It often occurs in the mouth and throat and is related to smoking. In a study done in 1997, researchers tested the effects of the retinyl palmitate form of vitamin A on leukoplakia of the larynx. The treatment period was five weeks and the doses used ranged from 90 000 mcg RE per day (300 000 IU) to 270 000 mcg (1 500 000 IU) per day. Complete remission was observed in 15 out of 20 patients and partial response was seen in the remaining five patients.[40]

Carotenes

Beta carotene supplements have been used in cancer and cardiovascular disease prevention trials including the Finnish Alpha Tocopherol Beta Carotene Cancer (ATBC) Prevention Study, the US Carotene and Retinol Efficacy Trial (CARET) and the US Physicians Health Study. In 1996, these studies reported results which received wide publicity. Results from the ATBC study showed an 18 per cent increase in lung cancer deaths in men who took daily supplements of 20 mg of beta carotene.[41]

The CARET study, which involved 18 000 smokers and people who had been exposed to asbestos was stopped 21 months early due to a 28 per cent increased risk of lung cancer, a 26 per cent increase in the risk of death from cardiovascular disease and a 17 per cent increase in overall deaths in the group receiving the supplements.[42] Results from the 12-year Physicians Health Study suggest that beta carotene supplements have no effect on the risk of cancer.[43] Further analyses of these results support the suggestion that beta carotene is susceptible to oxidative damage by alcohol and the gases in cigarette smoke.[44] Other antioxidants, such as vitamins C and E may help to exert protective effects against this damage. In smokers, dietary vitamin C supplementation should accompany beta carotene supplementation.[45] (See page 55 for more information.)

Vitamin C

Vitamin C supplements may have a part to play in cancer prevention.

Stomach cancer

Vitamin C supplements may be useful in helping to prevent stomach cancer. In a 1996 study, researchers gave 32 patients 500 mg of vitamin C twice daily for two weeks. Levels in gastric juices and gut tissues were increased, raising the possibility of increased protection against free radicals.[46]

A 1997 Japanese study suggests that vitamin C may inhibit the growth of *Helicobacter pylori*, a stomach bacterium that increases the risk of ulcers and stomach cancer. Vitamin C-rich diets have been found to decrease the risk of stomach cancer. This has been attributed to the antioxidant ability of vitamin C. However, vitamin E, which is also an antioxidant, does not inhibit the growth of *Helicobacter pylori*. This suggests that vitamin C may exert its protective effects through a biochemical mechanism. This research suggests the possibility of a safe, side effect-free alternative to antibiotics for the treatment of ulcers.[47]

Colon cancer

Vitamin C supplements may also help to prevent colon cancer. In a 1992 study, twenty patients with colorectal cancer were given vitamins A, C, and E for six months and 21 patients with adenomas received placebo. The results showed that supplementation with vitamins A, C, and E was effective in reducing precancerous abnormalities.[48] Vitamin C supplements may also be beneficial in the treatment of prostate cancer.[49]

Vitamin C and cancer treatment

Controversy surrounds the use of vitamin C in the treatment of cancer. The Nobel Prize winner, Linus Pauling and his colleagues have used vitamin C to improve survival times in cancer patients but these results have not been repeated in other studies. Vitamin C may also benefit cancer patients who are undergoing radiation treatment by enabling them to withstand greater doses of radiation with fewer side effects.[50]

Vitamin E

Vitamin E supplements, especially when combined with selenium, have shown beneficial effects in the prevention of certain types of cancer, including breast cancer. Analysis of results from a 1996 US National Institute on Aging study showed a 22 per cent decrease in the risk of death from cancer in those taking vitamin E supplements.[51]

Prostate cancer

According to more results from the ATBC study published in 1998 in the *Journal of the National Cancer Institute*, vitamin E reduces the risk of prostate cancer among smokers. Researchers studied the effects of 50 mg (75 IU) in Finnish men and the results showed a 32 per cent decrease in the incidence of prostate cancer and a 41 per cent decrease in prostate cancer deaths among the men taking vitamin E, compared with those who took no vitamin E.[52]

Selenium

Recent large scale studies in Linxian, China found reduced risk of cancer when selenium supplements were given to those living in selenium-deficient areas.[53] Other studies have shown that selenium supplements protect against some types of cancer such as rectal, ovarian, colon, lung and cervical cancers. However, there are also studies, including the Harvard Nurses Health Study which do not show a protective role for selenium against cancers at any major site. Laboratory studies have shown that selenium can slow tumor cell growth.

Results of a 1996 study showed that selenium supplements were associated with a 50 per cent reduction in deaths from cancer. Researchers at the Arizona Cancer Center set out to test the effectiveness of selenium supplements on the prevention of skin cancer in over 1300 patients. Participants received a placebo or 200 mcg selenium per day over a period of 4.5 years and a total follow-up of 6.4 years. While the results did not show any reduction in skin cancer risk, the selenium group had a 37 per cent reduction in cancer incidence and a 50 per cent reduction in cancer mortality. The effects appeared strongest for prostate (63 per cent lower risk), colorectal (58 per cent lower risk) and lung (53 per cent lower risk) cancers.[54]

Suggested doses of supplements

The doses of antioxidants used in cancer prevention trials are, in many cases, higher than those which could be obtained from the diet. Many nutrition experts recommend taking high daily doses of supplements to help prevent cancer. This may be particularly important in anyone who has a family history of disease or is often exposed to risk factors.

Suggested doses are:

Beta carotene	10 to 30 mg
Vitamin E	200 to 800 IU (134 to 536 mg alpha TE)
Vitamin C	1000-2000 mg
Selenium	200 mcg

Vitamin D

Vitamin D is involved in normal cell growth and maturation, and so may play a part in cancer prevention. Laboratory experiments show that vitamin D can inhibit the growth of human prostate cancer[55] and breast cancer cells.[56] Lung cancer and pancreatic cancer[57] cells may also be susceptible to the effects of vitamin D. Sunlight also seems to be protective against several types of cancer including ovarian,[58] breast and prostate cancers; and this effect may be mediated by vitamin D levels. Synthetic vitamin D-type compounds are being investigated for their potential as anticancer drugs.

Colorectal cancer

In a 1996 study, researchers conducted a population-based case-control study to examine the relationship between vitamin D intake and disease among 352 people with colon cancer, 217 people with rectal cancer and 512 healthy people in Stockholm, Sweden. The researchers used questionnaires to assess the vitamin D intake for the preceding five years. The results showed that those with the highest vitamin D intakes were around half as likely to get cancers of the colon or rectum than those with the lowest intakes.[59]

Results from the Harvard Nurses Health Study published in 1996 suggest a link between vitamin D and colorectal cancer. The study involved 89 448 female nurses and covered the time period from 1980 to 1992 during which 501 cases of colorectal cancer were documented. The results showed a link between intake of total vitamin D and risk of colorectal cancer.[60]

Prostate cancer

In a study published in 1996, researchers in a Boston hospital collected blood plasma samples from 14 916 participants in the Physicians' Health Study and measured vitamin D levels. Their analysis included 232 cases diagnosed up to 1992 and 414 age-matched control participants. Their results showed a slightly reduced risk of prostate cancer in those with high vitamin D levels.[61]

Genes affecting the way a man's body utilizes vitamin D could affect his risk of prostate cancer. A 1996 National Institute of Environmental Health Sciences study found that men with a particular type of vitamin D receptor gene are less likely than others to develop the type of prostate cancer that requires surgery. Researchers looked at the receptor genes in 108 cancer patients and 170 men without cancer. The results showed that 22 per cent of cancer patients had a particular gene while only eight per cent of the cancer-free men did. These findings support the theory that vitamin D plays an important role in prostate cancer development.[62]

Folic acid

Those with diets low in folic acid may have a higher risk of cancer than those who eat large amounts, particularly cancers of the cervix, lung and colon. Folic acid is vital for the maintenance of the genetic code and regulation of cell division in both healthy and tumor tissues. Folic acid deficiency leads to changes similar to those seen in cancer and may affect the repair of DNA and increase chromosome fragility. It may also diminish the ability of the immune system to fight cancer cells and viruses. Deficiency has been shown to affect a gene involved in suppressing tumor formation.[63]

Colorectal cancer

Results from the Alpha-Tocopherol Beta carotene Study published in 1996 suggest a relationship between folate status and colorectal cancer. The study involved male smokers aged from 50 to 69. The researchers measured folate levels in 144 cases of colorectal cancer and 276 healthy people. Those with higher dietary folate intakes had a reduced risk of colon cancer. Men with a high alcohol, low folate, low protein diet were at higher risk for colon cancer than men who consumed a low alcohol, high folate, high protein diet.[64]

Cervical dysplasia

Low blood levels of folic acid may increase the risk of cervical dysplasia (pre-cancerous changes in the cells lining the cervix), possibly by enhancing the effect of other risk factors. Researchers from the University of Alabama investigated the links between folate deficiency and cervical dysplasia in 294 women with the disorder and 170 healthy women. They also assessed the impact of factors such as smoking, oral contraceptive use, human papillomavirus (HPV) infection, and number of sexual partners. The results showed that at low folate levels the risk of dysplasia caused by HPV infection was increased.[65]

Supplements

Folic acid supplements can help to reduce the risk of cancerous changes in several areas such as the cervix, lung and gastrointestinal tract. In a 1997 study, researchers at the Cleveland Clinic investigated the links between folate supplements and cancerous changes in 98 patients with ulcerative colitis. Patients taking the supplements had a 30 per cent lower risk of developing cancerous changes in the bowel. The lower the folate levels the more advanced the degree of cancerous changes in the cells.[66] In a 1997 Italian study researchers also studied the effects of folate supplements on pre-cancerous cell changes in ulcerative colitis. The results showed that folate reduced these changes.[67] Folic acid may also help to prevent the pre-cancerous changes in lung tissue caused by smoking.[68]

Folic acid supplementation may protect abnormal cells from becoming cancerous and may reverse cervical dysplasia in some cases. A 1996 study done at the University of Alabama suggests that supplements may be useful in preventing the initial changes but do not appear to affect the progress of established disease.[69] Some researchers have found a higher risk of abnormalities in cervical tissue in women using oral contraceptives and suggest that folic acid supplements are beneficial in preventing cervical dysplasia in these women.[70]

Vitamin K

Vitamin K injections are often given to babies after birth to reduce the risk of internal bleeding. In the early 1990s, researchers reported a possible increase in the risk of childhood cancers in those who were given these injections. However, the results of studies are inconclusive. This link was examined in four studies published in the *British Medical Journal* in 1998. The results of two of the four studies suggest that there is no association between vitamin K injections and cancer; one could not exclude the possibility; and the fourth suggested a possible increase in the risk of leukemia. (See page 177 for more information.)

Calcium

High intakes of calcium-containing foods are linked to a lower risk of developing colon cancer, although the latest research suggests that the protective effect is not very marked. Calcium may exert its protective effects by binding to cancer-causing fats and bile acids in the intestine and normalizing the growth of cells in the intestinal wall. Calcium may also normalize the growth of cells in the intestinal wall, thus protecting against cancerous changes. Low calcium intake may also increase the risk of breast and cervical cancers.

Results from the Health Professionals Study, involving almost 48 000 men aged from 40 to 75 also suggest that a higher intake of calcium from foods and supplements slightly reduces the risk of colon cancer.[71] Data from the Nurses Health Study which involved over 89 000 nurses also showed a small reduced risk.[72] Results from the Iowa Women's Health Study published in 1998 suggest that calcium can decrease the risk of rectal cancer. Researchers analyzed information from 34 702 postmenopausal women who responded to a mailed survey in 1986. After nine years of follow-up, 144 rectal cancer cases were identified. The results showed that high total calcium intake reduced the risk of rectal cancer.[73] Other results from this study show a reduced risk of colon cancer in women with high intakes of calcium and vitamin D.

Copper

Copper may act to prevent cancer. Animal studies have shown that copper has a protective role and this may be due to its antioxidant properties as part of copper-zinc superoxide dismutase.

Fluoride

Some evidence suggests that water fluoridation may be linked to some types of cancer, although this is controversial. A study published in 1996 reported on the relationship between fluoride concentration in drinking water and deaths from uterine cancer in Okinawa, Japan. Fluoride was added to the water supplies in the region in the period from 1945 to 1972. The results showed significant links between the time of water fluoridation and deaths from uterine cancer.[74]

Iodine

Hypothyroidism and iodine deficiency are associated with a higher incidence of breast cancer.

Iron

In some population studies, high iron levels have been associated with an increased risk of throat and gastrointestinal cancers while others have not shown links.[75] Results from a study assessing the links between body iron stores and cancer in 3287 men and 5269 women participating in the first National Health and Nutrition Examination Survey found an increased risk with high iron levels.[76] Some experts believe that the findings of increased risk are due to causes such as defects in iron metabolism, rather than diet alone. Some studies have shown that iron can inhibit tumor development while others have shown that it might enhance it. Iron may increase the risk of cancer through its effect on free radical formation.

Manganese

A form of the antioxidant enzyme, superoxide dismutase, contains manganese. Proper function of this enzyme helps protect against free radical damage which can cause cancer.

Molybdenum

Population studies show that people living in areas where the soil is molybdenum-deficient have been found to have an increased risk of stomach and esophageal cancers.[3] This may be because molybdenum-deficient plants are unable to metabolize carcinogenic compounds known as nitrosamines, which are present in high levels in food.

Zinc

Zinc supplements have been used to improve taste perception in people taking medications which reduce taste sensation, and in cancer patients undergoing radiation therapy.[77] This can be valuable in helping to maintain normal weight and nutrient intake during treatment.

Vanadium

Some evidence suggests that vanadium may limit the initiation and frequency of tumors in animals. Its role in humans is unclear.

Other nutrients

Essential fatty acids

The levels and types of fat in the diet seem to influence cancer risk, and disease progression. High intakes of omega-6 polyunsaturated fatty acids seem to increase the risk of cancers while high intakes of omega-3 fatty acids may provide protection. Animal studies have demonstrated that polyunsaturated omega-6 fatty acids stimulate carcinogenesis and tumor growth and metastasis, whereas long-chain omega-3 fatty acids inhibit these processes. Reducing total fat intake and increasing the ratio of omega-3 to omega-6 fatty acids in the diet may be particularly useful for groups at a relatively high risk for breast or prostate cancer, and may also be useful after surgery to help prevent disease recurrence.[78]

Dietary intake of essential fatty acids may play a role in prostate cancer cell proliferation. Epidemiological studies have demonstrated that men whose dietary intake is high in omega-6 fatty acids have a higher incidence of clinical prostate cancer.[79] Diets high in omega-3 fatty acids may have protective effects. Other research suggests that omega-3 fatty acids inhibit breast cancer and that the degree of this inhibition depends on background levels of omega-6 fatty acids. Results from the European Community Multicenter Study on Antioxidants, Myocardial Infarction, and Cancer (EURAMIC) study published in 1998, suggest that an increase in the ratio of omega-3 fatty acids to total omega-6 fatty acids in fat tissue decreases the risk of breast cancer. In this study, total levels of omega-3 or omega-6 fat were not consistently associated with breast cancer.[80]

Population and laboratory studies suggest that omega-3 fatty acids may help to prevent and inhibit colon cancer. In a study published in 1995, death rates for colorectal cancer in 24 European countries were correlated with current fish and fish oil consumption, and with consumption ten and 23 years previously.

In men, there was a reduced risk of death from colorectal cancer and current intake of fish, a weaker link with fish consumption ten years earlier, and none with consumption 23 years earlier. The researchers concluded that fish consumption is associated with protection against the later stages of colorectal cancer, but not with the early initiation stages.[81]

Omega-3 fatty acid supplements

Omega-3 fatty acids may be beneficial in preventing as treating cancer as they seem to exert tumor-suppressive effects.[82] In a study published in 1997, Norwegian researchers studied the relationship between incidence of lung cancer and intake of dietary fats, high fat foods, fish, and fish products in 25 956 men and 25 496 women aged from 16 to 56. During the follow-up period, 153 cases of lung cancer were identified. The results showed that those who took cod liver oil supplements had around half the risk of those who did not.[83]

Essential fatty acids may also boost immune function which may help in cancer prevention and treatment. Studies on the immune T cells in cancer patients taking fish oil capsules suggest that omega-3 fatty acids bring about beneficial changes. In a Greek study published in 1998, researchers investigated the effect of dietary omega-3 polyunsaturated fatty acids and vitamin E on the immune status and survival in both well-nourished and malnourished cancer patients. The study involved 60 patients with solid tumors who were randomized to receive dietary supplementation with either fish oil (18 g of omega-3 fatty acids) or placebo daily. The authors measured various indicators of immune function. The results showed that omega-3 fatty acids had a significant immune-enhancing effect and seemed to prolong the survival of malnourished patients.[84]

Gamma-linolenic acid

Gamma-linolenic acid has been shown to be effective in killing cancer cells and is well-established as a topical treatment for some types of cancer, including bladder cancer.[85] It has also been shown to kill various other types of cancer cells.[86]

There are many other compounds under investigation for their anticancer potential, including soybeans, tea and garlic. Bioflavonoids, colored pigments from fruit and vegetables, may also have anticancer properties. Cruciferous vegetables such as broccoli, cauliflower and cabbage also contain anticancer compounds.

Cardiovascular disease

Cardiovascular disease is the general term for heart ("cardio") and blood vessel ("vascular") diseases. These include atherosclerosis, coronary heart disease, heart attack, stroke, high blood pressure, peripheral vascular diseases and congestive heart failure. Cardiovascular disease accounts for one in every two deaths in developed countries. Coronary heart disease causes 36 per cent of all deaths in the USA and is the number one killer disease. Stroke, another type of cardiovascular disease, is the third most common cause of death.

Causes of cardiovascular disease

Risk factors for cardiovascular disease include high cholesterol, smoking, high blood triglyceride levels, excess weight, stress, drinking too much alcohol and lack of exercise. Diabetics are also at increased risk of cardiovascular disease.

Heredity also plays a part in cardiovascular disease. Both men and women are more likely to develop heart disease if close blood relatives have had it. Screening, dietary intervention and possibly drugs may be useful in treating those in the early stages of disease. Being overweight in the first ten years of life also increases the risk of heart disease. The disorder is twice as likely to develop in those who are inactive as in those who are active.

Coronary heart disease strikes hardest at men in their mid-fifties. Men are more likely than women to suffer from heart attacks, and they also tend to have them earlier in life. However, after menopause more women die from heart attacks. Studies show that women's cholesterol is higher than men's from age 55 onwards.

Atherosclerosis

The underlying cause of cardiovascular disease is atherosclerosis. The general term arteriosclerosis is used to describe the thickening and hardening of the arteries that occurs as people get older. Atherosclerosis occurs when deposits of fatty substances, cholesterol, cell waste products, calcium and fibrin (a clotting material from blood) build up in the inner lining of the artery. The build-up is known as plaque and as it increases bleeding can occur, eventually leading to the formation of blood clots. If a clot blocks a whole artery, a heart attack or stroke can occur.

The development of atherosclerosis can begin at a very early age and is usually not noticed until serious health problems such as a heart attack or stroke occur. About 13.5 million Americans know that they have the disease.

Atherosclerosis is a complex process and exactly how it begins or what causes it, is unknown. However, it seems likely that damage to the inner lining of blood vessels starts the process. Considerable evidence suggests that a high level of cholesterol is the most important factor contributing to the disease process. Certain types of cholesterol are vulnerable to oxidative damage by free radicals, and oxidized cholesterol is more damaging to arteries than unoxidized cholesterol. New research suggests that other compounds are also vulnerable to oxidation, including those in white blood cells known as macrophages, which can promote plaque formation by causing inflammation and the release of toxic substances that can damage cells.

Atherosclerosis can affect any area of the body. Blocked coronary arteries affect the heart, while narrowing of the carotid arteries of the neck may reduce mental functioning. Atherosclerosis of the leg arteries leads to intermittent claudication in which it is difficult to walk without pain; and clogging of the pelvic arteries affects sexual performance.

Coronary heart disease

The coronary arteries are those that supply blood to the heart. They are attached directly to the wall of the heart and are squeezed and expanded as the heart muscle contracts and relaxes. This contraction occurs 100 000 times a day, placing the coronary arteries under considerable stress and causing them to be especially vulnerable to damage and disease. Coronary heart disease is also known as ischemic heart disease and its most common forms are myocardial infarction (heart attack) and angina pectoris (chest pain).

Angina

Angina pectoris has symptoms of a squeezing or pressure-like chest pain, which usually occurs after physical exertion. The pain can be severe or mild and usually lasts from one to 20 minutes. Angina is caused by an insufficient supply of oxygen to the heart, usually because of the build-up of atherosclerotic plaque.

A special type of angina, known as variant angina, occurs when the coronary arteries go into spasm. This type of angina can occur at rest, at odd times during the day or night, and is more common in women under the age of 50.

Heart attack

A heart attack occurs when the blood supply to the heart muscle is sharply reduced or stopped, after one of the coronary arteries is blocked. If the blood supply is cut off for a long period, death may result. About 1.5 million Americans suffer from a heart attack in any one year. Coronary artery disease, in which the arteries supplying blood to the heart become blocked by the build-up of atherosclerotic plaque, is the underlying cause of heart attacks.

Lifestyle changes such as stopping smoking, eating a healthy diet and an appropriate exercise program can help to prevent heart attacks, even in those who may have already suffered. Drug therapy including aspirin, ACE inhibitors, beta blockers and cholesterol-lowering drugs may also play a part. Hormone replacement therapy in postmenopausal women can also reduce the risk as estrogen protects the heart.

Risk factors for cardiovascular disease

Cholesterol

Cholesterol is a type of fat that has many vital functions in the body. It is part of cell membranes and is necessary for the manufacture of bile acids and many hormones. Cholesterol is manufactured in the body and is also found in foods of animal origin. Plant foods do not contain cholesterol.

As cholesterol is a fat-soluble molecule it cannot dissolve in the blood. It is therefore attached to compounds known as lipoproteins, which transport it to different places in the body. There are several types of lipoprotein cholesterol compounds. These include LDL (low density lipoprotein) cholesterol, which transports cholesterol to the tissues; and HDL (high density lipoprotein) cholesterol, which transports it to the liver for metabolism and excretion.

High levels of LDL cholesterol promote build-up in atherosclerotic plaques in the artery walls while HDL cholesterol reduces this. Hence LDL cholesterol is often referred to as bad cholesterol while HDL cholesterol is referred to as good cholesterol. The ratio of LDL to HDL cholesterol is an important factor in disease development as it determines whether cholesterol is being deposited into the arteries or taken to the liver to be excreted.

Cholesterol levels are influenced by genetic make up and by diet. For years it was thought that foods high in cholesterol raised blood cholesterol. Further research has shown that while high cholesterol foods can raise blood cholesterol levels, the saturated fat content of foods has a greater effect. It is currently recommended that total blood cholesterol should be less than 200 mg per deciliter of blood. LDL cholesterol should be less than 130 mg per deciliter and HDL cholesterol more than 35 mg per deciliter. At these levels, a person's risk of heart disease is low.

Recently, a compound called lipoprotein(a) or Lp(a) has been found to be an independent risk factor for heart disease. When Lp(a) levels are above 30

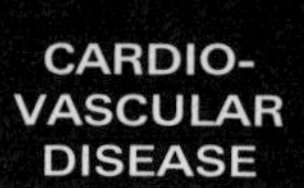

mg per deciliter, the risk of heart disease is increased. Lp(a) may act by delaying the breakdown of blood clots.

Triglycerides

Triglycerides are the chemical form in which most fats exist in food and in the body. Calories not used by the body immediately are converted to triglycerides and transported to fat cells. Hormones regulate the release to meet energy needs between meals. An excess of triglycerides in the blood is linked to an increased risk of heart disease. It is currently recommended that triglyceride levels should be lower than 150 mg per deciliter.

Blood platelets

Blood cell fragments known as platelets play an important role in the process of atherosclerosis. The gathering together or 'aggregation' of platelets is essential for the formation of blood clots in wound-healing. However, excessive platelet aggregation increases the risk of cardiovascular diseases such as heart attack and stroke. When platelets clump together around atherosclerotic plaques, they release compounds which cause the plaques to grow further and eventually block the artery. There are many chemicals in food which affect platelet function and these can either have beneficial or harmful effects depending on whether they increase or decrease aggregation.

High homocysteine levels

Several studies have found a link between high levels of a substance called homocysteine and cardiovascular disease. Homocysteine forms when the body breaks down protein. Enzymes either turn homocysteine back into the amino acid methionine, which can then be used to build protein, or break it down for excretion in the urine. High levels of homocysteine may be toxic to the cells that line blood vessels and may also increase the adhesiveness of platelets and other clotting factors.

Homocysteine levels are influenced by dietary intakes of folate, vitamin B6 and vitamin B12. They also vary according to race, gender, age and certain disease conditions. A dangerous cause of high blood pressure known as isolated systolic hypertension has also been found to be linked to homocysteine levels. Homocysteine may cause excessive stiffening of the aorta and other blood vessels thus forcing the heart to pump harder and thereby increasing the risk of heart and blood vessel diseases.

Obesity

Being overweight increases the risk of cardiovascular disease by raising blood pressure, increasing blood fats, reducing HDL cholesterol and raising the risk of diabetes. This is particularly the case when the excess body fat is stored in the chest and abdomen.

Smoking

Smoking increases the risk of cardiovascular disease. Smoking reduces the ability of the blood to deliver oxygen to the heart, stiffens arteries, damages blood vessel linings, promotes clotting, increases cholesterol levels and makes LDL cholesterol more susceptible to oxidative damage by free radicals. Even nonsmokers who live with heavy smokers have an increased risk of heart disease, and women may be more susceptible to the risks of smoking than men.

Stress

Stress increases the risk of heart disease and those who have high levels of hostility and unexpressed anger are also at higher risk. Sudden psychological stress may also trigger heart attacks. Depression also seems to be linked to heart disease, particularly new depression. Effective relaxation techniques such as meditation have been found to reduce stress and prevent heart attacks.

Preventing cardiovascular disease

Eating a healthy diet, not smoking, maintaining a healthy body weight, limiting alcohol consumption and practising effective stress reduction techniques are very important in the prevention of cardiovascular disease. Exercise is also a vital part of any prevention program and many studies have shown reduced risk in men and women who exercise regularly. Exercise can reduce blood cholesterol, blood pressure and lead to a reduced risk of obesity and diabetes. Vigorous exercise is good for the heart, lungs and circulation. Activities such as brisk walking, jogging, cycling and swimming for at least 30 minutes three to four days per week at 50 to 75 per cent of maximum heart rate bring the most beneficial effects. For elderly people, moderate or low intensity exercise may be more suitable.

Diet and cardiovascular disease

The link between diet and cardiovascular disease is a strong one. Diets high in saturated fats, salt, cholesterol and sugar increase the risk of heart disease; and diets high in fresh fruit, vegetables and fiber decrease it. Many population studies show that a 'Mediterranean diet' that is high in olive oil, fresh and dried fruit, grains, legumes and nuts appears to lower both cholesterol levels and heart disease risk.

Fiber

Fiber in the diet reduces the risk of heart disease. Daily intake should be around 35 grams. Fiber binds cholesterol and fats and lessens their absorption. It also decreases total and LDL cholesterol levels and increases protective HDL cholesterol levels. Results of studies such as the Physicians Health Study show that fewer heart attacks occur in those that eat more fiber, particularly the soluble type found in oat bran, fruit and vegetables.[1]

Fat

Reducing dietary fat has the greatest impact on lowering blood cholesterol and lowering the risk of cardiovascular disease. However, it is not only the amount of fat in the diet that affects the risk of heart disease, but also the type.

Saturated fats are found in animal foods such as meat, butter and cheese; and plant foods such as coconut oil and palm oil. Trans fats are unsaturated fats, which have undergone a chemical process called hydrogenation to turn them into saturated fats. They are found in packaged foods such as pastries, cookies, crackers and baked goods. High consumption of these fats increases cholesterol and triglyceride levels, and increases platelet aggregation. This contributes to atherosclerosis. Polyunsaturated fats which are found in oils of plant origin such as safflower, sesame, sunflower and corn may help to lower cholesterol and decrease platelet aggregation, thus reducing the risk of heart disease. However, polyunsaturated oils are susceptible to oxidation and may also lower HDL cholesterol. Monounsaturated fats such as those found in canola, olive and peanut oils may also help to lower cholesterol and decrease platelet aggregation. They are also less susceptible to oxidation. Adequate intakes of the essential fatty acids are important in the prevention of heart disease.

The results of a 1997 study published in the *New England Journal of Medicine* suggest that replacing saturated and trans-unsaturated fats with unhydrogenated monounsaturated and polyunsaturated fats is more effective in preventing coronary heart disease in women than reducing overall fat intake.[2]

The American Heart Association (AHA) recommends that 15 to 30 per cent of calories in the diet come from fat. Of this, a maximum of 10 per cent should come from saturated fats and also no more than 10 per cent from polyunsaturated fatty acids. The AHA also recommends that intake of dietary cholesterol, which is only found in animal foods, should be no more than 300 mg per day. Only saturated fatty acids and dietary cholesterol raise blood cholesterol. Some experts recommend very low fat diets to reduce the risk of, and even actually reverse damage caused by atherosclerosis. One such diet, which is known as the Ornish diet, recommends limiting fat intake to 10 per cent of calories.

Carbohydrate

The AHA recommends that 50 to 55 per cent, or more, of calories should come from carbohydrates, with the emphasis mainly on complex carbohydrates such as vegetables, beans and grains. Complex carbohydrates are absorbed more slowly into the blood than simple carbohydrates. This avoids the sharp rises and falls in insulin that a diet high in simple sugars can cause. Refined sugar also seems to cause a greater increase in blood fat levels than more complex carbohydrates.

In fat tissue, insulin facilitates the storage of glucose and its conversion to fatty acids, and also slows the breakdown of fatty acids. Thus sharp rises in insulin may contribute to obesity and heart disease, and it seems that blood insulin stores correspond to body fat stores. The longer and more often insulin levels are high the more likely sugars are to be converted to and stored as fat. This increases the risk of obesity and cardiovascular disease. Eating large amounts of foods high in both fat and sugar further increases the risk.

Protein

Diets high in animal protein seem to raise the risk of cardiovascular disease while diets high in vegetable proteins lower it.

Vitamins, minerals and cardiovascular disease

Antioxidants

Data from many sources, including laboratory experiments, epidemiology, animal studies and some clinical trials suggest that antioxidants may protect against the development of cardiovascular disease. The evidence is strongest for vitamin E and weakest for vitamin C.

Antioxidants may help prevent heart disease in a number of ways. They improve blood cholesterol levels and protect LDL cholesterol from oxidation. Oxidized LDL cholesterol is more likely to block arteries than unoxidized LDL cholesterol. Oxidized LDL cholesterol can also impair the action of nitric oxide, a chemical secreted by the blood vessel wall which dilates arteries. Levels of beneficial HDL cholesterol may be lowered by free radical activity. Antioxidants also help prevent the aggregation of blood platelets which can stick to blood vessel walls and cause blockages.

It is not yet clear what dose or in what combination, antioxidants provide the best protection. At the very least, it is important to consume the recommended dietary allowances for all antioxidants, especially from food which contains many other heart protective chemicals.

Carotenes

Many large population studies show that the risk of heart disease decreases with increasing beta carotene intake. Researchers involved in the Massachusetts Health Care Panel Study examined the links between consumption of carotene-containing fruits and vegetables, and death from cardiovascular disease among 1299 elderly people. The results of the study, which were published in the *Annals of Epidemiology* in 1995 showed that during the follow-up period of almost five years, there were 161 deaths from cardiovascular disease. The risk of death in the group who ate the most carotene-containing foods was almost half that of those people whose carotene consumption was low.[3]

Results from the EURAMIC study suggest that antioxidants protect heart attacks. Researchers studied people from ten European countries and analyzed for levels of carotenes in those who had suffered heart attacks and those who had not. They found protective effects of alpha carotene, beta carotene, and lycopene. Lycopene was particularly protective, with those in the highest intake group having around half the risk of heart attack of those in the lowest intake group.[4]

In a 1997 study, researchers in Italy investigated the relationship between nonfatal heart attacks and dietary intake of beta carotene. The study involved 433 heart attack patients and 869 women without cardiovascular disease. The results showed that women with high beta carotene intakes had around half the risk of heart attack of those with low intakes.[5] The relationship between intake of dietary antioxidants and risk of stroke was investigated as part of the Chicago Western Electric Study. The researchers found a moderately reduced risk in those with high beta carotene intakes.[6]

Supplements

Beta carotene supplements have been used in cancer and cardiovascular disease prevention trials including the Finnish Alpha Tocopherol Beta Carotene Cancer (ATBC) Prevention Study, the US Carotene and Retinol Efficacy Trial (CARET) and the US Physicians Health Study. In 1996 these studies reported results which received wide publicity. The ATBC Prevention group studied 29 000 men who smoked and drank alcohol. The results showed an 18 per cent increase in lung cancer deaths and an 11 per cent increase in ischemic heart disease deaths in men who took daily supplements of 20 mg beta carotene.[7] The CARET study was stopped 21 months early. This study was examining the effect of beta carotene (30 mg daily) and retinol (7500 mcg RE daily) supplementation on the prevention of cancer and heart disease in over 18 000 smokers and people who had been exposed to asbestos. The trial was stopped when the results showed a 28 per cent increased risk of lung cancer, a 26 per cent increase in the risk of death from cardiovascular disease and a 17 per cent increase in overall deaths in the group receiving the supplements.[8]

It seems likely that smoking and alcohol consumption contribute to the adverse effects of beta carotene supplements. The CARET results showed greater risk in current smokers than former smokers and also in those who drank alcohol. Recent laboratory research suggests that vitamin C protects against the harmful effects of beta carotene in smokers. Smokers tend to have low levels of vitamin C and this may allow a build-up of a harmful form of beta carotene called the carotene free radical which is formed when beta carotene acts to regenerate vitamin E. These results suggest that in smokers, dietary vitamin C supplementation should accompany beta carotene supplementation.[9]

Vitamin C

Low vitamin C intake is linked to an increased risk of cardiovascular disease. As well as exerting beneficial effects on cholesterol levels, vitamin C also increases the production of prostacyclin, a prostaglandin which decreases the clumping of blood platelets and dilates blood vessels, therefore reducing the risk of heart disease, atherosclerosis and stroke.

In a study begun in 1981, USDA researchers assessed the health and nutrition status of 747 elderly people aged 60 years and over. Particular attention was paid to the foods the participants usually ate their blood levels of the antioxidant vitamins C, E and beta carotene. The researchers following up the subjects from nine to 12 years later found that among people who ate lots of dark green and orange vegetables, there were fewer deaths from heart disease and other causes. The results showed that a daily intake of more than 400 mg and higher blood levels of vitamin C were linked to reduced risk of death from heart disease.[10]

In a study published in the *British Medical Journal* in 1995, UK researchers assessed the links between dietary intake and blood levels of vitamin C, and death from stroke and coronary heart disease in people aged 65 and over. The study involved 730 men and women who were followed up for a 20-year period. The results showed that those with the highest intakes had around half the risk of death from stroke when compared to those with the lowest intakes. However, in this study, no link was found between vitamin C status and risk of death from coronary heart disease.[11]

Low vitamin C levels are also associated with an increased risk of heart attack. In a 1997 study, Finnish researchers examined this link in 1605 men aged between 42 and 60 who were free from heart disease when they entered the study. During the follow-up period there were 70 heart attacks. The results showed that men with vitamin C deficiency were three-and-a-half times more likely to have a heart attack than those who were not deficient.[12] However, not all studies have shown protective effects of vitamin C. These include the large Nurses and Health Professionals Studies.[13,14]

Researchers from Cambridge University in the UK examined the relationship between blood levels of vitamin C status and angina in women aged from 45 to 74. Forty-two women with previously undiagnosed angina were compared with 877 women with no disease. Those with higher vitamin C levels had a 66 per cent reduced risk of angina.[15] The same researchers examined the link between blood levels of vitamin C and blood fat levels. Their results showed that a high intake of vitamin C from food raises beneficial HDL cholesterol and lowers serum triglyceride.[16]

Supplements

Vitamin C supplements may help protect against the development of cardiovascular disease. The results of a 1996 study showed that those taking vitamin E supplements had a 47 per cent lower risk of death from heart disease and those taking both vitamin C and vitamin E had a 53 per cent reduced risk.[17]

High fat meals cause damage to artery linings, which may contribute to the development of atherosclerosis. Research suggests that taking the antioxidant vitamins C and E before a meal may help to prevent this damage.[18] Vitamin C may also improve artery function in those with coronary artery disease[19], high cholesterol levels[20] and chronic heart failure.[21] When blood is re-supplied to an organ from which it was previously cut off, oxidative damage can occur. This has been found in many types of surgery; for example, in heart bypass operations.

Vitamin C has been shown to protect against this reperfusion injury.[22]

Vitamin C also seems to protect against smoking-related damage, possibly by decreasing the smoking-related build-up of atherosclerotic plaque and by improving artery function.[23]

Vitamin E

High intakes of vitamin E may reduce the risk of heart disease. Some studies have only shown benefit from the amount of vitamin E that can be obtained in the diet, whereas others suggest that the amount of vitamin E needed to show protective effects is considerably more than a typical diet provides.

Results from the Iowa Women's Health Study suggest a link between low vitamin E intake and heart disease. Researchers studied 34 486 postmenopausal women with no cardiovascular disease who in early 1986 completed a questionnaire that assessed, among other factors, their intake of vitamins A, E, and C from food sources and supplements. During seven years of follow-up, 242 women died of coronary heart disease. The results showed that high vitamin E consumption reduced the risk of death from coronary heart disease. This association was particularly striking in the subgroup of 21 809 women who did not consume vitamin supplements.[24]

Similar results have been seen in men. Harvard School of Public Health researchers have assessed the links between diet and heart disease in 39 910 US male health professionals aged between 40 to 75 years of age. Participants responded to a questionnaire in 1986 and were then followed up for four years, during which time there were 667 cases of coronary disease. The results showed a lower risk of disease among men with higher intakes of vitamin E. Men consuming more than 40 mg (60 IU) per day had a 36 per cent lower risk than those consuming less than 5 mg (7.5 IU) per day. Men who took at least 67 mg (100 IU) per day for at least two years had a 37 per cent lower risk than those who did not take supplements.[25]

Vitamin E appears to play a part in decreasing the risk of angina. The results of a 1996 study done in Japan suggest that low vitamin E levels increase the risk of a variant angina, a form of the disease caused by coronary artery spasm.[26] Results of the Finnish ATBC Prevention Study found a slightly reduced risk in those taking vitamin E supplements.[27]

Supplements

Results from the Nurses Health Study provide evidence for the protective effects of vitamin E supplements. Researchers assessed the links between vitamin E and heart disease in 87 245 female nurses aged from 34 to 59. During the follow-up period of eight years, there were 552 cases of major coronary disease

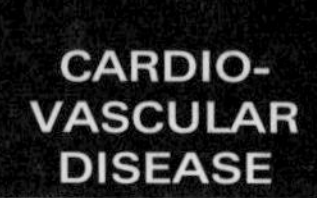

(437 nonfatal heart attacks and 115 deaths due to coronary disease). The results showed that women with the highest vitamin E intakes had 34 per cent less risk of major coronary disease compared to those with the lowest intakes. Most of the reduction in risk was attributable to vitamin E consumed as supplements, a finding which conflicts with some other studies which only show benefit from high dietary intakes. Women who took vitamin E supplements for short periods had little apparent benefit, but those who took them for more than two years had an even lower risk of disease.[28]

Results from a British study known as the Cambridge Heart Antioxidant Study (CHAOS) which were published in *The Lancet* in 1996 provide further evidence of a link between vitamin E supplements and reduction in heart disease risk. In this double-blind, placebo-controlled study, 2002 patients with coronary atherosclerosis were enrolled and followed up for 510 days. 546 patients were given 536 mg (800 IU) daily; 589 patients were given 268 mg (400 IU) per day; and 967 received identical placebo capsules. The results showed that those who received vitamin E supplements had a 75 per cent reduction in the risk of fatal heart attacks. However, when nonfatal events were included, there did not appear to be any benefit from the vitamin E supplements.[29]

B vitamins

Thiamin

Marginal thiamin deficiency may contribute to heart disease as those with heart disease have been found to have lower than normal levels of thiamin in their heart muscle.

Niacin

Large doses of the nicotinic acid form of niacin are used to lower harmful LDL blood cholesterol and triglyceride levels, and raise levels of beneficial HDL cholesterol. Niacin also favorably influences other lipid levels including lipoprotein (a). Doses used range from 1500 to 2500 mg. The increase of HDL cholesterol seems to occur at a lower dose (1500 mg per day) than the reduction of LDL cholesterol. In general, it is usual to start taking lower doses (around 50 to 100 mg) and then gradually increase to the higher doses over a period of two to three weeks.

Researchers involved in a 1997 study done in Minneapolis compared blood lipid levels in 244 patients treated with niacin and 160 treated with lovastatin, a widely used cholesterol-lowering drug. The results showed that both lovastatin and niacin effectively reduced LDL cholesterol levels with a greater drop seen in those taking lovastatin. Niacin use was associated with a 16.3 per cent improvement in HDL cholesterol, while HDL cholesterol levels in the lovastatin group improved 1.5 per cent. The improvement in triglyceride levels was also much greater in the niacin group.[35]

Nicotinic acid can also enhance the effects of other cholesterol-lowering medications. This may mean that the doses of these drugs can be reduced, thus lessening the possibility of undesirable side effects. In a recent US study researchers found that combination therapy with niacin and low dose lovastatin was as effective as high dose lovastatin.[36]

Nicotinic acid has also been shown to have favorable effects on the blood clotting system which can reduce the build-up of atherosclerotic plaque.[37] It has also been used to treat peripheral vascular disease and circulatory disorders such as Raynaud's disease, as it dilates blood vessels thereby increasing blood flow to certain areas of the body.

Vitamin B6

Vitamin B6 deficiency seems to increase the risk of developing heart disease, most likely because of increased homocysteine levels. In a study published in 1998, researchers involved in a study done in several centers in Europe compared 750 patients with vascular disease and 800 control subjects of the same ages and sex. They measured blood levels of homocysteine, folate, vitamin B12, and vitamin B6. The results showed that those with high blood homocysteine concentrations had a high risk of vascular disease. In addition, low concentrations of folate and vitamin B6 were also associated with increased risk. In this study, the relationship between vitamin B6 and atherosclerosis did not appear to be solely due to increased homocysteine levels, suggesting that vitamin B6 may have other important roles in heart disease prevention.[38]

Researchers involved in the Framingham Heart Study analyzed blood samples from the study participants to assess levels of homocysteine and the relationship between B vitamins and carotid artery narrowing, which increases the risk of heart attack. The results showed that low intakes of folate and vitamin B6 were associated with high homocysteine levels.[39]

Intake of folate and vitamin B6 above the current recommended dietary allowance seems to be important in the prevention of coronary heart disease among women. Researchers from the Harvard School of Public Health investigated the links between intakes of folate and vitamin B6 and the incidence of heart attacks in 80 082 women taking part in the Nurses Health Study. The women had no previous history of cardiovascular disease, cancer, high cholesterol levels or diabetes when they entered the study. During the 14 years of follow-up, there were 658 nonfatal heart attacks and 281 fatal ones. The results showed that those with the highest intakes of vitamin B6 had just over 30 per cent less risk of heart attack than those in the low intake group. Women in the group with the highest intakes of both folate and vitamin B6 had just less than half the risk of women in the lowest intake group. Risk of coronary heart disease was reduced among women who regularly used multiple vitamins, the major source of folate and vitamin B6.[40]

Supplements

In a study published in 1998, Irish researchers screened a group of clinically healthy working men aged 30 to 49 years and selected 132 with mildly raised homocysteine concentrations. They then assessed the effects of eight weeks of supplementation with B group vitamins and antioxidant vitamins on homocysteine concentrations. The men were randomly assigned to one of four groups: supplementation with B group vitamins alone (1 mg folic acid, 7.2 mg pyridoxine, and 0.02 mg vitamin B12); antioxidant vitamins alone; B-group vitamins with antioxidant vitamins; or placebo. The results showed significant decreases in both groups receiving B group vitamins either with or without antioxidants. The effect of the B group vitamins alone was a reduction in homocysteine concentrations of almost 30 per cent.[41]

Vitamin B6 may also exert beneficial effects on the cardiovascular system by protecting against the aggregation of blood platelets. This prolongs clotting time and helps to reduce atherosclerotic plaque build-up.[42] Vitamin B6 has also been shown to lower blood pressure and blood cholesterol levels. In a Swedish study published in 1990, researchers assessed the effect of 120 mg a day of vitamin B6 on seventeen 88 year-old men with low vitamin B6 levels. After supplementation for eight weeks, the average plasma total cholesterol and LDL cholesterol concentrations were decreased by 10 per cent and 17 per cent respectively.[43]

Folic acid

Diets high in folic acid seem to reduce the risk of heart disease. As with vitamin B6, this is likely to be due to the relationship with homocysteine levels. In a study published in 1998, researchers at the Cleveland Clinic conducted a study to investigate the relationships between homocysteine, B vitamins, and vascular diseases. The study involved 750 patients with documented vascular disease and 800 control patients matched for age and sex. The results showed that those in the lowest 10 per cent of folate intakes had an increased risk of disease.[44]

A 1996 Canadian study of the relationship between fatal coronary heart disease and folic acid levels in 5000 men and women found that the risk of coronary heart disease increased as folic acid levels decreased. Those in the lowest intake group were 69 per cent more likely to die of heart disease than those with the highest intakes.[45]

Low blood folic acid levels also seem to increase heart attack risk in young women. In a 1997 study, researchers at the University of Washington measured the homocysteine, folic acid and vitamin B12 levels in 79 heart attack survivors under 45 and compared these with levels in 386 healthy control subjects. Those with the highest homocysteine levels had 2.3 times the risk of heart attack compared to those with the lowest levels. Those with the highest levels of folic acid had around half the risk of heart attack compared to those with the lowest levels.[46]

Supplements

Several studies have examined the homocysteine-lowering effects of folate supplements. In a 1998 paper, researchers analyzed the results of randomized controlled trials that assessed the effects of folic acid-based supplements on blood homocysteine concentrations. The data included that from 1114 people in 12 trials. They found that 0.5 to 5 mg folic acid daily reduced blood homocysteine concentrations by 25 per cent.[47] Those with the highest homocysteine levels may respond best to increases in folic acid intake; and above a certain level of intake, increasing folic acid may not affect homocysteine levels. In a 1997 Irish study, researchers assessed the effects of various doses of supplements on homocysteine levels. Of the three folic acid doses, 200 mcg appeared to be as effective as 400 mcg, while 100 did not lower levels sufficiently.[48]

Vitamin B12

Vitamin B12 may also be important in maintaining normal levels of homocysteine.[49]

Vitamin D

Low vitamin D levels may also increase the risk of atherosclerosis. Research suggests that a low level of vitamin D increases the risk of calcium build-up in atherosclerotic plaques, and that higher levels reduce the risk of build-up. Researchers at UCLA School of Medicine measured the vitamin D levels in the blood of 173 men and women at risk of heart disease and also measured the build-up of calcium in coronary arteries (a common finding in coronary artery disease). The results suggest that calcium may regulate calcium deposition in the arteries as well as in the bone.[50]

Minerals and cardiovascular disease

Although there is no evidence for a direct cause and effect relationship between mineral and trace element status and atherosclerosis in humans, many elements exert a strong influence on individual risk factors for cardiovascular disease, such as disorders of blood fats, blood pressure and blood clotting. Epidemiological studies have shown that high intakes of minerals such as sodium, magnesium, calcium, chromium, copper, zinc, and iodine lead to a reduced risk of cardiovascular disease. The local environment, which influences the mineral content of food and dietary practices, can result in mineral and trace element imbalances. Deficiencies of chromium, iron, copper, zinc, selenium, and iodine are relatively common. Detection and correction of such imbalances in people may diminish risk factors and reduce the incidence of atherosclerotic heart disease.

Calcium

Calcium plays an important role in heart health. It is essential for heart muscle contraction, nerve impulse conduction, blood pressure regulation, and is involved in the control of blood cholesterol levels. Increasing calcium may normalize heart rhythm in arrhythmia sufferers. Calcium supplements can be useful in congestive heart failure as they increase the contractility of heart muscle. Calcium salts are used intravenously to treat heart attack associated with high potassium and magnesium levels and low calcium levels.

Chromium

Chromium deficiency may play a role in heart disease. On a population level, decreased chromium levels correlate with increased prevalence of heart disease. Recent studies have demonstrated that plasma chromium levels in patients with coronary artery disease are very much lower than in normal subjects. Chromium deficiency leads to impaired lipid and glucose metabolism and results in high cholesterol levels.

In a study published in 1996, researchers assessed the effects of daily supplements of 200 mcg of chromium and nicotinic acid on blood glucose and lipids, including total cholesterol, HDL cholesterol, LDL cholesterol, and triglycerides. The patients were 14 healthy adults and five adults with Type II diabetes mellitus. The results showed lowered total and LDL cholesterol, triglycerides, and glucose concentrations in patients with Type II diabetes.[51]

Copper

A deficiency of copper may contribute to heart disease. It may lead to a drop in beneficial HDL cholesterol and an increase in harmful LDL cholesterol. In animals, copper intake has also been associated with weakening of heart connective tissue and rupture of heart muscle. However, high copper levels may also be a risk factor for heart disease. The ratio of zinc to copper may be important in the regulation of blood cholesterol.

Copper supplements have been shown to have beneficial effects on the oxidation of blood fats. A 1997 study done over four weeks at Ohio State University found that 2 mg per day of copper increased the time taken for LDL cholesterol to become oxidized.[52] This helps to reduce the damage these fats do to arteries, and limits the build-up of atherosclerotic plaque.

Iron

Iron deficiency can adversely affect the heart, leading to abnormal heartbeat and heart function. However, the evidence from many scientific studies suggests that high iron levels (above 200 mcg per liter blood ferritin) may lead to an increase in the risk of cardiovascular disease. The increased risk may be due to oxidative damage to the heart and blood vessels, and increased oxidation of LDL cholesterol.

A study published in 1998 in the *American Journal of Epidemiology* suggests that men and women, particularly those over 60, are at increased risk of heart disease if they have high levels of iron in their diets. The study, which was conducted in Greece, involved 329 patients with heart disease and 570 people of similar age who were admitted to hospital with minor conditions believed to be unrelated to diet. Results showed that for every 50 mg increase in iron intake per month, men over 60 were 1.47 times more likely to have heart disease than their peers. In women over 60, the risk was even higher; with a 3.61-fold risk for every 50 mg increase.[53]

Another study published in 1998 in the journal *Circulation* suggests that men with high levels of stored iron in the body have an increased risk of heart attack. The study, which was done in Finland, involved 99 men who had had at least one heart attack and 99 healthy men matched for background and age. The results showed that those men with the highest iron levels had almost three times the risk of heart attack when compared to those with the lowest levels.[54] Further research is needed to confirm this link and to establish whether this applies to women whose blood ferritin levels are typically much lower (20 to 120 mcg per liter). Some experts believe that women are protected from heart disease until after menopause due to iron losses during menstruation.

However, a National Institute of Aging study suggests that low iron levels are linked to an increased likelihood of death in elderly people. Researchers looked at the iron status of nearly 4000 men and women aged 71 and over. Results of the five-year study showed that low iron levels increased the risk of total and coronary heart disease deaths. Those with higher iron levels had decreased risk. Men with the highest iron levels had only 20 per cent of the risk of dying of heart disease of those with the lowest levels. Women with the highest levels were about half as likely to die of heart disease compared to those with the lowest levels.[55]

Magnesium

High magnesium intake seems to protect against several types of cardiovascular disease, including atherosclerosis, heart attack, angina, ischemic heart disease and cardiac arrhythmias. Magnesium deficiency may increase the risk of cardiovascular disease in several ways. Chronic magnesium deficiency in animals has been shown to result in microscopic changes in the heart arteries and the development of atherosclerosis. Deficiency also leads to changes in the heart muscle itself, including cell degeneration, fibrosis, necrosis and calcification. Blood fat levels are also affected by magnesium dietary intake. Cholesterol may be more susceptible to oxidative damage when magnesium levels are low.

Studies show that death rates from coronary heart disease are higher in areas where the water is low in magnesium. In a 1996 study, Swedish researchers investigated these links in 17 municipalities in the southern part of the country which had differing water magnesium concentrations. The study included 854 men who had died of heart attacks between the ages of 50 and 69, and 989 men of the same age in the same area who had died from cancer during the same time period. The results showed that men living in high magnesium water areas had a 35 per cent lower chance of death from heart attack than those who drank low magnesium water.[56]

Results from the Atherosclerosis Risk in Communities (ARIC) Study support the association between low serum and dietary magnesium and various types of cardiovascular disease including high blood pressure. A total of 15 248 people took part, male and female, black and white, aged 45 to 64 years. The results showed that serum magnesium levels were significantly lower in participants with cardiovascular disease, high blood pressure, and diabetes than in those free of these diseases. Low dietary intake was linked to lower beneficial HDL cholesterol levels and thicker carotid artery walls, both of which increase the risk of cardiovascular disease.[57]

Magnesium deficiency is also linked to variant angina, a disorder in which coronary heart vessels go into spasm.[58] A 1996 Japanese study found that men with lower magnesium levels had more frequent and severe angina attacks.[59] Magnesium-deficient heart muscle is more vulnerable to lack of oxygen.

Magnesium deficiency also contributes to cardiac arrhythmias, possibly because magnesium is responsible for maintaining potassium concentrations inside muscle cells. Potassium plays a role in heart muscle contraction. Magnesium deficiency has been implicated in mitral valve prolapse, a disorder in which the mitral valve in the heart fails to properly close off the heart chambers from each other during contraction. As many as 85 per cent of sufferers may have chronic magnesium deficiency.

Supplements

Low magnesium levels have been found in the blood and cardiac muscle of heart attack victims, and several small studies have shown that magnesium sulfate injections can reduce death rates in heart attack patients, both in the short term and for longer periods.[60] It may act by improving energy production, inhibiting platelet aggregation, reducing vascular resistance, promoting clot breakdown, dilating blood vessels and improving the function of heart muscle. It also protects the damaged heart muscle against calcium overload and reduces free radical damage.

However, two recently published studies showed different results, although similar doses of magnesium were used. The LIMIT-2-study was a double-blind, placebo-controlled investigation of over 2300 patients with suspected heart attack. Magnesium infusion reduced 28-day death risk by 24 per cent.[61] The ISIS-4-study on over 50 000 patients with suspected heart attack did not show any positive effect of magnesium on death rate.[62]

Magnesium supplements are often used to treat angina, both that caused by atherosclerosis and variant angina caused by coronary artery spasm. In a 1997 study UK researchers assessed the effects of a 24-hour infusion of magnesium in patients with unstable angina. Thirty-one patients received magnesium sulfate and 31 placebo. After treatment, there were fewer ischemic episodes in the magnesium group and duration of ischemia in the placebo group was longer than that in the magnesium group.[63]

Magnesium supplements have also been used to treat cardiomyopathy, a weakening of heart muscle which leads to reduced efficiency of blood circulation and congestive heart failure. Sufferers of intermittent claudication, a painful condition caused by reduced blood flow to the legs, often have low magnesium levels and may be helped by supplements. Magnesium supplements have been

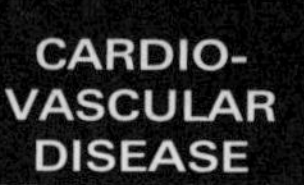

successfully used to treat mitral valve prolapse.[64] Magnesium supplements have been shown to reduce cholesterol and triglyceride levels.

Potassium

High potassium intake is associated with protection from cardiovascular disease and several studies have shown that increasing potassium intake can lower blood pressure. Potassium may protect against cardiovascular diseases in a number of ways: by reducing free radical formation; proliferation of vascular smooth muscle cells; platelet aggregation; and blood clotting.[65] Potassium supplements are used to treat heart arrhythmias.

Sodium

High sodium intake is linked to an increased risk of high blood pressure and other cardiovascular diseases. The American Heart Association recommends that the daily sodium intake for healthy American adults should not be more than 2.4 g per day. This is about one teaspoon of salt.

Selenium

Low selenium levels are linked to an increased risk of heart disease. Severe deficiency leads to weakened and damaged heart muscle and a type of congestive heart failure known as Keshan disease. As part of glutathione peroxidase, selenium takes part in the reduction of hydrogen peroxides and lipid peroxides. The concentration of these peroxides, in turn, affects platelet aggregation. Blood platelets of selenium-deficient people show increased aggregation, which selenium administration inhibits. Thus long-term supplementation with low doses of selenium could have a beneficial effect on the prevention of both thrombosis and coronary heart disease in people who are selenium-deficient.[30]

Dutch researchers studying the association between selenium status and the risk of heart attack, compared plasma, red blood cell, and toenail selenium levels and the activity of red blood cell glutathione peroxidase among 84 heart attack patients and 84 healthy people. They found lower selenium levels in all the heart attack patients. Because the toenail selenium level reflects blood levels up to one year before sampling, the results suggest that low selenium levels were present before the heart attacks, and may have played a role in their cause.[31]

However, results from the Physicians Health Study published in 1995 do not suggest a link between selenium levels and heart attack risk. Researchers analyzed blood selenium levels in 251 subjects who had heart attacks and an equal number of healthy people, matched by age and smoking status. The results did not show significant differences.[32]

Supplements

Finnish researchers evaluated the effect of selenium supplementation on 81 patients with heart attacks. Patients received either selenium-rich yeast (100 mcg per day) or placebo in addition to conventional drug therapy for a six-month period. During the follow-up period there were four cardiac deaths in the placebo group but none in the selenium group. There were two nonfatal heart attacks in the placebo group and one nonfatal attack in the selenium group.[33] A small 1997 German study showed that patients who were given selenium supplements after heart attacks showed greater improvements in heart function than patients not given supplements.[34]

Zinc

Low blood zinc levels may be associated with an increased risk of cardiovascular disease. The results of a recent study done over a period of ten years in Finland, which involved 230 men dying from cardiovascular diseases and 298 controls matched for age, place of residence and smoking found an increased risk of disease in those with low zinc levels.[66] This may be due to an imbalance in the copper-to-zinc ratio.

There is evidence that zinc can protect the inner lining of blood vessels from damage thus helping to prevent atherosclerosis. This may be due to its membrane-stabilizing, antioxidant and anti-inflammatory properties.[67] Some studies have shown that zinc supplements can reduce free radical damage to blood fats. In a 1996 Italian study, 25 mg zinc sulfate in 136 elderly people decreased plasma lipid peroxides.[68] This can help to reduce the risk of cardiovascular disease.

Other nutrients

Essential fatty acids

Some studies have shown that those who regularly eat fish have lower rates of heart disease. Fish are rich in omega-3 fatty acids, which can lower blood levels of triglycerides and LDL cholesterol. Fish oils can also interfere with the ability of blood to clot, which also protects against cardiovascular disease.

There are many population studies demonstrating that people who consume omega-3 fatty acid-rich diets have a reduced risk of heart disease. This was first noticed in countries such as Greenland and Japan where fish consumption is particularly high. Studies in other countries have found similar effects. In a study reported in the *New England Journal of Medicine*, researchers in Holland investigated the relationship between fish consumption and coronary heart disease in a group of men in the town of Zutphen. Information about the fish consumption of 852 middle-aged men without coronary heart disease was collected in 1960. During 20 years of follow-up, 78 men died from coronary heart disease. The results showed that compared to those who did not eat fish, death from coronary heart disease was more than 50 per cent lower in those who ate at least 30 g of fish per day.[69] However, not all studies have shown a reduced risk in those who regularly eat fish.

In a study reported in 1989, researchers examined the effects of dietary changes in the prevention of further heart attacks in 2033 men who had recovered from one attack. Some of the men were given various pieces of dietary advice, one of which was to increase the consumption of fatty fish to around two or three portions per week. Those advised to do this had a 29 per cent reduction in death from all causes and a 33 per cent reduction in death from heart attack compared with those who were not advised to eat fish.[70] These beneficial effects may be due to the anti-arrhythmic effects of omega-3 fatty acids.

Researchers involved in the US Physicians Health Study investigated the links between fish consumption and the risk of sudden death from heart attack in 20 551 US male physicians aged from 40 to 84. The follow-up period was 11 years, and in that time there were 133 sudden deaths. The results showed that men who ate fish at least once per week had around half the risk of sudden cardiac death when compared with men who consumed fish less than once a month. Neither dietary fish consumption nor omega-3 fatty acid intake was associated with a reduced risk of total heart attack, nonsudden cardiac death, or total cardiovascular mortality. However, fish consumption was associated with a significantly reduced risk of death from all causes.[71]

In a 1995 study, researchers at the University of Washington examined the links between risk of heart attack and the consumption of fatty acids from seafood, and assessed both directly and indirectly through examination of blood samples. The study involved 334 patients with primary cardiac arrest and 493 population-based control cases, matched for age and sex. The results showed that an intake of 5.5 g of omega-3 fatty acids (equivalent to one fish-containing meal a week) reduced the risk of heart attack by 50 per cent. Their results also showed a correlation between higher red blood cell levels of omega-3 fatty acids and reduction in risk of heart attack. Those with the highest levels had a 70 per cent reduction in risk compared to those with the lowest levels.[72]

Supplements
Omega-3 fatty acid supplements have been used to treat and prevent various types of cardiovascular disease. Supplements have been shown to have beneficial effects on cholesterol and triglyceride levels. In a 1994 study, researchers assessed the effects of fish oil supplements on 350 men and women aged from 30 to 54 years who were enrolled in a hypertension prevention trial. Once a day for six months, the participants received either a placebo or 6 g of purified fish oil, which supplied 3 g of omega-3 fatty acids. The results showed that the fish oil increased HDL cholesterol levels significantly. The effect was more marked in the women.[73]

Supplements have also been shown to affect blood clotting through effects on platelets and to lead to a reduction in production of prostaglandins and other substances that damage artery walls.[74] Other studies have shown that omega-3 fatty acids reduce the build-up of white blood cells in atherosclerotic plaque. A 1997 Australian study showed that flaxseed oil improved the elasticity of artery walls. This tends to decrease with increasing cardiovascular risk and has also been shown to improve with increasing intake of omega-3 fatty acids from fish.[75]

Choline

Choline helps to lower cholesterol levels as a choline-containing enzyme helps to remove cholesterol from tissues. In a 1995 study, researchers gave lecithin supplements to 32 patients with high cholesterol and triglyceride levels. The dosage used was 3.5 g three times daily before meals. After 30 days of treatment, total cholesterol and triglycerides levels decreased significantly and beneficial HDL cholesterol levels rose.[76] Choline has also been used to lower homocysteine concentrations.

Coenzyme Q10

Increasing scientific evidence suggests that coenzyme Q10 is a safe and effective therapy for a wide range of cardiovascular diseases such as congestive heart failure, cardiomyopathy, high blood pressure, mitral valve prolapse and angina. It has also been used to treat patients undergoing coronary artery bypass surgery. Coenzyme Q10 appears to exert its beneficial effects both by improving energy production and by acting as an antioxidant.

Coenzyme Q10 may help prevent atherosclerosis as it can protect against oxidative damage to fats. In a 1993 Japanese study, researchers measured levels of coenzyme Q10 and also levels of various types of cholesterol and other blood fats in 378 people. These included 249 people with no coronary artery disease, 29 patients with the disease who were receiving pravastatin, (a cholesterol-lowering drug) and 104 patients with the disease who were not receiving pravastatin. In the patient groups, the plasma total cholesterol and LDL cholesterol levels were higher and the plasma coenzyme Q10 level lower than in those with no disease. The results showed that coenzyme Q10 levels, either alone or when expressed in relation to LDL levels, were significantly lower in the patient groups compared with those with no disease. They concluded that coenzyme Q10 therapy would be beneficial in patients with atherosclerosis.[77]

In a study published in 1994, researchers at the University of Texas looked at the usefulness of long-term coenzyme Q10 therapy in clinical cardiology. Over an eight-year period, they treated 424 patients with various forms of cardiovascular disease by adding coenzyme Q10, in amounts ranging from 75 to 600 mg/day to their treatment programs. Patients were divided into six diagnostic categories including ischemic cardiomyopathy, dilated cardiomyopathy, primary diastolic dysfunction, hypertension, mitral valve prolapse and valvular heart disease.

The patients were followed for an average of 17.8 months. The researchers evaluated clinical response according to the New York Heart Association (NYHA) functional scale and found significant improvements in all the patients. Out of 424 patients, 58 per cent improved by one NYHA class, 28 per cent by two classes and 1.2 per cent by three classes. Statistically significant improvements in heart muscle function were shown using a variety of laboratory tests. Before treatment with coenzyme Q10, most patients were taking from one to five cardiac medications and during the study, overall medication requirements dropped considerably with 43 per cent of patients stopping between one and three drugs. Only 6 per cent of the patients required the addition of one drug. No apparent side effects from coenzyme Q10 treatment were noted other than a single case of transient nausea. The researchers concluded that coenzyme Q10 is a safe and effective treatment for a broad range of cardiovascular diseases, often in combination with other medications, as it produces improvements in a variety of symptoms and reduces medication needs.[78]

Coenzyme Q10 has also been used during heart surgery and to treat heart failure, cardiomyopathy and angina (See page 355 for more information.)

Carnitine

Carnitine can be used to treat several types of cardiovascular disease including cardiomyopathy, angina, heart attack and arrhythmias. It can also be used to lower blood fat levels, aid in weight loss, and improve muscle strength in some cases of weakness.

Herbal medicine and cardiovascular disease

There are many herbs used in the treatment of cardiovascular conditions. These include hawthorn (*Crataegus oxyacantha*), motherwort (*Leonurus cardiaca*), garlic (Allium sativum), onions (Allium cepa), ginger (*Zingiber officinale*), gugulipid (*Commiphora mukul*), cayenne (*Capsicum annuum*), ginkgo (*Ginkgo biloba*), yarrow *(Achillea millefolium*), linden blossom (*Tilia europea*) and cramp bark (*Viburnum opulus*). See page 384 for more information on these herbs and the precautions that may be necessary.

Carpal tunnel syndrome

Carpal tunnel syndrome is a painful disorder of the wrist and hand which is caused by irritation of the median nerve at the wrist. The carpal tunnel is a small circular structure located on the palm side of the wrist. Blood vessels, tendons and nerves travel through the tunnel and fan out to supply the palm and fingers of the hand. If this tunnel becomes inflamed and exerts pressure it causes numbness, tingling and pain in the hands and wrists.

Symptoms of carpal tunnel syndrome

Sufferers of carpal tunnel syndrome initially feel numbness and tingling of the hand in the thumb, index, middle and part of the fourth fingers. These sensations are often worse at night or on waking in the morning. As the disease progresses, patients can develop a burning sensation, cramping and weakness of the hand, and sharp shooting pains in the forearm. It may be difficult to clench the fist or grasp small objects.

Diagnosis of carpal tunnel syndrome

Symptoms may appear, or be worsened when the wrist is flexed for more than 60 seconds and then extended. This is known as the Phalen wrist flexion test. Carpal tunnel syndrome is strongly suggested when a nerve conduction test is abnormal. This test involves measuring the rate of speed of electrical impulses as they travel down a nerve. In carpal tunnel syndrome, the impulse slows as it goes through the carpal tunnel.

Causes of carpal tunnel syndrome

Any condition that exerts pressure on the median nerve can cause carpal tunnel syndrome. These include tendon inflammation resulting from repetitive work such as prolonged typing or assembly line work. Carpal tunnel syndrome is particularly common in those whose work requires grasping, twisting and turning, particularly if this involves repetitive vibration. Office workers who use excessive force while typing on their computer keyboards are at increased risk of carpal tunnel syndrome. Some sports such as rowing, golf, tennis, skiing and archery may also cause carpal tunnel syndrome, as can any condition which causes swelling or compression on nerves. These include sprains, obesity, pregnancy, hypothyroidism, arthritis and diabetes.

Carpal tunnel syndrome may also be referred to as cumulative trauma disorder, repetitive stress injury or overuse injury. It is most common in middle age and tends to affect women more than men, especially those who are overweight, pregnant or menopausal.

Treatment of carpal tunnel syndrome

Initial treatment of carpal tunnel syndrome involves rest and stopping or modifying the activities which worsen symptoms. Immobilization of the wrist in a splint, cool baths or cold compresses may also be useful. In cases where obesity, arthritis or other conditions are involved, treatment of the underlying cause is important.

Several types of medication can be used to treat carpal tunnel syndrome including nonsteroidal anti-inflammatory drugs and corticosteroids. Complete immobilization of the wrist in a cast or surgery to relieve compression may be necessary in severe cases. Physical therapies such as massage, stretching and gentle exercises are also useful and are particularly important after surgery in order to regain full hand use. Acupuncture and chiropractic treatments have also been used with some success.

Vitamins, minerals and carpal tunnel syndrome

B vitamins

A vitamin B6 deficiency may play a part in the development of carpal tunnel syndrome. Several small scale studies have found low vitamin B6 levels in sufferers of the disease.[1] Some research suggests that treatment with supplements can improve symptoms which may reduce the necessity of surgery in some patients.[2]

Some recent studies have cast doubt on these results. In a study of 125 randomly selected industrial plant workers, vitamin B6 levels were measured and the subjects filled out questionnaires and underwent nerve function tests. The researchers did not find a link between vitamin B6 and carpal tunnel syndrome.[3] Vitamin B6 has been shown to change pain thresholds in clinical and laboratory studies which may explain studies which have shown significant improvements in pain scores when nerve conduction test results showed only mild improvements.

Vitamin B6 supplements may be useful in the treatment of carpal tunnel syndrome but intake should not exceed 100 mg per day as large doses can cause nerve damage. Some practitioners use higher doses but this should only be done under supervision. Some experts believe that a therapeutic effect may take at least three months to become apparent.

Riboflavin may also help to relieve the symptoms of carpal tunnel syndrome. Combining riboflavin and vitamin B6 may be more effective than treatment with B6 alone. [4,5] Riboflavin is involved in the conversion of vitamin B6 to its active form.

Other nutrients and carpal tunnel syndrome

Other nutrients such as antioxidants and essential fatty acids may be useful in the treatment of carpal tunnel syndrome as they have anti-inflammatory effects.

Herbal medicine and carpal tunnel syndrome

St. John's wort (*Hypericum perforatum*) is a useful herb for joint, muscle, or nerve trauma and it has demonstrated anti-inflammatory effects in scientific studies. Rubbing oil of St. John's wort on the wrist may be useful in relieving the symptoms of carpal tunnel syndrome. Ginger (*Zingiber officinale*) is also anti-inflammatory and may also be useful if applied to the affected area. See page 384 for more information on these herbs and the precautions that may be necessary.

Cervical dysplasia

Cervical dysplasia is an abnormal growth of tissue in the cervix (the neck or opening of the uterus). Most cases are harmless but sometimes the abnormal cells may become cancerous. In such cases, the average time for progression to cervical cancer is from one to seven years.

Causes of cervical dysplasia

There are several lifestyle and nutritional factors that increase the risk of cervical dysplasia. These include viral infections such as herpes simplex and human papillomavirus (HPV), smoking, lowered immunity and oral contraceptive use. Lower socio-economic status, multiple sexual partners and early age of first intercourse also increase the risks.

Regular gynecological examination decreases cervical cancer mortality as cervical dysplasia can be caught in the early stages before it progresses to cancer. This examination, known as a Pap test, can accurately detect up to 90 per cent of cervical cancers, even before symptoms develop. Since its introduction, the number of deaths from cervical cancer has been reduced by more than 50 per cent. It is usually recommended that women have their first Pap test when they become sexually active or reach the age of 18. Tests can be performed annually but women who have had a normal test for three consecutive years, may wait for two to three years.

Nutrition and cervical dysplasia

As cervical dysplasia is a pre-cancerous condition, an anticancer diet may help to lower the risk of disease occurrence and progression. Diets high in saturated and polyunsaturated fats are likely to promote cancerous changes while a diet high in fruit, vegetables and fiber may help to reduce the risks.

Vitamins, minerals and cervical dysplasia

Several vitamin deficiencies may play a role in cervical dysplasia. A 1993 study of the links between diet and cervical dysplasia found a relationship between low folate, vitamin E, vitamin C and riboflavin intakes and the disease.[1]

Folate

The risk of cervical dysplasia appears to increase as folate intake decreases. It is possible that localized changes in folate levels contribute to cervical dysplasia. Some women appear to have normal levels of blood folate while concentrations in the cervical tissues are low. This may be due to use of oral contraceptives, which alter folate metabolism. Some researchers have found a higher risk of abnormalities in cervical tissue in women using oral contraceptives and suggest that folic acid supplements are beneficial in preventing cervical dysplasia in these women.[2]

Low red blood cell folate levels may increase the effect of other risk factors for cervical dysplasia; in particular, that of HPV infection. In a 1992 study, researchers from the University of Alabama in Birmingham investigated the links between folate deficiency and cervical dysplasia in 294 young women with the disorder and 170 healthy women. They also assessed the impact of factors such as smoking, oral contraceptive use, HPV infection, and number of sexual partners. The results showed that at low folate levels, the risk of dysplasia caused by HPV infection was increased.[3]

Even a marginal folic acid deficiency causes breaks and damage to the genetic material of the cell that resembles cervical dysplasia and, as this deficiency is common, some abnormal Pap smears may reflect folic acid deficiency rather than true dysplasia. However, it is also possible that such alteration in genetic material is an integral component of the dysplastic process that may be stopped, or in some cases reversed by oral folic acid supplementation. Several clinical studies have shown improvements in Pap smears in those with cervical dysplasia when they are given folic acid supplements. Folic acid supplementation may protect abnormal cells from becoming cancerous and may reverse cervical dysplasia in some cases. A 1996 study suggests that supplements may be useful in preventing the initial changes but do not appear to affect the progress of established disease.[4]

Antioxidants

Several studies have found links between low antioxidant levels and cervical dysplasia,[5] including carotenes[6] and vitamin E.[7]

Vitamin A

Epidemiological studies have links between low dietary intake or blood levels of vitamin A and the development of cervical dysplasia and/or cervical cancer. A 1996 Japanese study involving 137 women found a higher risk in women with low vitamin A levels.[8]

Some clinical investigations have examined the use of local application of a form of vitamin A to the cervix. In a 1994 placebo-controlled study, researchers examined the effects of this in 301 women with cervical dysplasia. The results showed that the treatment reversed mild dysplasia, but was not effective in more advanced cases.[9]

Vitamin C

Vitamin C levels have been shown to be lower in women suffering from cervical dysplasia. A 1981 US study measured nutrient intake in 87 women with cervical dysplasia and 82 women with no symptoms. Average vitamin C intake for those with cervical dysplasia was 80 mg and for healthy women, 107 mg. Women with intakes of less than 50 per cent of the RDA may have ten times the risk of cervical dysplasia than those with high intakes.[10]

Zinc

Some studies have shown that zinc levels may be low in cervical dysplasia.[11] Zinc is vital for many immune functions and can be protective against precancerous changes.[12]

Common cold

The common cold is one of the most frequently occurring illnesses in the world. It is caused by more than 200 known viruses that infect the upper respiratory tract. Symptoms include congestion in the nose, sore throat, headache, nasal discharge and sneezing. The larynx and lungs can also be affected. The average person catches a cold three times a year. Young children are particularly susceptible as their immune systems are still developing and may catch colds as often as eight times a year. Although most cases are mild and usually last about a week, colds are the leading cause of visits to the doctor and days off work and school.

Treatment of the common cold

In spite of the fact that it is a very common infection, both the causes and symptoms of the common cold are complicated and difficult to treat. There are still no cures for the many viruses that cause the common cold and the medicines available in local pharmacies may help relieve the symptoms but they cannot cure the cold, which has to run its course. Antibiotics are not effective against cold viruses and do not improve cold symptoms. Taking antibiotics unnecessarily can lead to antibiotic resistance, a potentially dangerous situation in which infection-causing bacteria become immune to the effects of certain antibiotics. Relaxation, enough sleep, water, staying warm and aspirin may be useful in treating cold symptoms.

Maintaining a strong immune system is important in avoiding colds. Stress and a poor diet can damage the immune system; and nutrients such as antioxidants, which enhance immunity, are important for the prevention of any infection. Research into the effects of specific nutrients in preventing and treating colds has focused on vitamin C and zinc.

Vitamins, minerals and the common cold

Vitamin C

In 1970, Nobel Prize winner Linus Pauling wrote a book called *Vitamin C and the Common Cold* in which he claimed that vitamin C was effective in reducing the severity of symptoms and the duration of a cold. These claims have caused much controversy in the medical community. Since 1971, many studies have investigated the ability of vitamin C in doses of 1 g per day or greater to affect the common cold. These studies have produced conflicting results with large variations in the benefits observed, and many doctors feel that the results are not clinically significant. There does not seem to be consistent evidence that vitamin C supplementation reduces the incidence of the common cold in the general population. Most studies show that the doses of vitamin C which are effective against colds are much higher than typical dietary intakes and at least 1 g per day may be necessary to show benefits.

Vitamin C treatment seems to have several effects, including reducing blood levels of histamine which can trigger tissue inflammation and a runny nose. As an antioxidant, Vitamin C may also protect the immune cells and surrounding tissue from damaging oxidative reactions that occur when white blood cells become activated and release oxidizing compounds to fight bacteria.[1]

It seems likely that the effects of supplementation are greater in those with low dietary vitamin C intake. In general, men have lower vitamin C levels than women. In four studies with British girls and women, vitamin C supplementation had no marked effect on the common cold. However, in four studies with British male schoolchildren and students, a reduction in common cold occurrence was found in groups supplemented with vitamin C.[2]

Some research suggests that vitamin C supplementation may be beneficial for people who do heavy exercise and who have problems with frequent upper respiratory infections. Three placebo-controlled studies have examined the effect of vitamin C supplementation on common cold occurrence in people under acute physical stress. In one study the subjects were school children at a skiing camp in the Swiss Alps; in another they were military troops training in Northern Canada; and in the third they were participants in a 90 km running race. In each of the three studies, a considerable reduction in common cold incidence in the group supplemented with vitamin C at levels of 600 mg to 1000 mg per day was seen.[3]

Zinc

Zinc may be effective in treating the common cold due to its antiviral and antibacterial effects and its ability to enhance immune system function. There have been several studies of the effects of zinc lozenges on the common cold. Some studies have shown benefit while others have not. The authors of a 1998 review of the trials concluded that treatment of the common cold with zinc gluconate lozenges, using adequate doses of elemental zinc, is likely to be effective in reducing duration and severity of cold symptoms. Most benefit is seen if the lozenges are started immediately after the onset of symptoms.[4]

In a 1996 randomized, double-blind, placebo-controlled study, researchers tested the effect of zinc gluconate lozenges on the common cold. The study involved 100 participants, and patients in the zinc group received a lozenge containing 13.3 mg of zinc every two hours. The lozenges reduced the duration of cold symptoms from 7.6 days to 4.4 days. However, some people did not like the taste of the lozenges.[5]

The type of zinc salts used in the lozenges also appears to be important, and the addition of citric or tartaric acids seems to reduce the benefit as these substances bind to zinc ions. A 1997 study suggests that zinc acetate lozenges may be more effective in treating colds than zinc gluconate. More zinc ions are released from zinc acetate under physiological conditions.[6]

The most recent study, published in the *Journal of the American Medical Association* in 1998 did not find zinc lozenges to be effective. The study involved 249 students in grades one through 12, some of whom were given 10 mg zinc lozenges five or six times a day for three weeks, and some of whom were given placebo lozenges containing no zinc. The study showed that it took children taking zinc lozenges an average of nine days to get over all their cold symptoms, which was the same amount of time for children who took placebo lozenges. The study also found that children who took zinc lozenges had a higher rate of adverse effects: bad taste reactions; nausea; mouth, tongue, or throat irritation; and diarrhea.[7]

Herbal medicine and the common cold

Useful herbs for cold prevention include those used to boost immunity such as echinacea (*Echinacea angustifolia)* and astragalus *(Astragalus membranaceus)*. Echinacea can also be useful at the onset of a cold as can elderflowers (*Sambucus nigra*), cayenne (*Capsicum spp.*), garlic (*Allium sativum*), goldenseal (*Hydrastis canadensis*). Other herbs that are useful include sage (*Salvia officinalis*), thyme (*Thymus vulgaris*), horseradish (*Armoracia spp.*), peppermint (*Mentha piperita*), *yarrow (Achillea millefolium*) and limeflowers (*Tilia europea*). See page 384 for more information on these herbs and the precautions that may be necessary.

Diabetes is a group of conditions in which sugar levels in the blood are abnormally high. During digestion the body converts sugars, starches and other carbohydrates into glucose which is carried in the bloodstream to cells throughout the body. Glucose is then used for energy release or stored for later use. The hormone, insulin, which is manufactured in the beta cells of the pancreas, is necessary for this process and therefore for the control of blood sugar levels. Diabetes can occur when the body attacks and destroys the cells in the pancreas that produce insulin or when the body is unable to use the insulin the pancreas produces. Sugar then collects in the blood and in the urine. Fat metabolism is also disturbed in diabetes, with high blood levels of cholesterol and triglycerides. As many as 120 million people worldwide have diabetes and the World Health Organization estimates that by the year 2025 this number will rise to 250 million.

Types of diabetes

Type I (insulin-dependent diabetes)

Type I diabetes accounts for around 5 to 10 per cent of cases and is most often seen in children and young adults. It occurs when the body attacks and destroys the cells in the pancreas that make insulin. Insulin production either stops altogether or only a tiny amount is made. Type I diabetes begins suddenly and symptoms quickly become severe. It is treated with insulin injections, regular exercise and a diet low in sugar and fat. Control of Type I diabetes requires a person to balance the intake of food and the entry of insulin into the blood.

Type II (non-insulin-dependent diabetes)

This type of diabetes, which accounts for around 90 per cent of cases, is also known as maturity onset diabetes and occurs most often in adults aged over 40, especially in those who are obese. In Type II diabetes the pancreas produces some insulin but it is not used effectively. The progression of the disease is slow and symptoms are mild in the beginning. Type II diabetes can often be controlled by diet and exercise, which can improve a person's blood glucose response. Overweight people may need to slim down and some people may need medication or insulin injections to control blood sugar.

Other types of diabetes

There are other kinds of diabetes, such as gestational diabetes, which occurs in around 2 to 3 per cent of pregnant women and usually disappears after the birth of the baby. Such women are at increased risk of developing Type II diabetes later in life. Secondary diabetes is caused by damage to the pancreas from chemicals, certain medicines, or diseases such as cancer.

Symptoms of diabetes

Symptoms of Type I diabetes, which usually occur suddenly, include frequent urination, excessive thirst, extreme hunger, dramatic weight loss, weakness, fatigue, blurred vision, nausea and vomiting. The symptoms of Type II diabetes usually occur less suddenly and include any of the above Type I symptoms and others such as recurring skin, gum or bladder infections; drowsiness; blurred vision; itching and tingling; or numbness in the hands and feet.

Causes of diabetes

The exact causes of both types of diabetes are still unknown and there may be several factors that play a part, although how important each factor is remains unclear. In Type I diabetes, the body's immune system attacks the beta cells of the pancreas and it is likely that genetic factors play a role in this. It is also possible that a viral infection that causes the immune system to destroy pancreatic cells instead of the virus may be involved. Cow's milk in the first few months of life may increase the risk of developing Type I diabetes, possibly due to the immune system recognizing the similarity between a protein in milk and a protein on the surface of the body's beta cells.[1]

Those who are overweight, do not exercise, eat a poor diet, suffer from hypertension, have high cholesterol and triglyceride levels, are aged over 40, and who have a family history of diabetes, are at particular risk of Type II diabetes. In this disorder the pancreas may produce enough insulin, but excess fat may prevent the insulin from working properly. This is known as insulin resistance and is often reversible with weight loss. Women with unexplained miscarriages, stillbirths, or who have had babies weighing nine pounds or more at birth also seem to be at increased risk of Type II diabetes.

Diet also influences the development of diabetes. Recent research suggests that those who eat an Asian diet have less risk of developing Type II diabetes.

In a 1996 study, Japanese American men in Hawaii who had a more Japanese lifestyle with a higher carbohydrate, lower fat, less animal protein-based diet had a lower risk of diabetes than Japanese American men who had a Western lifestyle.[2] A 1997 study published in the *Journal of the American Medical Association* showed that women who ate diets low in cereal fiber and high in foods which cause sharp rises in blood sugar are at increased risk of Type II diabetes.[3] Similar results have been seen in men.[4] Exercise also appears to decrease the risk of Type II diabetes.

Managing diabetes

Diabetes is a manageable condition, and with proper care, most people can live as they did before developing the disease. Successful management involves following a daily routine, which may include monitoring blood sugar levels, taking insulin or other medications, following a healthy diet and exercising regularly. Diabetics must avoid hypoglycemia (low blood sugar) and hyperglycemia (high blood sugar) as both can lead to coma if left untreated. Many experts now believe that keeping blood sugar levels tightly controlled can help prevent complications. Monitoring metabolic parameters including blood glucose, glycated hemoglobin, lipids, blood pressure and body weight is crucial to ensuring good control of the disease.

Diabetic complications

Diabetics are at increased risk of developing certain disorders such as heart, eye and kidney diseases; foot infections; and stroke. Increasing evidence suggests that many of these disorders arise as a result of oxidative damage to tissues. In diabetes, there may be an overproduction of free radicals and decreased efficiency of antioxidant defenses. Studies have shown lower levels of antioxidant vitamins and minerals in diabetic patients, especially those with complications.

Diabetics are at increased risk of cardiovascular disease as they have higher levels of harmful LDL cholesterol, which is more easily oxidized than other forms. The rate of this oxidation also appears to be higher in diabetics. This combination increases the risk of damage to arteries.

There are other compounds and processes that lead to diabetic complications. When glucose is metabolized, one of the compounds formed is sorbitol, which in nondiabetics is then converted to fructose and excreted.

However, in diabetics, who often have high blood sugar, sorbitol accumulates and may lead to complications. Prolonged periods of high blood sugar cause glucose molecules to become attached to proteins, causing changes in structure and function. This is known as glycation. Proteins commonly affected include those in red blood cells, the lens of the eye and the myelin sheath that surrounds nerve cells. Vitamins and minerals play an important part in protecting against these alterations in metabolism.

Diabetes and diet

It is vital for diabetics to maintain a desirable body weight and stabilize blood sugar and fat levels within a normal range in order to prevent or delay diabetic complications. The most important principle of diabetic diets is that they should be low in fat, especially saturated fat. They are also low in simple sugars and high in fiber. The American Diabetes Association (ADA) recommends that complex carbohydrates such as bread, pasta, potatoes and legumes make up 55 to 60 per cent of total calories; protein makes up around 20 per cent; and fat makes up 15 to 30 per cent.

The same food eaten by different people can produce different responses in blood sugar levels. It seems that the response is dependent upon the proportions of carbohydrate, protein and fat. A rating system known as the glycemic index (GI) ranks foods according to how fast their carbohydrate content is converted to glucose and enters the bloodstream. The lower the number, the slower the action. It may be advisable for people with diabetes to choose low GI foods wherever possible.

For many people, six small meals are easier to digest than three larger ones, as it is easier to dispose of smaller amounts of glucose because less insulin is needed. Sometimes eating meals and snacks at regular times will improve glucose levels.

A diet diary and glucose self-monitoring can be useful in helping a diabetic person to devise a diet appropriate for their lifestyle. Glucose meter readings indicate the body's response to meals, snacks, exercise, stress, illness and general habits. Many diabetics use the 'exchange list' system of food choices, in which foods are placed on one of six lists based upon their nutrient content. The six groups are: starch/bread, meat/substitutes, vegetables, fruit, milk, and fats. Portion sizes are also indicated to keep caloric value very close for all foods on the list. Meal plans usually indicate how many choices may be taken from a list for a meal or a snack.

Some diet plans involve the carbohydrate counting method. This involves making food choices so that an optimal amount of carbohydrate is present in the meal, the remainder of the calories are then allotted for protein and fat. Many vegetarians prefer to use carbohydrate counting, as animal products that appear on the meat and milk exchange lists are usually left out of the diet.

Vitamins, minerals and diabetes

Antioxidant vitamins

Diabetes is associated with higher levels of oxidized blood fats, which can increase the risk of diabetic complications such as cardiovascular disease. Oxidative stress may be increased because of glucose attachment to proteins. Levels of antioxidants are also lower in diabetics, and this lower level of antioxidant protection is likely to contribute to the development of diabetic complications.[5]

Regular consumption of adequate amounts of antioxidant-rich foods, such as fruits and vegetables, is important in the prevention of diabetic complications. Antioxidant supplements may also be beneficial, as the amounts needed to give protection may be higher than those that can easily be obtained from the diet. Multivitamin mixtures with trace elements have been shown to protect diabetic patients against free radical damage.[6]

Vitamin C

Vitamin C metabolism is altered in diabetics. The cellular uptake of vitamin C is promoted by insulin and inhibited by high blood sugar; and as diabetics have low insulin levels, they are at greater risk of vitamin C deficiency. Most studies have found people with diabetes to have at least 30 per cent lower vitamin C concentrations than people without the disease. Levels seem to be lower in diabetic people as a result of the disease rather than as a result of poor dietary intake.[7] This deficiency can lead to increased capillary permeability, poor wound-healing, increased cholesterol levels, and immune suppression; which all contribute to diabetic complications.

Several studies suggest that chronic vitamin C administration has beneficial effects on glucose and lipid metabolism in Type II diabetic patients. In a 1995 study, the effect of magnesium and vitamin C supplements on metabolic control was assessed in 56 diabetics. The study involved a 90-day run-in period followed by two 90-day treatment periods, during which patients received 600 mg of magnesium and 2 g of vitamin C per day. The results showed that vitamin C supplementation improved glycemic control, fasting blood glucose, cholesterol and triglycerides.[8]

Vitamin C supplementation is effective in reducing sorbitol accumulation in the red blood cells of diabetics. In a 58-day study carried out in 1994, researchers investigated the effect of two different doses of vitamin C supplements (100 or 600 mg) on young adults with Type I diabetes. The results showed that within 30 days, vitamin C supplementation at either dose normalized sorbitol levels in those with diabetes.[9] Vitamin C may also help to reduce capillary fragility, which also contributes to complications. The ability of the arteries to dilate is impaired in diabetics. Vitamin C supplements improve the response.[10] Drugs which are used to reduce sorbitol have many toxic side effects, and vitamin C therapy is beneficial in reducing sorbitol accumulation without the toxicity. Vitamin C has also been shown to reduce thc attachment of glucose to proteins, and the damage this causes.

Vitamin E

Vitamin E supplements have been shown to have beneficial effects in diabetics. As an antioxidant, vitamin E reduces damage to cell membranes, improving glucose metabolism and enabling insulin to act more efficiently. It also reduces the attachment of glucose to proteins.[11] Vitamin E has also been shown to have beneficial effects on cholesterol levels in diabetics by reducing the susceptibility of LDL to oxidative damage, thus limiting damage to arteries. Vitamin E also reduces blood clotting, another contributory factor to heart disease.

In a study published in 1996, Louisiana researchers examined whether 67 mg (100 IU) per day had any effect on blood lipid oxidation products and blood lipid profiles of 35 diabetic patients over a three-month period. The results showed that vitamin E supplementation significantly lowered lipid peroxidation products and lipid levels in diabetic patients.[12]

Type I diabetes

The results of a 1997 study done in Italy show that vitamin E can protect against damage to beta cells which produce insulin in Type I diabetes patients. The one-year study involved 84 patients between 5 and 35 years of age. One group was treated with vitamin E supplements and the other group received nicotinic acid which has been shown to protect pancreatic beta cell function (See page 80 for more information.) All patients were under intensive insulin therapy with three to four injections a day. The results showed that vitamin E was as effective as nicotinic acid in protecting the beta cells.[13]

Nicotinamide

The nicotinamide form of niacin may prevent or delay clinical onset of Type I diabetes. Nicotinamide appears to interfere with the immune-mediated beta cell destruction by reducing production of harmful compounds and increasing the energy metabolism of the cell.

New Zealand researchers have carried out a controlled trial of oral nicotinamide in the prevention of the onset of diabetes mellitus in a group of high risk children. All eight of the untreated children developed diabetes during the follow-up period of the study, whereas only one of 14 treated children did.[14] In 1996, the same researchers published the findings of a population-based diabetes prevention trial involving nicotinamide treatment of 173 children aged 5 to 8 at risk of Type I diabetes. The results showed a 50 per cent reduction in the development of diabetes in a five-year period, and suggest a protective effect of nicotinamide.[15]

Vitamin B6

Vitamin B6 deficiency causes symptoms such as low blood sugar, low insulin levels, degeneration of beta cells and an altered insulin response to sugar. Insulin sensitivity increases when vitamin B6 intake increases in people who are deficient.

Vitamin B12

The vitamin B12 deficiency disease, pernicious anemia, is not uncommon in Type I diabetics. Researchers have studied the effects of vitamin B12 on patients with diabetic nerve disease. Treatment has been shown to improve some of the symptoms.

Biotin

Biotin supplements may help to improve blood glucose control in diabetics by enhancing insulin sensitivity and increasing the activity of enzymes involved in glucose metabolism.[16] Biotin in high doses may also be useful in the treatment of diabetic neuropathy.[17]

Vitamin D

The alterations in mineral metabolism seen in diabetics may lead to changes in the vitamin D function. Vitamin D deficiency also impairs glucose metabolism by reducing insulin secretion which may increase the risk of diabetes. Vitamin D supplements are likely to be useful in preventing diabetes in areas where vitamin D deficiency is common.[18]

In a 1997 study looking at the links between environmental factors and Type II diabetes, vitamin D levels were assessed in 142 Dutch men aged from 70 to 88 years of age. Thirty-nine per cent were found to have low vitamin D levels and tests showed that low vitamin D levels increased the risk of glucose intolerance.[19]

Changes in mineral metabolism

There is evidence that the metabolism of several trace elements is altered in diabetes and that these nutrients might have specific roles in the progress of this disease. Diabetes can alter copper, zinc and magnesium status; and these changes in mineral metabolism are more pronounced in diabetic populations with specific complications. It is always clear whether differences in trace element status are a consequence of diabetes or, alternatively, whether they contribute to the disease. Recently, some essential trace elements such as vanadium and selenium have been shown to have insulin-like effects. It is very likely that chromium, manganese, vanadium, and selenium have a favorable effect on carbohydrate metabolism.

Magnesium

Magnesium deficiency is the most evident disturbance of mineral metabolism in both Type I and Type II diabetes, with up to 30 per cent of diabetics showing some evidence of magnesium depletion. The clinical consequences of magnesium deficiency include impaired insulin secretion and reduced tissue sensitivity to insulin, and increased risk of damage to blood vessels.

Magnesium excretion is increased in children with Type I diabetes, especially when the levels of glucose in the urine are high, as blood plasma magnesium levels in diabetes are closely dependent on blood glucose concentration. In Type II diabetes, magnesium deficiency seems to be associated with insulin resistance. It may also be involved in the development of diabetes complications and may contribute to the increased risk of sudden death associated with diabetes. Some studies suggest that magnesium deficiency may play a role in spontaneous abortion and birth defects in diabetic women.

Results from the ARIC study suggest that serum magnesium levels are low in those suffering from diabetes, and that intake is related to insulin levels. This study involved over 15 248 people, male and female, black and white, aged 45 to 64 years.[20] Magnesium plays a role in the insulin-mediated uptake of glucose into cells, and deficiency may worsen control of diabetes.[21] Low magnesium levels increase the risk of several disorders; including heart disease, eye disease and bone problems.

According to research presented at the 1997 annual meeting of the American Diabetes Association, low magnesium levels predict Type II diabetes in whites. Researchers from Johns Hopkins University Medical School examined blood levels of magnesium in over 12 000 nondiabetic, middle-aged African American and white subjects and monitored them for six years. No relationship was found between magnesium levels and diabetes in African Americans, but a relationship was seen in whites.

The ADA has recommended that diabetics with low magnesium levels should take supplements as they have been shown to improve glucose tolerance and insulin response and action. They may also help protect against diabetic complications including heart disease and eye disorders. In a 1994 study, Italian researchers investigated the effects of magnesium supplementation on glucose uptake and use in nine elderly Type II diabetic patients. Each patient was followed up for a period of three weeks before the study, and was then given either a placebo or a magnesium supplement for four weeks. At the end of this time, improvements in insulin sensitivity and glucose oxidation were seen in those taking magnesium.[22] Magnesium supplements have also been shown to lower blood pressure in Type II diabetics.[23]

Chromium

Chromium, as part of a compound known as glucose tolerance factor (GTF), plays a role in blood sugar control primarily by increasing tissue sensitivity to insulin. When sufficient levels of chromium are present much lower amounts of insulin are required. Diabetes has been shown to develop as a consequence of chromium deficiency in experimental animals and in humans sustained by prolonged total parenteral nutrition.

Chromium deficiency is relatively common in patients with Type II diabetes and may impair the function of GTF, causing the uptake of glucose into cells to become less efficient. Impaired chromium metabolism may also play a role in diabetes of pregnancy.[24] High insulin levels also seem to increase chromium excretion. Chromium deficiency may also lead to hypoglycemia or low blood sugar.

Chromium supplements have been successfully used to treat Type I and Type II diabetes, diabetes in pregnancy, and hypoglycemia. Chromium supplementation has been shown to lower fasting glucose levels, improve glucose tolerance and lower insulin levels in Type II diabetics. This helps to keep blood levels stable, thereby preventing damage to blood vessels and organs caused by high levels of blood sugar. The greatest benefits are seen in those who have severe deficiencies. Chromium acts to increase insulin sensitivity by improving insulin binding, insulin receptor number, insulin internalization, beta cell sensitivity and insulin receptor enzymes.[25]

According to the results of a Chinese study published in 1997, daily chromium supplements may help control blood sugar levels and insulin activity in Type II diabetics. The study, conducted by researchers at the US Department of Agriculture and Beijing Medical University, involved 180 Type II diabetics. Chinese subjects were chosen because of the likelihood that they had not previously used supplements. The subjects were divided into three groups: one group was given 1000 mcg of chromium picolinate, the second was given 200 mcg and the third group was given a placebo. After two months, the researchers assessed blood sugar and cholesterol levels. In the 1000 mcg group, levels were significantly reduced. In the 200 mcg group, it took four months to see a reduction in blood sugar levels, and this was not as significant as that seen in the first group.[26]

In a study published in 1996, researchers assessed the effects of daily supplements of 200 mcg of chromium and nicotinic acid on blood glucose and lipids, including total cholesterol, HDL cholesterol, LDL cholesterol, and triglycerides. The patients were 14 healthy adults and five adults with Type II diabetes mellitus. The results showed lowered total and LDL cholesterol, triglycerides, and glucose concentrations in patients with Type II diabetes.[27]

Selenium

A selenium deficiency may reduce insulin secretion. As part of the antioxidant enzyme, glutathione peroxidase, selenium is important in protecting against oxidative damage.

Vanadium

Vanadium can mimic the effects of insulin on cells in laboratory experiments and reduce the blood sugar levels in rats from high to normal. These benefits are seen with low doses. There have been limited clinical trials with vanadium salts in Type II diabetics, indicating that vanadium may have therapeutic potential in the treatment of diabetes.[28]

In a study published in 1996, researchers at the Albert Einstein College of Medicine in New York compared the effects of 100 mg/day of oral vanadyl sulfate in moderately obese diabetic and nondiabetic people. The results showed improvements in both liver and skeletal muscle insulin sensitivity in diabetics. Blood fat levels and oxidation were also reduced. Thus vanadium may also be useful in reducing the risk of atherosclerosis in diabetic people.[29]

Zinc

Alterations in zinc metabolism are seen in people with both Type I and Type II diabetes. Response to insulin may be decreased and excretion in the urine is increased, thus exacerbating the risk of deficiency with all the associated risks such as poor immune function and increased risk of birth defects.

Zinc deficiency has been shown to increase the risk for diabetes in diabetes-prone experimental animals, and low concentrations of zinc have also been shown in the blood of people recently diagnosed with Type I diabetes. The results of a 1995 Swedish study suggest that a low concentration of zinc in drinking water can increase the risk of childhood onset of the disease.[30]

Diabetics often excrete excess zinc in their urine and studies have shown beneficial effects of zinc supplementation. Zinc supplementation in animals improves glucose tolerance; and in a French study carried out in 1995, zinc gluconate supplements were shown to improve glucose assimilation in humans.[31]

Zinc deficiency may lead to slower growth in diabetic children, who may benefit from supplements. Zinc supplements may also be useful in protecting against pregnancy complications in diabetic women who are at risk, and may also improve wound-healing.

Other nutrients

Essential fatty acids

Increased intakes of omega-3 oils may be beneficial in helping to reduce the risk of cardiovascular disease in diabetics. There were some concerns that omega-3 fatty acid supplements would worsen blood sugar control in diabetics but more recent studies suggest that this is not the case. In a 1997 Italian study, researchers evaluated the effect of omega-3 fatty acid supplements on 935 patients with high blood fat levels, both with and without glucose intolerance or diabetes. The results showed improvements in blood fat levels and no worsening of blood sugar control.[32]

Diabetics seem to have a reduced ability to convert linoleic acid to GLA. This may lead to defective nerve function as metabolites of GLA are known to be important in nerve membrane structure, nerve blood flow, and nerve conduction. In a 1993 double-blind, placebo-controlled study, UK researchers compared the effects of placebo and GLA (480 mg per day) on the course of mild diabetic neuropathy in 111 patients over a one-year period. They used various nerve conduction, sensation and reflex tests, and the results of these showed that the change over one year in response to GLA was more favorable than the change with placebo.[33]

Lipoic acid

Lipoic acid has been used to treat diabetics by improving glucose transport and metabolism.[34] High intakes may increase the absorption of glucose into muscle tissue in Type II diabetes.[35] Lipoic acid may also decrease the damaging effects on proteins of high glucose levels.

Lipoic acid may be beneficial in improving nerve blood flow, reducing oxidative stress, and improving nerve conduction in diabetic neuropathy.[36] The effects of lipoic acid on diabetic neuropathy have been studied in two German randomized, double-blind placebo-controlled trials. In the first of these, 328 patients with Type II diabetes and symptoms of peripheral neuropathy were treated with either intravenous infusion of lipoic acid or placebo for three weeks. The results showed improvements in symptoms. In another study, patients with NIDDM and cardiac autonomic neuropathy were treated with a daily oral dose of 800 mg lipoic acid or placebo for four months. Two out of four symptoms test measurements were significantly improved in those taking the lipoic acid compared with placebo.[37]

Herbal medicine and diabetes

Herbal medicines will not replace insulin therapy where it is necessary, and anyone who is thinking of or is currently using herbs to control blood sugar should consult their health practitioner. However, there are many herbs which have been used to treat diabetes and its complications. These include gymnena (*Gymnema sylvestre*), fenugreek (*Trigonella foenum-graecum*), garlic (*Allium sativum*), onion (*Allium cepa*). Other herbs such as ginkgo (*Ginkgo biloba*), hawthorn (*Crataegus oxyacantha*) and bilberry (*Vaccinium myrtillus*) may be useful in preventing the vascular complications commonly seen in diabetic patients. See page 384 for more information on these herbs and the precautions that may be necessary.

Eye disorders

There are many disorders that affect the eyes. Some are localized problems while others are a sign of disease elsewhere in the body. Eye diseases are particularly common in elderly people. Cataracts are the most prevalent eye disease in the world and are a major cause of visual loss in developing and developed countries. Other common eye diseases include age-related macular degeneration, glaucoma, and diabetic retinopathy. There are a number of risk factors for these diseases; including age, high blood pressure, prolonged exposure to sunlight, and nutritional deficiencies.

Cataracts

A cataract is a cloudy or opaque area in the lens of the eye. As this cloudy area thickens, it prevents light from passing through the lens and focusing on the retina. Early changes may not affect vision but increasingly blurred vision, sensitivity to light and glare, increased shortsightedness or distorted images may develop. In the late stages, the lens becomes visibly opaque or white. Cataracts can occur in different places in the lens: nuclear cataracts occur in the center of the lens and are most commonly associated with aging. Other types include cortical cataracts and subcapsular cataracts, which are more commonly associated with diabetes. Although cataracts usually aren't painful, they may sometimes cause swelling in the lens and increased pressure in the eye.

Between the ages of 52 and 64, there is a 50 per cent chance of having a cataract. By age 75 most people have had a cataract and 50 per cent of people aged between 75 and 85 have lost some vision as a result. Cataract surgery is the number one therapeutic surgical procedure performed on Americans aged 65 and older.

Causes of cataracts

Cataracts occur when certain proteins within the lens become damaged. Damage to the enzymes necessary to eliminate the abnormal proteins may also occur. This damage is probably caused by free radicals generated by repeated exposure to ultraviolet light and oxygen. Cataracts may form when the oxidative stress on the lens exceeds the capacity of the antioxidant systems to protect against it, which occurs increasingly with age. Other causes include exposure to X-rays or strong sunlight, inflammatory eye diseases, certain drugs (such as corticosteroids), or complications of other diseases such as diabetes. They're more common in older people but babies can be born with cataracts. Heredity may play a part in the susceptibility to cataracts.

Macular degeneration

Macular degeneration is a condition in which the macula, the central part of the retina, degenerates. This is where most of the images formed by the lens are sent and it is much more sensitive to detail than the peripheral retina. The macula provides the central or close up vision necessary for detailed activities such as reading. Yellowish deposits called drusen accumulate beneath the retina of the eye. Loss of vision can start at the edge of the visual field and work its way towards the center or it may start in the center and work its way outwards.

There are two kinds of macular degeneration: dry and wet. Dry macular degeneration accounts for 85 to 90 per cent of cases and wet macular degeneration accounts for approximately 10 per cent. In dry macular degeneration, drusen is deposited in the macula without any evidence of scars, blood, or other fluid leakage. In wet macular degeneration, leaked material forms a mound, often surrounded by small hemorrhages. Eventually the mound contracts, leaving a scar. Both forms of macular degeneration usually affect both eyes at the same time. The dry form develops slowly and usually causes mild vision loss. The wet form is a much greater threat to vision and is indicated by a large blind spot in the middle of the visual field.

Age-related macular degeneration is the most common cause of blindness in developed countries and affects about 6 per cent of Americans between the ages of 65 and 75 and almost 20 per cent of those aged over 75.

Symptoms

Macular degeneration leads to a painless loss of vision. Symptoms include night blindness, blurry or fuzzy vision, straight lines appearing as wavy ones, a dark or empty area in the center of vision, narrowed blood vessels in the retina and gradual development of poor vision that can lead to total blindness.

Causes

It is unclear exactly why macular degeneration develops and there is currently no cure. Risk factors for the disorder include high blood pressure, cardiovascular disease, nutritional deficiencies, exposure to certain chemicals, and heredity. Light eye pigmentation and cigarette smoking may also be risk factors. Some experts believe that long-term exposure to light causes free radical damage to the retina, and that this contributes to the development of macular degeneration.

Treatment

Some forms of macular degeneration can be treated with laser surgery and low vision aids can be useful in allowing people to continue normal activities. Sunglasses may be useful in preventing light damage.

Nutrition and the eye

Nutrient deficiencies can either directly affect eye function or increase the susceptibility to degenerative problems such as cataracts and macular degeneration.

Vitamin A

Vitamin A deficiency is the leading preventable cause of blindness in the world. Vitamin A plays a role in maintaining the cornea and enhancing night vision through a compound known as visual purple. One of the first symptoms of vitamin A deficiency is night blindness, and prolonged deficiency leads to xerophthalmia, a condition in which eyes become dry, ulcers appear on the cornea, and the eyelids become swollen and sticky. This condition eventually leads to blindness.

B vitamins

Several B vitamin deficiencies can lead to abnormal eye function. Riboflavin deficiency can cause aversion to bright light, dimness of vision and a burning and itching in the eyes. Low intake must occur for several months before these symptoms appear. A low level of riboflavin may also contribute to cataracts and macular degeneration. Low levels of vitamin B12 can also lead to poor vision.

Antioxidants

As oxidative damage is believed to play a role in the development of eye diseases, and in particular cataract and macular degeneration, many research studies have investigated the ability of antioxidant vitamins and trace minerals to prevent the onset or progression of the disorders. Basic research studies have shown that antioxidants can protect against the cumulative effects of oxidative stress in animal models of cataract and macular degeneration. Epidemiological evidence in humans suggests that people with comparatively higher intakes or blood concentrations of antioxidant vitamins are at a reduced risk of cataract and macular degeneration.

Vitamins, minerals and cataracts

Carotenes

Researchers involved in the Nurses Health Study examined the link between cataract development and intake of various foods and antioxidant vitamins in over 50 000 women. The results of their studies showed that those with high beta carotene and vitamin A intakes were less likely to develop cataracts. Those whose diets contained spinach also seemed to have a lower risk. The researchers concluded that dietary carotenes, although not necessarily beta carotene, can decrease the risk of cataracts severe enough to require extraction.[1]

In a 1992 study, Finnish researchers compared the differences in beta carotene levels between patients admitted to eye wards for senile cataract and those without eye disorders. The results showed that those with low concentrations of beta carotene were 1.7 times as likely to suffer from cataract.[2] As well as protecting against free radical damage, beta carotene may also act as a filter and protect against light-induced damage to the fiber portion of the eye lens.

Other carotenes may also exert protective effects. In a 1997 study, researchers at Arizona State University assessed the relationship between carotenoid pigments in the retina of the eye, including lutein and zeaxanthin, and the density of clouding in the lens. The study involved younger people (ages 24 to 36 years) and older people (aged 48 to 82 years). The results showed that lens density increased with age, and that the increase was related to lower macular pigment carotenes.[3]

Vitamin C

The vitamin C content of the eye is 20 times greater than that in the blood. Results from some studies, including the Beaver Dam Eye Study, suggest that people with high levels of vitamin C are at less risk of cataracts than those with low levels of vitamin C.[4] Vitamin C causes more iron-binding protein, ferritin, to be produced which may reduce the oxidative damage done by iron. Vitamin C may act to protect enzymes within the lens that remove oxidation-damaged proteins.

Results from the Nurses Health Study previously mentioned showed that the risk of cataract was 45 per cent lower among women who used vitamin C supplements for ten or more years.[1]

Further results from this study reported in 1997 in the *American Journal of Clinical Nutrition* also suggests that vitamin C supplements taken for long periods can reduce the development of cataracts. Researchers from the US Department of Agriculture and Harvard School of Public Health examined the link between cataract development and vitamin C supplement use over a ten to 12-year period. The subjects were 247 Boston area nurses aged from 56 to 71. The researchers performed detailed eye examinations to determine the degree of opacity (clouding) of the eye lenses of the subjects. Results showed that use of vitamin C supplements for over ten years was associated with a 77 per cent lower prevalence of early lens opacities and an 83 per cent lower prevalence of moderate lens opacities.[5]

Vitamin E

Recent research suggests that cortical cataracts are more likely when plasma vitamin E concentrations are low. A 1996 Finnish study of over 400 men found an increased risk of cataracts in those with low vitamin E levels. The researchers evaluated the link between vitamin E levels and progression of eye lens opacities in 410 men with high cholesterol. The results showed that those with low vitamin E levels had almost four times the risk of lens opacities when compared with those in the highest intake group.[6]

Riboflavin

Riboflavin deficiency may be associated with the development of cataracts. Researchers involved in the New York State Lens Opacities Case-Control Study assessed the risk factors for various types of cataract among 1380 participants aged 40 to 79 years. They found an increased risk with low levels of several nutrients including riboflavin.[7] Riboflavin is necessary for the activity of an enzyme that exerts protective effects on the eye.

Diet and macular degeneration

Several studies suggest that increasing the consumption of foods rich in vitamin A, carotenes and other antioxidants; in particular dark green, leafy vegetables; may decrease the risk of developing advanced macular degeneration.

As part of the Eye Disease Case-Control Study, researchers compared blood levels of carotenes, vitamins C and E, and selenium in 421 patients with macular degeneration and 615 people without the disorder. The results showed that people with high carotenoid intakes had a lower risk of macular degeneration.

Results also showed that those with high intakes of all the antioxidants had significantly reduced risk of the disorder.[8]

Carotenes

The carotenes, lutein and zeaxanthin, may also have protective effects. Lutein and zeaxanthin are constituents of the pigment of the eye. A low density of this pigment in the macula of the eye may increase the risk of the disorder, macular degeneration, possibly because it permits greater blue light damage.

In a study published in 1997, researchers at Florida International University in Miami tested the effects of 30 mg of lutein on eye pigment in two people for a period of 140 days. The results showed that 20 to 40 days after the people started taking the lutein supplement, the density of the pigment in their eyes started to increase. This amount of blue light reaching thc vulnerable eye tissues that are damaged in macular degeneration was reduced by around 30 to 40 per cent.[9]

Zinc

Zinc is highly concentrated in the eye, particularly in the retina and tissues surrounding the macula. Zinc deficiency can lead to loss of eye function as several zinc-dependent enzymes play important roles in eye function. Levels of these enzymes decline with age. Zinc deficiency may contribute to macular degeneration of the central part of the retina. Results from the Beaver Dam Eye Study, published in 1996, suggest a link between low zinc intakes and risk of macular degeneration.[10]

Selenium

As part of the enzyme, glutathione peroxidase, selenium may be important in protecting the eye from oxidative damage. A recent study found an association between macular degeneration and low selenium levels.[11]

Fibrocystic breast disease

Fibrocystic breast disease is the most common benign breast disorder, affecting around 30 per cent of premenopausal women. It is most common in women aged from 30 to 50. Symptoms are tender breasts containing lumps and benign cysts. These may be mildly uncomfortable to severely painful. Fibrocystic breast disease usually affects both breasts and worsens premenstrually. It may be associated with an increased risk of breast cancer.

Causes of fibrocystic breast disease

Fibrocystic breast disease may be due to imbalances in female sex hormones, specifically an increase in the estrogen to progesterone ratio. Prolactin, the milk release hormone secreted by the pituitary gland, may also play a role. Oral contraceptives relieve the symptoms of fibrocystic breast disease in most women, and diuretic drugs may also be effective.

Fibrocystic breast disease and diet

A diet high in fiber and unrefined foods, and low in saturated fat and salt, plays a role in reducing the symptoms of fibrocystic breast disease. Soy foods may also be beneficial as they contain high levels of estrogen-like compounds and may improve hormonal balance. Regular consumption of oily fish, which contain anti-inflammatory omega-3 fatty acids, may also be useful. Caffeine, theophylline and theobromine; which are found in coffee, tea, cola and chocolate; may play a role in stimulating overproduction of fibrous tissue and cyst fluid, and should be avoided. Obesity may also exacerbate fibrocystic breast disease.

Vitamins, minerals and fibrocystic breast disease

Vitamin A

In a 1984 study, 12 twelve patients with benign breast disease were treated with daily doses of 150,000 IU of vitamin A. After three months of treatment, nine of the women experienced marked pain reduction and five patients had at least a 50 per cent decrease in the size of their breast lumps.[1] The lessening of breast pain was still evident eight months after the study ended. However, vitamin A in high doses can cause toxic symptoms, and several women in this study had severe headaches during treatment, while several other women had milder side effects.

Vitamin E

Some research suggests that vitamin E levels may be lower in fibrocystic breast disease sufferers. In a 1985 double-blind, randomized dose-response study, 75 women with benign breast disease were treated for two months with placebo or vitamin E in doses of 150, 300, or 600 IU per day. The results showed that vitamin E was significantly more effective than placebo.[2]

In a 1981 study, 17 young women with fibrocystic breast disease and six age-matched controls were treated with vitamin E for four months. Blood samples collected at monthly intervals were analyzed for various hormone and blood fat levels. Fifteen patients showed improvements in symptoms and laboratory measurements showed normalization of abnormal hormone and lipid levels in the patients.[3] Other studies also suggest that vitamin E supplements may correct the hormonal imbalances seen in fibrocystic breast disease patients.[4] However, not all studies have shown beneficial effects.[5]

Iodine

Iodine deficiency may play a role in fibrocystic breast disease, possibly by increasing the susceptibility of the tissue to estrogen stimulation. Some studies have shown that iodine treatment can relieve the symptoms, although the forms of iodine used in the studies are not available commercially.[6]

Essential fatty acids

Fatty acid profiles may be abnormal in women with fibrocystic breast disease. Treatment with essential fatty acids may help to normalize this.[7] Some studies have looked at the beneficial effects of evening primrose oil on fibrocystic breast disease. Evening primrose contains the essential fatty acids, linoleic acid and gamma linolenic acid (GLA), which has beneficial effects in reducing inflammation.

Headache and migraine

Headaches occur when the pain-sensitive nerves in head muscles and blood vessels are stimulated. The Headache Classification Committee of the International Headache Society currently recognizes more than 100 types of headaches. As many as 50 million Americans experience chronic headaches.

Types of headache

Headaches can be divided into several different types:

- Vascular headaches, which include migraine headaches, and are thought to involve abnormal function of blood vessels.
- Muscle contraction headaches.
- Traction headaches, which occur when pain sensitive parts of the head are pulled, stretched or displaced.
- Inflammatory headaches, which are symptoms of other diseases such as those of the sinuses, spine, neck, ears and teeth.

Causes of headache

There are many causes of headache but most are caused by fatigue, emotional disorders, or allergies. Other causes include diseases of the eye, ear, nose, throat, and sinuses; brain tumors; thyroid disease; high blood pressure; low blood sugar; dental problmes; head injuries; aneurysm (ruptured blood vessel); and nutrient deficiencies and toxicities. Alcohol; cigarette smoke; exposure to chemicals and pollution; and some medications, including oral contraceptives; may also cause headaches.

Headache prevention

Regular exercise seems to help prevent some types of headache. If headaches are caused by reactions to certain foods, it is obviously advisable to avoid these foods. Common triggers include alcoholic beverages, especially red wine; the artificial sweetener, aspartame; bananas; caffeine from coffee, tea, cola soft drinks, or some medications; chocolate; citrus fruits; cured meats; food additives such as monosodium glutamate (MSG); hard cheeses; nuts and peanut butter; onions; sour cream; fermented foods such as soy sauce and pickles; and vinegar.

MSG is found in hydrolyzed protein, autolyzed yeast, sodium caseinate and calcium caseinate.

Headache treatment

Rest in a quiet, dark room; massaging the base of the skull, temples, shoulders, neck and jaw; a warm bath or shower; a cold or warm washcloth placed over the area that aches; ice packs; relaxation techniques; acupuncture and biofeedback techniques may all be useful in treating headaches. Painkillers such as aspirin and ibuprofen are more effective if taken as soon as a headache starts to develop.

Muscle contraction headaches

A muscle contraction headache involves the tightening or tensing of the facial, scalp and neck muscles. This is the most common type of headache, accounting for around 60 per cent of those suffered. The pain is mild to moderate and usually steady. Chronic muscle contraction headaches can last for weeks or months.

Muscle contraction headaches can develop for a number of reasons, including poor sleep patterns, depression, anxiety and stress. Certain physical postures such as holding the head to one side while using a phone may aggravate muscle tension and cause chronic headaches.

Migraine

A migraine headache usually has the following symptoms: one-sided headache pain; pulsating or throbbing pain; intense attacks with moderate to severe pain that can inhibit daily activity; worsening routine physical activity; and possibly nausea and/or vomiting; and sensitivity to light and sound. Some migraine sufferers experience an aura before a migraine attack. These nervous system disturbances include symptoms such as flashing lights, bright spots, blurry vision, or blind spots. Aura may also involve anxiety, fatigue and numbness or tingling on one side of the body.

Migraine headaches are caused by the inability of the blood vessels in the membrane covering the brain to expand and contract at uniform rates. When the blood flow increases through the larger vessels, the pressure on the smaller ones causes painful stretching as they unsuccessfully try to expand to allow for the heavier flow. As the vessels undergo this stretching and constricting, the nerve cells register a throbbing pain, which is often accompanied by nausea; distortions of speech, hearing and vision; and clamminess of the skin.

As many as 15 to 20 per cent of men and 25 to 30 per cent of women suffer from migraine headaches. Migraines can occur as often as several times a week or once every few years. Some people experience migraines at predictable times; in women they often occur premenstrually.

Causes of migraine

The causes of migraine are not well understood, and triggers tend to be different for everyone. Common ones include stress, fatigue, bright light, loud noises, weather changes, changes in sleeping patterns or diet, low blood sugar, certain foods and chemicals.

Treatment of migraine

Regular exercise, stress reduction and elimination of certain foods from the diet are the most common methods of preventing migraine and other vascular headaches. Migraine medications include aspirin and caffeine which act to reduce blood vessel dilation and inflammation. A relatively new drug, sumatriptan, is effective in alleviating severe migraine attacks. It binds to serotonin receptors in the brain and causes blood vessels to return to their normal diameter. Side effects include increased heart rate, elevated blood pressure, and a feeling of tightness in the chest, jaw, or neck.

Diet and migraine

There are several dietary factors, which may contribute to headaches and migraine. These include the foods listed above. Recent research indicates that a low fat, high complex carbohydrate diet may be effective in reducing the frequency, intensity and duration of migraine headaches in sufferers. As low blood sugar may provoke a migraine, eating regular meals and avoiding sugary foods, which cause blood sugar levels to crash, may be a useful preventive measure. High fat foods, which are difficult to digest and can lead to a stomach-ache and headache, should be avoided. Identifying and avoiding allergenic foods is important in migraine prevention.

Vitamins, minerals and headaches

B vitamins

A deficiency of any B vitamin may lead to headache. Both vitamin B12 and folic acid deficiencies eventually lead to anemia, one of the symptoms of which is headache. Supplements are useful in these cases. Niacin is sometimes used to treat headaches and migraines. It is given at the onset of a migraine and its effect may be due to its ability to dilate blood vessels. Vitamin B6 may be useful for treating headaches associated with premenstrual syndrome and estrogen-related headaches that occur in the early stages of pregnancy.

Riboflavin

High doses of riboflavin may be effective in the treatment of migraine. In a 1998 study done in Belgium, researchers tested the effects of either 400 mg of riboflavin or a placebo on 55 patients with migraine in a randomized trial lasting three months. The results showed reductions in attack-frequency and headache days. Fifty-nine per cent of patients in the riboflavin group improved compared to 15 per cent in the placebo group. No serious side effects occurred. The researchers concluded that because of its effectiveness, excellent tolerability, and low cost, riboflavin is a valuable option for migraine prevention.[1]

Magnesium

Several studies suggest that magnesium metabolism is altered in some migraine sufferers. Low magnesium levels may contribute to migraine in a number of ways, including increased muscle and blood vessel contraction, which may lead to reduced blood flow to the brain. The activity of serotonin receptors can also be affected by changes in magnesium levels.[2]

Supplements may be beneficial in the treatment and prevention of migraine. In a 1996 study, Belgian researchers assessed the effect of oral magnesium on the prevention of migraine in 81 patients aged from 18 to 65. They were either given a placebo or a daily supplement of 600 mg of magnesium for 12 weeks. In weeks nine to12 the attack frequency was reduced by 42 per cent in the magnesium group and by 16 per cent in the placebo group. The number of days with migraine and the drug consumption for symptomatic treatment per patient also decreased significantly in the magnesium group.[3] Supplements may also be useful in the treatment of menstrual migraine.[4]

Calcium and vitamin D

In a 1994 study, researchers treated two premenopausal women with a history of menstrually-related migraines with a combination of vitamin D and calcium. Both women experienced reductions in their headache attacks as well as premenstrual symptoms within two months of therapy.[5] In another study, the same researchers successfully treated two postmenopausal women with frequent and excruciating migraine headaches with vitamin D and calcium.[6]

Essential fatty acids

GLA and alpha-linolenic acid have been used to prevent migraine. In a 1997 study, EFAs were administered to 168 patients over a period of six months. In 129 patients available for the study, 86 per cent experienced reductions in severity, frequency and duration of migraine attacks; 22 per cent became free of migraine; and more than 90 per cent had reduced nausea and vomiting.[7]

Herbal medicine and headache

Herbal treatment of headaches focuses on treating the underlying cause whether it be muscle tension, poor liver function or sinus infection. Commonly used herbs include black cohosh (*Cimicifuga racemosa*), chamomile (*Matricaria recutita*), skullcap (*Scutellaria laterifolia*), white willow (*Salix alba*) and valerian (*Valeriana officinalis*). Feverfew (*Tanacetum parthenium*) is a very useful herb in the prevention of migraine. See page 384 for more information on these herbs and the precautions that may be necessary.

Acquired immune deficiency syndrome (AIDS) is a condition in which there is a serious defect in the immune system, the body's natural defense against disease. This increases susceptibility to opportunistic infections, cancer, nerve disorders, and a variety of other syndromes. Since it was first described in 1981, AIDS has been the cause of much fear and controversy. It is now known to occur as a result of infection with the human immunodeficiency virus (HIV). The World Health Organization (WHO) estimates that some 30 million people worldwide are infected with HIV. More than 90 per cent of these are in developing countries and most do not know that they are infected. In 1997 alone, there were over 2.3 million deaths from the disorder.

HIV infection

HIV was first isolated in the laboratory in 1983, and shown to be the likely cause of AIDS in 1984. The virus is transmitted through certain body fluids including blood, semen, vaginal secretions and breast milk. It is not transmitted by air, saliva, tears or sweat so there is no danger of infection with casual contact.

After HIV enters the body, it becomes incorporated into the genetic material of the body cells and affects the production of a number of different cells of the immune and nervous systems. This eventually reduces the ability of the immune system to fight bacterial, viral and fungal infections, and detect cancerous changes in cells. Nervous system function may also be affected.

Symptoms of AIDS

The spectrum of conditions related to AIDS ranges from the presence of HIV with no symptoms to severe immune deficiency with life-threatening secondary infections. It is still unclear how many people infected with HIV will progress to AIDS or how long this process takes. The period between infection with HIV and the onset of AIDS averages ten years in adults in the USA.

As AIDS is not a disease in itself, but rather, an increased susceptibility to infection, the symptoms vary widely. In some cases, HIV infection is followed by flu-like symptoms which may persist for two weeks to a few months. After this, symptoms may disappear for several years. The most common symptoms of AIDS include long-term fatigue, swollen lymph nodes, weight loss, persistent infections, diarrhea, yeast infections and easy bruising.

As the immune system weakens further, an HIV-infected person becomes vulnerable to more serious infections and cancer. Among the more serious disorders are pneumonia, which affects approximately 60 per cent of patients; tuberculosis; and Kaposi's sarcoma, a connective tissue cancer. Even with treatment, most people with AIDS die within a few years of developing infections or cancers that take advantage of their weakened immune systems.

HIV diagnosis and laboratory measurements

Infection with the virus is diagnosed by the presence of antibodies to HIV in the blood. These antibodies are usually present in the blood a few weeks after infection. However, in some cases the body may take as long as 35 months to produce detectable antibody levels. Regular testing is recommended for anyone in a high risk group.

While HIV affects a number of different immune cells, it has been found that much of the immune system dysfunction can be explained by the effects of HIV on a certain type of cells called CD4+ lymphocytes (CD4+ T cells). These cells play a crucial role in the immune response, signaling other cells in the immune system to perform their special defensive functions. During the course of infection, the number of these cells progressively declines. The level of CD4+ lymphocytes in the blood has been shown to predict the onset of AIDS symptoms.

A healthy, uninfected person usually has around 800 to 1300 CD4+ lymphocytes per microliter (one millionth of a liter) of blood. Vulnerability to opportunistic infections and cancer increases when an HIV-infected person's CD4+ lymphocyte count falls below 200 to 300 cells per microliter.

Prevention of HIV infection

Large scale public awareness campaigns have been conducted to inform people about the prevention of HIV infection, particularly those in high risk groups. Higher rates of HIV infection were originally seen in homosexual or bisexual men who had many sex partners, intravenous drug users, heterosexual partners of infected persons, and those who had received blood transfusions. Practising safe sex and avoiding used injection needles are very important in preventing HIV infection.

Treatment of those infected with HIV

As there is no known cure for full-blown AIDS, the aim of therapy is to affect the action of HIV and reduce the immune suppression it causes. With improving treatment, fewer people should develop AIDS and it is possible that HIV infection may one day be a manageable chronic illness.

Managing patients with HIV infection and AIDS is becoming increasingly more complex as new medications and technologies are approved. Recent research shows that therapy which combines more than one type of antiviral drug offers the best chance of managing HIV and AIDS progression. As the majority of AIDS patients die because of opportunistic infections, advances in the prevention and treatment of these has helped to decrease mortality rates in AIDS patients.

Enhancing immune function plays an important role in delaying the onset of AIDS. A healthy diet; nutritional supplements; avoiding smoking, alcohol and caffeine; adequate sleep; and exercise all play an important role in helping the immune system to work well. Stress reduction is also very important. Research has shown that severe life stress increases the risk of early progression of disease in those who are HIV-positive.[1]

Many HIV-positive people use alternative treatments such as relaxation, touch, spiritual and self help therapies. Herbal medicine, acupuncture, homeopathy and dietary therapies are also popular.

Diet and HIV

The progression and physical symptoms of HIV disease are affected by diet. It is very important to eat foods which enhance immune function and to avoid foods and other substances which may cause damage. (See page 422 for more information.)

Medical treatments are more effective in a well-nourished person due to improved drug response and tolerance, and reduced risk of toxicity and adverse reactions. It is important to consult a dietitian or nutritionist knowledgeable in HIV as a lot of general nutrition advice is aimed at people who are overweight, and the needs of an HIV-positive person may be different.

Malnutrition can occur early in HIV infection and nutritional status progressively deteriorates, resulting in weight loss, muscle tissue loss and reduced immune function. The HIV-wasting syndrome may occur because of loss of appetite, increased nutrient needs, altered ability to process nutrients, and decreased absorption. Clinical nutrient deficiencies develop as the disease progresses, and supplements may be very useful. Malnutrition is common in AIDS patients, and those patients in whom it is more severe tend to die sooner.

It is important to eat enough calories to maintain a healthy body weight and to eat enough protein to build muscle and repair any damage that occurs. In those who are infected with HIV but have no signs of the disease, eating a wide variety of healthy foods every day is vital as nutrient and calorie requirements are increased. Diets high in protein, complex carbohydrates and fiber; and low in fat, are usually recommended. Foods which are high in sugar and fat should not replace nutritious foods but can be enjoyed along with these foods and can be useful to help with maintaining or gaining weight. However, large amounts of sugar may suppress immunity and should be avoided.

Food safety can be very important for people with HIV; and handling, cooking and storing food safely are very important to prevent infection. In a 1998 study, New York researchers advised HIV-infected people to boil tap water before drinking. Even at low levels, the water-borne parasite cryptosporidium represents a threat to those with weakened immune systems.[2]

When and if AIDS develops, specialized dietary approaches are necessary. AIDS sufferers experience various physical disturbances due to the disease or the various medications used to treat it. These include diarrhea, nausea, mouth ulcers, painful swallowing, poor appetite and fatigue. Choosing carefully the types of foods to be eaten and the times and ways to eat them can help deal with these effects.

Vitamins, minerals and AIDS

HIV-positive people may be deficient in vitamins A, C, E, B6, B12, folic acid, selenium, zinc and beta carotene. Nutrient deficiencies are often the result of inadequate dietary intake and intestinal malabsorption but it is not well known how individual nutrients are affected by the disease. As any nutrient deficiency leads to lower immune function, it is very likely that deficiencies affect progression to AIDS in HIV-positive people.[3]

RDA levels are almost certainly inadequate for people with HIV. Optimal dietary intake of all vitamins and minerals is essential and most experts recommend supplements which supply at least 100 per cent of the RDA for all nutrients. It is particularly important to consume adequate amounts of nutrients which strengthen immune function, including antioxidants, B vitamins and trace elements such as selenium and zinc.

Antioxidants

Blood levels of antioxidants are often low in AIDS patients. This leads to increased oxidative and inflammatory damage which can adversely affect the immune system. Increased oxidative damage also affects the nervous system and leads to mental problems. Recent studies have found that HIV patients with the lowest levels of antioxidants may progress to AIDS more quickly than those with high levels. Multiplication of HIV may also be affected by the concentration of antioxidants, and low levels of antioxidants may shorten the time taken for those who are HIV-positive to develop AIDS.[4]

Vitamin A

Vitamin A deficiency is often seen in HIV-positive people.[5] It may be due to metabolic changes associated with HIV infection.[6] A 1995 study done on HIV-infected drug users in the US found that there was a higher risk of death in those with vitamin A deficiency.[7] Research has shown that development of a deficiency of vitamin A is associated with lower CD4+ lymphocyte counts, and there is some evidence that returning vitamin A levels to normal can increase CD4+ lymphocyte counts.[8]

Vitamin A deficiency is often seen in HIV-positive pregnant women. This is particularly common in developing countries, although it has been seen in the USA.[9] Severe deficiency increases infant mortality and the risk of mother-to-child transmission of HIV. This may be due to impaired immune responses in both mother and baby; an increase in the amount of HIV breast milk and blood; and abnormalities in placental and vaginal tissues.[9]A 1997 study done on HIV-positive pregnant women in New York State did not find a link between vitamin A levels and transmission of the virus.[10]

Beta carotene

Beta carotene levels have been shown to be deficient in HIV-positive patients.[11,12] Research has shown that large doses of beta carotene may boost immune function. In a Yale University study done in 1995, researchers found that daily supplements of 60 mg beta carotene given to seven AIDS patients for a period of four weeks increased CD4+ lymphocyte cell counts.[13] A 1996 double-blind study which looked at the effect of oral beta carotene supplements over a three-month period did not find the same effects. However, both groups in the study were given multivitamin supplements which may have masked any beneficial effect.[14] It is possible that natural carotene supplements or increasing intake of carotene-rich foods may be more beneficial than using synthetic beta carotene supplements.[15]

Vitamin C

Vitamin C supplements are likely to be useful in HIV-positive individuals as they have been shown to boost the immune system and prevent damage to nerves. However, caution should be used with very high doses as they can cause diarrhea. Vitamin C has been shown to inhibit HIV in the laboratory and may also kill HIV-infected cells.[16]

Vitamin E

Research has shown that many HIV-positive people have a deficiency in blood levels of vitamin E early in the course of their disease. In a 1997 study involving 121 people, researchers showed that these levels decreased significantly over a 12-month period.[17]

High levels of vitamin E seem to be linked to slower disease progression. In a study published in 1997, researchers at Johns Hopkins University working on the Multicenter AIDS Cohort Study found that those patients with the highest vitamin E intakes had a 35 per cent decrease in risk of progression to AIDS when compared to those in the lowest intake group. The study involved 311 patients followed for a period of nine years.[18]

B vitamins

Recent research from the US Multicenter AIDS Cohort Study suggests that high intakes of B group vitamin supplements may be associated with improved survival in HIV patients. The average increased survival time was up to 1.3 years. In particular, vitamin B6 intake of more than twice the recommended dietary allowance was associated with longer survival. Vitamin B1 and B2 intakes of more than five times the RDA were also associated with improved survival.[19]

Vitamin B12

Vitamin B12 is vital for healthy nerve and immune system function. Low blood vitamin B12 levels are common in HIV infection and may help predict those patients in whom the disease will progress most rapidly. Results from the Multicenter AIDS Cohort Study showed that HIV-positive individuals with low serum B12 levels had around four years AIDS-free time whereas those with higher levels were free of the disease for around eight years.[20]

AIDS patients often show signs of nerve damage, including numbness and tingling in the hands and toes. These symptoms may be due to vitamin B12 deficiency and may lessen after treatment with supplements.[21] Even marginal vitamin B12 deficiency is likely to contribute to impairments in mental function. Normalization of vitamin B12 levels seems to improve this.[22]

Vitamin B6

Vitamin B6 deficiency is common in HIV-infected people. In a 1991 study, University of Miami researchers examined the relationship between deficiency and immune dysfunction. The results showed that while CD4+ and CD8+ cell numbers were not be affected, other measures of immune system function were.[23]

Selenium

As part of the antioxidant enzyme, glutathione peroxidase, selenium is necessary to help prevent oxidative damage. Levels of this enzyme have been shown to be low in some HIV-positive patients which may increase immune suppression and nerve damage. In a 1997 study done in Germany, blood serum selenium levels were determined in 104 HIV-positive patients at various disease stages. Results showed that both selenium levels and glutathione peroxidase activity in hospitalized AIDS patients were significantly lower compared to healthy subjects and patients with no symptoms.[24] Low selenium levels appear to be associated with low CD4+ lymphocyte counts[25] and with higher death rates in AIDS patients.[26] The results of a 1997 study suggest that deaths from AIDS are higher in areas where soil selenium is low.[27]

Iron

Anemia is often seen in HIV-positive people, but why this happens is not well understood. Iron deficiency may be associated with reduced immune response in HIV-positive people. However, as HIV disease progresses, body iron stores increase. This enhances oxidative damage, impairs the function of the immune system, and directly promotes the growth of micro-organisms. Some experts believe that reducing the amount of iron in the diet may help minimize the adverse effects of excess iron.[28]

Zinc

Zinc is probably the most important mineral for immune function. It strengthens the immune system, is vital for cell-mediated immunity, and acts as an antiviral agent. It is also necessary for transport of other nutrients such as vitamin A. The antioxidant enzyme, copper-zinc superoxide dismutase, has been shown in laboratory experiments to inhibit the replication of HIV.[29]

AIDS patients may suffer from zinc deficiency, which may adversely affect immune function. In a 1995 Italian study, zinc sulfate supplements (200 mg per day for 30 days) were given to patients receiving the medication, azathioprine (AZT). Results showed stabilization in body weight and increases in CD4+ lymphocytes and the immune stimulating hormone levels.[30]

Low zinc levels have been shown to increase the risk of opportunistic infection in AIDS patients. In a recent study, researchers at the San Francisco General Hospital measured zinc levels in 228 patients with AIDS. They found that those with zinc deficiency had a significantly higher incidence of bacterial infections than did patients with normal zinc levels.[31] The frequency of some opportunistic infections was also reduced after zinc supplementation.

Herbal medicine and HIV/AIDS

There are many herbal medicines which have demonstrated antiviral effects and/or stimulatory effects on the immune system. Some of these and compounds extracted from them have been used to treat those with HIV/AIDS. These include cat's claw (*Uncaria tomentosa*), echinacea (*Echinacea purpurea)*, ginseng (*Panax ginseng*), St John's wort (*Hypericum perforatum*), reishi and shiitake mushrooms, licorice (*Glycyrrhiza glabra*), turmeric (*Curcuma longa*), astragalus (*Astragalus membranaceus*), aloe vera (*Aloe vera*) and mistletoe (*Viscum album*). Many patients have also used traditional Chinese herbal treatments. See page 384 for more information on these herbs and the precautions that may be necessary.

Hypertension

Hypertension is when blood pressure, the blood's force against the walls of the arteries, is consistently abnormally high in relation to age. It is a major public health problem that often requires long-term medication. More than one in four American adults have high blood pressure and more than 50 per cent of Americans over the age of 65 may be affected. It is the most prevalent form of cardiovascular disease and, if left untreated, can lead to heart attack, stroke and kidney disease.

Diagnosis of hypertension

A normal blood pressure reading for adults is considered to be around 120/80 mmHg. The first number represents the systolic pressure (the pressure when the heart is contracting) and the second number is the diastolic pressure (the pressure when the heart is relaxed). A high blood pressure is 140/90 mmHg or above.

High blood pressure can be divided into two major categories. When high blood pressure occurs without apparent cause, it is known as primary or essential hypertension; and when it occurs because of another disease, such as poor kidney function, it is known as secondary hypertension. Anyone can have temporary high blood pressure, resulting from excitement, nervousness, exertion, anger, fatigue, cold or smoking. In hypertension, high blood pressure is sustained over a period of time.

Blood pressure tends to rise with age but hypertension can also occur in children and teenagers, with increased risk of disease later in life. Most younger sufferers have a family history of hypertension and tend to be overweight.

Symptoms of hypertension

When high blood pressure is mild it usually has no symptoms. In more severe cases, it can cause headaches, fatigue, dizziness, heart palpitations, nosebleeds and blurred vision.

Causes of hypertension

The causes of primary hypertension remain unclear, although there are several risk factors. These include heredity, diet, environmental factors, smoking, alcohol, drinking large amounts of coffee, lack of exercise, obesity and stress. Hypertension may occur due to a combination of factors, and these may vary from person to person. Hypertension is twice as common in African Americans than Caucasians. The reasons for this are not known. Hypertension is rare in cultures that are relatively untouched by the Western life-style.

Treatment of hypertension

Because lifestyle plays a major role in causing and maintaining hypertension, effective treatment often involves changes in dietary, psychological and social factors. Exercise, relaxation techniques and meditation have all shown beneficial effects. In some cases, hypertension can be controlled by lifestyle changes; in other cases medications may be used.

There are several different types of drugs that are used to treat hypertension. These include diuretics, which act by forcing the kidneys to excrete water and sodium at a faster rate; and beta blockers, which lower heart rate and cardiac output. Other drugs known as ACE inhibitors affect the levels of hormones that constrict blood vessels.

Another major class of drugs used to lower high blood pressure blocks the channels which transport calcium across muscle cell membranes. There is currently an ongoing debate as to whether these calcium channel blockers increase the risk of heart attacks.

Diet and hypertension

Because hypertension is currently a chronic incurable disease, prevention is more important than cure. Diet is strongly linked to the prevention and treatment of hypertension.

Obesity increases the risk of hypertension. About one-third of people with hypertension are overweight, and even a small decrease in weight can reduce the risk of hypertension. Many studies indicate that exercise and keeping to a reasonable weight may be the best way to control hypertension. Effective stress management, watching salt intake, limiting coffee intake and drinking alcohol in moderation may also help to prevent high blood pressure.

High intakes of fruit and vegetables seem to be linked to lower blood pressure as they contain so many beneficial nutrients. An effective diet for blood pressure reduction is low in fat, particularly saturated fat; high in essential fatty acids; low in sugar, especially refined sugar; low in cholesterol; high in fiber; low in salt and high in potassium, magnesium, calcium and vitamin C.

Minerals and blood pressure

Blood pressure is regulated by a balance of the minerals sodium, potassium, calcium and magnesium. Hypertension appears to be associated with an imbalance of these minerals where sodium and possibly chloride are too high, and potassium, calcium and magnesium are too low.

Increasing dietary intakes of potassium, calcium, and magnesium have each been reported to lower blood pressure, but the extent of blood pressure reduction in epidemiological studies and clinical trials has varied. Studies in China have shown that multivitamin and mineral supplements lower the risk of hypertension in a population with a vitamin/mineral-poor diet.[1]

Sodium

Epidemiological studies suggest that high sodium intakes are linked to high blood pressure. As a person ages, changes in the hormonal systems that regulate the control of water and sodium balance lead to changes in blood pressure. The evidence for the role of sodium is strongest in those subjects with impaired ability to excrete sodium because of kidney disease or hormonal abnormalities. In these cases, restriction of dietary sodium promptly lowers blood pressure. The role of sodium in causing primary hypertension is more controversial.

The Intersalt study

Most studies find that high salt diets accelerate the increase in blood pressure that occurs with age. These include the Intersalt study, which is an international epidemiological study covering 32 countries and including 10 000 subjects. This study has shown a relationship between blood pressure and body mass index and alcohol consumption, but the data on salt has been interpreted differently by different researchers. The results suggest that dietary salt restriction has more effect on blood pressure in those aged 45 and older. In young people diet and exercise may play a more important part. Some patients with mild to moderate primary hypertension respond to moderate sodium restriction with a fall in blood pressure. This restriction also seems to reduce the amount of medication needed to keep blood pressure under control.[2]

Salt-sensitivity

Some people are more susceptible than others to the blood pressure-raising effects of salt. This is known as salt-sensitivity. About 30 per cent of people and as many as 40 to 50 per cent of those suffering from hypertension may be salt-sensitive and respond favorably when salt is restricted. Salt-sensitivity is more common among certain population groups including black people, diabetics and the elderly. Reduction of salt intake is generally recommended to reduce the risk of developing high blood pressure as most Western diets are very high in salt.

A review published in 1997 in the *American Journal of Clinical Nutrition* showed that experimental data support the view that when adults meet or exceed the recommended dietary allowances of calcium, potassium, and magnesium, high sodium intakes are not associated with high blood pressure. Thus adequate mineral intake may protect against salt-sensitivity.[3]

Salt restriction

A new study of almost 1500 British people has found that those who eat the most salt tend to have the highest blood pressure. The study, which involved men and women aged 16 to 64 found that as daily salt intakes rose from 1600 mg to 9200 mg, so did blood pressures. A rise in salt consumption from 2300 mg to 4600 mg led to a 7.1 mmHg rise in systolic blood pressure for women and a 4.9 mmHg rise for men.[4]

In a two-month double-blind, randomized, placebo-controlled crossover study published in 1997 in *The Lancet*, researchers found that modest reduction in salt in the diets of elderly people led to lower blood pressure. The study involved 29 patients with high blood pressure and 18 with normal blood pressure. The average blood pressure fall was 8.2/3.9 mmHg in the normal subjects and 6.6/2.7 mmHg in those with high blood pressure.[5] In those with normal blood pressure, cutting salt may have little effect, according to an analysis of 83 studies published in the *Journal of the American Medical Association* in 1998.[6]

Dietary sodium restriction is used to control pregnancy-related high blood pressure. It does not seem to lead to any adverse effects on other minerals or the baby. In fact, increasing evidence suggests that the amount of salt in a baby's diet affects blood pressure later in life. In a study published in 1997, Dutch researchers compared the effects of low salt and normal salt diets in 476 children born in 1980. They measured blood pressures in the first week of life and every four weeks after that for a six-month period. Fifteen years later, the study participants had their blood pressures measured again and the results showed that children who had been in the low salt group had lower blood pressures than those in the normal salt group.[7]

Stress and sodium

Stress may affect sodium excretion. In certain people, stress seems to contribute to high blood pressure, and this may be mediated via effects on sodium excretion. In a 1995 German study, researchers tested the effects of stress on 27 people with normal blood pressure and 21 with high blood pressure. The participants in the study took part in a 30-minute video game after which their excretion of sodium was measured. Seventy per cent of the people showed increased sodium excretion and 30 per cent showed decreased excretion. Those who excreted more sodium showed less stress-associated increases in blood pressure and greater expression of anger.[8]

Chloride

Some evidence indicates that when sodium is combined with chloride, it exerts greater effects on raising blood pressure than when it is combined with other compounds such as phosphate. Dietary intake of both sodium and chloride may be necessary for the development of hypertension.

Potassium

Population studies suggest that a low intake of potassium may be linked to an increase in blood pressure, and increasing potassium-rich foods in the diet can lead to a reduction in high blood pressure. The typical Western diet is low in potassium relative to sodium, and the ratio of sodium to potassium in the diet may be more important than sodium alone. Studies suggest that the most beneficial effects on blood pressure are seen when sodium intake is reduced and potassium intake is increased.

Potassium depletion causes the body to retain more fluid in response to a large dose of salt. Potassium may help to lower blood pressure in several ways, including enhancing sodium excretion, by directly dilating blood vessels, or lowering cardiovascular reactivity to body chemicals which constrict blood vessels.

Potassium supplements may be useful in the treatment of high blood pressure. Doses involved usually range from 2.5 to 5 g. In people with normal blood pressure, those who are salt-sensitive or who have a family history of hypertension appear to benefit most from potassium supplementation. The greatest blood pressure-lowering effect of potassium supplements occurs in those with severe hypertension. Beneficial effects are more pronounced with long-term supplementation.

A 1997 analysis of studies on the effects of potassium supplementation on blood pressure confirms that low intake of the mineral is linked to high blood pressure and increasing intake is a beneficial part of treatment. Researchers at Johns Hopkins University looked at 33 randomized controlled trials with over 2069 participants in which potassium supplements were used. Positive effects were seen with a decrease in mean systolic pressure of 3.11 mmHg and in diastolic pressure of 1.97 mmHg. The effects were enhanced in those exposed to a high intake of sodium.[9]

In a study published in 1998 in the American Heart Association journal *Hypertension*, researchers at the Harvard School of Public health tested the effects of potassium, calcium and magnesium supplements on 300 women (average age 39 years) whose dietary intakes of those minerals were low. The participants had blood pressure in the normal range. The women were divided into five groups: the calcium (1200 mg per day), magnesium (336 mg per day) and potassium (1600 mg per day) groups; a group who received all three supplements; and a placebo group. The result showed that potassium supplements lowered blood pressure whereas calcium and magnesium supplements did not. The results also showed that those in the three supplements group had smaller falls in blood pressure than those in the potassium group. The researchers speculate that calcium and magnesium might in some way interfere with the blood pressure-lowering effect of potassium.[10]

Calcium

Low dietary calcium may increase the risk of high blood pressure. Data from the US Health and Nutrition Examination Survey (NHANES I) show that hypertensive people consume 18 per cent less dietary calcium than those with normal blood pressure.[11]

Disturbances in calcium metabolism have been found in people suffering from primary hypertension. These include reduced blood calcium levels, increased urinary excretion of calcium, raised intracellular calcium levels, reduced cell membrane calcium binding, and other indicators of higher calcium needs. Some of these changes, however, may be secondary to blood pressure elevation. Some research suggests that alterations in calcium-regulating hormones in general, and vitamin D in particular, contribute to essential hypertension, especially salt-sensitive forms.

Researchers involved in the Dutch Hypertension and Offspring Study studied young people with normal blood pressure. Some of them had a family history of high blood pressure while others did not. The findings showed that disturbances in calcium metabolism are present in the early phase of primary hypertension and may precede the development of high blood pressure. Changes in calcium metabolism may reflect a genetic basis for calcium-sensitive hypertension.[12]

Increasing calcium intake has been shown to lower blood pressure in some cases. Supplemental dietary calcium may affect blood pressure by a number of mechanisms. It may affect smooth muscle cell contraction, hormone action, nervous system function and increase sodium excretion. In an eight week randomized, placebo-controlled study done in 1985 in the US, researchers assessed the effect of 1000 mg per day of calcium supplements on the blood pressure of 48 people with hypertension and 32 without. Compared with placebo, calcium significantly lowered both systolic and diastolic blood pressures, but only in those with high blood pressure.[13]

Whether calcium can lower blood pressure in cases where there is no apparent deficiency is not clear. Increasing calcium intake may lower blood pressure by increasing the excretion of sodium, and calcium supplements may be most useful in those who are salt-sensitive. Results from the University of Pittsburgh Trials of Hypertension Prevention (TOHP) showed calcium supplements (100 mg per day) to have little effect on blood pressure. The participants were healthy adult men and women (both white and African American) aged 30 to 54 years with high-normal diastolic blood pressure. However, the supplements did seem to lower blood pressure in white women, who are at particular risk of low calcium intakes.[14] Supplements may be beneficial in cases where calcium intake is insufficient, which may be relatively common.

Pregnancy

The results of a study reported in 1997 in the *British Medical Journal* suggest that women who take calcium supplements in pregnancy have children with lower blood pressures. Researchers measured the blood pressures of almost 600 children of women who had previously been involved in a double-blind trial of the effects of calcium on blood pressure during pregnancy. The results showed that, overall, systolic blood pressure was lower in the calcium group, particularly among overweight children.[15]

Use of calcium supplements during pregnancy may lower a woman's risk of pre-eclampsia, a disorder which occurs in one in every 20 pregnant women. Symptoms of pre-eclampsia are high blood pressure, headache, protein in the urine, blurred vision and anxiety. It can lead to eclampsia, a seizure disorder which can cause complications with pregnancy, and even death. There is some evidence that abnormalities in calcium metabolism are involved in pre-eclampsia. Many pregnant women do not consume enough calcium to ensure optimal blood pressure regulation, and the results of several clinical trials have suggested that calcium supplements reduce the incidence of pre-eclampsia.[16]

A 1996 analysis of clinical trials which looked at the effects of calcium intake on pre-eclampsia and pregnancy outcomes in 2500 women found that those who consumed 1500 to 2000 mg of calcium supplements per day were 70 per cent less likely to suffer from high blood pressure in pregnancy.[17]

However, in a study published in 1997 in the *New England Journal of Medicine*, researchers found that calcium supplements did not prevent pre-eclampsia. The study, the largest ever done on the subject, involved 4589 healthy, first-time mothers. Half of the subjects received 2000 mg of calcium per day and the other half received a placebo. The researchers then assessed the incidence of high blood pressure and protein excretion in the urine. No significant differences in the groups were found. Supplements did not reduce other complications associated with childbirth or increase the incidence of kidney stones.[18] The results of this study still leave open the possibility that calcium supplements may be useful as the women included in the study were already consuming higher than average levels of calcium than is typical even before they took the supplements. Women at high risk of pre-eclampsia were also not included in the investigation.

Magnesium

Magnesium deficiency may contribute to high blood pressure. Studies suggest that around 30 per cent of high blood pressure sufferers consume inadequate amounts of magnesium, and high blood pressure is more common in areas where the water is low in magnesium. Magnesium can affect blood pressure by directly exerting effects on blood vessels and by indirectly affecting potassium balance in the body.

Intravenous magnesium has been shown to reduce blood pressure by relaxing constricted blood vessel walls. Changes in magnesium levels may contribute to altered cell membrane calcium binding seen in essential hypertension.

The Honolulu Heart Study, which looked at the relationship between dietary magnesium intake and blood pressure, found that those in the high intake group had, on average, systolic blood pressures 6.4 mmHg lower and diastolic pressures 3.1 mmHg lower than those in the low intake group.[19] In another survey of over 58 000 women, researchers found that those with magnesium intakes of less than 200 mg per day had a significantly higher risk of developing high blood pressure than women whose intakes were over 300 mg per day.[20] In a study published in 1992, researchers also found that low dietary intakes of magnesium were linked to an increased risk of high blood pressure in over 30 000 men.[21]

Magnesium supplements may be useful in the treatment of high blood pressure, although the results of studies have been mixed. Intravenous magnesium has been shown to reduce blood pressure, possibly by relaxing constricted blood vessels. Those with high sodium and low potassium levels and those taking diuretic drugs may benefit from magnesium supplements. These drugs can decrease the amount of magnesium in the body as they increase fluid excretion.

In a 1997 double-blind, placebo-controlled study carried out in Japan, 33 people received either a four-week treatment with oral magnesium supplementation (411 to 548 mg per day) or a placebo. The results showed that the systolic and diastolic blood pressure values decreased significantly in the magnesium group, but not in the placebo group. Measurements made during the study suggest that magnesium may lower blood pressure through its effects on the secretion of adrenal hormones and resulting increase in sodium excretion.[22]

In a 1994 study, 91 middle-aged and elderly women with mild to moderate hypertension who were not on anti-hypertenstive medication were treated with either magnesium supplements or placebo for six months. At the end of the study, both systolic and diastolic pressures had fallen in both groups but the falls in the magnesium group were significantly greater.[23]

Vitamins and blood pressure

Vitamin D

Vitamin D deficiency may play a role in the development of high blood pressure, possibly via effects on calcium metabolism.

Vitamin C

Hypertension sufferers often have low blood levels of vitamin C and increasing intake may help to lower blood pressure. In a study done in Cambridge, UK researchers examined the relationship between blood pressure and vitamin C levels in the blood in 835 men and 1025 women aged from 45 to75. The results showed that low vitamin C levels were associated with higher systolic and diastolic blood pressures.[24]

Some research suggests that vitamin C supplements may have beneficial effects in lowering high blood pressure.[25] They have been shown to improve abnormal artery lining function in hypertensive people.[26] Vitamin C supplements may be useful in combination with other treatments.

Other nutrients

Omega-3 fatty acid supplements may be effective in treating mild hypertension. In a 1996 study of 78 patients with untreated mild hypertension, Norwegian researchers found that overall blood pressure was reduced by about six points in people who took fish oil supplements, compared with those who took a corn-oil placebo.[27] In some cases, it may also be an effective addition to drug treatment.[28] In a 1996 study, 21 men whose blood pressure was not successfully controlled with anti-hypertenstive medications were randomized to receive either fish oil (4.5 g omega-3 fatty acids per day) or a placebo. Blood pressure readings were taken at the start of the study and at four and eight weeks. Both systolic and diastolic blood pressures were significantly reduced in the fish oil group at both week four and at week eight.[29] Supplements have also been useful in preventing high blood pressure in heart transplant patients. [31] However, not all studies have shown beneficial effects. [31]

Herbal medicine and hypertension

Herbs used to treat hypertension include hawthorn (*Crataegus oxyacantha*), linden (*Tilia europea*), yarrow (*Achillea millefolium*), garlic (*Allium sativum*) and wild celery (*Apium graveolens*). See page 384 for more information on these herbs and the precautions that may be necessary.

Inflammatory bowel disease

Inflammatory bowel disease (IBD) is the term given to a group of disorders that cause inflammation or ulceration in the small and large intestines. IBD is divided into two major categories: ulcerative colitis and Crohn's disease. Ulcerative colitis appears to be slightly more common than Crohn's disease. The rate of IBD is increasing in Western cultures whereas it is virtually unknown in countries where people eat less refined foods. IBD can occur at any age but it is most common in those aged from 15 to 35.

Symptoms

Ulcerative colitis causes inflammation and ulceration of the inner lining of the large bowel. The most common early symptoms are constipation with passage of blood or mucus in the stools. It may be months or years before diarrhea and abdominal pains develop.

Crohn's disease may affect any part of the upper and lower intestine, but most commonly the last part of the small intestine and/or parts of the large bowel. In Crohn's disease, the inflammatory reaction spreads throughout the entire thickness of the bowel wall. The symptoms of Crohn's disease are abdominal pain, especially in the right lower area of the abdomen, and diarrhea. There may also be rectal bleeding, weight loss and fever. The onset of Crohn's disease is often slow and insidious.

The most common complication of Crohn's disease is blockage of the intestine due to thickening of the bowel wall. In more severe cases, communicating passages known as fistulas, may develop between the affected bowel and other parts of the bowel, bladder, vagina or skin. Other complications include arthritis, skin problems, inflammation in the eyes and mouth, kidney stones and gallstones. Inflammatory bowel disease is a chronic condition that can recur at various times during a person's life. Some people have periods of remission, which can last for years, when they are free of the symptoms; and there is often no way to predict when the symptoms will return. IBD can be particularly serious in children as it can severely affect growth and development. Crohn's disease is also likely to increase the risk of gastrointestinal cancer.

Causes

There are various theories about the causes of IBD. Genetic factors, modern diets high in sugar and refined foods, and viral and bacterial triggers may contribute to the disease. Smoking may also play a role. As IBD is increasingly prevalent in countries where diets are high in refined foods and low in fruit, vegetables and fiber, diet is likely to play a part in the cause and progression of the disease.

In an effort to understand some of the dietary factors which may be involved in the development of IBD, researchers involved in a 1997 study examined the pre-illness diets of 87 patients with recent IBD (54 ulcerative colitis and 33 Crohn's disease) and compared these with 144 healthy people. The results showed that a high sucrose consumption was associated with an increased risk for IBD. Lactose consumption showed no effect while fructose intake decreased the risk of IBD. A high fat intake was associated with an increased risk for UC; this was particularly marked for animal fat and cholesterol. A high intake of fluids, magnesium, vitamin C, and fruits also decreased the risk. Most of the findings were similar in ulcerative colitis and Crohn's disease except for potassium and vegetable consumption, which only seemed to decrease the risk for Crohn's disease.[1] Increased sensitivity to yeast, food intolerances and immune abnormalities may play a role; although it is often unclear whether these are a cause or a result of the disease. Psychological factors are said to play a part in the progression of the disease.

Treatment of IBD

Therapy for Crohn's disease aims to correct nutritional deficiencies and control inflammation, abdominal pain, diarrhea and rectal bleeding. Drugs are often used to control symptoms such as abdominal cramps and diarrhea. These include sulfasalazine drugs, corticosteroids and immunosuppressive drugs, many of which have adverse side effects if taken for long periods. The wide variety of treatments gives an indication of the inadequacy of drug therapy for curing the disease. In severe cases, surgery may be used to remove diseased sections of bowel and 50 per cent of people need more than one operation. Parenteral nutrition may also be used in severe cases.

Dietary therapy in IBD

Nutritional deficiencies are common in sufferers of IBD. In a 1998 study, Dutch researchers evaluated nutritional status in 32 patients with Crohn's disease. They measured body composition, dietary intake, biochemical indexes of nutrition, and muscle strength. The results showed that daily intakes of fiber and phosphorus were significantly lower in Crohn's disease patients than in healthy people. Serum concentrations of beta carotene, vitamin C, vitamin E, selenium, magnesium, vitamin D and zinc, and activity of the enzyme, glutathione peroxidase were also significantly lower in Crohn's disease patients. Percentage body fat and hamstring muscle strength were significantly lower in male Crohn's disease patients than in healthy people.[2]

The aim of dietary therapy in IBD is to improve nutritional support and diminish inflammatory processes. It centers around high fiber and low refined sugar diets. However, wheat is a common allergen and wheat fiber may not be suitable for use in IBD patients. It is important to be aware that raw fruit and vegetables may be irritating during an active phase of the disease.

It is very likely that food allergies and intolerances play a role in IBD, and identifying and eliminating offending foods is likely to be useful in any treatment program. This applies particularly to wheat and dairy products. Lactose intolerance may be particularly prevalent in IBD sufferers. Elemental diets are often used to treat Crohn's disease and consist of all the essential nutrients, with protein provided as pre-digested or free-form amino acids. However, most patients relapse when they return to a normal diet. Along with an increase in fiber, elemental and elimination diets seem to alter the gut environment favorably, resulting in a healthier balance of micro-organisms and a decrease of toxin production. This contributes to clinical improvement.

There has been considerable interest in recent years on the influence of fat on the occurrence of IBD and it is possible that elemental diets produce beneficial effects because of their fat composition.[3] Increases in recent years in the frequency of Crohn's disease in Japan have been correlated with increased dietary fat intake and fatty acid deficiencies; omega-3 fatty acid deficiencies in particular, have been seen in Crohn's patients.[4]

IBD sufferers should also avoid food additives such as carrageenan and sorbitol. Carrageenan, a compound extracted from seaweed, is used as a stabilizing and suspending agent and is often found in milk and chocolate milk products. The alterations in gut bacteria which are often seen in Crohn's disease patients may make them particularly susceptible to carrageenan-induced damage. Caffeine and stimulant drugs should also be avoided. Some patients have benefited from macrobiotic diets and fasting.

Nutritional supplements

IBD impairs digestion and absorption, and because of this a high percentage of sufferers are malnourished. This malnutrition may in turn worsen bowel function, leading to further problems. Many sufferers are deficient in protein and calories and have a fat intolerance which results in fat-soluble vitamin deficiencies. Diarrhea promotes depletion of water-soluble B vitamins and essential minerals like zinc and magnesium. Vitamin and mineral supplements are extremely useful in the treatment of IBD; with zinc, magnesium, folic acid and antioxidants being particularly beneficial. Nutritional supplements are also important when patients need extra nutrients; for example, in children with growth retardation.

However, problems can arise from large doses of supplements as high doses of vitamin C, magnesium, zinc and iron can irritate the digestive tract and worsen diarrhea. Slow gradual repletion of nutrients by mouth may be the most effective way to supplement in IBD.

Vitamins, minerals and IBD

Antioxidants

Inflammatory damage in IBD may be mediated by free radicals and sufferers may be deficient in antioxidant vitamins. Increasing intake of antioxidants may protect against this damage. In a 1996 study published in the *American Journal of Clinical Nutrition*, researchers at the University of Colorado investigated antioxidant concentrations in the blood plasma of children with IBD. The study involved 12 children with Crohn's disease and 12 with ulcerative colitis. Their blood levels of vitamin C, glutathione, glutathione peroxidase and vitamin E were compared with those of 23 healthy children. The results showed that levels were lower in IBD sufferers, particularly those with Crohn's disease.[5] Other studies have shown low levels of vitamin A in children suffering from the disorder.[6]

Vitamin A

Low serum vitamin A levels are found in many Crohn's disease patients. Vitamin A is important for maintaining a healthy gut lining.

B vitamins

Folic acid

Some of the drugs used to treat IBD, such as sulfasalazine, may deplete folic acid. Folic acid is essential for tissue regeneration and to protect against genetic damage which may possibly lead to cancer. As there may be an increased risk of developing cancer in those who have ulcerative colitis, folic acid supplements may be useful in preventing this. A woman taking sulfasalazine drugs who plans to get pregnant should take folic acid supplements to help prevent neural tube defects.

Vitamin B12

Vitamin B12 supplements may be useful in sufferers of Crohn's disease as this vitamin is absorbed in the area of the intestine most commonly affected by Crohn's disease.[7]

Vitamin D

Reduced fat absorption can lead to vitamin D deficiency. Patients with IBD may have lower serum levels of vitamin D than healthy controls, despite normal intake. This may increase the risk of osteoporosis. Anti-inflammatory corticosteroid drugs, which are often given to IBD sufferers, may also increase the risk of osteoporosis, and vitamin D and calcium supplements may help to decrease this risk.

Iron

The gastrointestinal bleeding seen in IBD commonly leads to iron deficiency and anemia. However, large doses of iron may increase oxidative damage and promote intestinal infection, and should be avoided by IBD sufferers.

Magnesium

Magnesium deficiency is often found in IBD sufferers. However, large doses of magnesium supplements may have a laxative effect and should be taken with care.

Zinc

Disturbances in zinc metabolism have been shown in patients with inflammatory bowel disease. Several studies have found decreases in absorption and serum zinc levels, and increased excretion. The copper-to-zinc ratio appears to be higher in those with active disease. Zinc deficiency may be due to low intake, poor absorption and excess losses in the feces.[8] The concentration of superoxide dismutase, a copper and zinc-containing protein involved in the scavenging of free radicals, may be decreased in the gut lining of patients with IBD, which could contribute to inflammation.

Other nutrients

Essential fatty acids

Essential fatty acid supplements have been shown to have beneficial effects in the treatment of IBD as they may correct abnormalities in fatty acid and prostaglandin metabolism, and act to reduce inflammation. A 1996 Italian study published in the *New England Journal of Medicine* showed beneficial effects of fish oil in treating Crohn's disease. Researchers involved in the one-year, double-blind, placebo-controlled study investigated the effects of an enteric fish oil preparation on the maintenance of remission in 78 patients with Crohn's disease who had a high risk of relapse. Every day, the patients received either nine fish oil capsules containing a total of 2.7 g of omega-3 fatty acids or placebo. The proportion of patients in the treatment group who remained in remission after a year was 59 per cent, compared to only 26 per cent of patients in the placebo group. Enteric-coated capsules may be particularly useful as side effects such as unpleasant taste, bad breath and diarrhea are minimized.[9]

Probiotics

The composition of gut bacteria is often unfavorable in Crohn's disease and probiotic supplements may be useful in correcting these abnormalities and improving gut function.[10] Researchers involved in a 1996 study found improvements in the function of the immunological barrier of the gut in patients given Lactobacillus supplements.[11]

Herbal medicine and IBD

Herbal treatment of IBD involves the use of plants which soothe irritated mucous membranes such as slippery elm bark (*Ulmus fulva*), marshmallow (*Althaea officinalis*) and aloe vera (*Aloe vera*). Other herbs that may be useful include echinacea, (*Echinacea angustifolia* or *E purpurea*) and goldenseal (*Hydrastis canadensis*). See page 384 for more information on these herbs and the precautions that may be necessary.

Insomnia

Insomnia is a common sleep disorder suffered by up to 50 per cent of people in any one year. It can mean difficulty falling asleep, difficulty staying asleep, or waking too early in the morning.

Causes of insomnia

Insomnia is caused by many disorders, with psychological factors probably accounting for around half of all types. Depression, anxiety and stress are closely associated with insomnia, and other causes include chronic pain, disease, lack of physical exercise, nutrient deficiencies and stimulants such as caffeine, tobacco, chocolate and alcohol. Sensitive people should avoid these, particularly late at night. Some medications cause insomnia. Sleep requirements lessen with age and elderly people experiencing changes in sleep patterns may need reassurance that these changes are normal.

Treatment and prevention of insomnia

This depends on the underlying cause. There are several measures that may be useful. These include regular exercise (but not before bed), avoidance of stimulants, developing a regular bedtime routine, warm baths before bedtime; and avoidance of distractions that promote wakefulness. Drinking warm milk, or eating a high carbohydrate snack before bed also helps some people sleep. Medications such as sedatives and hypnotics are sometimes prescribed for people suffering from insomnia. These are potentially addictive and should only be taken for short periods.

Vitamins, minerals and insomnia

B vitamins

B vitamins are involved in the metabolism of neurotransmitters such as serotonin, which aids in the regulation of sleep. Deficiencies may lead to insomnia, and vitamin B6, niacin and folic acid are sometimes used to treat the disorder. Increasing intake of these vitamins is most likely to be effective in cases of deficiency.

Vitamin B12 injections have been used to treat insomnia and have had beneficial effects on the sleep-wake cycles in some patients. Some research suggests that vitamin B12 might affect sleep quality and performance. In a 1996 study, German researchers explored the effects of 3 mg of vitamin B12 on the quality of sleep and work performance of ten healthy, male staff members of an Austrian industrial plant. The results showed better sleep quality and shorter total sleep time in those taking supplements.[1]

Iron

Sleeping difficulties may be exacerbated by iron deficiency. Studies suggest that restless legs syndrome caused by iron deficiency, is relatively common in the elderly and causes significant discomfort and sleep disturbance. Iron supplements can help reduce the symptoms and lead to improvements in sleeping patterns.

Calcium and magnesium

Magnesium supplements have muscle relaxant effects and may be beneficial if taken at night.

Other nutrients

Melatonin

Melatonin is a hormone involved in the regulation of the sleep-wake cycle. Supplements have been used to treat insomnia. They may be useful in improving sleep duration and quality in those in whom the normal cycle is disrupted, such as people with jet lag and shift workers.

In a 1997 placebo-controlled, double-blind, cross-over study, researchers assessed the effects of melatonin in eight males. Following a 7-hour night-time sleep, the participants were given either a placebo or one of three doses of melatonin (1 mg, 10 mg, and 40 mg) at 10 am. All doses of melatonin significantly shortened the time taken to go to sleep. Melatonin also significantly increased total sleep time and decreased wake after sleep onset.[2]

In another placebo-controlled study, researchers studied the effects of single evening doses of melatonin on sleep in 15 healthy middle-aged volunteers. Compared to placebo, the 1.0 mg dose of melatonin significantly increased sleep time, sleep efficiency, non-REM Sleep and REM sleep latency.[3]

Jet lag

Melatonin use in jet lag appears to decrease jet lag symptoms and hasten the return to normal energy levels. In a double-blind placebo-controlled study published in 1993, New Zealand researchers investigated the efficacy of melatonin in alleviating jet lag in 52 flight crew members after a series of international flights. The optimal time for taking melatonin in this group was also investigated. The participants were randomly assigned to three groups; early melatonin (5 mg started three days prior to arrival until five days after return home); late melatonin (placebo for three days, then 5 mg melatonin for five days); and placebo. The results showed that the late melatonin group reported significantly less jet lag and sleep disturbance following the flight compared to placebo. The late melatonin group also showed a significantly faster recovery of energy and alertness than the early melatonin group, which reported a worse overall recovery than placebo.[4]

Herbal medicine and insomnia

Herbs, which act as relaxants and nervine tonics, are beneficial in the treatment of insomnia. These include valerian (*Valeriana officinalis*), passion flower (*Passiflora incarnata*), chamomile (*Matricaria recutita*), vervain (*Verbena officinalis*), hops (*Humulus lupulus*), kava (*Piper methysticum*) and oatstraw (*Avena sativa*). Other herbs that may be useful in helping the body adapt to stress include ginseng (*Eleutherococcus senticosus* and *Panax ginseng*). See page 384 for more information on these herbs and the precautions that may be necessary.

Kidney stones

Kidney stones are usually made up of crystals of calcium oxalate, either alone or in combination with calcium phosphate. They can be found in the kidney itself or anywhere in the duct (ureter) that carries urine from the kidney to the bladder. Kidney stones can be as small as a tiny pebble or an inch or more in diameter. The compounds from which stones are formed are normally present in human urine but remain in solution due to control of acidity and the presence of various protective compounds. When these protective mechanisms are overwhelmed, stones may be allowed to form. There are usually no symptoms until the stone blocks the urinary tract resulting in excruciating pain until the stone passes. The rate of occurrence of kidney stones is increasing, and over 10 per cent of men and 5 per cent of women experience at least one kidney stone during their lifetime.

Causes of kidney stones

Although there are many types of kidney stones, the most common type contains calcium and occurs due to alterations in calcium metabolism, including absorption from the intestine, filtering from the kidneys or abnormalities in the hormones that regulate the use of calcium in the body.

Treatment of kidney stones

Treatment depends on the size, symptoms, location and cause of the kidney stone. If the stone is small and can be passed, drinking plenty of fluids may be enough. For kidney stones too large to be passed, a procedure known as lithotripsy is often used. During this procedure, shock waves are directed to the areas where the stone is located. The shock waves break it into fragments. After the treatment, the patient drinks a lot of water to flush out the stone fragments.

Diet and kidney stones

Diets which are low in fiber and high in refined carbohydrates, alcohol, animal protein, fat and salt lead to an increased risk of kidney stones. High intakes of calcium and vitamin D-enriched foods may also increase the risk. Vegetarians appear to have a decreased risk of developing kidney stones, as their diets are usually lower in protein and higher in green vegetables and grains. Drinking plenty of water can be a useful preventive measure.

Eating an alkaline diet that includes potatoes, vegetables and fruit (but not citrus fruit), and reducing protein intake will help to reduce the risk of uric acid stone recurrence. Some experts advise limiting intake of liver, kidneys, fish roe and sardines as these foods are high in purines which may contribute to stone formation.

To reduce the risk of calcium oxalate stones, it is helpful to avoid foods containing oxalates, such as spinach, rhubarb, beet, parsley, sorrel, and chocolate. People who have a tendency to form oxalate stones often secrete too much calcium in their urine, which reacts with oxalic acids to form the stones. In such people, calcium and sodium intakes should not be too high and restricting intake of dairy products is likely to be beneficial.

Vitamins, minerals and kidney stones

Vitamin B6

Vitamin B6 deficiency may also play a role in the development of some kinds of kidney stones. Combined magnesium and vitamin B6 treatment may bring more beneficial results in the treatment of kidney stones than the use of magnesium alone. Vitamin B6 reduces the production and excretion of oxalates, compounds that combine with calcium to form some types of kidney stones.[1]

Vitamin C

There have been reports that excess vitamin C may increase the risk of kidney stone formation as large doses may raise blood levels of oxalates and lead to increased excretion. However, healthy people do not seem to be at risk.[2] Those suffering from kidney disease, gout, or who are on hemodialysis may be at increased risk and should avoid large doses of vitamin C.

Vitamin K

Vitamin K is necessary for the production of a urinary protein involved in kidney function that inhibits the formation of calcium oxalate kidney stones.[3] This may account for the fact that vegetarians, whose diets are often high in vitamin K, have a low incidence of kidney stones.

Calcium

Some forms of calcium supplements may lead to an increased risk of kidney stones. This risk can be lowered by using supplements in calcium citrate form.

Citrate levels are lower in kidney stone patients, and citrate supplementation has been shown to reduce stone crystallization.

Magnesium

Magnesium deficiency may play a role in kidney stone formation as magnesium increases the solubility of calcium oxalate and inhibits the precipitation of calcium phosphate and calcium oxalate. Kidney stones are frequently associated with low levels of magnesium in the urine, although the exact effects of this abnormality are not well understood. Magnesium citrate supplements may be the most beneficial type to use to reduce the incidence of kidney stones.

The results of a 1997 study suggest that magnesium supplements may be beneficial in preventing kidney stones. Researchers found that giving potassium-magnesium citrate to calcium oxalate kidney stone sufferers reduced the risk of them developing further stones. In the double-blind study reported in the *Journal of Urology*, 64 patients were given either a placebo or the potassium-magnesium citrate compound for up to three years. New kidney stones occurred in 63.6 per cent of the patients taking placebo but in only 12.9 per cent of those taking the potassium-magnesium citrate compound.[4]

Herbal medicine and kidney stones

Useful herbs include pellitory of the wall (*Parietaria officinalis*), couch grass (*Agropyron repens*), nettles (*Urtica dioica*), gravel root (*Eupatorium purpureum*), corn silk (*Zea mays*), golden rod (*Solidago virgaurea*) and stone root (*Collinsonia canadensis*). See page 384 for more information on these herbs and the precautions that may be necessary.

Mood disorders

For psychiatric purposes, a mood is defined as a sustained emotion. Depression and elation are the types of moods most commonly seen in mood disorders; others include anxiety and anger. Clinical depression and mania are diagnosed when feelings of sadness or elation are overly intense, continue beyond the expected impact of a stressful life event, or arise without apparent or significant life stress. Difficulty in functioning in everyday life is another characteristic differentiating mood disorders from normal emotional reactions.

Depression

Originally a strictly medical term, the word 'depression' has become common in everyday speech and is regularly used to refer to feelings ranging from everyday disappointments to major loss. However, it is important to distinguish between this understandable reaction to life events, and clinical depression. The dividing line is not a clear one as not everyone who is depressed experiences every symptom of the illness, and the severity of symptoms can vary according to the individual involved.

Clinical depression is the most common psychiatric problem in our society and takes several forms including major depression, dysthymia, cyclothymia, bipolar disorder and seasonal affective disorder (SAD). Research suggests that as many as 10 per cent of patients who visit a doctor are experiencing depression serious enough to affect their physical condition. The rate of major depression may be as high as one in four women and one in eight men. Sometimes depression is appropriate to a life event, such as bereavement, and does not need medical treatment.

Diagnosis of mood disorders

In an effort to build a framework for the study and treatment of mental illness, psychiatrists have defined criteria for diagnosing disorders such as clinical depression. One of the best known sets of criteria is contained in the *Diagnostic and Statistical Manual of Mental Disorders* published by the American Psychiatric Association. It is now in its fourth edition and is known as DSM-IV.

Symptoms of depression include persistent sad or empty mood, loss of interest or pleasure in everyday activities, decreased energy, fatigue, poor appetite with weight loss, increased appetite with weight gain, altered sleeping patterns, physical hyperactivity or inactivity, feelings of worthlessness, diminished ability to think or concentrate, aches and pains, and recurrent thoughts of death or suicide.

At least two weeks of lowered mood is considered to be the minimum period to warrant a diagnosis of major depression. Someone with minor depression may not feel bad all the time but may still feel a sense of gloom, and minor disappointments may affect them deeply. Major depression is more severe and health may be affected by self-neglect. The risk of suicide is high.

Causes of mood disorders

Depression and other mood disorders are complex problems, the causes of which are not well understood. It seems likely that any explanation or approach that emphasizes only one factor as the cause of depression is misleading and simplistic. However, sometimes depression can occur due to another disorder or as a drug side effect, and in these cases it is known as secondary depression. Where there is no clear physiological cause, the disorder is known as primary depression and it seems likely that the disorder will have several contributory causes. Research has focussed on biological factors such as heredity, hormonal abnormalities, medication side effects, disease-related effects, nutritional deficiencies and psychological and social causes. Changes in brain levels of neurotransmitters, chemicals which serve as communication links between nerve cells, are often seen in depressed patients. For example, levels of noradrenaline and serotonin are reduced.

Treatment of mood disorders

Treatment of mood disorders such as depression is a complex process and may involve psychotherapy and drug treatment. Drugs which have antidepressant effects usually alter levels of neurotransmitters, serotonin and noradrenaline, which are involved in the transmission of nerve impulses in the brain. There are several types and they have slightly different effects in the body. People respond differently to the various types of antidepressant drugs; and a person's symptoms, age, whether or not they have a physical illness, suicide risk, and response to previous medication may help to play a role in deciding what drugs are given. Types of antidepressant drugs include heterocyclic antidepressants, monoamine oxidase inhibitors and selective serotonin re-uptake inhibitors.

An appropriate exercise program is an important part of any treatment of depression. The effects of exercise in improving the symptoms of depression are well-documented. Several studies have shown that exercise can improve mood and increase the ability to handle stress. A nutritious diet, exercise, limiting alcohol and tobacco, and effective stress reduction techniques are also important in the treatment of depression.

Food and mental function

Many substances in food may affect mood by altering the levels of various neurotransmitters in the brain. It is possible that nutritional factors play a part in many mental illnesses and even marginal nutrient deficiencies can change the structure and function of the brain and nervous system, and affect behavior. Memory loss, confusion and fatigue can be the consequences of a poor diet. Nutrient intake may have a powerful effect on a person's mood, behavior and ability to learn before the better known physical symptoms of deficiency are obvious.

Almost any nutrient deficiency can result in depression. Many depressed people show signs of nutrient deficiencies but it is unclear in many cases whether these deficiencies are an actual feature of the disease or are secondary to malnutrition. When a mood disorder is caused by a nutrient deficiency, increased intake usually reverses the symptoms; although in certain cases, permanent damage may occur.

Food allergies may also be linked to depression, and eliminating offending foods from the diet may help to relieve symptoms. Avoiding caffeine-containing drinks and food additives is also advisable.

Carbohydrates and protein

Carbohydrate-rich foods raise brain levels of tryptophan and therefore serotonin, which can lead to feelings of wellbeing. It is no coincidence that people often crave carbohydrate-rich foods when they are feeling sad. This is particularly common in those suffering from SAD and premenstrual syndrome. In contrast to carbohydrates, high protein foods seem to decrease the levels of serotonin in the brain. Some research suggests that the amino acids, tyrosine and phenylalanine can help to improve the symptoms of depression. Foods high in these amino acids include turkey, chicken, and milk; and they are also available as supplements.

There is some research to suggest that diets high in sugar can aggravate depression. It may be that some people are particularly susceptible to the effects of sugar on mood while others are relatively unaffected. It is unclear exactly how sugar exerts these effects but anyone suffering from depression may find it helpful to try and cut down or eliminate sugary foods.

B vitamins

Inadequate intake of zinc, vitamin B6, iodine, vitamin B12 and folic acid during early life may impair nervous system development and permanently alter function and behavior. Deficiencies of folic acid and vitamin B12 cause defects in red blood cell production and function, which can lead to a reduction in the amount of oxygen reaching the brain. This can lead to fatigue, depression and mental problems.

Serotonin is manufactured in the brain from the amino acid, tryptophan with the help of vitamin B6, vitamin B12 and folic acid. Thus serotonin levels are related to the availability of tryptophan and these vitamins.

While virtually any vitamin or mineral deficiency can affect mood, and many depressed people show signs of nutrient deficiencies, B vitamin deficiencies may be particularly common and are often found in psychiatric patients. Researchers involved in a 1991 study measured the B complex vitamin status at time of admission of 20 geriatric and 16 young adult nonalcoholic patients with major depression. Twenty-eight per cent of the patients were deficient in riboflavin, vitamin B6, and/or vitamin B12. However, the degree of vitamin deficiency did not appear to be related to the severity of the disorder.[1]

In a randomized placebo-controlled study published in 1992, researchers at Harvard Medical School assessed the effects of 10 mg each of vitamins B1, B2, and B6 in 14 geriatric inpatients with depression who were taking antidepressant drugs. The results showed that those patients taking the vitamins showed greater improvement in scores on ratings of depression and cognitive function when compared with placebo-treated patients.[2]

Thiamin

Thiamin plays an important role in nerve function and release of the neurotransmitter, acetylcholine, which affects several brain functions. Thiamin deficiency can lead to depression, psychosis, apathy, anxiety and irritability. Alcoholics and binge drinkers are especially prone to thiamin deficiency as alcohol depletes body stores. Thiamin has been used to treat some of the symptoms associated with alcohol abuse; such as the reduction in certain brain chemicals involved with memory and thought processes.

In a study done in Wales in 1997, researchers gave 120 young adult women either a placebo or 50 mg thiamin, each day for two months. The women were not thiamin-deficient. Before and after taking the tablets, mood, memory and reaction times were assessed. The women taking the thiamin reported that they felt more clearheaded, composed and energetic.[3]

Riboflavin

Riboflavin is essential for the proper development of nerves and blood cells, iron metabolism, the activation of vitamin B6 and the conversion of tryptophan to niacin. Deficiency may contribute to depression.[4]

Niacin

Niacin deficiency leads to anxiety, depression, insomnia, and eventually dementia. Niacin may exert beneficial effects due to increases in levels of the amino acid, tryptophan, which is a building block for both niacin and serotonin. Niacin supplements have been used with tryptophan to treat depression and some researchers report improvement in symptoms.

The psychiatric symptoms of the niacin deficiency disease, pellagra resemble the symptoms of schizophrenia and large doses of niacin have been used to treat schizophrenia. Studies have shown mixed results.

Vitamin B6

Vitamin B6 deficiency can cause the mental symptoms of irritability and depression. Vitamin B6 is vital for the healthy development and function of the nervous system. It is necessary for the conversion of tryptophan to serotonin, and even a marginal deficiency may affect neurotransmitter levels.

Vitamin B6 deficiency is often found in depressed people and several studies have shown that mood improves when vitamin B6 supplements are given. As estrogen may suppress vitamin B6 metabolism, supplements may be beneficial for pregnant women, and for those on the contraceptive pill or hormone replacement therapy (HRT) who suffer from mood swings and depression. Vitamin B6 is also used to treat stress conditions.

Folate

Folate deficiency leads to confusion, forgetfulness, insomnia, irritability, depression and mood changes. It is often seen in those affected by psychiatric disorders, particularly depressive illness, and may play a part in causing or aggravating psychiatric disturbances.

Borderline low or deficient folate levels have been detected in as many as 38 per cent of adults diagnosed with depressive disorders.[5] Low folate levels have also been linked to poorer response to the antidepressant drug, Prozac. In a study published in 1997, researchers examined the relationships between levels of folate, vitamin B12, and homocysteine in 213 depressed patients taking Prozac. The results showed that people with low folate levels were more likely to have melancholic depression and were significantly less likely to respond to the drug.[6] Folic acid supplements may improve mood in depressed people, especially those who are taking drugs which interfere with folic acid metabolism.

Vitamin B12

Vitamin B12 deficiency eventually leads to a deterioration in mental functioning, to neurological damage, and to a number of psychological disturbances including memory loss, dementia, moodiness, confusion and delusions. Vitamin B12 is involved in the manufacture of myelin, the fatty sheath protein which insulates the nerves. It is also essential in the formation of neurotransmitters and in the normal functioning of blood cells.

Vitamin B12 deficiency is more common in the elderly than in younger people, with around 15 per cent of elderly men and women affected. Supplementation can prevent irreversible neurological damage if started early, and have been shown to improve mental function. Elderly people with vitamin B12 deficiency may show psychiatric or metabolic deficiency symptoms even before anemia is diagnosed. Screening for low vitamin B12 levels is necessary in elderly people with mental impairment, although it has also been found that deficiency states can still exist even when blood levels are higher than the traditional lower reference limit for vitamin B12.

Iron

Iron deficiency is associated with fatigue and depression and has also been implicated in emotional, social and learning difficulties in children and adults. Iron is also involved in the production of several brain neurotransmitters.

Selenium

Selenium supplements may improve mood and reduce anxiety, fatigue and depression in those whose intake is low. A 1996 study done at the USDA Human Nutrition Research Center in San Francisco suggests that people with low selenium levels might experience depressed moods, supporting the idea that selenium plays a special role in the brain. However, the study did not find improvements with selenium supplementation in people eating a typical American diet.[7]

Herbal medicine and depression

St John's wort (*Hypericum perforatum*) is a well-known herbal treatment for depression. In a study published in 1996 in the *British Medical Journal,* researchers from Germany and America analysed the results of 23 clinical trials that looked at St John's wort in the treatment of depression.[8] The trials involved 1757 patients with mild to moderately severe depression. They specifically investigated whether St John's wort was more effective than a placebo, whether it was as effective as standard antidepressant drugs, and whether it had fewer side effects than those drugs. When the results of the trials were put together, they showed that St John's wort extracts were significantly better than placebo. Fifty-five per cent of patients given St John's wort found that their symptoms improved, whereas only 22 per cent of patients in the placebo group showed improvement. Other herbs that can be used to treat depression and strengthen the nervous system include vervain (*Verbena officinalis*), oat straw (*Avena sativa*), skullcap (*Scutellaria laterifolia*) and lemon balm (*Melissa officinalis*). Kava (*Piper methysticum*) has been used to treat anxiety. See page 384 for more information on these herbs and the precautions that may be necessary.

Osteoporosis

Osteoporosis, which literally means "porous bones", is the result of a long-term decline in bone mass which, in severe cases, causes the bones to break under the weight of the body. Particularly badly affected bones include the spinal vertebrae, the thigh bone and the radius (shorter arm bone). Over 25 million Americans may be affected by osteoporosis and 80 per cent of those are women. Although the problem also occurs in men, postmenopausal women are particularly susceptible, with around 35 per cent of women suffering from osteoporosis after menopause.

Symptoms of osteoporosis

The symptoms of osteoporosis are often absent until fractures occur, although in some cases there may be a loss of height, a hunched back or back pain. Osteoporotic fractures affect 50 per cent of women and 30 per cent of men over 50. These fractures are particularly serious as demineralized bones shatter when they break and usually take longer to heal. Radiological examination can be used to measure bone mineral density and assess the risk of fracture.

Causes of osteoporosis

Around 35 per cent of women suffer from osteoporosis after menopause and, although it is less common, the problem occurs in a similar way in men. Osteoporosis is more common in Caucasians and Asians because they are often smaller boned.

Most of the bone loss seen in osteoporosis in women occurs in the first five to six years after menopause due to a decline in circulating female hormones and an age-related reduction in vitamin D production. Genetic factors seem to play a part in osteoporosis but behavioral and hormonal factors may be more important. Sufficient body fat and muscle are necessary to keep hormone levels high enough to maintain bone mineral content. Athletes and premenopausal women whose menstrual periods have stopped may also be at increased risk of osteoporosis due to alterations in their hormone levels.

Adequate intakes of calcium, vitamin D, magnesium and boron are also necessary. Diets high in dairy products, protein, sugar, alcohol, salt, caffeine-containing drinks and very high in fiber also seem to increase the risk of the disorder, most likely due to effects on mineral absorption and metabolism. People on weight-reducing diets are also at risk as they avoid foods high in bone-building nutrients.

Inactivity leads to an increased risk of osteoporosis, as does gastric surgery and certain types of medications such as corticosteroids.

Treatment of osteoporosis

The conventional treatment for osteoporosis is estrogen therapy but this is not suitable for some women due to the increased risk of breast cancer. Some women are treated with calcitonin, a hormone that inhibits removal and promotes formation of bone. It is available in injection forms and as a nasal spray. Intake of calcium and vitamin D must also be adequate. Newer osteoporosis drugs include alendronate, which inhibits bone breakdown; and raloxifene, a selective estrogen receptor modifier.

Osteoporosis prevention

Exercise

Regular exercise plays a vital part in preventing loss of bone mass. Weight-bearing exercises such as walking, jogging and yoga contribute to increases in bone density and prevention of bone loss. Exercise also helps build muscle mass which can help protect bones from injury. It also improves strength and flexibility, decreasing susceptibility to falls.

Diet

A healthy diet can reduce the incidence of osteoporosis by ensuring the development of a favorable peak bone mass during the first 30 to 40 years of life. Adequate nutrient intake early in life is vital for bones to reach their maximum density so that they are strong enough to support the body even when they lose mass later in life. However, it is never too late to slow the bone loss seen in osteoporosis, and early postmenopausal years are an important time to ensure optimal intake of nutrients including calcium, magnesium, boron and vitamin D.

Recent research suggests that including soybeans in the diets of postmenopausal women may decrease the risk of osteoporosis. Soybeans contain compounds called phytoestrogens which act in a similar way to estrogen and have beneficial effects on bone mineral density.

Caffeine-containing drinks can increase the loss of calcium in the urine. Diet soda drinks which contain phosphoric acid can alter the calcium phosphorus balance and contribute to calcium loss from the bones. Consuming large amounts of these drinks can increase the risk of osteoporosis. Nicotine and alcohol also adversely affect bone mineral density. High salt intakes seem to increase calcium excretion, lowering bone mineral density and increasing the risk of osteoporosis. In a study published in 1995, Australian researchers investigated the influence of urinary sodium excretion on bone density in a 2 year study of 124 postmenopausal women. The results showed that increased sodium excretion was linked to decreases in bone density.[1]

While dairy products are good sources of calcium, there is concern that their protein content can actually increase the loss of calcium from bone. Researchers involved in the Nurses Health Study analyzed the diets of over 77 000 participants in the study and looked at the rates of bone fractures. Results showed that women who drank two or more glasses of milk per day had around a 45 per cent increased risk of hip fracture and a 5 per cent increased risk of forearm fracture compared to women who drank one glass or less per week. There was also no drop in risk with intake of calcium from other dairy foods.[2] A varied diet which includes nondairy sources of calcium is likely to be more beneficial in protecting against osteoporosis.

Vitamins, minerals and osteoporosis

B vitamins

B vitamin deficiencies may contribute to osteoporosis, particularly those of folate, vitamin B12 and vitamin B6. This may be partly due to the effects of increased homocysteine levels on bone metabolism.

Vitamin D

Vitamin D regulates the absorption and use of calcium and phosphorus, which are vital for normal growth and development of bones. Vitamin D is necessary for calcium absorption and increases the deposition of calcium into bones. In cases of vitamin D deficiency, the body increases production of parathyroid hormone which removes calcium from the bones and leads to bone thinning.

Research suggests that there may be a genetic link between vitamin D receptor types and osteoporosis. It is also possible that patients with osteoporosis have impaired conversion of vitamin D to its most active form. The ability to produce vitamin D in the skin may decline with age and bone loss may increase in the winter months when people have less exposure to sunshine. People with a certain type of vitamin D receptor may be more susceptible to osteoporosis, and research suggests that women with different types of vitamin D receptors respond differently to vitamin D supplements.[3]

A study done in 1997 at Tufts University in Boston showed reduced rates of bone loss and fractures in men and women over 65 who took calcium and vitamin D supplements. Researchers assessed the effects of calcium (500 mg per day) and vitamin D (700 IU per day) on 176 men and 213 women aged 65 years or older. After a three-year period, those taking the supplements had higher bone density at all body sites measured. The fracture rate was also reduced by 50 per cent in those taking the supplements.[4]

Vitamin D supplements may also be useful in preventing bone loss in patients taking corticosteroid drugs. In a study published in 1996, researchers at the University of Virginia found that calcium and vitamin D supplements helped prevent the loss of bone mineral density in those taking the drugs for arthritis, asthma and other chronic diseases.[5] Vitamin D supplements may also be useful in reducing the risk of osteoporosis due to long-term use of anticonvulsant drugs.

However, other studies have not shown any reduction in fracture rates in those taking vitamin D supplements. A 1996 study which was carried out in Amsterdam looked at the effects of either vitamin D or a placebo on 2500 healthy men and women over the age of 70 who were living independently. The participants received a placebo or a daily dose of 400 IU of vitamin D for a three-and-a-half year period. Dietary calcium intake was the same in both groups. Forty-eight fractures were observed in the placebo group and 58 in the vitamin D group.[6]

Vitamin K

Low levels of vitamin K have been seen in sufferers of osteoporosis. In a Japanese study published in 1997, researchers investigated the relationship between bone mineral density, vitamin K levels and other biological parameters of bone metabolism in 71 postmenopausal women and 24 women with menopausal symptoms receiving hormone replacement therapy. The results showed that women with reduced bone mineral density had lower levels of vitamin K1 and K2 than those with normal bone mineral density.[7] Low levels have also been seen in osteoporotic men.[8]

Boron

Boron acts with calcium, magnesium and phosphorus in the metabolism of bone. Deficiency seems to affect calcium and magnesium metabolism and affects the composition, structure and strength of bone, leading to changes similar to those seen in osteoporosis.[9] Combined boron and magnesium deficiency seems to worsen osteoporosis, suppress bone building and cause decreased magnesium concentrations in bone.[10] Supplements of around 3 mg per day have been shown to enhance the effects of estrogen in postmenopausal women. This is likely to contribute to its beneficial effects on bone health.[11] Studies done in 1994 in athletic college women suggest that boron supplements decrease blood phosphorus concentration and increase magnesium concentration. Both of these changes are beneficial to bone building.[12]

Calcium

Osteoporosis is not merely a loss of calcium from bone, although calcium deficiency does contribute to osteoporosis. The National Osteoporosis Foundation estimates that the average adult in the US gets only 500 to 700 mg per day. The US government has recently raised its recommendation for daily calcium intake. For men and women aged from 19 to 50, the RDA is now 1000 mg, and for those over 50 it is 1200 mg.

The new RDA for adolescents is 1300 mg and adequate calcium intake during this time of life plays a vital part in allowing bones to reach their maximum density so that they are strong enough to support the body even when they lose density later in life. Studies suggest that calcium intake in adolescence is often below the recommended levels. Researchers involved in a 1994 USDA study measured calcium intake in 51 girls aged 5 to16 years old. They found calcium intake to be below the recommended dietary allowance for 21 out of 25 girls aged 11 or over. These studies suggest that the current calcium intake of American girls during puberty is not enough to enable bones to develop maximum strength, and that increased intakes may be necessary.[13] A 1993 study published in the *Journal of the American Medical Association* suggests that calcium supplements may be beneficial in adolescent girls. Researchers gave daily calcium doses of 500 mg or placebo to 94 girls and then measured bone mineral density and bone mineral content at the lumbar spine. The results showed that increasing calcium intake led to significant gains in bone mass.[14]

However, it is never too late to slow the bone loss seen in osteoporosis, and early postmenopausal years are also an important time to ensure optimal intake. A 1997 study done at King's College Hospital in London suggests that high calcium intakes are linked to bone mineral density in elderly women. Researchers assessed calcium intake in 124 women aged from 52 to 62 and also measured bone mineral density at the spine, hip and the os calcis bone in the foot. Results showed that women with high calcium intakes had higher bone mineral density.[15] Results from the Rotterdam Study, which involved 1856 men and 2452 women aged 55 years and over, show that high calcium intakes also protect against bone loss in men.[16]

Taking calcium supplements later in life can slow the bone loss associated with osteoporosis, and treatment which combines calcium and estrogen is likely to be better at building bone than treatment with estrogen alone. In a 1998 study, researchers analyzed the results of 31 studies and found that the postmenopausal women who took estrogen alone had an average increase in spinal bone mass of 1.3 per cent per year, while those who took estrogen and calcium supplements had an average increase of 3.3 per cent. Increases in bone mass in the forearm and upper thigh were also greater in women taking supplements. The added benefit from the calcium was seen when the women increased their intake from an average of 563 mg per day to 1200 mg per day.[17]

It is recommended that postmenopausal women who are not on estrogen therapy consume 1500 mg calcium per day. Multivitamin supplements often do not provide enough calcium and separate supplements may be necessary. Supplements should be taken in divided doses throughout the day, with a maximum of 500 mg being taken at any one time.

Fluoride

Bones seem to be more stable and resistant to degeneration when the diet is adequate in fluoride. Sodium fluoride supplements have been used to treat osteoporosis.[3] Researchers involved in a 1998 study published in the *Annals of Internal Medicine* compared the vertebral fracture rates in 200 women over a four-year period. One group was given 20 mg of fluoride and 1000 mg of calcium daily, and the other group received only calcium. The rate of new fractures in the fluoride group was 2.4 per cent compared to 10 per cent in the calcium only group.[18] Sustained release of fluoride in doses of 23 mg per day appears to be more beneficial than forms which are quickly absorbed from the gut.[19] However, a 1996 study done in Argentina suggests that the increases in bone mineral density are not maintained after sodium fluoride therapy is stopped.[20]

The treatment of osteoporosis with fluoride supplements is controversial as there is the possibility that fluoride bone is not always stronger than normal bone. There may be an increase in the number of hairline fractures in the hips, knees, feet and ankles. In 1983/1984, a study of bone mass and fractures was begun in 827 women aged 20-80 years in three rural Iowa communities selected for the fluoride and calcium content of their community water supplies. Residence in the higher-fluoride community was associated with a significantly lower radial bone mass in premenopausal and postmenopausal women, an increased rate of radial bone mass loss in premenopausal women, and significantly more fractures among postmenopausal women.[21] Fluoride therapy may increase the requirement for calcium as more is needed for bone formation.

Magnesium

Magnesium and calcium interact in many body functions including that of bone formation. Women with osteoporosis may have lower magnesium levels than women without the disorder. In a 1995 study, results showed that women whose dietary intakes were less than 187 mg per day had a lower bone mineral density than women whose average intakes were more than 187 mg.[22]

Magnesium is essential for the normal function of the parathyroid glands, metabolism of vitamin D, and adequate sensitivity of bone to parathyroid hormone and vitamin D. Magnesium deficiency may impair vitamin D metabolism which adversely affects bone building.[23] Magnesium deficiency is also known to cause resistance to parathyroid hormone action which affects calcium balance and may cause abnormal bone formation.[24] However, magnesium excess inhibits parathyroid hormone secretion which means that bone metabolism is impaired under positive as well as under negative magnesium balance.[25] Maintaining normal calcium-to-magnesium balance is very important in the prevention of osteoporosis.

Supplements may help to increase bone mineral density in postmenopausal women, thus reducing the risk of osteoporosis. In a 1990 study, US researchers investigated the effect of a dietary program emphasizing magnesium instead of calcium for the management of postmenopausal osteoporosis. Nineteen women on hormone replacement therapy (HRT) received 500 mg magnesium and 600 mg calcium, and seven other women on HRT did not receive supplements. The results showed that in one year, those women given the supplements had greater increases in bone mineral density than those who were not. Fifteen of the 19 women had had bone mineral density below the spine fracture threshold before treatment; within one year, only seven of them still had values below that threshold.[26]

In a 1993 study, Israeli researchers assessed the effects of supplemental magnesium in 31 postmenopausal women who received six 125 mg tablets daily for six months and two tablets for another 18 months in a two-year trial. Twenty-three symptom-free postmenopausal women were assessed as controls. The results showed that 22 patients responded with a 1 to 8 per cent rise of bone density. The mean bone density of all treated patients increased significantly after one year and remained unchanged after two years. In control patients, the mean bone density decreased significantly.[27]

Zinc

Zinc accompanies calcium in the mineralization of bone, and is lost when calcium is lost from bone. Recent research in monkeys suggests that diets low in zinc during adolescence may increase the risk of osteoporosis later in life, as bones may not develop properly.

In a 1996 study, researchers studied zinc deficiency in two groups of ten monkeys. Both groups were given nutritionally balanced diets but one group received 50 mg of zinc per gram of food while the other group only received 2 mg of zinc per gram of food. Eight of the monkeys were then studied throughout their lives to ages equivalent to that of ages 10 to 16 in human girls. The researchers found that the monkeys on low zinc diets had slower skeletal growth, maturation and less bone mass than the other monkeys, with substantial differences noticed in the lumbar spine. The differences were only apparent during rapid growth phases in the monkeys, especially during pregnancy.[28]

Other minerals

Chromium may help to boost the bone-building effects of insulin and may have a role in the maintenance of bone density and prevention of osteoporosis.[29] Copper is necessary for bone formation, and inadequate intake can cause the loss of calcium from bones, reduced bone formation and deformities. Manganese deficiency may also increase loss of calcium from the bone. Silicon may have a role in the prevention and treatment of osteoporosis, and supplements are used to increase bone mineral density.

Herbal medicine and osteoporosis

Herbs used to treat osteoporosis include horsetail (*Equisetum arvense*), oat straw *(Avena sativa*), alfalfa (*Medicago sativa*) and hawthorn (*Crataegus oxyacantha*). Herbs commonly used to alleviate the side effects of menopause include black cohosh (*Cimicifuga racemosa*) and dong quai (*Angelica sinensis*). See page 384 for more information on these herbs and the precautions that may be necessary.

Periodontal disease

Periodontal disease is an inflammation and degeneration of the bone and gum structures that support the teeth. It starts when a bacterial infection attacks the gums, bone and ligaments that support the teeth and hold them in the jaw. The initial damage is painless and a person may not be aware of the disease until severe damage is done, making tooth loss inevitable. The early stages of periodontal disease are seen in as many as 50 per cent of adults. By age 35, about 75 per cent of people are affected; and by age 65, as many as 90 per cent suffer from the disease. Even children aged as young as five or six can have signs of periodontal disease.

Causes of periodontal disease

Periodontal disease is caused by bacteria in plaque – the sticky, colorless film that constantly forms on teeth. The bacteria create toxins that irritate the gums, causing breakdown of gum tissue. As periodontal disease develops, the gums become detached from the teeth. The tooth roots are then susceptible to decay and sensitive to cold and touch. As the disease progresses further, it becomes more painful; and in the advanced stages, the supporting bone is destroyed, causing the teeth to become loose and fall out.

Gingivitis, in which the gums become red, swollen, tender and likely to bleed easily, almost always precedes periodontal disease but does not always lead to it. In gingivitis, small gaps open up giving bacteria access to teeth and gums. Regular brushing and flossing can help to treat gingivitis and thus lessen the risk of periodontal disease. Smoking, poor dental work, some medications, clenching or grinding teeth, and diseases such as diabetes may contribute to periodontal disease.

Prevention

Regular dental check ups and good dental hygiene may help to prevent periodontal disease. A healthy diet also plays a role in slowing the progress of the disease. Avoiding simple sugars, eating plenty of whole grains and other high fiber foods, and thoroughly chewing food are important preventive measures.

Vitamins, minerals and periodontal disease

Antioxidants

Antioxidants protect against free radical damage to connective tissue that may contribute to periodontal disease.

Vitamin C

Vitamin C is necessary for the production of collagen in the gums. Deficiency affects this process and leads to increased redness and swelling. Vitamin C deficiency may also impair immune function, affecting the body's ability to fight plaque bacteria which cause periodontal disease.[1]

A weak association between periodontal disease and vitamin C deficiency has been shown in the analysis of data collected from population studies.[2] In a 1993 Finnish study, low vitamin C levels did correlate with disease severity.[3] Adequate dietary intake of vitamin C is important in protecting against gum and tooth disorders but there does not seem to be any evidence that supplementation is beneficial when the diet contains healthy levels of vitamin C.

Folic acid

Topical or internal folic acid has been shown to reduce plaque and gum inflammation and bleeding in periodontal disease. Folate mouthwash seems to be more effective than oral supplements, suggesting a local effect.[4]

Calcium

Calcium is vital for the formation and maintenance of healthy teeth, and inadequate intake throughout life may contribute to periodontal disease. Low intakes are often seen in those with the disease but calcium supplements do not seem to produce improvement. It may be that the damage is too late to repair or that factors other than calcium deficiency are more important for the development of periodontal disease.

Fluoride

Fluoride has been shown to protect against dental caries but the relationship between fluoride and periodontal health and disease is not clear. Some studies suggest that fluoride should be used with conventional periodontal therapy while other studies suggest that it should be avoided.[5]

Zinc

Mouthwashes containing zinc salts may be useful in the treatment of periodontal disease. Zinc levels may be decreased and copper levels increased in sufferers. Zinc is essential for collagen synthesis, a healthy immune system, and for wound-healing.

Coenzyme Q10

Coenzyme Q10 may be beneficial in the treatment of periodontal disease. It acts as an antioxidant and may improve tissue repair and healing. Topical application may also be useful.

Herbal medicine and periodontal disease

Useful herbs treat periodontal disease include echinacea (*Echinacea angustifolia and E. purpurea*), hawthorn (*Crataegus oxyacantha*), aloe vera (*Aloe vera*), goldenseal (*Hydrastis canadensis*), myrrh (*Commiphora molmol*) and bilberry (*Vaccinium myrtillus*). See page 384 for more information on these herbs and the precautions that may be necessary.

Premenstrual syndrome

Premenstrual syndrome (PMS) refers to a variety of symptoms experienced by women one to ten days before the beginning of a menstrual period. These symptoms disappear with the onset of menstruation and include physical discomforts and mood disorders. PMS is particularly common in women who are over 30 years of age.

Symptoms of PMS

There are more than 150 identified symptoms of PMS and these have been divided into four subgroups, each subgroup being linked to particular symptoms, hormonal and metabolic changes. These are:
PMS-A: Anxiety, irritability, mood swings and nervous tension.
PMS-D: Depression, insomnia, lethargy and confusion.
PMS-H: Bloating, weight gain, headaches and breast tenderness.
PMS-C: Increase in appetite, cravings for sugar and/or salt and fatigue.

Other symptoms include crying spells, constipation, muscle aches and pains, and acne. In some women, respiratory problems such as allergies, and infections and eye complaints may be worse. Most women experience some emotional and physical changes premenstrually, and the severity of PMS varies. Some women experience only a few symptoms, while others have many. Also, the discomfort felt as a result of PMS symptoms ranges from mild to so severe that it may interfere with everyday activities such as performance at work and/or relationships with others.

Causes of PMS

There are many theories as to the causes of PMS but none are universally agreed upon. Estrogen-progesterone ratio imbalance, excessive aldosterone or anti-diuretic hormone levels, carbohydrate metabolism changes, low blood sugar, high prolactin levels, allergy to progesterone, retention of sodium and water by the kidneys, psychological factors, alterations in neurotransmitters and prostaglandin levels, and nutritional inadequacies or excesses may all play a part.

Treatment of PMS

Oral contraceptives help relieve the symptoms of PMS in some women. Painkillers, diuretics and tranquilizers are also sometimes used. Regular exercise and good stress-reduction techniques are also beneficial.

Diet and PMS

A healthy diet is essential to help minimize the symptoms of PMS. Reducing refined sugar intake and limiting alcohol, caffeine and salt are particularly beneficial. Eating several regular small meals that include complex carbohydrates may also be helpful.

Researchers involved in a 1991 double-blind randomized study looked at the effects of a vitamin and mineral supplement on premenstrual symptoms in 44 women. The women took either six tablets, 12 tablets or a placebo for three menstrual cycles. Significant effects were seen in three symptom subgroups for the six-tablet group, and in all four subgroups for the 12-tablet group.[1]

Vitamins, minerals and PMS

Vitamin B6

Several studies have looked at the effects of vitamin B6 on premenstrual syndrome symptoms, although most of these trials have involved a limited number of patients. Some have shown positive effects. Many experts recommend doses of 50 mg to 150 mg per day started on day ten of the menstrual cycle and continued until day three of the next cycle.

Researchers in Oxford, UK conducted a double-blind trial to study the effects of 50 mg of vitamin B6 per day on premenstrual syndrome symptoms. The trial involved 63 women aged 18 to 49 years old who had noticed moderate to severe premenstrual symptoms during the previous year. Thirty-two women completed the full seven months of the study and the results showed a significant beneficial effect of vitamin B6 on emotional-type symptoms such as depression, irritability and tiredness.[2] Vitamin B6 is necessary for the production of serotonin and dopamine, and a deficiency may lead to or aggravate the effects of PMS through effects on these neurotransmitters.

Magnesium

Red blood cell concentrations of magnesium are low in women with PMS and this may play a role in the development of symptoms. The calcium to magnesium ratio also seems to be affected by hormonal fluctuations, which may affect neurotransmitter levels and lead to premenstrual symptoms.[3]

Magnesium supplements have been shown to relieve menstrual and premenstrual symptoms, including mood changes and breast tenderness. In a 1991 study, Italian researchers investigated the effects of a two-month period of magnesium supplementation on premenstrual symptoms in 32 women. The dose used was 360 mg three times a day, from the 15th day of the menstrual cycle to the onset of menstrual flow. The results showed that supplementation was effective in the treatment of premenstrual symptoms related to mood changes.[4]

Calcium

Calcium supplements may help to reduce the physical and psychological symptoms of premenstrual syndrome. In a 1998 randomized, double-blind, placebo-controlled clinical trial, 720 healthy, premenopausal women between the ages of 18 and 45 years were screened for premenstrual symptoms. Of these women, 466 were randomly assigned to receive 1200 mg of calcium per day or placebo for 3 menstrual cycles. After three months, the results showed that during the luteal phase of the treatment cycle, women who took calcium experienced significantly fewer symptoms than those in the placebo group. Mood swings and depression were reduced by 45 per cent (compared to 28 per cent in the placebo group), while generalized aches and pains, back pains and cramping reduced by 54 per cent in three months.[5]

Vitamin E

Vitamin E may be useful in reducing breast tenderness and other symptoms of PMS, possibly via effects of prostaglandins.[6]

Sodium

Most experts recommend avoiding salt and salt-rich foods as they may cause fluid retention and worsen the symptoms of PMS.

Zinc

Zinc deficiency may exacerbate the symptoms of premenstrual syndrome. In a study published in 1994, researchers assessed copper and zinc levels in ten PMS sufferers and compared these to those in nonsufferers. Results showed lower zinc levels in the luteal phase (latter half) of the menstrual cycle in PMS sufferers.[7]

Essential fatty acids

Essential fatty acid supplements may be useful in the treatment of PMS. Evening primrose and blackcurrant oils contain the fatty acid, GLA, which may affect prostaglandin production and improve breast tenderness, irritability and depression.

Essential fatty acids may also be effective in treating menstrual pain. In a 1996 study, researchers assessed the effects of fish oil supplements on girls aged from 15 to 18 who reported suffering from period pain. Twenty-one girls received fish oil supplements (1,080 mg EPA, 720 mg DHA and 1.5 mg vitamin E) and the other 21 received a placebo. After two months, the groups switched treatments for another two months. The amount of painkillers that the girls took during each menstrual period was also compared over the four months. After two months of treatment with fish oil, there were marked reductions in symptoms and painkiller use. Placebo treatment did not ease pain.[8]

Herbal medicine and PMS

Herbal treatment of PMS aims to rectify the hormonal imbalances and other underlying causes of the symptoms. Commonly used herbs include chaste tree (*Vitex agnus castus*), licorice (*Glycyrrhiza glabra*), dong quai *(Angelica sinensis*), raspberry (*Rubus idaeus*), black haw *(Viburnum prunifolium*) and milk thistle (*Silybum marianum*).See page 384 for more information on these herbs and the precautions that may be necessary.

Skin disorders

The skin is the largest organ in the human body. It acts as a barrier between the body and the environment and prevents harmful substances and micro-organisms from entering. Other skin functions include excretion of waste, temperature regulation, vitamin D production and sensation. The skin consists of three layers; the epidermis (outer layer), the dermis (middle layer) and the subcutaneous layer (inner layer).

Nutrition and the skin

Good nourishment is vital for healthy skin. Due to their short lifespan and rapid growth and division, skin cells need a steady supply of nutrients to stay healthy. Good circulation, a healthy nerve supply and optimal intake of all nutrients, including water, all play a part in the maintenance of healthy skin.

Drinking plenty of water is vital for healthy skin and most experts recommend at least eight glasses a day. Smoking tobacco should also be avoided, as this is very damaging for skin, possibly due to a toxic chemical-induced increase in free radical production. Ultraviolet light causes skin to dry out, lose elasticity and age more rapidly. Sunlight exposure should be minimized to prevent these adverse effects. Regular aerobic exercise and good stress relief also help to maintain healthy skin.

In addition to its other health benefits, a diet high in fruits and vegetables helps to maintain healthy skin. These foods are high in fiber, which helps to keep the bowel functioning well and avoid a build-up of toxins, which can lead to skin problems. Foods rich in essential fatty acids are also important to prevent dry skin. Adequate but not excessive protein intake is also essential. Because of its rapid growth, the effect of nutrient deficiencies shows quickly in the skin.

Antioxidants

Antioxidants help to protect against free radical damage to skin, which is caused by the effects of chemicals or age. Antioxidants may also help to protect skin from sun damage. In a study published in 1998, German dermatologists found that people who took these vitamins had a higher threshold for sunburn reaction. The researchers tested ultraviolet sensitivity in two groups of ten Caucasian people by exposing a section of skin to UV light. Subjects in one of the groups then took 2 g of vitamin C and 1000 IU of vitamin E for 8 days. The UV test was then re-done. Those taking the vitamins showed increased tolerance, particularly at higher UV doses. However, in comparison with the protection afforded by topical sunscreens, this level of protection is small.[1]

Vitamin C-containing cosmetic skin creams such as Cellex-C have also become extremely popular in the last few years. They are designed to protect against pollutants and to promote healing.

Vitamin A

Vitamin A-containing treatments are used in a cosmetic procedure known as skin peels, in which the top layer of skin is removed to reveal younger skin underneath. Creams containing the vitamin A-derivative, tretinoin, may help to retard skin aging, according to a 1997 report in the *New England Journal of Medicine*. Researchers studied the activity of enzymes known as metalloproteinases, which break down collagen, and found that exposure to ultraviolet light increased the activity of these enzymes. Even a small amount of ultraviolet light, although not sufficient to cause redness, was enough to increase enzyme activity. This suggests that exposure to a few minutes of sunlight periodically over several years may lead to premature skin aging.

This increase in enzyme activity was blocked by treatment with tretinoin before radiation. The researchers concluded that tretinoin may be useful in treating patients with signs of premature skin aging but noted that careful monitoring of tretinoin use is essential as over-treatment can cause irritation and reddening of skin. The results of this study may lead to the development of new sunscreens and anti-aging creams containing vitamin A derivatives.[2]

B vitamins

Optimal intakes of all the B vitamins are essential for healthy skin. Deficiencies may cause dermatitis, and supplements may be useful in treating various skin conditions.

Zinc

Adequate zinc intake is vital for maintaining healthy skin. Zinc is involved in oil gland function, local hormone activation, vitamin A-binding protein formation, wound-healing, inflammation control, and tissue regeneration.

Dermatitis

Dermatitis is the term used to refer to inflammation of the skin. Symptoms include rash, itching, burning, dryness, blemishes or other skin disorders. The treatment depends on the cause.

There are many causes of dermatitis, including chafing of the skin, allergies, side effects of long-term medication, nutrient deficiencies or nervous irritability.

Contact dermatitis can occur when the skin is touched by irritating substances such as industrial solvents, dyes, nickel and other metals, and some soaps.

Vitamins, minerals and dermatitis

B vitamins

A symptom of all B vitamin deficiencies is dermatitis. Symptoms of severe riboflavin deficiency include greasy, scaly skin on the nose, eyebrows, hairline, trunk and limbs. It may also lead to red, swollen, cracked lips, mouth and tongue.

Early signs of niacin deficiency include skin eruptions and dermatitis. Severe deficiency causes the disease known as pellagra, in which a reddish skin rash on the face, hands and feet becomes rough and dark when exposed to sunlight.

Vitamin B6 deficiency can lead to greasy inflammation of the skin around the nose, eyebrows and hairline. Vitamin B12 deficiency can lead to reduced tissue repair and dermatitis.

Biotin deficiency in children can lead to skin disorders such as seborrheic dermatitis, which has symptoms of reddened bumps and scaly eruptions on the scalp, cheeks, armpits, groin and neck. Supplements have been shown to improve these symptoms and may be given either directly to the infant or to the mother if she is breastfeeding. Intravenous administration of biotin is less painful and less dangerous than multiple intramuscular injections.

Vitamin A

Vitamin A is involved in the growth and repair of epithelial cells. These cells cover the internal and external surfaces of the body and are found in the skin. Prolonged vitamin A deficiency leads to thickened dry skin which is prone to infections. Small hardened bumps of a protein known as keratin may develop around the hair follicles. Because of its important role in the formation of healthy skin vitamin A is used to treat skin disorders including rashes, ulcers and wounds. However, excess vitamin A can lead to hair loss, skin dryness, itching and flaking.

Vitamin C

Vitamin C is vital for the production of collagen, and inadequate intake may affect the skin. Small hemorrhages under the skin and poor wound-healing are symptoms of deficiency. A 1980 study tested the therapeutic effect of a combination preparation of vitamins E and C in the treatment of pigmented contact dermatitis. The results showed that symptoms improved.[3]

Eczema

Eczema, which is also known as atopic dermatitis, is a common skin condition, affecting about 3 per cent of the US population. Symptoms of eczema include superficial inflammation of the skin, redness, edema, oozing, crusting, scaling and vesicles in acute cases. The inflamed areas are intensely itchy which can lead to uncontrollable, subconscious scratching. Excessive scratching can cause the skin to thicken and develop flakes, crusts and breaks, which can bleed and become infected.

Although eczema can occur at any age, it is most common in infants, children and young adults. It is a chronic disease with periods of flare up and remission and often begins in childhood where it is typically found on the face or groin. It can also affect the hands, feet and ankles. Asthma is often associated with eczema. Hereditary factors are likely to contribute to the occurrence of eczema.

Eczema may fluctuate seasonally and over the course of a day. Blood tests reveal increased levels of cells and chemicals associated with allergic reactions. A number of factors may aggravate eczema; including stress, mechanical irritation, heat, sweat retention, excessive moisture or dryness of the skin, and dietary triggers.

Treatment of eczema

The main goal of eczema treatment is to stop the itch-scratch cycle. Good general health and minimizing stress are very important. Wearing loose clothing, preferably cotton, which allows the skin to breathe; and avoiding harsh soaps, chemicals and detergents can help to manage eczema. Medicated baths and nongreasy moisturizers may also be useful.

The symptoms of eczema are often treated with topical, or in more severe cases, oral steroids. However, these drugs have several undesirable side effects, including thinning of the skin, reductions in bone mineral density, adrenal suppression and immune system suppression. Antihistamines may also be prescribed to suppress itching.

Diet and eczema

Dietary triggers such as milk, eggs, fish, milk products and food additives may also aggravate eczema, and it is currently estimated that 15 to 30 per cent of children with eczema are affected by food allergies. In cases where food allergies cause eczema it is very important to eliminate the offending foods.

Low stomach acid is often found in eczema sufferers, and is likely to contribute to the development of food allergies. Improving digestive function may help to relieve the symptoms of eczema.

Vitamins, minerals and eczema

Antioxidants

As they protect against free radical damage and have anti-inflammatory effects, antioxidants may be beneficial in the treatment of eczema.

Zinc

Zinc levels may be lower in eczema sufferers, although this may be due to nonspecific inflammatory effects.[4] Clinical trials have not shown clear benefits of zinc supplementation.[5]

Selenium

Reduced concentrations of selenium in whole blood, plasma and white cells; and reduced activity of the selenium-dependent enzyme, glutathione peroxidase, have been found in eczema sufferers. However, few studies have shown an improvement in symptoms with selenium supplements.[6]

Essential fatty acids

Essential fatty acids have anti-inflammatory effects and have been shown to have beneficial effects in the treatment of eczema. This is likely to be due to effects on prostaglandin metabolism. In a 1997 Italian study, researchers treated 30 eczema patients with gamma-linolenic acid (GLA) (274 mg twice a day), and 30 with placebo for 12 weeks. During this time, the patients assessed their own symptoms and they were also assessed by a dermatologist every four weeks. The patients who received GLA showed gradual improvements in itching, redness, vesicle formation and oozing, which were statistically significant compared with the control group.[7] Borage seed oil capsules have also shown beneficial effects in the treatment of eczema,[8] as have evening primrose oil capsules.[9]

Psoriasis

Psoriasis is a skin disorder which takes its name from the Greek word for 'itch', and usually appears as inflamed swollen skin lesions covered with silvery white scales. It commonly affects the scalp, knees, elbows, hands and feet. Psoriasis affects over six million people in the USA, particularly those between the ages of 15 and 35. The disorder comes in many forms which differ in severity, duration, location and in the shape and pattern of the lesions.

Skin cells in a normal growth pattern are created in the basal cell layer and move up to the outermost layer, where they are shed at about the same rate as new ones are produced. This process normally takes about 28 days. When skin is injured, the cells are produced at a faster rate to replace and repair the wound. There is also an increased blood supply and localized inflammation. In psoriasis, the growth and maturation rate of skin cells is increased and the whole process can occur in as little as three to six days. The skin cannot shed the dead cells fast enough and they build up and form scaly lesions.

The cause of psoriasis is unknown, although it may have a genetic component and may be an autoimmune disorder. A trigger, such as a medication or an injury to the skin, may cause psoriasis to develop. Nutritional factors, stress and psychological factors may also play a part. It is common for a flare up of symptoms to accompany an infection, especially a respiratory one. Environmental factors such as stress, and climate (usually cold) are important in some patients. About a third of patients have spontaneous remissions of their disease. Some cases are associated with severe arthritis, called psoriatic arthritis.

Treatment of psoriasis

Although there is no cure, there are several treatments for psoriasis. Therapy aims to reduce inflammation and slow down the rapid cell division. Treatment is based on the severity of the disease and the health, lifestyle and age of the person being treated.

Each person may benefit from a different therapy or combination of therapies. Therapies for mild psoriasis include exposure to sunlight, coal tar medications, anthralin, and steroids; either topical, injected or oral. Other treatments include the drugs, methotrexate and cyclosporin; and medically supervised administration of ultraviolet light with or without the drug, psoralen. Many of these treatments have adverse side effects.

Vitamins, minerals and psoriasis

Vitamin D derivatives

Synthetic vitamin D analogs known as calcipotriene and calcipotriol are used to treat psoriasis. These drugs affect immune response and skin cell proliferation and differentiation. Treatment with calcipotriene results in decreased redness, scaling and thickness of skin plaques. Irritant dermatitis is a common side effect of calcipotriene, especially when it is applied to the face. Careful patient monitoring is recommended because alterations in calcium metabolism have been reported to occur with use of calcipotriene. Calcipotriol may not have adverse effects on calcium metabolism and still has the beneficial effects against psoriasis.[10] Ordinary vitamin D is not particularly effective in treating psoriasis.

Vitamin A derivatives

Vitamin A levels may be lower in psoriasis sufferers. The vitamin A derivatives, etretinate and isotretinoin, are widely used in psoriasis. Etretinate in combination with ultraviolet B and psoralen-ultraviolet A (PUVA) has shown beneficial effects. Vitamin A-derivative drugs help to normalize skin development by reducing the increased growth, turnover and keratinization of skin which occurs in the disorder.

However, long-term administration of vitamin A derivatives may lead to toxic effects, including headaches, inflammation of the lips, conjunctivitis, photosensitivity, and arthritis and bone abnormalities. These drugs can cause birth defects if taken during pregnancy and should also be avoided by breastfeeding women.

Zinc

Zinc metabolism may be abnormal in psoriasis, and copper-to-zinc ratio may also be high. There may also be a relationship between the total body area covered by the lesions and the plasma zinc level; those with more widespread lesions having lower levels than those with less.[11] Oral zinc sulfate may be useful in the treatment of psoriatic arthritis, which accompanies the skin disease in approximately 10 to 20 per cent of cases.[12]

Selenium

Selenium levels may be low in psoriasis and this may affect the immune system. A 1993 study showed improvement in some measurements of immune system effectiveness when selenium-rich yeast was given to psoriasis patients.[13] Blood levels of the selenium-containing enzyme, glutathione peroxidase, may be low in psoriasis sufferers. In one study, 50 patients with low glutathione peroxidase levels were treated with tablets containing 0.2 mg selenium and 10 mg vitamin E.[14] The glutathione peroxidase levels increased slowly within six to eight weeks of treatment, and some improvement in symptoms was seen. However, other studies have not shown benefits with selenium supplements.[15]

Essential fatty acids

Essential fatty acid supplements may be beneficial in psoriasis sufferers. Analysis of blood and fat tissue has shown that the amount of anti-inflammatory alpha-linolenic acid decreases, while the level of arachidonic acid, which has inflammatory effects, increases. These changes may be more pronounced in patients with severe psoriasis than in those with a milder form of the disease.[16] The results of a 1993 study suggest that eating oily fish may help reduce the symptoms of psoriasis.[17] Some small studies suggest that fish oil supplementation may be beneficial in psoriasis. In a 1998 study, researchers from several European centers treated 83 patients with either a with either an omega-3 fatty acid-based lipid emulsion or a placebo. There were significant improvements in symptoms, as assessed both by the patients and the researchers.[18] Topical fish oils have also shown some beneficial effects.[19] Essential fatty acid supplements also help to reduce the toxicity of immune suppressant and vitamin A-derivative drugs.[20]

Herbal medicine and skin disorders

Herbal treatment of eczema and psoriasis involves the use of blood cleansing remedies and diuretics such as figwort (*Scrophularia nodosa*), cleavers (*Galium aparine*), nettles (*Urtica dioica*), burdock (*Arctium lappa*), red clover (*Trifolium pratense*) and yellow dock (*Rumex crispus*). Liver herbs, such as Oregon grape root (*Mahonia aquifolium*), may be used to improve detoxification. Other remedies, such as chickweed (*Stellaria media*), can be used to reduce itching while others act as antiseptics and anti-inflammatories. Nervine relaxants are sometimes used to help treat stress associated with eczema. See page 384 for more information on these herbs and the precautions that may be necessary.

Glossary

Acetylcholine: a chemical involved in the transmission of nerve impulses.

Acrodermatitis enteropathica: an inherited zinc deficiency disorder in infants.

Adrenal glands: a pair of glands positioned above the kidneys, which are responsible for production of stress hormones including adrenaline and cortisone.

Adrenaline: a stress hormone which aids in the release of stored sugar in the liver, increased muscle contraction and increased blood supply to the muscles. Also known as epinephrine.

Aerobic exercise: exercise that requires additional effort by the heart and lungs to meet the increased demand by the skeletal muscles for oxygen.

Aldosterone: an adrenal hormone that increases the reabsorption of sodium and excretion of potassium.

Allergen: a substance that provokes an allergic response.

Alzheimer's disease: a form of dementia. Symptoms include memory loss, disorientation and speech disturbances.

Amenorrhea: cessation of menstruation.

Amino acid: a nitrogen containing organic acid that is used as a building block for protein.

Anaerobic exercise: high intensity exercise performed without a sufficient oxygen supply to the tissues.

Analgesic: a substance that relieves pain.

Anencephaly: a birth defect in which the brain and spinal cord fail to develop.

Anesthetic: a substance that causes loss of sensation.

Angina: angina pectoris. Chest pain brought on by exertion, caused by inadequate blood supply to the heart.

Anion: a negatively charged ion.

Anorexia: lack or loss of appetite resulting in the inability to eat. Anorexia nervosa is a disorder characterized by a prolonged refusal to eat.

Antacid: a substance that neutralizes stomach acid.

Antibiotic: a substance that inhibits or destroys susceptible microorganisms, particularly bacteria.

Antibody: a blood protein produced by the immune system in response to a foreign organism or substance.

Anticonvulsant: a substance that prevents or relieves convulsions.

Antigen: a foreign substance that causes the body to produce antibodies.

Antihistamine: a substance that counteracts the effects of histamine.

Antioxidant: a substance that protects other compounds from damaging oxidation reactions caused by free radicals.

Arginine: an amino acid.

Artery: a blood vessel that supplies blood, oxygen and nutrients to the tissues.

Arrhythmia: cardiac arrhythmia. Abnormal heartbeat.

Arteriosclerosis: thickening and stiffening of artery walls.

Ascorbic acid: vitamin C.

Atherosclerosis: arteriosclerosis caused by the accumulation of fat in the inner linings of the arteries.

Atopic dermatitis: eczema.

ATP: adenosine triphosphate. An energy storage molecule.

Autoimmune disease: a disorder in which the immune system attacks the body's own tissues.

Bell's palsy: a paralysis of the facial nerve. The person may not be able to close an eye or control salivation on the affected side

Benign: harmless. Usually used to refer to cells growing in inappropriate locations but which are not cancerous.

Benign prostatic hyperplasia (BPH): enlargement of the prostate gland.

Beriberi: thiamin deficiency disease.

Bile: a substance secreted by the liver for the digestion of fats.

Bioavailability: the amount of a substance such as a vitamin or mineral that is available to a target tissue after administration.

Biofeedback: a technique in which a person becomes aware of usually unconscious body processes and can affect these processes.

Bioflavonoid: a biologically active plant compound thought to enhance the activity of vitamin C and exert antioxidant effects.

Body Mass Index (BMI): a term used to define nutritional status. It is derived from the formula: weight (kg)/height(m)^2. The acceptable range is 20-25. Obesity is taken to start at a BMI of 30 and gross obesity at 40. A BMI of 18-20 is defined as mild starvation.

Bulimia nervosa: an eating disorder characterized by excessive food intake followed by vomiting, fasting or laxative use.

Calcitonin: a hormone that reduces the release of calcium from bone thus lowering blood calcium concentration.

Calorie: a measurement of the energy in food. Used interchangeably with kilocalorie.

Candida albicans: a fungus that can cause an infection known as a yeast infection or "thrush".

Capillaries: tiny blood vessels connecting arteries and veins that allow the exchange of nutrients and wastes between the blood and the tissues.

Carbohydrate: an energy-producing organic compound composed of carbon, hydrogen and oxygen.

Carcinogen: a substance that causes cancer.

Cardiac: relating to the heart.

Cardiomyopathy: damage to the heart.

Carotene: a plant pigment that is converted to vitamin A in the body and which also has antioxidant properties.

Cation: a positively charged ion.

Celiac disease: a metabolic disease characterized by sensitivity to the wheat protein, gluten.

Cell: a very small organic unit that is composed of cytoplasm and a nucleus enclosed in a cell membrane.

Cellulose: an indigestible carbohydrate found in plant cell walls.

Cerebral: relating to the brain.

Cerebrospinal fluid (CSF): the fluid that flows through and protects the brain and spinal canal.

Cerebrovascular: relating to the blood vessels in the brain.

Ceruloplasmin: a copper-containing enzyme.

Cervix: the neck of the uterus.

Chelation: the combination of a mineral with a larger molecule.

Chemotherapy: the treatment of disease with chemical substances. Usually used to refer to cancer therapy.

Chlorophyll: a green pigment found in plant tissues.

Cholesterol: a type of fat found in animal foods and produced by the liver.

Clinical trial: a study in which human subjects receive treatment.

Coenzyme: a molecule that works with an enzyme to enable it to fulfil its function in the body.

Cold pressed: a term used to describe a process of extracting oils from food without using heat.

Collagen: a connective tissue protein.

Complete protein: a source of protein that supplies all eight essential amino acids.

Complex carbohydrate: carbohydrates such as starch and cellulose that contain more than 10 linked glucose units.

Congenital: present from birth.

Congestive heart failure: a condition in which the heart fails to pump properly.

Connective tissue: a tissue that supports and binds other body tissue and parts.

Contraceptive: a substance, method or device that prevents conception.

Cornea: the curved, exposed, transparent part of the eyeball.

Coronary artery: an artery that supplies blood to the heart.

Crohn's disease: an inflammatory disease of the bowel.

Cruciferous: cross-shaped. Used to refer to a group of vegetables that include broccoli, cabbage and cauliflower.

Cutaneous: relating to the skin.

Cystic fibrosis: a genetic disorder characterized by exocrine and endocrine dysfunction which results in abnormally thick mucus secretions, increased electrolyte concentrations and overactivity of parts of the nervous system.

Cytochromes: proteins involved in the transport of electrons and associated with energy production.

Dehydration: excessive loss of water from the body.

Dermis: the layer of skin below the epidermis.

Diastolic blood pressure: the minimum level of blood pressure measured between heart contractions.

Dietary Reference Intakes (DRI): new set of dietary guidelines that provide sets of measures for each nutrient, including Adequate Intake (AI), Estimated Average Requirement (EAR), Tolerable Upper Intake Level (UL) and Recommended Dietary Allowance (RDA).

Diuretic: a substance that increases the formation and excretion of urine.

DNA: deoxyribonucleic acid. Substance in the nucleus of a cell that carries genetic information.

Docosahexaenoic acid: an omega-3 fatty acid.

Dopamine: a chemical involved in the transmission of nerve impulses.

Down syndrome: a genetic disorder characterized by varying degrees of mental retardation.

Drusen: white deposits that develop beneath the retina of the eye.

Dysplasia: abnormal tissue or organ development.

ECG: electrocardiogram. A record of the electrical activity associated with the heart.

Eclampsia: pregnancy induced high blood pressure.

Edema: abnormal accumulation of fluid in tissues.

Eicosapentaenoic acid: an omega-3 fatty acid found in fish oils.

Elastin: a protein found in elastic tissue fibers.

Electrolyte: an element or compound that, when dissolved in water, dissociates into positive and negative ions and can conduct an electric current.

Emulsification: the dispersal of one liquid into another liquid.

Enamel: the hard outer layer of the teeth.

Endocrine system: the network of glands that secrete hormones directly into the bloodstream.

Endorphin: a neurotransmitter-like substance that reduces pain.

Enteric coated: a coating added to some vitamins and drugs which stops them from being broken down by stomach juices. This enables the substances to be absorbed in the intestine.

Enzyme: a protein produced by living organisms that catalyzes chemical reactions.

Epidemiology: the study of distribution, occurrence and causes of disease in humans. An epidemiological study is an analysis of large populations that looks at patterns of disease and the factors that influence them.

Epidermis: the outer layer of the skin.

Epithelium: the cells that cover the internal and external surfaces of the body.

Erythropoietic protoporphyria: a disorder in which large quantities of compounds known as porphyrins are produced in the blood producing bone marrow. Symptoms include photosensitivity, abdominal pain and nerve damage.

Esophagus: the tube connecting the throat and stomach.

Essential nutrients: nutrients which must be supplied in the diet as they cannot be made in the body in the quantities required for normal health.

Estimated Average Requirement (EAR): the nutrient intake value that is estimated to meet the requirement in 50 per cent of people in a specific group, usually defined by age and sex.

Estrogen: a family of female sex hormones.

Extracellular: outside the cells.

Fatty acid: a fat-soluble organic acid.

Ferritin: an iron compound formed in the intestine and stored in the liver, spleen and bone marrow.

Ferrous: a form of iron.

Fiber: the indigestible residue found mainly in fruits, vegetables and cereals.

Food intolerance: the inability to absorb or metabolize a particular nutrient or drug.

Free radicals: atoms or groups of atoms that are chemically reactive because of an unpaired electron or proton. They attack cells and damage tissues contributing to heart disease, cancer, cataracts, arthritis and premature aging.

Fructose: a simple carbohydrate sometimes known as fruit sugar.

Gastrointestinal tract: the digestive tract, a tube extending from the mouth to the anus.

Glaucoma: an abnormal condition of increased pressure within the eye.

Gingivitis: inflammation of the gums.

Glucose: a simple sugar that is a major source of energy in the human body.

Glucose tolerance factor: a compound containing chromium that helps in blood sugar regulation.

Glutathione peroxidase: an antioxidant enzyme.

Gluten: an insoluble protein found in wheat.

Glycogen: a carbohydrate formed from glucose and the main form of stored energy in animal cells.

Glycoprotein: a compound containing a protein and a carbohydrate.

Goiter: enlargement of the thyroid gland.

Goitrogen: a substance that causes goiter.

Gram (g): a unit of weight measurement. 100 g is equal to 3.53 ounces. One ounce is equal to 28.35 g.

Granulocyte: a type of white blood cell.

Graves disease: a disorder characterized by an overactive thyroid gland.

GTF: see glucose tolerance factor.

HDL: high density lipoprotein. A protein made in the liver which is responsible for transporting cholesterol and other lipids from the body.

Hematocrit: a measure of the red blood cell volume expressed as a percentage of the total blood volume.

Heme: the non-protein part of the hemoglobin molecule that contains iron.

Hemochromatosis: a disease of iron metabolism in which iron accumulates in the body.

Hemodialysis: a procedure in which impurities are removed from the blood.

Hemoglobin: an iron-containing protein that carries oxygen in the blood.

Hemolytic anemia: anemia in which the red blood cells are destroyed prematurely.

Hemorrhage: the loss of a large amount of blood in a short period of time.

Hepatitis: an inflammatory condition of the liver.

Hesperidin: a bioflavonoid.

Histamine: a compound found in all cells and released in allergic and inflammatory reactions.

HIV: human immunodeficiency virus. The virus associated with AIDS.

Homocysteine: a product of protein breakdown that is considered to be an independent risk factor for cardiovascular disease.

Hormone: a substance produced in one part of the body that initiates or regulates the activity of an organ or group of cells in another part.

HRT: hormone replacement therapy. The administration of estrogen to postmenopausal women.

Huntington's chorea: a rare hereditary condition characterized by mental deterioration that ends in dementia.

Hydrochloric acid: stomach acid.

Hydrogenation: the addition of hydrogen to a substance. A process used to turn liquid oils into more solid form.

Hyperglycemia: abnormally high blood sugar levels.

Hyperkalemia: abnormally high potassium levels.

Hyperplasia: an increase in the number of cells in a body part.

Hyperreactivity: an exaggerated response to stimuli.

Hypertension: persistent abnormally high blood pressure.

Hypoglycemia: abnormally low blood sugar levels.

Hypoparathyroidism: diminished parathyroid gland function.

Hypotension: abnormally low blood pressure.

Hypothalamus: a portion of the brain that regulates several hormone functions and other functions including body temperature, sleep and appetite.

Idiopathic: without a known cause.

Immune system: the tissues, substances and organs that protect the body against disease and infection.

Immunotherapy: treatment of allergy by giving increasingly large doses of the allergen to gradually develop immunity.

Insulin: a hormone secreted by the pancreas that regulates the metabolism of glucose.

Interferon: a protein produced when cells are exposed to a virus or other foreign genetic material which protects uninfected cells from infection.

Intermittent claudication: intermittent cramp-like pains in the calves caused by poor circulation of the blood to the leg muscles.

International unit (IU): A measure of vitamin potency based on an internationally accepted system of units.

Intracellular: inside the cell.

Intramuscular injection: an injection into a muscle.

Intravenous: relating to the inside of a vein.

Intrinsic factor: a substance secreted by the gastrointestinal tract that is necessary for the absorption of vitamin B12.

In vitro: a process occurring in laboratory apparatus.

In vivo: a reaction occurring in a living organism.

Ischemia: a decreased supply of oxygenated blood to a body organ or part.

IU: see international unit.

Jaundice: a yellow discoloration of the skin and eyes due to the accumulation of the bile pigment bilirubin in the blood.

Kaposi's sarcoma: a type of cancer commonly seen in AIDS patients.

Keratin: a fibrous protein that is the primary component of the skin, hair and nails.

Keratinization: a process in which epithelial cells are replaced by horny tissue.

Keratinocytes: a skin cell that synthesizes the protein keratin.

Kilogram: unit of measurement of mass. 1 kilogram is equivalent to 2.2 pounds.

Kilojoule: a measurement of the energy in food. 1 Calorie is equal to 4.2 kilojoules.

kg: see kilogram.

kJ: see kilojoule.

Lactation: breast-feeding.

Lacto-ovo vegetarian diet: a diet that omits meat, chicken and fish but includes dairy products and eggs.

LDL: low density lipoprotein. A blood protein that delivers fats to body tissues.

Lecithin: any of a group of phospholipids found in plants and animals which are essential for fat metabolism.

Leukocyte: or leucocyte. A type of white blood cell.

Legumes: dried beans and peas.

Leukemia: a cancer of the blood forming tissues.

Leukotrienes: compounds produced by leucocytes that produce allergic and inflammatory reactions.

Linoleic acid: an essential fatty acid.

Linolenic acid: an essential fatty acid.

Lipid: any of the free fatty acid fractions found in the blood.

Lipoprotein: a type of protein molecule that contains a lipid.

Lipoprotein (a): a lipoprotein considered to be an independent risk factor for cardiovascular disease.

Liter: a unit of measurement of liquid.

Luteal phase: the phase of the menstrual cycle after the release of an egg from the follicle.

Lycopene: a carotenoid pigment.

Lymph: a fluid produced in organs and tissues that circulates through the lymphatic vessels and eventually joins blood circulation.

Lymphocyte: a type of white blood cell.

Lysine: an amino acid.

Lysosome: a cell particle that contains digestive enzymes.

Macrocytic anemia: a blood disorder where the cells are larger than normal.

Macronutrients: a nutrient required in large quantities for normal body function.

Macrophage: a white blood cell.

Macula: macula lutea. A spot at the center of the retina where vision is clearest.

Malabsorption: impaired absorption of nutrients from the intestines.

Malignant: "evil". Used to refer to cells that are cancerous and likely to spread.

mcg: see microgram.

Megadose: a dose much greater than the amount usually taken.

Megaloblastic anemia: anemia characterized by large, irregularly shaped red blood cells.

Menkes syndrome: a genetic disorder characterized by defects in copper absorption.

Menopause: cessation of menstruation that occurs with a decrease in female sex hormones production.

Metabolism: the chemical processes that takes place in living organisms.

Metastasis: the spreading of disease from one site to another in the body.

Methionine: an amino acid.

Microgram (mcg or mg): one millionth of a gram.

Microliter: one millionth of a liter.

Micronutrient: an organic compound needed in very small quantities for normal body function.

Microvascular: the part of the circulation that is composed of the capillary network.

Milligram: one thousandth of a gram.

Milliliter: one thousandth of a liter.

Mineral: an inorganic substance occurring naturally in the earth's crust which has a characteristic chemical composition. Many minerals are essential nutrients.

Mineralization: the addition of any mineral to the body.

Mitochondria: a part of a cell involved in cell metabolism, respiration and energy production.

ml: see milliliter.

Monocyte: a type of white blood cell.

Monounsaturated fat: a type of fat that has one site for the addition of a hydrogen atom.

Mucous membranes: thin sheets of tissue that cover cavities and canals of the body that are open to the air.

Multiple sclerosis: a progressive disease characterized by a loss of myelin from nerves in the brain and spinal cord. Symptoms include abnormal sensations, muscle weakness and visual disturbances.

Myelin: a fatty sheath surrounding the nerve cells.

Myocardial infarction: damage or death to a part of the heart resulting from reduced blood supply.

Myoglobin: an iron containing molecule that stores oxygen in the tissues.

Natural killer cell: a type of white blood cell.

Nephropathy: any disorder of the kidney.

Neural tube defects: birth defects involving malformations in the skull and spinal column.

Neuron: a nerve cell.

Neuropathy: inflammation or degeneration of the peripheral nerves.

Neurotransmitter: a chemical that modifies or results in the transmission of nerve impulses.

Neutrophil: a type of white blood cell.

Nitrosamine: potentially carcinogenic compounds formed by the reactions of nitrites with amines or amides normally present in the body.

Noradrenaline: also known as norepinephrine. A chemical involved in the transmission of nerve impulses.

Nucleic acids: chemical compounds found in plant and animal cells which are involved in the transmission of genetic characteristics.

Omega-3 fatty acids: fatty acids which may have health benefits including protection against heart disease, asthma, cancer, arthritis and other disorders.

Organic: any chemical compound containing carbon.

Ovary: the female sex organ that produces eggs and hormones.

Osteoarthritis: a form of arthritis where the joints undergo degenerative changes.

Osteomalacia: a disorder in which the bones become soft resulting in fracture and pain.

Osteosclerosis: an abnormal increase in the density of bone tissue.

Otosclerosis: deafness due to abnormal bone formation in the ear.

Ovulation: expulsion of an egg from the ovary.

Oxalate: a compound found in plants that binds to minerals such as calcium and reduces their absorption.

Oxidation: a chemical reaction that increases the oxygen content of a compound or in which there is a loss of electrons.

Oxidative damage: free radical damage to tissues.

Paget's disease: a disorder characterized by excessive bone destruction and unorganized bone repair.

Pancreas: an organ responsible for the production of digestive enzymes and the hormones insulin and glucagon.

Pancreatitis: an inflammatory condition of the pancreas.

Pap test or Pap smear: Papanicolaou test. A test used to detect cancers of the cervix.

Papillomavirus: the virus that causes warts in humans.

Parathyroid gland: a gland that secretes hormones that regulate blood calcium levels.

Parenteral: not in or through the digestive system. Parenteral nutrition refers to the administration of nutrients through a route other than the gastrointestinal tract, for example intravenously.

Parkinson's disease: a progressive, degenerative neurological disorder. Symptoms include tremors, shuffling gait, muscle rigidity and weakness.

Pellagra: niacin deficiency disease.

Pernicious anemia: anemia caused by vitamin B12 deficiency.

Peroxide: a free radical.

Phospholipids: compounds that contains phosphoric acid, fatty acids and a nitrogenous base.

Phytate: a compound found in plant fibers that binds to minerals such as calcium, iron and zinc and prevents their absorption.

Phytochemical: a plant compound that has health-promoting properties.

Phytoestrogen: a plant compound with estrogen-like activity.

Pica: the eating of non-food items such as ice or clay.

Placebo: an inactive substance used in medical experiments to provide a basis of comparison with the effects of an experimental drug.

Plaque: a deposit of a substance on body tissues, such as a patch of atherosclerosis or a deposit in the brain of an Alzheimer's disease sufferer.

Platelets: blood cell fragments that play a role in blood clotting.

Polyunsaturated fat: a fat in which there are two or more links in the chain of carbon atoms that can be opened to accept hydrogen atoms.

Postmenopause: the period after menopause.

Precancerous: abnormal tissue that is likely to become cancerous.

Precursor: a substance used as a building block for another substance.

Pre-eclampsia: a disorder associated with the later stages of pregnancy. Symptoms include high blood pressure, edema and protein in the urine.

Premenopause: the period before menopause.

Prolactin: a female hormone involved in milk production.

Prolapse: the falling, sinking or sliding of an organ from its normal position.

Prophylaxis: prevention of or protection against disease.

Prostacyclin: a prostaglandin.

Prostaglandin: a hormone-like compound with many effects including effects on the secretion of hormones and enzymes, inflammatory response, blood pressure and blood clotting.

Pulmonary: relating to the lungs.

RDA: recommended dietary allowance. The amount of a nutrient necessary to prevent deficiency symptoms (USA old definition). The dietary intake level that is sufficient to meet the nutrient requirements of nearly all the people in the group. (USA new definition)

RDI: recommended dietary intake. The amount of a nutrient necessary to prevent deficiency symptoms (Australia) or Reference daily intakes, a new term used to refer to the US RDAs (see US RDA).

RE: see Retinol equivalent.

Reflux: abnormal backward flow of a fluid. Often used to refer to the inflammation resulting from the backward flow of the stomach contents into the esophagus.

Resorption: the loss of a substance, such as bone, by physiological or pathological means.

Respiratory tract: the lungs and associated passageways.

Retina: the part of the eye that receives images and transmits visual impulses to the brain.

Retinal: a form of vitamin A.

Retinoic acid: a form of vitamin A.

Retinol: vitamin A.

Retinol equivalents: a unit of measurement for vitamin A.

Retinopathy: an eye disorder resulting from changes in the retinal blood vessels.

Rickets: abnormal bone development caused by a vitamin D deficiency.

RNA: ribonucleic acid. Substance in the nucleus of a cell which carries genetic information.

RNI: recommended nutrient intake. The amount of a nutrient necessary to prevent deficiency symptoms (UK).

Rosacea: a form of acne seen in adults.

Saturated fat: a fat in which all the atoms are joined by single bonds.

Schilling test: a diagnostic test for vitamin B12 deficiency.

Scoliosis: lateral curvature of the spine.

Scurvy: vitamin C deficiency disease.

Seborrhea: a condition in which there is an overproduction of sebum.

Sebum: the oily secretion of certain glands in the skin.

Serotonin: a chemical involved in the transmission of nerve impulses.

Serum: the fluid part of the blood.

Sickle cell anemia: a severe, chronic type of anemia characterized by abnormal hemoglobin and red blood cell formation.

Simple carbohydrate: a type of carbohydrate, for example lactose, fructose and glucose.

Sorbitol: a by-product of glucose metabolism which, in diabetics, can accumulate and lead to complications.

Spina bifida: a neural tube defect.

Steroid: any fat-soluble organic substance with a certain basic chemical structure. Several different hormones, drugs and other substances are classed as steroids.

Subclinical deficiency: a deficiency so mild it produces no obvious symptoms.

Superoxide dismutase: an antioxidant enzyme.

Systolic blood pressure: the blood pressure measured when the heart is contracting.

T cell: a type of white blood cell involved in immune function.

TE: see tocopherol equivalents.

Tetany: a condition involving cramps, convulsion and twitching of the muscles.

TIBC: total iron binding capacity. A test to measure iron in the blood.

Thalassemia: a type of anemia.

Thromboxane: a prostaglandin.

Thymus gland: a gland in the upper part of the chest that is involved in the maturation and development of the immune system.

Thyroid gland: a gland at the front of the neck involved in growth and metabolism.

Thioctic acid: lipoic acid.

Thyroxin: a hormone produced by the thyroid gland.

Tocopherol: vitamin E.

Tocopherol equivalents: a unit of measurement for vitamin E.

Tolerable Upper Intake Level (UL): the upper limit of nutrient intake associated with a low risk of adverse effects in most people.

Topical: relating to the surface of the body.

Trace element: an element essential for human health in minute quantities.

Trans fatty acids: a type of fat formed when unsaturated vegetable oils are hydrogenated. These forms are more stable but do not occur in nature.

Transferrin: a protein involved in iron transport.

Triglyceride: the major type of fat molecule found in the blood.

Triiodothyronine: a thyroid hormone involved in the regulation of growth, development, metabolism and body temperature.

Tryptophan: an amino acid that can be converted to niacin and serotonin.

Ubiquinone: coenzyme Q10.

Ulcerative colitis: an inflammatory disorder of the large intestine and rectum.

Unsaturated fat: a type of fat in which some of the links are triple or double bonds.

Urea: the main excretion product of metabolism.

Urogenital: relating to the urinary and reproductive systems.

US RDA: The highest recommended dietary allowance values (see RDA).

Vasoconstrictor: a substance that constricts blood vessels.

Vasodilator: a substance that acts to dilate blood vessels.

Vegan: a strict vegetarian who eats no foods of animal origin.

Visual purple: a purple pigmented compound in the retina that is involved in the adaptation of the eye to low density light.

Vitamin: an organic compound essential in small quantities for normal body function. With few exceptions vitamins cannot be synthesized by the body and must be obtained from the diet.

Vitiligo: a skin pigmentation disorder.

Wernicke Korsakoff syndrome: brain damage caused by thiamin deficiency. It is often seen in chronic alcoholics.

Wilson's disease: an inherited disorder of copper metabolism in which copper accumulates in the liver.

Xerophthalmia: an eye condition caused by vitamin A deficiency.

Imperial Measurements and Equivalents

LENGTH

IMPERIAL	METRIC*
1 inch (in) (")	2.54 centimeter (cm)
1 foot (ft) (') (12 inch)	30.5 cm
1 yard (yd) (3 feet)	91.5 cm (.915 m)
1 mile (m) (1760 yards)	1.6 km (1600m)

WEIGHT

IMPERIAL	METRIC*
1 ounce (oz)	30 gram (g)
6 oz	170 g
8 oz (½ lb)	230 g
16 oz (1lb)	455 g
2 pounds (lb)	950 g
10 lb	4.6 kg (4500 g)
1 stone (14lb)	6.5 kilograms (kg)

LIQUID WEIGHT

IMPERIAL	METRIC*
¼ teaspoon	1.25 millileter (ml)
½ teaspoon	2.5 ml
1 teaspoon	5 ml
1 tablespoon	20 ml
1 oz	30 ml
4 oz (½ cup)	120 ml
8 oz (1 cup)	240 ml
10 oz (½ pint)	300 ml
16 oz (2 cups)	475 ml
20 oz (1 pint)	600 ml
1 quart	1 litre (l) (1000 ml)

** For ease of use, volume measurements have been rounded off.*

References

Vitamin A

1 Arrieta AC; Zaleska M; Stutman HR; Marks MI. Vitamin A levels in children with measles in Long Beach, California. J Pediatr, 1992 Jul, 121:1, 75-8

2 Zhang S; Tang G; Russell RM; Mayzel KA; Stampfer MJ; Willett WC; Hunter DJ. Measurement of retinoids and carotenoids in breast adipose tissue and a comparison of concentrations in breast cancer cases and control subjects. Am J Clin Nutr, 1997 Sep, 66:3, 626-32

3 Ruiz Rejón F; Martín Pena G; López Manglano C; Seijas Martínez V; Ruiz Galiana J. Plasma levels of vitamins A and E and the risk of acute myocardial infarct. Rev Clin Esp, 1997 Jun, 197:6, 411-6

4 Rothman KJ; Moore LL; Singer MR; Nguyen US; Mannino S; Milunsky A Teratogenicity of high vitamin A intake. N Engl J Med, 1995 Nov, 333:21, 1369-73

5 Mills JL; Simpson JL; Cunningham GC; Conley MR; Rhoads GG. Vitamin A and birth defects. Am J Obstet Gynecol, 1997 Jul, 177:1, 31-6

6 Glasziou P, Mackerras D. Vitamin A supplementation in infectious diseases. Br Med J. 1993;306: 366-370

7 Coutsoudis A et al. The effects of vitamin A supplementation on the morbidity of children born to HIV-infected women. Am J Public Health, 85: 8 Pt 1, 1995 Aug, 1076-81

8 Pastorino U; Infante M; Maioli M; Chiesa G; Buyse M; Firket P; Rosmentz N; Clerici M; Soresi E; Valente M; et al Adjuvant treatment of stage I lung cancer with high-dose vitamin A. J Clin Oncol, 1993 Jul, 11:7, 1216-22

9 de Klerk NH; Musk AW; Ambrosini GL; Eccles JL; Hansen J; Olsen N; Watts VL; Lund HG; Pang SC; Beilby J; Hobbs MS. Vitamin A and cancer prevention II: comparison of the effects of retinol and beta-carotene. Int J Cancer, 1998 Jan, 75:3, 362-7

10 Musk AW; de Klerk NH; Ambrosini GL; Eccles JL; Hansen J; Olsen NJ; Watts VL; Lund HG; Pang SC; Beilby J; Hobbs MS. Vitamin A and cancer prevention I: observations in workers previously exposed to asbestos at Wittenoom, Western Australia. Int J Cancer, 1998 Jan, 75:3, 355-61

11 Issing WJ; Struck R; Naumann A. Positive impact of retinyl palmitate in leukoplakia of the larynx. Eur Arch Otorhinolaryngol Suppl, 1997, 1:, S105-9

12 Xu XC; Sozzi G; Lee JS; Lee JJ; Pastorino U; Pilotti S; Kurie JM; Hong WK; Lotan R. Suppression of retinoic acid receptor beta in non-small-cell lung cancer in vivo: implications for lung cancer development. J Natl Cancer Inst, 1997 May, 89:9, 624-9

13 Paiva SA; Godoy I; Vannucchi H; Fávaro RM; Geraldo RR; Campana AO Assessment of vitamin A status in chronic obstructive pulmonary disease patients and healthy smokers. Am J Clin Nutr, 1996 Dec, 64:6, 928-34

14 Massaro GD; Massaro D. Retinoic acid treatment abrogates elastase-induced pulmonary emphysema in rats. Nat Med, 1997 Jun, 3:6, 675-7

15 DiGiovanna JJ; Sollitto RB; Abangan DL; Steinberg SM; Reynolds JC. Osteoporosis is a toxic effect of long-term etretinate therapy. Arch Dermatol, 1995 Nov, 131:11, 1263-7

16 Fisher GJ; Wang ZQ; Datta SC; Varani J; Kang S; Voorhees JJ. Pathophysiology of premature skin aging induced by ultraviolet light. N Engl J Med, 1997 Nov, 337:20, 1419-28

17 Aldoori WH; Giovannucci EL; Stampfer MJ; Rimm EB; Wing AL; Willett WC. Prospective study of diet and the risk of duodenal ulcer in men. Am J Epidemiol, 1997 Jan, 145:1, 42-50

18 Ribaya-Mercado JD Importance of adequate vitamin A status during iron supplementation. Nutr Rev, 1997 Aug, 55:8, 306-7

Carotenes

1 Pappalardo G; Maiani G; Mobarhan S; Guadalaxara A; Azzini E; Raguzzini A; Salucci M; Serafini M; Trifero M; Illomei G; Ferro Luzzi A. Plasma (carotenoids, retinol, alpha-tocopherol) and tissue (carotenoids) levels after supplementation with beta-carotene in subjects with precancerous and cancerous lesions of sigmoid colon. Eur J Clin Nutr, 1997 Oct, 51:10, 661-6

2 Freudenheim JL; Marshall JR; Vena JE; Laughlin R; Brasure JR; Swanson MK; Nemoto T; Graham S. Premenopausal breast cancer risk and intake of vegetables, fruits, and related nutrients. J Natl Cancer Inst, 1996 Mar, 88:6, 340-

3 Dorgan JF; Sowell A; Swanson CA; Potischman N; Miller R; Schussler N; Stephenson HE Jr Relationships of serum carotenoids, retinol, alpha-tocopherol, and selenium with breast cancer risk: results from a prospective study in Columbia, Missouri (United States) Cancer Causes Control, 1998 Jan, 9:1, 89-97

4 Zhang S; Tang G; Russell RM; Mayzel KA; Stampfer MJ; Willett WC; Hunter DJ. Measurement of retinoids and carotenoids in breast adipose tissue and a comparison of concentrations in breast cancer cases and control subjects. Am J Clin Nutr, 1997 Sep, 66:3, 626-32

5 Comstock GW; Alberg AJ; Huang HY; Wu K; Burke AE; Hoffman SC; Norkus EP; Gross M; Cutler RG; Morris JS; Spate VL; Helzlsouer KJ. The risk of developing lung cancer associated with antioxidants in the blood: ascorbic acid, carotenoids, alpha-tocopherol, selenium, and total peroxyl radical absorbing capacity. Cancer Epidemiol Biomarkers Prev, 1997 Nov, 6:11, 907-16

6 Gaziano JM; Manson JE; Branch LG; Colditz GA; Willett WC; Buring JE. A prospective study of consumption of carotenoids in fruits and vegetables and decreased cardiovascular mortality in the elderly. Ann Epidemiol, 1995 Jul, 5:4, 255-60

7 Howard AN; Williams NR; Palmer CR; Cambou JP; Evans AE; Foote JW; Marques Vidal P; McCrum EE; Ruidavets JB; Nigdikar SV; Rajput Williams J; Thurnham DI. Do hydroxy-carotenoids prevent coronary heart disease? A comparison between Belfast and Toulouse. Int J Vitam Nutr Res, 1996, 66:2, 113-8

8 Hankinson SE; Stampfer MJ; Seddon JM; Colditz GA; Rosner B; Speizer FE; Willett WC Nutrient intake and cataract extraction in women: a prospective study. BMJ, 1992 Aug 8, 305:6849, 335-9

9 Bohne M; Struy H; Gerber A; Gollnick H Protection against UVA damage and effects on neutrophil-derived reactive oxygen species by beta-carotene. Inflamm Res, 1997 Oct, 46:10, 425-6

10 Smith AH; Waller KD. Serum beta-carotene in persons with cancer and their immediate families. Am J Epidemiol, 1991 Apr 1, 133:7, 661-71

11 Mayne ST; Janerich DT; Greenwald P; Chorost S; Tucci C; Zaman MB; Melamed MR; Kiely M; McKneally MF Dietary beta carotene and lung cancer risk in U.S. nonsmokers. J Natl Cancer Inst, 1994 Jan, 86:1, 33-8

12 Negri E; La Vecchia C; Franceschi S; DAvanzo B; Talamini R; Parpinel M; Ferraroni M; Filiberti R; Montella M; Falcini F; Conti E; Decarli A. Intake of selected micronutrients and the risk of breast cancer. Int J Cancer, 1996 Jan, 65:2, 140-4

13 Ingram D. Diet and subsequent survival in women with breast cancer. Br J Cancer, 1994 Mar, 69:3, 592-5

14 Daviglus ML; Dyer AR; Persky V; Chavez N; Drum M; Goldberg J; Liu K; Morris DK; Shekelle RB; Stamler J Dietary beta-carotene, vitamin C, and risk of prostate cancer: results from the Western Electric Study. Epidemiology, 1996 Sep, 7:5, 472-7

15 Muto Y; Fujii J; Shidoji Y; Moriwaki H; Kawaguchi T; Noda T Growth retardation in human cervical dysplasia-derived cell lines by beta-carotene through down-regulation of epidermal growth factor receptor. Am J Clin Nutr, 1995 Dec, 62:6 Suppl, 1535S-1540S

16 Palan PR; Mikhail MS; Basu J; Romney SL Beta-carotene levels in exfoliated cervicovaginal epithelial cells in cervical intraepithelial neoplasia and cervical cancer. Am J Obstet Gynecol, 1992 Dec, 167:6, 1899-903

17 Daviglus ML; Orencia AJ; Dyer AR; Liu K; Morris DK; Persky V; Chavez N; Goldberg J; Drum M; Shekelle RB; Stamler J Dietary vitamin C, beta-carotene and 30-year risk of stroke: results from the Western Electric Study. Neuroepidemiology, 1997, 16:2, 69-77

18 Tavani A; Negri E; DAvanzo B; La Vecchia C. Beta-carotene intake and risk of nonfatal acute myocardial infarction in women. Eur J Epidemiol, 1997 Sep, 13:6, 631-7

19 Comstock GW; Burke AE; Hoffman SC; Helzlsouer KJ; Bendich A; Masi AT; Norkus EP; Malamet RL; Gershwin ME. Serum concentrations of alpha tocopherol, beta carotene, and retinol preceding the diagnosis of rheumatoid arthritis and systemic lupus erythematosus. Ann Rheum Dis, 1997 May, 56:5, 323-5

20 Knekt P; Heliövaara M; Rissanen A; Aromaa A; Aaran RK. Serum antioxidant vitamins and risk of cataract. BMJ, 1992 Dec 5, 305:6866, 1392-4

21 Jama JW; Launer LJ; Witteman JC; den Breeijen JH; Breteler MM; Grobbee DE; Hofman A. Dietary antioxidants and cognitive function in a population-based sample of older persons. The Am J Epidemiol, 1996 Aug, 144:3, 275-80

22 Perrig WJ; Perrig P; Stähelin HB The relation between antioxidants and memory performance in the old and very old. J Am Geriatr Soc, 1997 Jun, 45:6, 718-24

23 Mikhail MS; Palan PR; Basu J; Anyaegbunam A; Romney SL Decreased beta-carotene levels in exfoliated vaginal epithelial cells in women with vaginal candidiasis. Am J Reprod Immunol, 1994 Oct, 32:3, 221-5

24 Ben Amotz A; Levy Y. Bioavailability of a natural isomer mixture compared with synthetic all-trans beta-carotene in human serum. Am J Clin Nutr, 1996 May, 63:5, 729-34

25 Albanes D et al; Alpha-Tocopherol and beta-carotene supplements and lung cancer incidence in the alpha-tocopherol, beta-carotene cancer prevention study: effects of base-line characteristics and study compliance J Natl Cancer Inst, 1996 Nov, 88:21, 1560-70

26 Omenn G et al. Effects of a combination of beta carotene and vitamin A on lung cancer and cardiovascular disease. N Engl J Med. 1996;334: 1150-5

27 Hennekens C H et al. Lack of effect of long term supplementation with beta carotene on the incidence of malignant neoplasms and cardiovascular disease. N Engl J Med. 1996;334: 1145-9 and 1189-90

28 Handelman GJ, Packer L and Cross C E. Destruction of tocopherols, carotenoids and retinol in human plasma by cigarette smoke. Am J Clin Nutr. 1996;63: 559-65

29 Journal of the American Chemical Society 1997;119:621-622

30 Hughes DA; Wright AJ; Finglas PM; Peerless AC; Bailey AL; Astley SB; Pinder AC; Southon S. The effect of beta-carotene supplementation on the immune function of blood monocytes from healthy male nonsmokers. J Lab Clin Med, 1997 Mar, 129:3, 309-17

31 Fryburg DA, Mark RJ, Griffith BP, Askenase PW, Patterson TF. The effect of supplemental beta-carotene on immunologic indices in patients with AIDS: a pilot study. Yale J Biol Med 1995 Jan;68(1-2):19-23

32 Cueto SM; Romney AD; Wang Y; Walsh SW. beta-Carotene attenuates peroxide-induced vasoconstriction in the human placenta. J Soc Gynecol Investig, 1997 Mar, 4:2, 64-71

33 Chuwers P; Barnhart S; Blanc P; Brodkin CA; Cullen M; Kelly T; Keogh J; Omenn G; Williams J; Balmes JR. The protective effect of beta-carotene and retinol on ventilatory function in an asbestos-exposed cohort. Am J Respir Crit Care Med, 1997 Mar, 155:3, 1066-71

34 García Casal MN; Layrisse M; Solano L; Barón MA; Arguello F; Llovera D; Ramírez J; Leets I; Tropper E Vitamin A and beta-carotene can improve nonheme iron absorption from rice, wheat and corn by humans. J Nutr, 1998 Mar, 128:3, 646-50

35 Berg G; Kohlmeier L; Brenner H. Use of oral contraceptives and serum beta-carotene. Eur J Clin Nutr, 1997 Mar, 51:3, 181-7

36 Kitamura Y; Tanaka K; Kiyohara C; Hirohata T; Tomita Y; Ishibashi M; Kido K Relationship of alcohol use, physical activity and dietary habits with serum carotenoids, retinol and alpha-tocopherol among male Japanese smokers. Int J Epidemiol, 1997 Apr, 26:2, 307-14

37 Granado F; Olmedilla B; Gil Martínez E; Blanco I; Millan I; Rojas Hidalgo E Carotenoids, retinol and tocopherols in patients with insulin-dependent diabetes mellitus and their immediate relatives. Clin Sci (Colch), 1998 Feb, 94:2, 189-95

38 Clinton SK. Lycopene: chemistry, biology, and implications for human health and disease. Nutr Rev, 1998 Feb, 56:2 Pt 1, 35-51

39 Gärtner C; Stahl W; Sies H Lycopene is more bioavailable from tomato paste than from fresh tomatoes. Am J Clin Nutr, 1997 Jul, 66:1, 116-22

40 Giovannucci E; Ascherio A; Rimm EB; Stampfer MJ; Colditz GA; Willett WC. Intake of carotenoids and retinol in relation to risk of prostate cancer. J Natl Cancer Inst, 1995 Dec, 87:23, 1767-76

41 Kohlmeier L et al; Lycopene and myocardial infarction risk in the EURAMIC Study. Am J Epidemiol, 1997 Oct, 146:8, 618-26

42 Landrum JT; Bone RA; Joa H; Kilburn MD; Moore LL; Sprague KE A one year study of the macular pigment: the

effect of 140 days of a lutein supplement. Exp Eye Res, 1997 Jul, 65:1, 57-62

43 Hammond BR Jr; Wooten BR; Snodderly DM. Density of the human crystalline lens is related to the macular pigment carotenoids, lutein and zeaxanthin. Optom Vis Sci, 1997 Jul, 74:7, 499-504

Thiamin

1 Haisraeli Shalish M; Livneh A; Katz J; Doolman R; Sela BA Recurrent aphthous stomatitis and thiamine deficiency. Oral Surg Oral Med Oral Pathol Oral Radiol Endod, 1996 Dec, 82:6, 634-6

2 Wilkinson TJ; Hanger HC; Elmslie J; George PM; Sainsbury R. The response to treatment of subclinical thiamine deficiency in the elderly. Am J Clin Nutr, 1997 Oct, 66:4, 925-8

3 Suzuki M; Itokawa Y Effects of thiamine supplementation on exercise-induced fatigue. Metab Brain Dis, 1996 Mar, 11:1, 95-106

4 Benton D; Griffiths R; Haller J Thiamine supplementation mood and cognitive functioning. Psychopharmacology (Berl), 1997 Jan, 129:1, 66-71

5 Easton CJ; Bauer LO Beneficial effects of thiamine on recognition memory and P300 in abstinent cocaine-dependent patients. Psychiatry Res, 1997 May, 70:3, 165-74

6 Meador K; Loring D; Nichols M; Zamrini E; Rivner M; Posas H; Thompson E; Moore E Preliminary findings of high-dose thiamine in dementia of Alzheimer's type. J Geriatr Psychiatry Neurol, 1993 Oct-Dec, 6:4, 222-9

7 Mimori Y; Katsuoka H; Nakamura S Thiamine therapy in Alzheimer's disease. Metab Brain Dis, 1996 Mar, 11:1, 89-94

Riboflavin

1 Leske MC et al; Biochemical factors in the lens opacities. Case-control study. The Lens Opacities Case-Control Study Group. Arch Ophthalmol, 1995 Sep, 113:9, 1113-9

2 Mulherin DM; Thurnham DI; Situnayake RD Glutathione reductase activity, riboflavin status, and disease activity in rheumatoid arthritis. Ann Rheum Dis, 1996 Nov, 55:11, 837-40

3 Schoenen J; Jacquy J; Lenaerts M. Effectiveness of high-dose riboflavin in migraine prophylaxis. A randomized controlled trial. Neurology, 1998 Feb, 50:2, 466-70

4 Folkers K; Ellis J Successful therapy with vitamin B6 and vitamin B2 of the carpal tunnel syndrome and need for determination of the RDAs for vitamins B6 and B2 for disease states. Ann N Y Acad Sci, 1990, 585:, 295-301

5 Folkers K; Wolaniuk A; Vadhanavikit S. Enzymology of the response of the carpal tunnel syndrome to riboflavin and to combined riboflavin and pyridoxine. Proc Natl Acad Sci U S A, 1984 Nov, 81:22, 7076-8

Niacin

1 O'Connor PJ; Rush WA; Trence DL. Relative effectiveness of niacin and lovastatin for treatment of dyslipidemias in a health maintenance organization. J Fam Pract, 1997 May, 44:5, 462-7

2 Gardner SF; Schneider EF; Granberry MC; Carter IR. Combination therapy with low-dose lovastatin and niacin is as effective as higher-dose lovastatin. Pharmacotherapy, 1996 May, 16:3, 419-23

3 Gardner SF; Marx MA; White LM; Granberry MC; Skelton DR; Fonseca VA. Combination of low-dose niacin and pravastatin improves the lipid profile in diabetic patients without compromising glycemic control. Ann Pharmacother, 1997 Jun, 31:6, 677-82

4 Johansson JO; Egberg N; Asplund Carlson A; Carlson LA. Nicotinic acid treatment shifts the fibrinolytic balance favourably and decreases plasma fibrinogen in hypertriglyceridaemic men. J Cardiovasc Risk, 1997 Jun, 4:3, 165-71

5 Elliott RB; Chase HP. Prevention or delay of type 1 (insulin-dependent) diabetes mellitus in children using nicotinamide. Diabetologia, 1991 May, 34:5, 362-5

6 Elliott RB; Pilcher CC; Fergusson DM; Stewart AW A population based strategy to prevent insulin-dependent diabetes using nicotinamide. Pediatr Endocrinol Metab, 1996 Sep, 9:5, 501-9

7 Agte VV; Paknikar KM; Chiplonkar SA. Effect of nicotinic acid on zinc and iron metabolism. Biometals, 1997 Oct, 10:4, 271-6

8 Volpi E; Lucidi P; Cruciani G; Monacchia F; Reboldi G; Brunetti P; Bolli GB; De Feo P Nicotinamide counteracts alcohol-induced impairment of hepatic protein metabolism in humans. J Nutr, 1997 Nov, 127:11, 2199-204

Vitamin B6

1 Riggs KM; Spiro A 3rd; Tucker K; Rush D Relations of vitamin B-12, vitamin B-6, folate, and homocysteine to cognitive performance in the Normative Aging Study. Am J Clin Nutr, 1996 Mar, 63:3, 306-14

2 Baum MK; Mantero-Atienza E; Shor-Posner G; Fletcher MA; Morgan R; Eisdorfer C; Sauberlich HE; Cornwell PE; Beach RS. Association of vitamin B6 status with parameters of immune function in early HIV-1 infection. J Acquir Immune Defic Syndr, 1991, 4:11, 1122-32

3 Selhub J; Jacques PF; Bostom AG; DAgostino RB; Wilson PW; Belanger AJ; OLeary DH; Wolf PA; Rush D; Schaefer EJ; Rosenberg IH. Relationship between plasma homocysteine, vitamin status and extracranial carotid-artery stenosis in the Framingham Study population. J Nutr, 1996 Apr, 126:4 Suppl, 1258S-65S

4 Robinson K; Arheart K; Refsum H; Brattström L; Boers G; Ueland P; Rubba P; Palma Reis R; Meleady R; Daly L; Witteman J; Graham I. Low circulating folate and vitamin B6 concentrations: risk factors for stroke, peripheral vascular disease, and coronary artery disease. European COMAC Group. Circulation, 1998 Feb, 97:5, 437-43

5 Rimm EB; Willett WC; Hu FB; Sampson L; Colditz GA; Manson JE; Hennekens C; Stampfer MJ Folate and vitamin B6 from diet and supplements in relation to risk of coronary heart disease among women. JAMA, 1998 Feb, 279:5, 359-64

6 Verhoef P; Stampfer MJ; Buring JE; Gaziano JM; Allen RH; Stabler SP; Reynolds RD; Kok FJ; Hennekens CH; Willett WC Homocysteine metabolism and risk of myocardial infarction: relation with vitamins B6, B12, and folate. Am J Epidemiol, 1996 May, 143:9, 845-59

7 21 Fuhr JE; Farrow A; Nelson HS Jr Vitamin B6 levels in patients with carpal tunnel syndrome. Arch Surg, 1989 Nov, 124:11, 1329-30

8 van der Wielen RP; Löwik MR; Haller J; van den Berg H; Ferry M; van Staveren WA Vitamin B-6 malnutrition among

elderly Europeans: the SENECA study. J Gerontol A Biol Sci Med Sci, 1996 Nov, 51:6, B417-24

9 Pfitzenmeyer P; Guilland JC; dAthis P. Vitamin B6 and vitamin C status in elderly patients with infections during hospitalization. Ann Nutr Metab, 1997, 41:6, 344-52

10 Huang YC; Chen W; Evans MA; Mitchell ME; Shultz TD. Vitamin B-6 requirement and status assessment of young women fed a high-protein diet with various levels of vitamin B-6. Am J Clin Nutr, 1998 Feb, 67:2, 208-20

11 Collipp PJ; Goldzier S 3d; Weiss N; Soleymani Y; Snyder R. Pyridoxine treatment of childhood bronchial asthma. Ann Allergy, 1975 Aug, 35:2, 93-7

12 Reynolds RD; Natta CL. Depressed plasma pyridoxal phosphate concentrations in adult asthmatics. Am J Clin Nutr, 1985 Apr, 41:4, 684-8

13 Sur S; Camara M; Buchmeier A; Morgan S; Nelson HS. Double-blind trial of pyridoxine (vitamin B6) in the treatment of steroid-dependent asthma. Ann Allergy, 1993 Feb, 70:2, 147-52

14 Shimizu T; Maeda S; Arakawa H; Mochizuki H; Tokuyama K; Morikawa A. Relation between theophylline and circulating vitamin levels in children with asthma. Pharmacology, 1996 Dec, 53:6, 384-9

15 Ubbink JB; Vermaak WJ; van der Merwe A; Becker PJ. Vitamin B-12, vitamin B-6, and folate nutritional status in men with hyperhomocysteinemia. Am J Clin Nutr, 1993 Jan, 57:1, 47-53

16 Woodside JV et al. Effect of B-group vitamins and antioxidant vitamins on hyperhomocysteinemia: a double-blind, randomized, factorial-design, controlled trial. Am J Clin Nutr, 1998 May, 67:5, 858-66

17 Sermet A; Aybak M; Ulak G; Güzel C; Denli O Effect of oral pyridoxine hydrochloride supplementation on in vitro platelet sensitivity to different agonists. Arzneimittelforschung, 1995 Jan, 45:1, 19-21

18 Brattström L; Stavenow L; Galvard H; Nilsson-Ehle P; Berntorp E; Jerntorp P; Elmståhl S; Pessah-Rasmussen H. Pyridoxine reduces cholesterol and low-density lipoprotein and increases antithrombin III activity in 80-year-old men with low plasma pyridoxal 5-phosphate. Scand J Clin Lab Invest, 1990 Dec, 50:8, 873-7

19 Bell IR; Edman JS; Morrow FD; Marby DW; Perrone G; Kayne HL; Greenwald M; Cole JO Brief communication. Vitamin B1, B2, and B6 augmentation of tricyclic antidepressant treatment in geriatric depression with cognitive dysfunction. J Am Coll Nutr, 1992 Apr, 11:2, 159-63

20 Doll H; Brown S; Thurston A; Vessey M. Pyridoxine (vitamin B6) and the premenstrual syndrome: a randomized crossover trial. J R Coll Gen Pract, 1989 Sep, 39:326, 364-8

21 Sahakian V; Rouse D; Sipes S; Rose N; Niebyl J Vitamin B6 is effective therapy for nausea and vomiting of pregnancy: a randomized, double-blind placebo-controlled study. Obstet Gynecol, 1991 Jul, 78:1, 33-6

22 Ellis JM; Folkers K; Levy M; Shizukuishi S; Lewandowski J; Nishii S; Schubert HA; Ulrich R. Response of vitamin B-6 deficiency and the carpal tunnel syndrome to pyridoxine. Proc Natl Acad Sci U S A, 1982 Dec, 79:23, 7494-8

23 Franzblau A; Rock CL; Werner RA; Albers JW; Kelly MP; Johnston EC . The relationship of vitamin B6 status to median nerve function and carpal tunnel syndrome among active industrial workers. J Occup Environ Med, 1996 May, 38:5, 485-91

24 Keniston RC; Nathan PA; Leklem JE; Lockwood RS Vitamin B6, vitamin C, and carpal tunnel syndrome. A cross-sectional study of 441 adults. J Occup Environ Med, 1997 Oct, 39:10, 949-59

25 Tang AM; Graham NM; Saah AJ. Effects of micronutrient intake on survival in human immunodeficiency virus type 1 infection. Am J Epidemiol, 1996 Jun, 143:12, 1244-56

26 Massé PG; van den Berg H; Duguay C; Beaulieu G; Simard JM. Early effect of a low dose (30 micrograms) ethinyl estradiol-containing Triphasil on vitamin B6 status. A follow-up study on six menstrual cycles. Int J Vitam Nutr Res, 1996, 66:1, 46-54

Folate

1 Pfeiffer CM; Rogers LM; Bailey LB; Gregory JF 3rd Absorption of folate from fortified cereal-grain products and of supplemental folate consumed with or without food determined by using a dual-label stable-isotope protocol. Am J Clin Nutr, 1997 Dec, 66:6, 1388-97

2 Jacques PF; Bostom AG; Williams RR; Ellison RC; Eckfeldt JH; Rosenberg IH; Selhub J; Rozen R. Relation between folate status, a common mutation in methylenetetrahydrofolate reductase, and plasma homocysteine concentrations. Circulation, 1996 Jan, 93:1, 7-9

3 Quinn K; Basu TK. Folate and vitamin B12 status of the elderly. Eur J Clin Nutr, 1996 Jun, 50:6, 340-2

4 Ortega RM; Mañas LR; Andrés P; Gaspar MJ; Agudo FR; Jiménez A; Pascual T Functional and psychic deterioration in elderly people may be aggravated by folate deficiency. J Nutr, 1996 Aug, 126:8, 1992-9

5 Tucker KL; Selhub J; Wilson PW; Rosenberg IH Dietary intake pattern relates to plasma folate and homocysteine concentrations in the Framingham Heart Study. J Nutr, 1996 Dec, 126:12, 3025-31

6 Robinson K; Arheart K; Refsum H; Brattström L; Boers G; Ueland P; Rubba P; Palma Reis R; Meleady R; Daly L; Witteman J; Graham I Low circulating folate and vitamin B6 concentrations: risk factors for stroke, peripheral vascular disease, and coronary artery disease. European COMAC Group. Circulation, 1998 Feb, 97:5, 437-43

7 Morrison HI; Schaubel D; Desmeules M; Wigle DT Serum folate and risk of fatal coronary heart disease. JAMA, 1996 Jun, 275:24, 1893-6

8 Schwartz SM et al. Myocardial infarction in young women in relation to plasma total homocysteine, folate, and a common variant in the methylenetetrahydrofolate reductase gene. Circulation, 1997 Jul, 96:2, 412-7

9 Chasan-Taber L, Selhub J, Rosenberg IH, Malinow MR, Terry P, Tishler PV, Willett W, Hennekens CH, Stampfer MJ. A prospective study of folate and vitamin B6 and risk of myocardial infarction in US physicians. J Am Coll Nutr 1996 Apr;15(2):136-143

10 Riggs KM; Spiro A 3rd; Tucker K; Rush D Relations of vitamin B-12, vitamin B-6, folate, and homocysteine to cognitive performance in the Normative Aging Study. Am J Clin Nutr, 1996 Mar, 63:3, 306-14

11 Alpert JE; Fava M Nutrition and depression: the role of folate. Nutr Rev, 1997 May, 55:5, 145-9

12 Fava M; Borus JS; Alpert JE; Nierenberg AA; Rosenbaum JF; Bottiglieri T Folate, vitamin B12, and homocysteine in major depressive disorder. Am J Psychiatry, 1997 Mar, 154:3, 426-8

13 Kim YI; Pogribny IP; Basnakian AG; Miller JW; Selhub J; James SJ; Mason JB Folate deficiency in rats induces DNA strand breaks and hypomethylation within the p53 tumor suppressor gene. Am J Clin Nutr, 1997 Jan, 65:1, 46-52

14 Glynn SA; Albanes D; Pietinen P; Brown CC; Rautalahti M; Tangrea JA; Gunter EW; Barrett MJ; Virtamo J; Taylor PR. Colorectal cancer and folate status: a nested case-control study among male smokers. Cancer Epidemiol Biomarkers Prev, 1996 Jul, 5:7, 487-94

15 Butterworth CE Jr; Hatch KD; Macaluso M; Cole P; Sauberlich HE; Soong SJ; Borst M; Baker VV. Folate deficiency and cervical dysplasia. JAMA, 1992 Jan 22-29, 267:4, 528-33

16 Tucker KL; Mahnken B; Wilson PW; Jacques P; Selhub J. Folic acid fortification of the food supply. Potential benefits and risks for the elderly population. JAMA, 1996 Dec, 276:23, 1879-85 1996;276:1879-85

17 Malinow MR; Duell PB; Hess DL; Anderson PH; Kruger WD; Phillipson BE; Gluckman RA; Block PC; Upson BM. Reduction of plasma homocyst(e)ine levels by breakfast cereal fortified with folic acid in patients with coronary heart disease. N Engl J Med, 1998 Apr, 338:15, 1009-15

18 Use of folic acid-containing supplements among women of childbearing age—United States, 1997. MMWR Morb Mortal Wkly Rep, 1998 Feb, 47:7, 131-4

19 Hoag SW; Ramachandruni H; Shangraw RF. Failure of prescription prenatal vitamin products to meet USP standards for folic acid dissolution. J Am Pharm Assoc (Wash), 1997 Jul, NS37:4, 397-400

20 Cuskelly GJ; McNulty H; Scott JM. Effect of increasing dietary folate on red-cell folate: implications for prevention of neural tube defects Lancet, 1996 Mar, 347:9002, 657-9

21 Daly S; Mills JL; Molloy AM; Conley M; Lee YJ; Kirke PN; Weir DG; Scott JM. Minimum effective dose of folic acid for food fortification to prevent neural-tube defects. Lancet, 1997 Dec, 350:9092, 1666-9 Lancet 1997; 350: 1666-69

22 Czeizel AE; Dudás I Prevention of the first occurrence of neural-tube defects by periconceptional vitamin supplementation. N Engl J Med, 1992 Dec 24, 327:26, 1832-5

23 Lowering blood homocysteine with folic acid based supplements: meta-analysis of randomised trials. Homocysteine Lowering Trialists' Collaboration. BMJ, 1998 Mar, 316:7135, 894-8

24 Rimm EB; Willett WC; Hu FB; Sampson L; Colditz GA; Manson JE; Hennekens C; Stampfer MJ Folate and vitamin B6 from diet and supplements in relation to risk of coronary heart disease among women. JAMA, 1998 Feb, 279:5, 359-64

25 Ward M, McNulty H, McPartlin J, Strain JJ, Weir DG, Scott JM. Plasma homocysteine, a risk factor for cardiovascular disease, is lowered by physiological doses of folic acid. QJM 1997;90:519-24.

26 Lashner BA; Provencher KS; Seidner DL; Knesebeck A; Brzezinski A The effect of folic acid supplementation on the risk for cancer or dysplasia in ulcerative colitis. Gastroenterology, 1997 Jan, 112:1, 29-32

27 Biasco G et al. Folic acid supplementation and cell kinetics of rectal mucosa in patients with ulcerative colitis. Cancer Epidemiol Biomarkers Prev, 1997 Jun, 6:6, 469-71

28 Saito M; Kato H; Tsuchida T; Konaka C Chemoprevention effects on bronchial squamous metaplasia by folate and vitamin B12 in heavy smokers. Chest, 1994 Aug, 106:2, 496-9

29 Butterworth CE Jr; Hatch KD; Soong SJ; Cole P; Tamura T; Sauberlich HE; Borst M; Macaluso M; Baker V. Oral folic acid supplementation for cervical dysplasia: a clinical intervention trial. Am J Obstet Gynecol, 1992 Mar, 166:3, 803-9

30 Harper JM; Levine AJ; Rosenthal DL; Wiesmeier E; Hunt IF; Swendseid ME; Haile RW. Acta Cytol, Erythrocyte folate levels, oral contraceptive use and abnormal cervical cytology. Author 1994 May, 38:3, 324-30

31 Morgan SL; Baggott JE; Lee JY; Alarcón GS Folic acid supplementation prevents deficient blood folate levels and hyperhomocysteinemia during longterm, low dose methotrexate therapy for rheumatoid arthritis: implications for cardiovascular disease prevention. J Rheumatol, 1998 Mar, 25:3, 441-6

32 Juhlin L; Olsson MJ Improvement of vitiligo after oral treatment with vitamin B12 and folic acid and the importance of sun exposure. Acta Derm Venereol, 1997 Nov, 77:6, 460-2

Vitamin B12

1 Nilsson Ehle H Age-related changes in cobalamin (vitamin B12) handling. Implications for therapy. Drugs Aging, 1998 Apr, 12:4, 277-92

2 Fata FT; Herzlich BC; Schiffman G; Ast AL. Impaired antibody responses to pneumococcal polysaccharide in elderly patients with low serum vitamin B12 levels. Ann Intern Med, 1996 Feb, 124:3, 299-304

3 Chadefaux B; Cooper BA; Gilfix BM; Lue Shing H; Carson W; Gavsie A; Rosenblatt DS. Homocysteine: relationship to serum cobalamin, serum folate, erythrocyte folate, and lobation of neutrophils. Clin Invest Med, 1994 Dec, 17:6, 540-50

4 Fenech MF; Dreosti IE; Rinaldi JR. Folate, vitamin B12, homocysteine status and chromosome damage rate in lymphocytes of older men. Carcinogenesis, 1997 Jul, 18:7, 1329-36

5 Kim GS; Kim CH; Park JY; Lee KU; Park CS Effects of vitamin B12 on cell proliferation and cellular alkaline phosphatase activity in human bone marrow stromal osteoprogenitor cells and UMR106 osteoblastic cells. Metabolism, 1996 Dec, 45:12, 1443-6

6 Lederly FA. Oral cobalamin for pernicious anemia: Medicine's best kept secret. JAMA. 1991;265:94,95

7 Tang AM; Graham NM; Chandra RK; Saah AJ. Low serum vitamin B-12 concentrations are associated with faster human immunodeficiency virus type 1 (HIV-1) disease progression. J Nutr, 1997 Feb, 127:2, 345-51

8 Kieburtz KD; Giang DW; Schiffer RB; Vakil N. Abnormal vitamin B12 metabolism in human immunodeficiency virus infection. Association with neurological dysfunction. Arch Neurol, 1991 Mar, 48:3, 312-4

9 Baum MK; Beach R; Morgan R; Mantero-Atienza A; Wilke F; Eisdorfer C. Vitamin B12 and cognitive function in HIV infection. Int Conf AIDS, 1990 Jun 20-23, 6:2, 97 (abstract no. F.B.32)

10 Bohr KC. Effect of vitamin B12 on sleep quality and performance of shift workers. Wien Med Wochenschr, 1996, 146:13-14, 289-91

Biotin

1 Báez-Saldaña A; Diaz G; Espinoza B; and Ortega E. Biotin deficiency induces changes in subpopulations of spleen lymphocytes in mice. Am J Clin Nutr 1998;67:431-7

2 Koutsikos D et al. Oral glucose tolerance test after high-dose i.v. biotin administration in normoglucemic hemodialysis patients. Ren Fail, 1996 Jan, 18:1, 131-7

3 Koutsikos D et al. Biotin for diabetic peripheral neuropathy. Biomed Pharmacother. 1990; 44: 511-514

4 Hochman LG et al. Brittle nails: Response to daily biotin supplementation. Cutis. 1993;51: 303-307

5 Honke K; Hasui M; Takano N. Abnormal metabolism of fatty acids and ketone bodies in Duchenne muscular dystrophy, and the effect of biotin on these abnormalities] No To Hattatsu, 1997 Jan, 29:1, 13-8

Pantothenic acid

1 Binaghi P; Cellina G; Lo Cicero G; Bruschi F; Porcaro E; Penotti M. Evaluation of the cholesterol-lowering effectiveness of pantethine in women in perimenopausal age. Minerva Med, 1990 Jun, 81:6, 475-9

2 Komar VI The use of pantothenic acid preparations in treating patients with viral hepatitis A. Ter Arkh, 1991, 63:11, 58-60

Vitamin C

1 Enstrom JE, Kanim LE, Klein MA. Vitamin C intake and mortality among a sample of the United States population. Epidemiology 1992 May; 3(3):194-202

2 Johnston CS, Thompson LL. Vitamin C status of an outpatient population. J Am Coll Nutr, 1998 Aug, 17:4, 366-70

3 Sahyoun NR; Jacques PF; Russell RM Carotenoids, vitamins C and E, and mortality in an elderly population. Am J Epidemiol, 1996 Sep, 144:5, 501-11

4 Gey KF; Stähelin HB; Eichholzer M Poor plasma status of carotene and vitamin C is associated with higher mortality from ischemic heart disease and stroke: Basel Prospective Study. Clin Investig, 1993 Jan, 71:1, 3-6

5 Gale CR; Martyn CN; Winter PD; Cooper C Vitamin C and risk of death from stroke and coronary heart disease in cohort of elderly people. BMJ, 1995 Jun, 310:6994, 1563-6

6 Nyyssönen K; Parviainen MT; Salonen R; Tuomilehto J; Salonen JT. Vitamin C deficiency and risk of myocardial infarction: prospective population study of men from eastern Finland. BMJ, 1997 Mar, 314:7081, 634-8

7 Rimm EB; Stampfer MJ; Ascherio A; Giovannucci E; Colditz GA; Willett WC Vitamin E consumption and the risk of coronary heart disease in men. N Engl J Med, 1993 May 20, 328:20, 1450-6

8 Stampfer MJ; Hennekens CH; Manson JE; Colditz GA; Rosner B; Willett WC Vitamin E consumption and the risk of coronary disease in women. N Engl J Med, 1993 May 20, 328:20, 1444-9

9 Ness AR; Khaw KT; Bingham S; Day NE Vitamin C status and undiagnosed angina. J Cardiovasc Risk, 1996 Aug, 3:4, 373-7

10 Ness AR; Khaw KT; Bingham S; Day NE Vitamin C status and serum lipids. Eur J Clin Nutr, 1996 Nov, 50:11, 724-9

11 Hallfrisch J; Singh VN; Muller DC; Baldwin H; Bannon ME; Andres R. High plasma vitamin C associated with high plasma HDL- and HDL2 cholesterol. Am J Clin Nutr, 1994 Jul, 60:1, 100-5

12 Ness AR; Khaw KT; Bingham S; Day NE Vitamin C status and blood pressure. J Hypertens, 1996 Apr, 14:4, 503-8

13 Block G Vitamin C and cancer prevention: the epidemiologic evidence. Am J Clin Nutr, 1991 Jan, 53:1 Suppl, 270S-282S

14 Pandey DK; Shekelle R; Selwyn BJ; Tangney C; Stamler J. Dietary vitamin C and beta-carotene and risk of death in middle-aged men. The Western Electric Study. Am J Epidemiol, 1995 Dec, 142:12, 1269-78

15 Daviglus ML; Dyer AR; Persky V; Chavez N; Drum M; Goldberg J; Liu K; Morris DK; Shekelle RB; Stamler J Dietary beta-carotene, vitamin C, and risk of prostate cancer: results from the Western Electric Study. Epidemiology, 1996 Sep, 7:5, 472-7

16 Ocké MC; Kromhout D; Menotti A; Aravanis C; Blackburn H; Buzina R; Fidanza F; Jansen A; Nedeljkovic S; Nissienen A; et al. Average intake of anti-oxidant (pro)vitamins and subsequent cancer mortality in the 16 cohorts of the Seven Countries Study. Int J Cancer, 1995 May, 61:4, 480-4

17 La Vecchia C; Ferraroni M; DAvanzo B; Decarli A; Franceschi S Selected micronutrient intake and the risk of gastric cancer. Cancer Epidemiol Biomarkers Prev, 1994 Jul, 3:5, 393-8

18 Ocké MC; Bueno de Mesquita HB; Feskens EJ; van Staveren WA; Kromhout D Repeated measurements of vegetables, fruits, beta-carotene, and vitamins C and E in relation to lung cancer. The Zutphen Study. Am J Epidemiol, 1997 Feb, 145:4, 358-65

19 Shibata A; Paganini-Hill A; Ross RK; Henderson BE Intake of vegetables, fruits, beta-carotene, vitamin C and vitamin supplements and cancer incidence among the elderly: a prospective study. Br J Cancer, 1992 Oct, 66:4, 673-9

20 Ferraroni M; La Vecchia C; DAvanzo B; Negri E; Franceschi S; Decarli A Selected micronutrient intake and the risk of colorectal cancer. Br J Cancer, 1994 Dec, 70:6, 1150-5

21 Jain M; Miller AB; To T. Premorbid diet and the prognosis of women with breast cancer. J Natl Cancer Inst, 1994 Sep, 86:18, 1390-7

22 Hunter DJ; Manson JE; Colditz GA; Stampfer MJ; Rosner B; Hennekens CH; Speizer FE; Willett WC A prospective study of the intake of vitamins C, E, and A and the risk of breast cancer. N Engl J Med, 1993 Jul 22, 329:4, 234-40

23 Mares Perlman JA; Brady WE; Klein BE; Klein R; Haus GJ; Palta M; Ritter LL; Shoff SM. Diet and nuclear lens opacities. Am J Epidemiol, 1995 Feb, 141:4, 322-34

24 Sinclair AJ; Taylor PB; Lunec J; Girling AJ; Barnett AH Low plasma ascorbate levels in patients with type 2 diabetes mellitus consuming adequate dietary vitamin C. Diabet Med, 1994 Nov, 11:9, 893-8

25 Mayer Davis EJ; Monaco JH; Marshall JA; Rushing J; Juhaeri Vitamin C intake and cardiovascular disease risk factors in persons with non-insulin-dependent diabetes mellitus. From the Insulin Resistance Atherosclerosis Study and the San Luis Valley Diabetes Study. Prev Med, 1997 May, 26:3, 277-83

26 Ness AR; Khaw KT; Bingham S; Day NE Vitamin C status and respiratory function. Eur J Clin Nutr, 1996 Sep, 50:9, 573-9

27 Hatch GE Asthma, inhaled oxidants, and dietary antioxidants. Am J Clin Nutr, 1995 Mar, 61:3 Suppl, 625S-630S

28 Soutar A; Seaton A; Brown K Bronchial reactivity and dietary antioxidants. Thorax, 1997 Feb, 52:2, 166-70

29 Pfitzenmeyer P; Guilland JC; dAthis P. Vitamin B6 and vitamin C status in elderly patients with infections during hospitalization. Ann Nutr Metab, 1997, 41:6, 344-52

30 Levine M et al. Vitamin C pharmacokinetics in healthy volunteers: evidence for a recommended dietary allowance. Proc Natl Acad Sci U S A, 1996 Apr, 93:8, 3704-9

31 Blanchard J; Tozer TN; Rowland M Pharmacokinetic perspectives on megadoses of ascorbic acid. Am J Clin Nutr, 1997 Nov, 66:5, 1165-71

32 Cathcart RF. The method of determining proper doses of vitamin C for the treatment of disease by titrating to bowel tolerance. J Orthomol Psychiat. 1981;10:125-132

33 Podmore ID; Griffiths HR; Herbert KE; Mistry N; Mistry P; Lunec J. Vitamin C exhibits pro-oxidant properties. Nature, 1998 Apr, 392:6676, 559

34 Losonczy KG; Harris TB; Havlik RJ Vitamin E and vitamin C supplement use and risk of all-cause and coronary heart disease mortality in older persons: the Established Populations for Epidemiologic Studies of the Elderly. Am J Clin Nutr, 1996 Aug, 64:2, 190-6

35 Plotnick GD; Corretti MC; Vogel RA Effect of antioxidant vitamins on the transient impairment of endothelium-dependent brachial artery vasoactivity following a single high-fat meal. JAMA 1997;278:1682-1686

36 Levine GN; Frei B; Koulouris SN; Gerhard MD; Keaney JF Jr; Vita JA Ascorbic acid reverses endothelial vasomotor dysfunction in patients with coronary artery disease. Circulation, 1996 Mar, 93:6, 1107-13

37 Ting HH; Timimi FK; Haley EA; Roddy MA; Ganz P; Creager MA Vitamin C improves endothelium-dependent vasodilation in forearm resistance vessels of humans with hypercholesterolemia. Circulation, 1997 Jun, 95:12, 2617-22

38 Hornig B; Arakawa N; Kohler C; Drexler H Vitamin C improves endothelial function of conduit arteries in patients with chronic heart failure. Circulation, 1998 Feb, 97:4, 363-8

39 Dingchao H; Zhiduan Q; Liye H; Xiaodong F The protective effects of high-dose ascorbic acid on myocardium against reperfusion injury during and after cardiopulmonary bypass. Thorac Cardiovasc Surg, 1994 Oct, 42:5, 276-8

40 Lehr HA; Weyrich AS; Saetzler RK; Jurek A; Arfors KE; Zimmerman GA; Prescott SM; McIntyre TM Vitamin C blocks inflammatory platelet-activating factor mimetics created by cigarette smoking. J Clin Invest, 1997 May, 99:10, 2358-64

41 Weber C; Erl W; Weber K; Weber PC Increased adhesiveness of isolated monocytes to endothelium is prevented by vitamin C intake in smokers. Circulation, 1996 Apr, 93:8, 1488-92

42 Motoyama T; Kawano H; Kugiyama K; Hirashima O; Ohgushi M; Yoshimura M; Ogawa H; Yasue H Endothelium-dependent vasodilation in the brachial artery is impaired in smokers: effect of vitamin C. Am J Physiol, 1997 Oct, 273:4 Pt 2, H1644-50

43 Ness AR; Chee D; Elliott P Vitamin C and blood pressure—an overview. J Hum Hypertens, 1997 Jun, 11:6, 343-50

44 Solzbach U; Hornig B; Jeserich M; Just H Vitamin C improves endothelial dysfunction of epicardial coronary arteries in hypertensive patients. Circulation, 1997 Sep, 96:5, 1513-9

45 Waring AJ; Drake IM; Schorah CJ; White KL; Lynch DA; Axon AT; Dixon MF Ascorbic acid and total vitamin C concentrations in plasma, gastric juice, and gastrointestinal mucosa: effects of gastritis and oral supplementation. Gut, 1996 Feb, 38:2, 171-6

46 Zhang HM; Wakisaka N; Maeda O; Yamamoto T. Vitamin C inhibits the growth of a bacterial risk factor for gastric carcinoma: *Helicobacter pylori*. Cancer, 1997 Nov, 80:10, 1897-903

47 Paganelli GM; Biasco G; Brandi G; Santucci R; Gizzi G; Villani V; Cianci M; Miglioli M; Barbara L Effect of vitamin A, C, and E supplementation on rectal cell proliferation in patients with colorectal adenomas. J Natl Cancer Inst, 1992 Jan 1, 84:1, 47-51

48 Maramag C; Menon M; Balaji KC; Reddy PG; Laxmanan S Effect of vitamin C on prostate cancer cells in vitro: effect on cell number, viability, and DNA synthesis. Prostate, 1997 Aug, 32:3, 188-95

49 Okunieff P. Interactions between ascorbic acid and the radiation of bone marrow, skin and tumor. Am J Clin Nutr 1991;54:1281S-1283S

50 Bielory L; Gandhi R Asthma and vitamin C. Ann Allergy, 1994 Aug, 73:2, 89-96; quiz 96-100

51 Cohen HA; Neuman I; Nahum H Blocking effect of vitamin C in exercise-induced asthma. Vitamin C supplements can also help to reduce exercise induced asthma by reducing airway hyperreactivity. Arch Pediatr Adolesc Med, 1997 Apr, 151:4, 367-70

52 Heuser G; Vojdani A Enhancement of natural killer cell activity and T and B cell function by buffered vitamin C in patients exposed to toxic chemicals: the role of protein kinase-C. Immunopharmacol Immunotoxicol, 1997 Aug, 19:3, 291-312

53 Rivas CI; Vera JC; Guaiquil VH; Velásquez FV; Bórquez-Ojeda OA; Cárcamo JG; Concha II; Golde DW Increased uptake and accumulation of vitamin C in human immunodeficiency virus 1-infected hematopoietic cell lines. J Biol Chem, 1997 Feb 28, 272:9, 5814-20

54 Hemilä H Vitamin C supplementation and common cold symptoms: problems with inaccurate reviews. Nutrition, 1996 Nov, 12:11-12, 804-9

55 Hemilä H Vitamin C intake and susceptibility to the common cold. Br J Nutr, 1997 Jan, 77:1, 59-72

56 Hemilä H Vitamin C and common cold incidence: a review of studies with subjects under heavy physical stress. Int J Sports Med, 1996 Jul, 17:5, 379-83

57 Hankinson SE; Stampfer MJ; Seddon JM; Colditz GA; Rosner B; Speizer FE; Willett WC. Nutrient intake and cataract extraction in women: a prospective study. BMJ, 1992 Aug 8, 305:6849, 335-9

58 Jacques PF; Taylor A; Hankinson SE; Willett WC; Mahnken B; Lee Y; Vaid K; Lahav M. Long-term vitamin C supplement use and prevalence of early age-related lens opacities. Am J Clin Nutr, 1997 Oct, 66:4, 911-6

59 Eriksson J; Kohvakka A Magnesium and ascorbic acid supplementation in diabetes mellitus. Ann Nutr Metab, 1995, 39:4, 217-23

60 Cunningham JJ; Mearkle PL; Brown RG Vitamin C: an aldose reductase inhibitor that normalizes erythrocyte sorbitol in insulin-dependent diabetes mellitus. J Am Coll Nutr, 1994 Aug, 13:4, 344-5

61 Timimi FK; Ting HH; Haley EA; Roddy MA; Ganz P; Creager MA Vitamin C improves endothelium-dependent vasodilation in patients with insulin-dependent diabetes mellitus. J Am Coll Cardiol, 1998 Mar, 31:3, 552-7

62 Eberlein König B; Placzek M; Przybilla B Protective effect against sunburn of combined systemic ascorbic acid (vitamin C) and d-alpha-tocopherol (vitamin E). Am Acad Dermatol, 1998 Jan, 38:1, 45-8

63 Simon JA; Grady D; Snabes MC; Fong J; Hunninghake DB. Ascorbic acid supplement use and the prevalence of gallbladder disease. Heart & Estrogen-Progestin Replacement Study (HERS) Research Group. J Clin Epidemiol, 1998 Mar, 51:3, 257-65

64 Gustafsson U; Wang FH; Axelson M; Kallner A; Sahlin S; Einarsson K The effect of vitamin C in high doses on plasma and biliary lipid composition in patients with cholesterol gallstones: prolongation of the nucleation time. Eur J Clin Invest, 1997 May, 27:5, 387-91

65 Alessio HM; Goldfarb AH; Cao G Exercise-induced oxidative stress before and after vitamin C supplementation. Int J Sport Nutr, 1997 Mar, 7:1, 1-9

66 Dawson EB; Harris WA; Teter MC; Powell LC. Effect of ascorbic acid supplementation on the sperm quality of smokers. Fertil Steril, 1992 Nov, 58:5, 1034-9

67 Böhm F et al.Carotenoids Enhance Vitamin E Antioxidant Efficiency. Journal of the American Chemical Society 1997;119:621-622

68 Watanabe H; Kakihana M; Ohtsuka S; Sugishita Y Randomized, double-blind, placebo-controlled study of the preventive effect of supplemental oral vitamin C on attenuation of development of nitrate tolerance. J Am Coll Cardiol, 1998 May, 31:6, 1323-9

69 Gerster H. No contribution of ascorbic acid to renal calcium oxalate stones. Ann Nutr Metab, 1997, 41:5, 269-82

Vitamin D

1 Thomas MK; Lloyd Jones DM; Thadhani RI; Shaw AC; Deraska DJ; Kitch BT; Vamvakas EC; Dick IM; Prince RL; Finkelstein JS. Hypovitaminosis D in medical inpatients. N Engl J Med, 1998 Mar, 338:12, 777-83

2 Dawson Hughes B; Harris SS; Dallal GE Plasma calcidiol, season, and serum parathyroid hormone concentrations in healthy elderly men and women. Am J Clin Nutr, 1997 Jan, 65:1, 67-71

3 Graafmans WC; Lips P; Ooms ME; van Leeuwen JP; Pols HA; Uitterlinden AG. The effect of vitamin D supplementation on the bone mineral density of the femoral neck is associated with vitamin D receptor genotype. J Bone Miner Res, 1997 Aug, 12:8, 1241-5

4 McAlindon TE; Felson DT; Zhang Y; Hannan MT; Aliabadi P; Weissman B; Rush D; Wilson PW. Relation of dietary intake and serum levels of vitamin D to progression of osteoarthritis of the knee among participants in the Framingham Study. Ann Intern Med, 1996 Sep, 125:5, 353-9

5 Oelzner P; Müller A; Deschner F; Hüller M; Abendroth K; Hein G; Stein G. Relationship between disease activity and serum levels of vitamin D metabolites and PTH in rheumatoid arthritis. Calcif Tissue Int, 1998 Mar, 62:3, 193-8

6 Feldman D; Skowronski RJ; Peehl DM Vitamin D and prostate cancer. Adv Exp Med Biol, 1995, 375:, 53-63

7 Brenner RV; Shabahang M; Schumaker LM; Nauta RJ; Uskokovic MR; Evans SR; Buras RR The antiproliferative effect of vitamin D analogs on MCF-7 human breast cancer cells. Cancer Lett, 1995 May, 92:1, 77-82

8 Colston KW; James SY; Ofori Kuragu EA; Binderup L; Grant AG. Vitamin D receptors and anti-proliferative effects of vitamin D derivatives in human pancreatic carcinoma cells in vivo and in vitro. Br J Cancer, 1997, 76:8, 1017-20

9 Lefkowitz ES; Garland CF Sunlight, vitamin D, and ovarian cancer mortality rates in US women. Int J Epidemiol, 1994 Dec, 23:6, 1133-6

10 Pritchard RS; Baron JA; Gerhardsson de Verdier M. Dietary calcium, vitamin D, and the risk of colorectal cancer in Stockholm, Sweden. Cancer Epidemiol Biomarkers Prev, 1996 Nov, 5:11, 897-900

11 Martínez ME; Giovannucci EL; Colditz GA; Stampfer MJ; Hunter DJ; Speizer FE; Wing A; Willett WC Calcium, vitamin D, and the occurrence of colorectal cancer among women. J Natl Cancer Inst, 1996 Oct, 88:19, 1375-82

12 Gann PH; Ma J; Hennekens CH; Hollis BW; Haddad JG; Stampfer MJ Circulating vitamin D metabolites in relation to subsequent development of prostate cancer. Cancer Epidemiol Biomarkers Prev, 1996 Feb, 5:2, 121-6

13 Taylor JA; Hirvonen A; Watson M; Pittman G; Mohler JL; Bell DA Association of prostate cancer with vitamin D receptor gene polymorphism. Cancer Res, 1996 Sep, 56:18, 4108-10

14 Hayes CE; Cantorna MT; DeLuca HF Vitamin D and multiple sclerosis. Proc Soc Exp Biol Med, 1997 Oct, 216:1, 21-7

15 Boucher BJ; Mannan N; Noonan K; Hales CN; Evans SJ Glucose intolerance and impairment of insulin secretion in relation to vitamin D deficiency in east London Asians. Diabetologia, 1995 Oct, 38:10, 1239-45

16 Baynes KC; Boucher BJ; Feskens EJ; Kromhout D Vitamin D, glucose tolerance and insulinaemia in elderly men. Diabetologia, 1997 Mar, 40:3, 344-7

17 Watson KE; Abrolat ML; Malone LL; Hoeg JM; Doherty T; Detrano R; Demer LL Active serum vitamin D levels are inversely correlated with coronary calcification. Circulation, 1997 Sep, 96:6, 1755-60

18 Adams JS; Lee G. Gains in bone mineral density with resolution of vitamin D intoxication. Ann Int Med, 1997 Aug; 127:3, 203-6

19 Dawson Hughes B; Harris SS; Krall EA; Dallal GE Effect of calcium and vitamin D supplementation on bone density in men and women 65 years of age or older. N Engl J Med, 1997 Sep, 337:10, 670-6

20 Buckley et al.Calcium and vitamin D3 supplementation prevents bone loss in the spine secondary to low-dose corticosteroids in patients with rheumatoid arthritis. A randomized, double-blind, placebo-controlled trial. Ann Intern Med 1996 Dec 15;125(12):961-968

21 Lips P, Graafmans WC, Ooms ME, Bezemer PD, Bouter LM. Vitamin D supplementation and fracture incidence in elderly persons. A randomized, placebo-controlled clinical trial. Ann Intern Med 1996 Feb 15;124(4):400-406

Vitamin E

1 Kushi LH; Fee RM; Sellers TA; Zheng W; Folsom AR. Intake of vitamins A, C, and E and postmenopausal breast cancer. The Iowa Women's Health Study. Am J Epidemiol, 1996 Jul, 144:2, 165-74

2 Rimm EB. Vitamin E consumption and the risk of coronary heart disease in men. N Engl J Med, 328: 20, 1993 May 20, 1450-6

3 Miwa K; Miyagi Y; Igawa A; Nakagawa K; Inoue H Vitamin E deficiency in variant angina. Circulation, 1996 Jul, 94:1, 14-8

4 Bostick RM; Potter JD; McKenzie DR; Sellers TA; Kushi LH; Steinmetz KA; Folsom AR. Reduced risk of colon cancer with high intake of vitamin E: the Iowa Women's Health Study. Cancer Res, 1993 Sep 15, 53:18, 4230-7

5 Zheng W; Sellers TA; Doyle TJ; Kushi LH; Potter JD; Folsom AR Retinol, antioxidant vitamins, and cancers of the upper digestive tract in a prospective cohort study of postmenopausal women. Am J Epidemiol, 1995 Nov, 142:9, 955-60

6 London SJ; Stein EA; Henderson IC; Stampfer MJ; Wood WC; Remine S; Dmochowski JR; Robert NJ; Willett WC. Carotenoids, retinol, and vitamin E and risk of proliferative benign breast disease and breast cancer. Cancer Causes Control, 1992 Nov, 3:6, 503-12

7 Hunter DJ; Manson JE; Colditz GA; Stampfer MJ; Rosner B; Hennekens CH; Speizer FE; Willett WC. A prospective study of the intake of vitamins C, E, and A and the risk of breast cancer. N Engl J Med, 1993 Jul 22, 329:4, 234-40

8 Slattery ML; Abbott TM; Overall JC Jr; Robison LM; French TK; Jolles C; Gardner JW; West DW. Dietary vitamins A, C, and E and selenium as risk factors for cervical cancer. Epidemiology, 1990 Jan, 1:1, 8-15

9 Palan PR; Mikhail MS; Basu J; Romney SL. Plasma levels of antioxidant beta-carotene and alpha-tocopherol in uterine cervix dysplasias and cancer. Nutr Cancer, 1991, 15:1, 13-20

10 Comstock GW; Helzlsouer KJ; Bush TL. Prediagnostic serum levels of carotenoids and vitamin E as related to subsequent cancer in Washington County, Maryland. Am J Clin Nutr, 1991 Jan, 53:1 Suppl, 260S-264S

11 Rouhiainen P; Rouhiainen H; Salonen JT. Association between low plasma vitamin E concentration and progression of early cortical lens opacities. Am J Epidemiol, 1996 Sep, 144:5, 496-500

12 de Rijk MC et al. Dietary antioxidants and Parkinson disease. The Rotterdam Study. Arch Neurol, 1997 Jun, 54:6, 762-5

13 Christen S; Woodall AA; Shigenaga MK; Southwell Keely PT; Duncan MW; Ames BN gamma-tocopherol traps mutagenic electrophiles such as NO(X) and complements alpha-tocopherol: physiological implications. Proc Natl Acad Sci U S A, 1997 Apr, 94:7, 3217-22

14 Brown KM; Morrice PC; Duthie GG Erythrocyte vitamin E and plasma ascorbate concentrations in relation to erythrocyte peroxidation in smokers and nonsmokers: dose response to vitamin E supplementation. Am J Clin Nutr, 1997 Feb, 65:2, 496-502

15 Losonczy KG; Harris TB; Havlik RJ. Vitamin E and vitamin C supplement use and risk of all-cause and coronary heart disease mortality in older persons: the Established Populations for Epidemiologic Studies of the Elderly. Am J Clin Nutr, 1996 Aug, 64:2, 190-6

16 Stampfer M et al. Vitamin E consumption and the risk of coronary disease in women. N Engl J Med. 1993;328:1450-1456

17 Stephens N G et al. Randomised controlled trial of vitamin E in patients with coronary disease: Cambridge Heart Antioxidant Study (CHAOS). Lancet, 347: 9004, 1996 Mar 23, 781-6

18 Virtamo J; Rapola JM; Ripatti S; Heinonen OP; Taylor PR; Albanes D; Huttunen JK. Vitamin E supplements are used in the treatment of the peripheral vascular disease, intermittent claudication. Arch Intern Med, 1998 Mar, 158:6, 668-75

19 Williams JC; Forster LA; Tull SP; Wong M; Bevan RJ; Ferns GA Dietary vitamin E supplementation inhibits thrombin-induced platelet aggregation, but not monocyte adhesiveness, in patients with hypercholesterolaemia. Int J Exp Pathol, 1997 Aug, 78:4, 259-66

20 Martin A; Foxall T; Blumberg JB; Meydani M. Vitamin E inhibits low-density lipoprotein-induced adhesion of monocytes to human aortic endothelial cells in vitro. Arterioscler Thromb Vasc Biol, 1997 Mar, 17:3, 429-36

21 Simons LA; Von Konigsmark M; Balasubramaniam S What dose of vitamin E is required to reduce susceptibility of LDL to oxidation? Aust N Z J Med, 1996 Aug, 26:4, 496-503

22 Rapola JM; Virtamo J; Haukka JK; Heinonen OP; Albanes D; Taylor PR; Huttunen JK Effect of vitamin E and beta carotene on the incidence of angina pectoris. A randomized, double-blind, controlled trial. JAMA, 1996 Mar, 275:9, 693-8

23 Heinonen OP et al. Prostate cancer and supplementation with alpha-tocopherol and beta-carotene: incidence and mortality in a controlled trial. J Natl Cancer Inst, 1998 Mar, 90:6, 440-6

24 Meydani SN; Meydani M; Blumberg JB; Leka LS; Siber G; Loszewski R; Thompson C; Pedrosa MC; Diamond RD; Stollar BD Vitamin E supplementation and in vivo immune response in healthy elderly subjects. A randomized controlled trial. JAMA, 1997 May, 277:17, 1380-6

25 Tang AM; Graham NM; Semba RD; Saah AJ. Association between serum vitamin A and E levels and HIV-1 disease progression. AIDS, 1997 Apr, 11:5, 613-20

26 Jain SK; McVie R; Jaramillo JJ; Palmer M; Smith T; Meachum ZD; Little RL The effect of modest vitamin E supplementation on lipid peroxidation products and other cardiovascular risk factors in diabetic patients. Lipids, 1996 Mar, 31 Suppl:, S87-90

27 Pozzilli P et al. Vitamin E and nicotinamide have similar effects in maintaining residual beta cell function in recent onset insulin-dependent diabetes (the IMDIAB IV study). Eur J Endocrinol, 1997 Sep, 137:3, 234-9

28 Ophthalmology 1998; 105:831-836

29 Vézina D; Mauffette F; Roberts KD; Bleau G. Selenium-vitamin E supplementation in infertile men. Effects on semen parameters and micronutrient levels and distribution. Biol Trace Elem Res, 1996 Sum, 53:1-3, 65-83

30 Edmonds SE; Winyard PG; Guo R; Kidd B; Merry P; Langrish Smith A; Hansen C; Ramm S; Blake DR. Putative analgesic activity of repeated oral doses of vitamin E in the treatment of rheumatoid arthritis. Results of a prospective placebo controlled double blind trial. Ann Rheum Dis, 1997 Nov, 56:11, 649-55

31 Sano M et al. A controlled trial of selegiline, alpha-tocopherol, or both as treatment for Alzheimer's disease. The Alzheimer's Disease Cooperative Study. N Engl J Med, 1997 Apr, 336:17, 1216-22

32 von Herbay A; Stahl W; Niederau C; Sies H. Vitamin E improves the aminotransferase status of patients suffering from viral hepatitis C: a randomized, double-blind, placebo-controlled study. Free Radic Res, 1997 Dec, 27:6, 599-605

33 Barton DL et al. Prospective evaluation of vitamin E for hot flashes in breast cancer survivors. J Clin Oncol, 1998 Feb, 16:2, 495-500

34 Eberlein König B; Placzek M; Przybilla B. Protective effect against sunburn of combined systemic ascorbic acid (vitamin C) and d-alpha-tocopherol (vitamin E). J Am Acad Dermatol, 1998 Jan, 38:1, 45-8

35 McBride JM; Kraemer WJ; Triplett McBride T; Sebastianelli W Effect of resistance exercise on free radical production. Med Sci Sports Exerc, 1998 Jan, 30:1, 67-72

36 Lohr JB; Caligiuri MP A double-blind placebo-controlled study of vitamin E treatment of tardive dyskinesia. J Clin Psychiatry, 1996 Apr, 57:4, 167-73

37 Novelli GP; Adembri C; Gandini E; Orlandini SZ; Papucci L; Formigli L; Manneschi LI; Quattrone A; Pratesi C; Capaccioli S. Vitamin E protects human skeletal muscle from damage during surgical ischemia-reperfusion. Am J Surg, 1997 Mar, 173:3, 206-9

38 Kim JM; White RH. Effect of vitamin E on the anticoagulant response to warfarin. Am J Cardiol, 1996 Mar, 77:7, 545-6

Vitamin K

1 Kanai T; Takagi T; Masuhiro K; Nakamura M; Iwata M; Saji F Serum vitamin K level and bone mineral density in post-menopausal women. Int J Gynaecol Obstet, 1997 Jan, 56:1, 25-30

2 Tamatani M; Morimoto S; Nakajima M; Fukuo K; Onishi T; Kitano S; Niinobu T; Ogihara T. Decreased circulating levels of vitamin K and 25-hydroxyvitamin D in osteopenic elderly men. Metabolism, 1998 Feb, 47:2, 195-9

3 McKinney PA; Juszczak E; Findlay E; Smith K. Case-control study of childhood leukaemia and cancer in Scotland: findings for neonatal intramuscular vitamin K. BMJ, 1998 Jan, 316:7126, 173-7

4 Passmore SJ; Draper G; Brownbill P; Kroll M Ecological studies of relation between hospital policies on neonatal vitamin K administration and subsequent occurrence of childhood cancer. BMJ, 1998 Jan, 316:7126, 184-9

5 Passmore SJ; Draper G; Brownbill P; Kroll M Case-control studies of relation between childhood cancer and neonatal vitamin K administration. BMJ, 1998 Jan, 316:7126, 178-84

6 Parker L; Cole M; Craft AW; Hey EN Neonatal vitamin K administration and childhood cancer in the north of England: retrospective case-control study. BMJ, 1998 Jan, 316:7126, 189-93

7 Hansen KN; Ebbesen F. Neonatal vitamin K prophylaxis in Denmark: three years' experience with oral administration during the first three months of life compared with one oral administration at birth. Acta Paediatr, 1996 Oct, 85:10, 1137-9

8 Greer FR; Marshall SP; Foley AL; Suttie JW. Improving the vitamin K status of breastfeeding infants with maternal vitamin K supplements. Pediatrics, 1997 Jan, 99:1, 88-92

Boron

1 McCoy H; Kenney MA; Montgomery C; Irwin A; Williams L; Orrell R. Relation of boron to the composition and mechanical properties of bone. Environ Health Perspect, 1994 Nov, 102 Suppl 7:, 49-53

2 Nielsen FH. Biochemical and physiologic consequences of boron deprivation in humans. Environ Health Perspect, 1994 Nov, 102 Suppl 7:, 59-63

3 Nielsen FH Studies on the relationship between boron and magnesium which possibly affects the formation and maintenance of bones. Magnes Trace Elem, 1990, 9:2, 61-9

4 Penland JG Dietary boron, brain function, and cognitive performance. Environ Health Perspect, 1994 Nov, 102 Suppl 7:, 65-72

5 Helliwell TR; Kelly SA; Walsh HP; Klenerman L; Haines J; Clark R; Roberts NB. Elemental analysis of femoral bone from patients with fractured neck of femur or osteoarthrosis. Bone, 1996 Feb, 18:2, 151-7

6 Hunt CD; Shuler TR; Mullen LM. Concentration of boron and other elements in human foods and personal-care products. J Am Diet Assoc, 1991 May, 91:5, 558-68

7 Hunt CD; Herbel JL; Nielsen FH Metabolic responses of postmenopausal women to supplemental dietary boron and aluminum during usual and low magnesium intake: boron, calcium, and magnesium absorption and retention and blood mineral concentrations. Am J Clin Nutr, 1997 Mar, 65:3, 803-13

8 Green NR; Ferrando AA Plasma boron and the effects of boron supplementation in males. Environ Health Perspect, 1994 Nov, 102 Suppl 7:, 73-7

9 Nielsen FH; Hunt CD; Mullen LM; Hunt JR. Effect of dietary boron on mineral, estrogen, and testosterone metabolism in postmenopausal women. FASEB J, 1987 Nov, 1:5, 394-7

10 Meacham SL; Taper LJ; Volpe SL Effects of boron supplementation on bone mineral density and dietary, blood, and urinary calcium, phosphorus, magnesium, and boron in female athletes. Environ Health Perspect, 1994 Nov, 102 Suppl 7:, 79-82

11 Naghii MR; Samman S The effect of boron supplementation on its urinary excretion and selected cardiovascular risk factors in healthy male subjects. Biol Trace Elem Res, 1997 Mar, 56:3, 273-86

12 Newnham RE. Essentiality of boron for healthy bones and joints. Environ Health Perspect, 1994 Nov, 102 Suppl 7:, 83-5

Calcium

1 OBrien KO; Abrams SA; Liang LK; Ellis KJ; Gagel RF Increased efficiency of calcium absorption during short periods of inadequate calcium intake in girls. Am J Clin Nutr, 1996 Apr, 63:4, 579-83

2 Heaney RP; Recker RR; Stegman MR; Moy AJ Calcium absorption in women: relationships to calcium intake, estrogen status, and age. J Bone Miner Res, 1989 Aug, 4:4, 469-75

3 Kalkwarf HJ; Specker BL; Heubi JE; Vieira NE; Yergey AL. Intestinal calcium absorption of women during lactation and after weaning. Am J Clin Nutr, 1996 Apr, 63:4, 526-31

4 Itoh R; Nishiyama N; Suyama Y. Dietary protein intake and urinary excretion of calcium: a cross-sectional study in a healthy Japanese population. Am J Clin Nutr 1998;67:438-44

5 Abrams SA; Stuff JE Calcium metabolism in girls: current dietary intakes lead to low rates of calcium absorption and retention during puberty. Am J Clin Nutr, 1994 Nov, 60:5, 739-43

6 Suleiman S, Nelson M, Li F, Buxton-Thomas M, Moniz C. Effect of calcium intake and physical activity level on bone mass and turnover in healthy, white, postmenopausal women. Am J Clin Nutr 1997 Oct;66(4):937-943

7 Burger H et al Risk Factors for Increased Bone Loss in an Elderly Population The Rotterdam Study. Am J Epidemiol 1998;147:871-9

8 Slob IC; Lambregts JL; Schuit AJ; Kok FJ. Calcium intake and 28-year gastro-intestinal cancer mortality in Dutch civil servants. Int J Cancer, 1993 Apr 22, 54:1, 20-5

9 Zheng W; Anderson KE; Kushi LH; Sellers TA; Greenstein J; Hong CP; Cerhan JR; Bostick RM; Folsom AR. A prospective cohort study of intake of calcium, vitamin D, and other micronutrients in relation to incidence of rectal cancer among postmenopausal women. Cancer Epidemiol Biomarkers Prev, 1998 Mar, 7:3, 221-5

10 Kearney J; Giovannucci E; Rimm EB; Ascherio A; Stampfer MJ; Colditz GA; Wing A; Kampman E; Willett WC. Calcium, vitamin D, and dairy foods and the occurrence of colon cancer in men. Am J Epidemiol, 1996 May, 143:9, 907-17

11 Martínez ME; Giovannucci EL; Colditz GA; Stampfer MJ; Hunter DJ; Speizer FE; Wing A; Willett WC. Calcium, vitamin D, and the occurrence of colorectal cancer among women. J Natl Cancer Inst, 1996 Oct, 88:19, 1375-82

12 Yang CY; Chiu HF; Chiu JF; Tsai SS; Cheng MF. Calcium and magnesium in drinking water and risk of death from colon cancer. Jpn J Cancer Res, 1997 Oct, 88:10, 928-33

13 Yang CY; Cheng MF; Tsai SS; Hsieh YL Calcium, magnesium, and nitrate in drinking water and gastric cancer mortality. Jpn J Cancer Res, 1998 Feb, 89:2, 124-30

14 McCarron DA Calcium and magnesium nutrition in human hypertension. Ann Intern Med, 1983 May, 98:5 Pt 2, 800-5

15 McCarron DA Role of adequate dietary calcium intake in the prevention and management of salt-sensitive hypertension. Am J Clin Nutr, 1997 Feb, 65:2 Suppl, 712S-716S

16 Wynckel A; Hanrotel C; Wuillai A; Chanard J Intestinal calcium absorption from mineral water. Miner Electrolyte Metab, 1997, 23:2, 88-92

17 Heaney RP; Weaver CM Calcium absorption from kale. Am J Clin Nutr, 1990 Apr, 51:4, 656-7

18 Heaney RP; Smith KT; Recker RR; Hinders SM. Meal effects on calcium absorption. Am J Clin Nutr, 1989 Feb, 49:2, 372-6

19 Feskanich D; Willett WC; Stampfer MJ; Colditz GA Milk, dietary calcium, and bone fractures in women: a 12-year prospective study. Am J Public Health, 1997 Jun, 87:6, 992-7

20 Richardson BE; Baird DD. A study of milk and calcium supplement intake and subsequent preeclampsia in a cohort of pregnant women. Am J Epidemiol, 1995 Apr, 141:7, 667-73

21 Laskey MA; Prentice A; Hanratty LA; Jarjou LMA; Dibba B; Beavan SR; Cole TJ. Bone changes after 3 mo of lactation: influence of calcium intake, breast-milk output, and vitamin D—receptor genotype. Am J Clin Nutr 1998;67:685-92.

22 Kalkwarf HJ, Specker BL, Bianchi DC, Ranz J, Ho M. The effect of calcium supplementation on bone density during lactation and after weaning. N Engl J Med 1997;337:523-8

23 Ritchie LD; Fung EB; Halloran BP; Turnlund JR; Van Loan MD; Cann CE; King JC. A longitudinal study of calcium homeostasis during human pregnancy and lactation and after resumption of menses. Am J Clin Nutr 1998;67:693-701.

24 Harvey JA; Kenny P; Poindexter J; Pak CY Superior calcium absorption from calcium citrate than calcium carbonate using external forearm counting. J Am Coll Nutr, 1990 Dec, 9:6, 583-7

25 Blanchard J; Aeschlimann JM. Calcium absorption in man: some dosing recommendations. J Pharmacokinet Biopharm, 1989 Dec, 17:6, 631-44

26 Heaney RP, Weaver CM. Effect of psyllium on absorption of co-ingested calcium. J Am Geriatr Soc 1995 Mar;43(3):261-263

27 Heaney RP. Calcium supplements: practical considerations. Osteoporos Int 1991 Feb;1(2):65-71

28 Giovannucci E; Rimm EB; Wolk A; Ascherio A; Stampfer MJ; Colditz GA; Willett WC. Calcium and fructose intake in relation to risk of prostate cancer. Cancer Res, 1998 Feb, 58:3, 442-7

29 Nieves JW, Komar L, Cosman F, Lindsay R. Calcium potentiates the effect of estrogen and calcitonin on bone mass: review and analysis. Am J Clin Nutr 1998;67:5-6, 18-24

30 Dawson-Hughes B, Harris SS, Krall EA, Dallal GE. Effect of calcium and vitamin D supplementation on bone density in men and women 65 years of age or older. N Engl J Med 1997 Sep 4;337(10):670-676

31 Lee WT, Leung SS, Leung DM, Cheng JC. A follow-up study on the effects of calcium-supplement withdrawal and puberty on bone acquisition of children. Am J Clin Nutr 1996 Jul;64(1):71-77

32 Buckley LM; Leib ES; Cartularo KS; Vacek PM; Cooper SM. Calcium and vitamin D3 supplementation prevents bone loss in the spine secondary to low-dose corticosteroids in patients with rheumatoid arthritis. A randomized, double-blind, placebo-controlled trial. Ann Intern Med, 1996 Dec, 125:12, 961-8

33 McCarron DA; Morris CD Blood pressure response to oral calcium in persons with mild to moderate hypertension. A randomized, double-blind, placebo-controlled, crossover trial. Ann Intern Med, 1985 Dec, 103:6 (Pt 1), 825-31

34 Yamamoto ME; Applegate WB; Klag MJ; Borhani NO; Cohen JD; Kirchner KA; Lakatos E; Sacks FM; Taylor JO; Hennekens CH Lack of blood pressure effect with calcium and magnesium supplementation in adults with high-normal blood pressure. Results from Phase I of the Trials of Hypertension Prevention (TOHP). Trials of Hypertension Prevention (TOHP) Collaborative Research Group. Ann Epidemiol, 1995 Mar, 5:2, 96-107

35 Belizán JM; Villar J; Bergel E; del Pino A; Di Fulvio S; Galliano SV; Kattan C. Long-term effect of calcium supplementation during pregnancy on the blood pressure of offspring: follow up of a randomised controlled trial. BMJ, 1997 Aug, 315:7103, 281-5

36 Herrera JA; Arevalo Herrera M; Herrera S. Prevention of preeclampsia by linoleic acid and calcium supplementation: a randomized controlled trial. Obstet Gynecol, 1998 Apr, 91:4, 585-90

37 Bucher HC; Guyatt GH; Cook RJ; Hatala R; Cook DJ; Lang JD; Hunt D. Effect of calcium supplementation on pregnancy-induced hypertension and preeclampsia: a meta-analysis of randomized controlled trials. JAMA, 1996 Apr, 275:14, 1113-7

38 Levine RJ; Hauth JC; Curet LB; Sibai BM; Catalano PM; Morris CD; DerSimonian R; Esterlitz JR; Raymond EG; Bild DE; Clemens JD; Cutler JA. Trial of calcium to prevent preeclampsia. N Engl J Med, 1997 Jul, 337:2, 69-76

39 Hallberg L; Brune M; Erlandsson M; Sandberg AS; Rossander-Hultén L. Calcium: effect of different amounts on nonheme- and heme-iron absorption in humans. Am J Clin Nutr, 1991 Jan, 53:1, 112-9

40 Pak CY; Stewart A; Haynes SD Effect of added citrate or malate on calcium absorption from calcium-fortified orange juice. J Am Coll Nutr, 1994 Dec, 13:6, 575-7

41 Hallberg L; Rossander-Hultén L; Brune M; Gleerup A Calcium and iron absorption: mechanism of action and nutritional importance. Eur J Clin Nutr, 1992 May, 46:5, 317-27

42 Deehr MS; Dallal GE; Smith KT; Taulbee JD; Dawson-Hughes B. Effects of different calcium sources on iron absorption in postmenopausal women. Am J Clin Nutr, 1990 Jan, 51:1, 95-9

43 Spencer H; Fuller H; Norris C; Williams D. Effect of magnesium on the intestinal absorption of calcium in man. J Am Coll Nutr, 1994 Oct, 13:5, 485-92

44 Argiratos V; Samman S. The effect of calcium carbonate and calcium citrate on the absorption of zinc in healthy female subjects. Eur J Clin Nutr, 1994 Mar, 48:3, 198-204

45 Wood RJ; Zheng JJ High dietary calcium intakes reduce zinc absorption and balance in humans. Am J Clin Nutr, 1997 Jun, 65:6, 1803-9

Chromium

1 Davies S; McLaren Howard J; Hunnisett A; Howard M. Age-related decreases in chromium levels in 51,665 hair, sweat, and serum samples from 40,872 patients—implications for the prevention of cardiovascular disease and type II diabetes mellitus. Metabolism, 1997 May, 46:5, 469-73

2 Aharoni A; Tesler B; Paltieli Y; Tal J; Dori Z; Sharf M Hair chromium content of women with gestational diabetes compared with nondiabetic pregnant women. Am J Clin Nutr, 1992 Jan, 55:1, 104-7

3 Stearns DM; Wise JP Sr; Patierno SR; Wetterhahn KE. Chromium(III) picolinate produces chromosome damage in Chinese hamster ovary cells. FASEB J, 1995 Dec, 9:15, 1643-8

4 Anderson RA Nutritional factors influencing the glucose/ insulin system: chromium. J Am Coll Nutr, 1997 Oct, 16:5, 404-10

5 Anderson RA; Cheng N; Bryden NA; Polansky MM; Cheng N; Chi J; Feng J. Elevated intakes of supplemental chromium improve glucose and insulin variables in individuals with type 2 diabetes. Diabetes, 1997 Nov, 46:11, 1786-91

6 Lee NA; Reasner CA Beneficial effect of chromium supplementation on serum triglyceride levels in NIDDM. Diabetes Care, 1994 Dec, 17:12, 1449-52

7 Clausen J Chromium induced clinical improvement in symptomatic hypoglycemia. Biol Trace Elem Res, 1988 Sep-Dec, 17:, 229-36

8 Thomas VL; Gropper SS. Effect of chromium nicotinic acid supplementation on selected cardiovascular disease risk factors. Biol Trace Elem Res, 1996 Dec, 55:3, 297-305

9 Bahadori B; Wallner S; Schneider H; Wascher TC; Toplak H. Effect of chromium yeast and chromium picolinate on body composition of obese, non-diabetic patients during and after a formula diet. Acta Med Austriaca, 1997, 24:5, 185-7

10 Grant KE; Chandler RM; Castle AL; Ivy JL. Chromium and exercise training: effect on obese women. Med Sci Sports Exerc, 1997 Aug, 29:8, 992-8

11 McCarty MF Anabolic effects of insulin on bone suggest a role for chromium picolinate in preservation of bone density. Med Hypotheses, 1995 Sep, 45:3, 241-6

12 McCarty M. High-chromium yeast for acne? Med Hypotheses, 1984 Jul, 14:3, 307-10

Copper

1 Schuschke DA. Dietary copper in the physiology of the microcirculation. Nutr, 1997 Dec, 127:12, 2274-81

2 Kremer JM; Bigaouette J Nutrient intake of patients with rheumatoid arthritis is deficient in pyridoxine, zinc, copper, and magnesium. J Rheumatol, 1996 Jun, 23:6, 990-4

3 Lukaski HC; Klevay LM; Milne DB Effects of dietary copper on human autonomic cardiovascular function. Eur J Appl Physiol, 1988, 58:1-2, 74-80

4 Knobeloch L; Schubert C; Hayes J; Clark J; Fitzgerald C; Fraundorff A Gastrointestinal upsets and new copper plumbing—is there a connection? WMJ, 1998 Jan, 97:1, 49-53

5 Jones AA; DiSilvestro RA; Coleman M; Wagner TL Copper supplementation of adult men: effects on blood copper enzyme activities and indicators of cardiovascular disease risk. Metabolism, 1997 Dec, 46:12, 1380-3

6 Serum copper/zinc superoxide dismutase levels in patients with rheumatoid arthritis. Mazzetti I; Grigolo B; Borzì RM; Meliconi R; Facchini A. Int J Clin Lab Res, 1996, 26:4, 245-9

Electrolytes

1 Whelton P K et al. Effects of oral potassium on blood pressure. JAMA 1997;277:1624-1632

2 Sacks FM, Willett WC, Smith A, Brown LE, Rosner B, Moore TJ. Effect on blood pressure of potassium, calcium, and magnesium in women with low habitual intake. Hypertension 1998 Jan;31(1):131-138

3 Young DB, Lin H, McCabe RD. Potassium's cardiovascular protective mechanisms. Am J Physiol 1995 Apr;268(4 Pt 2):R825-R837

4 Ettinger B et al. Potassium magnesium citrate is an effective prophylaxis against recurrent calcium oxalate nephrolithiasis. Journal of Urology 1997;158:2069-73

5 Beard TC; Blizzard L; OBrien DJ; Dwyer T. Association between blood pressure and dietary factors in the dietary and nutritional survey of British adults. Arch Intern Med 1997;157:234-238

6 Cappuccio FP; Markandu ND; Carney C; Sagnella GA; MacGregor GA. Double-blind randomised trial of modest salt restriction in older people. Lancet, 1997 Sep, 350:9081, 850-4

7 Graudal NA et al. Effects of Sodium Restriction on Blood Pressure, Renin, Aldosterone, Catecholamines, Cholesterols, and Triglyceride. JAMA. 1998;279:1383-1391

8 Geleijnse JM; Hofman A; Witteman JC; Hazebroek AA; Valkenburg HA; Grobbee DE. Long-term effects of neonatal sodium restriction on blood pressure. Hypertension, 1997 Apr, 29:4, 913-7

9 Rollnik JD; Mills PJ; Dimsdale JE. Characteristics of individuals who excrete versus retain sodium under stress. J Psychosom Res, 1995 May, 39:4, 499-505

10 Devine A; Criddle RA; Dick IM; Kerr DA; Prince RL. A longitudinal study of the effect of sodium and calcium intakes on regional bone density in postmenopausal women. Am J Clin Nutr, 1995 Oct, 62:4, 740-5

11 Carey OJ; Locke C; Cookson JB Effect of alterations of dietary sodium on the severity of asthma in men. Thorax, 1993 Jul, 48:7, 714-8

12 Cirillo M; Laurenzi M; Panarelli W; Stamler J. Urinary sodium to potassium ratio and urinary stone disease. The Gubbio Population Study Research Group. Kidney Int, 1994 Oct, 46:4, 1133-9

Fluoride

1 Tohyama E. Relationship between fluoride concentration in drinking water and mortality rate from uterine cancer in Okinawa prefecture, Japan. Epidemiol, 1996 Dec, 6:4, 184-91

2 Heilman JR; Kiritsy MC; Levy SM; Wefel JS Fluoride concentrations of infant foods. J Am Dent Assoc, 1997 Jul, 128:7, 857-63

3 Murray TM; Ste Marie LG Prevention and management of osteoporosis: consensus statements from the Scientific Advisory Board of the Osteoporosis Society of Canada. 7. Fluoride therapy for osteoporosis. CMAJ, 1996 Oct, 155:7, 949-54

4 Ann Int Med 1998;129:1-8

5 Pak CYC, et. al. Treatment of postmenopausal osteoporosis with slow-release sodium fluoride. Annals of Internal Medicine 1995 September 15;123(6):401-408.

6 Talbot JR; Fischer MM; Farley SM; Libanati C; Farley J; Tabuenca A; Baylink DJ. The increase in spinal bone density that occurs in response to fluoride therapy for osteoporosis is not maintained after the therapy is discontinued. Osteoporos Int, 1996, 6:6, 442-7

7 Sowers MF; Clark MK; Jannausch ML; Wallace RB A prospective study of bone mineral content and fracture in communities with differential fluoride exposure. Am J Epidemiol, 1991 Apr 1, 133:7, 649-60

8 Adachi JD et al. Fluoride therapy in prevention of rheumatoid arthritis induced bone loss. J Rheumatol, 1997 Dec, 24:12, 2308-13

Iodine

1 Smyth PP. Thyroid disease and breast cancer. J Endocrinol Invest, 1993 May, 16:5, 396-401

2 Ghent WR; Eskin BA; Low DA; Hill LP Iodine replacement in fibrocystic disease of the breast. Can J Surg, 1993 Oct, 36:5, 453-60

Iron

1 Uzel C; Conrad ME Absorption of heme iron. Semin Hematol, 1998 Jan, 35:1, 27-34

2 García Casal MN et al. Vitamin A and beta-carotene can improve nonheme iron absorption from rice, wheat and corn by humans. J Nutr, 1998 Mar, 128:3, 646-50

3 Looker AC; Dallman PR; Carroll MD; Gunter EW; Johnson CL. Prevalence of iron deficiency in the United States. JAMA, 1997 Mar, 277:12, 973-6

4 van Iperen CE; Kraaijenhagen RJ; Biesma DH; Beguin Y; Marx JJ; van de Wiel A. Iron metabolism and erythropoiesis after surgery. Br J Surg, 1998 Jan, 85:1, 41-5

5 Corti MC; Guralnik JM; Salive ME; Ferrucci L; Pahor M; Wallace RB; Hennekens CH. Serum iron level, coronary artery disease, and all-cause mortality in older men and women. Am J Cardiol, 1997 Jan, 79:2, 120-7

6 Innis SM; Nelson CM; Wadsworth LD; MacLaren IA; Lwanga D. Incidence of iron-deficiency anaemia and depleted iron stores among nine-month-old infants in Vancouver, Canada. Can J Public Health, 1997 Mar, 88:2, 80-4

7 Tzonou A; Lagiou P; Trichopoulou A; Tsoutsos V; Trichopoulos D. Dietary iron and coronary heart disease risk: a study from Greece. Am J Epidemiol, 1998 Jan, 147:2, 161-6

8 Kiechl S; Willeit J; Egger G; Poewe W; Oberhollenzer F. Body iron stores and the risk of carotid atherosclerosis: prospective results from the Bruneck study. Circulation, 1997 Nov, 96:10, 3300-7

9 Tuomainen TP; Punnonen K; Nyyssönen K; Salonen JT Association between body iron stores and the risk of acute myocardial infarction in men. Circulation, 1998 Apr, 97:15, 1461-6

10 Salonen et al. Am J Epidemiol. 1998;148:445-451

11 Tseng M; Sandler RS; Greenberg ER; Mandel JS; Haile RW; Baron JA. Dietary iron and recurrence of colorectal adenomas. Cancer Epidemiol Biomarkers Prev, 1997 Dec, 6:12, 1029-32

12 Stevens R et al. Moderate elevation of body iron level and increased risk of cancer occurrence and death. Int J Cancer 1994;56:364-369

13 Ribaya Mercado JD Importance of adequate vitamin A status during iron supplementation. Nutr Rev, 1997 Aug, 55:8, 306-7

14 Bruner A et al. Randomised study of cognitive effects of iron supplementation in non-anaemic iron-deficient adolescent girls. Lancet. 1996;348:973, 992-996

15 Agte VV; Paknikar KM; Chiplonkar SA. Effect of nicotinic acid on zinc and iron metabolism. Biometals, 1997 Oct, 10:4, 271-6

Magnesium

1 Spencer H; Fuller H; Norris C; Williams D Effect of magnesium on the intestinal absorption of calcium in man. J Am Coll Nutr, 1994 Oct, 13:5, 485-92

2 Rubenowitz E; Axelsson G; Rylander R. Magnesium in drinking water and death from acute myocardial infarction. Am J Epidemiol, 1996 Mar, 143:5, 456-62

3 Yang CY; Chiu HF; Chiu JF; Wang TN; Cheng MF Magnesium and calcium in drinking water and cerebrovascular mortality in Taiwan. Magnes Res, 1997 Mar, 10:1, 51-7

4 Ma J et al. Associations of serum and dietary magnesium with cardiovascular disease, hypertension, diabetes, insulin,

and carotid arterial wall thickness: the ARIC study. Atherosclerosis Risk in Communities. J Clin Epidemiol, 1995 Jul, 48:7, 927-40

5 Elwood PC; Fehily AM; Ising H; Poor DJ; Pickering J; Kamel F Dietary magnesium does not predict ischaemic heart disease in the Caerphilly cohort. Eur J Clin Nutr, 1996 Oct, 50:10, 694-7

6 Goto K; Yasue H; Okumura K; Matsuyama K; Kugiyama K; Miyagi H; Higashi T Magnesium deficiency detected by intravenous loading test in variant angina pectoris. Am J Cardiol, 1990 Mar 15, 65:11, 709-12

7 Satake K; Lee JD; Shimizu H; Ueda T; Nakamura T Relation between severity of magnesium deficiency and frequency of anginal attacks in men with variant angina. J Am Coll Cardiol, 1996 Oct, 28:4, 897-902

8 Joffres MR; Reed DM; Yano K. Relationship of magnesium intake and other dietary factors to blood pressure: the Honolulu heart study. Am J Clin Nutr, 1987 Feb, 45:2, 469-75

9 Witteman JC et al. A prospective study of nutritional factors and hypertension among US women. Circulation, 1989 Nov, 80:5, 1320-7

10 Ascherio A et al. A prospective study of nutritional factors and hypertension among US men. Circulation, 1992 Nov, 86:5, 1475-84

11 Paolisso G; Barbagallo M Hypertension, diabetes mellitus, and insulin resistance: the role of intracellular magnesium. Am J Hypertens, 1997 Mar, 10:3, 346-55

12 Tucker K et al. Magnesium intake is associated with bone mineral density (BMD) in elderly women. J Bone Miner Res, 1995, 10S:466

13 Rude RK et al. Low serum concentrations of 1,25-dihydroxyvitamin D in human magnesium deficiency. J Clin Endocrinol Metab, 1985 Nov, 61:5, 933-40

14 Fatemi S; Ryzen E; Flores J; Endres DB; Rude RK. Effect of experimental human magnesium depletion on parathyroid hormone secretion and 1,25-dihydroxyvitamin D metabolism. J Clin Endocrinol Metab, 1991 Nov, 73:5, 1067-72

15 Zofková I; Kancheva RL. The relationship between magnesium and calciotropic hormones. Magnes Res, 1995 Mar, 8:1, 77-84

16 Gallai V; Sarchielli P; Morucci P; Abbritti G. Red blood cell magnesium levels in migraine patients. Cephalalgia, 1993 Apr, 13:2, 94-81; discussion 73

17 Muneyvirci Delale O; Nacharaju VL; Altura BM; Altura BT. Sex steroid hormones modulate serum ionized magnesium and calcium levels throughout the menstrual cycle in women. Fertil Steril, 1998 May, 69:5, 958-62

18 Moreno Díaz MT et al. Magnesium deficiency in patients with HIV-AIDS. Nutr Hosp, 1997 Nov, 12:6, 304-8

19 J Am Coll Nutr 1998,17:124-27

20 Yang CY; Cheng MF; Tsai SS; Hsieh YL Calcium, magnesium, and nitrate in drinking water and gastric cancer mortality. Jpn J Cancer Res, 1998 Feb, 89:2, 124-30

21 Fine KD; Santa Ana CA; Porter JL; Fordtran JS Intestinal absorption of magnesium from food and supplements. J Clin Invest, 1991 Aug, 88:2, 396-402

22 Rabbani LE; Antman EM The role of magnesium therapy in acute myocardial infarction. Clin Cardiol, 1996 Nov, 19:11, 841-4

23 Woods KL; Fletcher S Long-term outcome after intravenous magnesium sulphate in suspected acute myocardial infarction: the second Leicester Intravenous Magnesium Intervention Trial (LIMIT-2). Lancet, 1994 Apr, 343:8901, 816-9

24 ISIS-4: a randomised factorial trial assessing early oral captopril, oral mononitrate, and intravenous magnesium sulphate in 58,050 patients with suspected acute myocardial infarction. ISIS-4 (Fourth International Study of Infarct Survival) Collaborative Group Lancet, 1995 Mar, 345:8951, 669-85

25 Zehender M; Meinertz T; Faber T; Caspary A; Jeron A; Bremm K; Just H Antiarrhythmic effects of increasing the daily intake of magnesium and potassium in patients with frequent ventricular arrhythmias. Magnesium in Cardiac Arrhythmias (MAGICA) Investigators. J Am Coll Cardiol, 1997 Apr, 29:5, 1028-34

26 Redwood SR; Bashir Y; Huang J; Leatham EW; Kaski JC; Camm AJ Effect of magnesium sulphate in patients with unstable angina. A double blind, randomized, placebo-controlled study. Eur Heart J, 1997 Aug, 18:8, 1269-77

27 Lichodziejewska B; K et al. Clinical symptoms of mitral valve prolapse are related to hypomagnesemia and attenuated by magnesium supplementation. Am J Cardiol, 1997 Mar, 79:6, 768-72

28 Itoh K; Kawasaka T; Nakamura M The effects of high oral magnesium supplementation on blood pressure, serum lipids and related variables in apparently healthy Japanese subjects. Br J Nutr, 1997 Nov, 78:5, 737-50

29 Witteman J et al. Reduction of blood pressure with oral magnesium supplementation in women with mild to moderate hypertension. Am J Clin Nutr. 1994;60:129-135

30 Ettinger B; Pak CY; Citron JT; Thomas C; Adams Huet B; Vangessel A. Potassium-magnesium citrate is an effective prophylaxis against recurrent calcium oxalate nephrolithiasis. J Urol, 1997 Dec, 158:6, 2069-73

31 Rodgers AL Effect of mineral water containing calcium and magnesium on calcium oxalate urolithiasis risk factors. Urol Int, 1997, 58:2, 93-9

32 Chien PF; Khan KS; Arnott N. Magnesium sulphate in the treatment of eclampsia and pre-eclampsia: an overview of the evidence from randomised trials. Br J Obstet Gynaecol, 1996 Nov, 103:11, 1085-91

33 Schendel DE; Berg CJ; Yeargin Allsopp M; Boyle CA; Decoufle P Prenatal magnesium sulfate exposure and the risk for cerebral palsy or mental retardation among very low-birth-weight children aged 3 to 5 years. JAMA, 1996 Dec, 276:22, 1805-10

34 Dahle LO; Berg G; Hammar M; Hurtig M; Larsson L The effect of oral magnesium substitution on pregnancy-induced leg cramps. Am J Obstet Gynecol, 1995 Jul, 173:1, 175-80

35 Paolisso G et al. Changes in glucose turnover parameters and improvement of glucose oxidation after 4-week magnesium administration in elderly noninsulin-dependent (type II) diabetic patients. J Clin Endocrinol Metab, 1994 Jun, 78:6, 1510-4

36 Gilleran G; OLeary M; Bartlett WA; Vinall H; Jones AF; Dodson PM Effects of dietary sodium substitution with potassium and magnesium in hypertensive type II diabetics: a randomised blind controlled parallel study. J Hum Hypertens, 1996 Aug, 10:8, 517-21

37 Hill J; Micklewright A; Lewis S; Britton J Investigation of the effect of short-term change in dietary magnesium intake in asthma. Eur Respir J, 1997 Oct, 10:10, 2225-9

38 Ciarallo L; Sauer AH; Shannon MW a Intravenous magnesium therapy for moderate to severe pediatric asthma: results of a randomized, placebo-controlled trial. J Pediatr, 1996 Dec, 129:6, 809-14

39 Emelianova AV; Goncharova VA; Sinitsina TM. Magnesium sulfate in management of bronchial asthma. Klin Med (Mosk), 1996, 74:8, 55-8

40 Peikert A; Wilimzig C; Köhne Volland R Prophylaxis of migraine with oral magnesium: results from a prospective, multi-center, placebo-controlled and double-blind randomized study. Cephalalgia, 1996 Jun, 16:4, 257-63

41 Facchinetti F; Sances G; Borella P; Genazzani AR; Nappi G Magnesium prophylaxis of menstrual migraine: effects on intracellular magnesium. Headache, 1991 May, 31:5, 298-301

42 Facchinetti F; Borella P; Sances G; Fioroni L; Nappi RE; Genazzani AR Oral magnesium successfully relieves premenstrual mood changes. Obstet Gynecol, 1991 Aug, 78:2, 177-81

43 Cox IM; Campbell MJ; Dowson D. Red blood cell magnesium and chronic fatigue syndrome. Lancet, 1991 Mar 30, 337:8744, 757-60

44 Abraham GE; Grewal H A total dietary program emphasizing magnesium instead of calcium. Effect on the mineral density of calcaneous bone in postmenopausal women on hormonal therapy. J Reprod Med, 1990 May, 35:5, 503-7

45 Stendig-Lindberg G; Tepper R; Leichter I. Trabecular bone density in a two year controlled trial of peroral magnesium in osteoporosis. Magnes Res, 1993 Jun, 6:2, 155-63

Manganese

1 Keller JN et al. Mitochondrial manganese superoxide dismutase prevents neural apoptosis and reduces ischemic brain injury: suppression of peroxynitrite production, lipid peroxidation, and mitochondrial dysfunction. J Neurosci, 1998 Jan, 18:2, 687-97

2 Thome J; Foley P; Gsell W; Davids E; Wodarz N; Wiesbeck GA; Böning J; Riederer P. Increased concentrations of manganese superoxide dismutase in serum of alcohol-dependent patients. Alcohol Alcohol, 1997 Jan, 32:1, 65-9

3 Baly D et al. Effect of manganese deficiency on insulin binding, glucose transport and metabolism in rat adipocytes. J Nutr. 1990;120:1075-1079

4 Pasquier C et al. Manganese containing superoxide dismutase deficiency in polymorphonuclear lymphocytes in rheumatoid arthritis. Inflammation. 1984;8:27-32

Molybdenum

1 Turnlund JR; Keyes WR; Peiffer GL. Molybdenum absorption, excretion, and retention studied with stable isotopes in young men at five intakes of dietary molybdenum. Am J Clin Nutr, 1995 Oct, 62:4, 790-6

2 Sardesai VM. Molybdenum: an essential trace element. Nutr Clin Pract, 1993 Dec, 8:6, 277-81

3 Nakadaira H; Endoh K; Yamamoto M; Katoh K Distribution of selenium and molybdenum and cancer mortality in Niigata, Japan. Arch Environ Health, 1995 Sep, 50:5, 374-80

4 Brewer G J. Practical recommendations and new therapies for Wilson's disease. Drugs. 1995;50:240-249

Nickel

1 Panzani RC; Schiavino D; Nucera E; Pellegrino S; Fais G; Schinco G; Patriarca G. Oral hyposensitization to nickel allergy: preliminary clinical results. Int Arch Allergy Immunol, 1995 May, 107:1-3, 251-4

Phosphorus

1 Grenby T H, Saldanha M G. The use of high-phosphorus supplements to inhibity dental enamel demineralisation by ice lollies. Int J Food Sci Nutr. 1995;46:275-9

2 Calvo MS; Park YK Changing phosphorus content of the U.S. diet: potential for adverse effects on bone. J Nutr, 1996 Apr, 126:4 Suppl, 1168S-80S

3 Portale AA; Halloran BP; Morris RC Jr; Lonergan ET Effect of aging on the metabolism of phosphorus and 1,25-dihydroxyvitamin D in healthy men. Am J Physiol, 1996 Mar, 270:3 Pt 1, E483-90

4 Narang R; Ridout D; Nonis C; Kooner JS Serum calcium, phosphorus and albumin levels in relation to the angiographic severity of coronary artery disease. Int J Cardiol, 1997 Jun, 60:1, 73-9

Selenium

1 Olivieri O; Girelli D; Stanzial AM; Rossi L; Bassi A; Corrocher R Selenium, zinc, and thyroid hormones in healthy subjects: low T3/T4 ratio in the elderly is related to impaired selenium status. Biol Trace Elem Res, 1996 Jan, 51:1, 31-41

2 Russo MW; Murray SC; Wurzelmann JI; Woosley JT; Sandler RS Plasma selenium levels and the risk of colorectal adenomas. Nutr Cancer, 1997, 28:2, 125-9

3 Psathakis D; Wedemeyer N; Oevermann E; Krug F; Siegers CP; Bruch HP Blood selenium and glutathione peroxidase status in patients with colorectal cancer. Dis Colon Rectum, 1998 Mar, 41:3, 328-35

4 van den Brandt PA; Goldbohm RA; van 't Veer P; Bode P; Dorant E; Hermus RJ; Sturmans F A prospective cohort study on selenium status and the risk of lung cancer. Cancer Res, 1993 Oct 15, 53:20, 4860-5

5 Vitoux D; Chappuis P; Arnaud J; Bost M; Accominotti M; Roussel AM Selenium, glutathione peroxidase, peroxides and platelet functions. Ann Biol Clin (Paris), 1996, 54:5, 181-7

6 Kok FJ; Hofman A; Witteman JC; de Bruijn AM; Kruyssen DH; de Bruin M; Valkenburg HA. Decreased selenium levels in acute myocardial infarction. JAMA, 1989 Feb 24, 261:8, 1161-4

7 Salvini S; Hennekens CH; Morris JS; Willett WC; Stampfer MJ. Plasma levels of the antioxidant selenium and risk of myocardial infarction among U.S. physicians. Am J Cardiol, 1995 Dec, 76:17, 1218-21

8 Barrington JW; Lindsay P; James D; Smith S; Roberts A Selenium deficiency and miscarriage: a possible link? Br J Obstet Gynaecol, 1996 Feb, 103:2, 130-2

9 Shaw R, Woodman K, Crane J, Moyes C, Kennedy J, Pearce N. Risk factors for asthma symptoms in Kawerau children. N Z Med J. 1994;107:387-391.

10 Flatt A, Pearce N, Thomson CD, Sears MR, Robinson MF, Beasley R. Reduced selenium in asthmatic subjects in New Zealand. Thorax. 1990;45:95-99

11 Karaküçük S et al. Selenium concentrations in serum, lens and aqueous humour of patients with senile cataract. Acta Ophthalmol Scand, 1995 Aug, 73:4, 329-32

12 Hawkes WC; Hornbostel L Effects of dietary selenium on mood in healthy men living in a metabolic research unit. Biol Psychiatry, 1996 Jan, 39:2, 121-8

13 Clark LC et al. Effects of selenium supplementation for cancer prevention in patients with carcinoma of the skin. A randomized controlled trial. Nutritional Prevention of Cancer Study Group. JAMA, 1996 Dec, 276:24, 1957-63

15 Korpela H; Kumpulainen J; Jussila E; Kemilä S; Kääriäinen M; Kääriäinen T; Sotaniemi EA Effect of selenium supplementation after acute myocardial infarction. Res Commun Chem Pathol Pharmacol, 1989 Aug, 65:2, 249-52

16 Thiele R; Wagner D; Gassel M; Winnefeld K; Pleissner J; Pfeifer R Selenium substitution in acute myocardial infarct. Med Klin, 1997 Sep, 92 Suppl 3:, 26-8

14 Reddy BS et al. Chemoprevention of colon cancer by organoselenium compounds and impact of high or low fat diets. J Natl Cancer Inst 1997, 89:506-12

17 Hasselmark L, Malmgren R, Zetterstrom O, Unge G. Selenium supplementation in intrinsic asthma. Allergy. 1993;48:3026.

18 Heinle K; Adam A; Gradl M; Wiseman M; Adam O. Selenium concentration in erythrocytes of patients with rheumatoid arthritis. Clinical and laboratory chemistry infection markers during administration of selenium. Med Klin, 1997 Sep, 92 Suppl 3:, 29-31

19 Robinson MF; Thomson CD; Huemmer PK. Effect of a megadose of ascorbic acid, a meal and orange juice on the absorption of selenium as sodium selenite. N Z Med J, 1985 Aug 14, 98:784, 627-9

Vanadium

1 Naylor GJ; Corrigan FM; Smith AH; Connelly P; Ward NI Further studies of vanadium in depressive psychosis. Br J Psychiatry, 1987 May, 150:, 656-61

2 Verma S; Cam MC; McNeill JH. Nutritional factors that can favorably influence the glucose/insulin system: vanadium. J Am Coll Nutr, 1998 Feb, 17:1, 11-8

3 Halberstam M; Cohen N; Shlimovich P; Rossetti L; Shamoon H Oral vanadyl sulfate improves insulin sensitivity in NIDDM but not in obese nondiabetic subjects. Diabetes, 1996 May, 45:5, 659-66

4 Hanauske U; Hanauske AR; Marshall MH; Muggia VA; Von Hoff DD. Biphasic effect of vanadium salts on in vitro tumor colony growth. Int J Cell Cloning, 1987 Mar, 5:2, 170-8

5 Fawcett JP; Farquhar SJ; Walker RJ; Thou T; Lowe G; Goulding A. The effect of oral vanadyl sulfate on body composition and performance in weight-training athletes. Int J Sport Nutr, 1996 Dec, 6:4, 382-90

Zinc

1 Fung EB; Ritchie LD; Woodhouse LR; Roehl R; King JC Zinc absorption in women during pregnancy and lactation: a longitudinal study. Am J Clin Nutr, 1997 Jul, 66:1, 80-8

2 Herzberg M; Lusky A; Blonder J; Frenkel Y. HRT appears to decrease zinc excretion. Title The effect of estrogen replacement therapy on zinc in serum and urine. Obstet Gynecol, 1996 Jun, 87:6, 1035-40

3 Mares Perlman JA; Subar AF; Block G; Greger JL; Luby MH. Zinc intake and sources in the US adult population: 1976-1980. J Am Coll Nutr, 1995 Aug, 14:4, 349-57

4 Haglund B; Ryckenberg K; Selinus O; Dahlquist G Evidence of a relationship between childhood-onset type I diabetes and low groundwater concentration of zinc. Diabetes Care, 1996 Aug, 19:8, 873-5

5 Reunanen A; Knekt P; Marniemi J; Mäki J; Maatela J; Aromaa A Serum calcium, magnesium, copper and zinc and risk of cardiovascular death. Eur J Clin Nutr, 1996 Jul, 50:7, 431-7

6 Hennig B; Toborek M; Mcclain CJ Antiatherogenic properties of zinc: implications in endothelial cell metabolism. Nutrition, 1996 Oct, 12:10, 711-7

7 Mares Perlman JA; Klein R; Klein BE; Greger JL; Brady WE; Palta M; Ritter LL. Association of zinc and antioxidant nutrients with age-related maculopathy. Arch Ophthalmol, 1996 Aug, 114:8, 991-7

8 Chuong CJ; Dawson EB Zinc and copper levels in premenstrual syndrome. Fertil Steril, 1994 Aug, 62:2, 313-20

9 Prasad AS; Mantzoros CS; Beck FW; Hess JW; Brewer GJ. Zinc status and serum testosterone levels of healthy adults. Nutrition, 1996 May, 12:5, 344-8

10 Golub MS; Keen CL; Gershwin ME; Styne DM; Takeuchi PT; Ontell F; Walter RM; and Hendrickx AG. Adolescent growth and maturation in zinc-deprived rhesus monkeys. Am J Clin Nutr 1996;64:274-82.

11 Naveh Y; Schapira D; Ravel Y; Geller E; Scharf Y Zinc metabolism in rheumatoid arthritis: plasma and urinary zinc and relationship to disease activity. J Rheumatol, 1997 Apr, 24:4, 643-6

12 Kadrabová J; Madaric A; Podivínsky F; Gazdík F; Ginter F Plasma zinc, copper and copper/zinc ratio in intrinsic asthma. J Trace Elem Med Biol, 1996 Apr, 10:1, 50-3

13 Rivera JA; Ruel MT; Santizo MC; Lönnerdal B; Brown KH. Zinc supplementation improves the growth of stunted rural Guatemalan infants. J Nutr, 1998 Mar, 128:3, 556-62

14 Cakman I; Kirchner H; Rink L. Zinc supplementation reconstitutes the production of interferon-alpha by leukocytes from elderly persons. J Interferon Cytokine Res, 1997 Aug, 17:8, 469-72

15 Bogden JD; Oleske JM; Lavenhar MA; Munves EM; Kemp FW; Bruening KS; Holding KJ; Denny TN; Guarino MA; Holland BK. J Am Coll Nutr, 1990 Jun, 9:3, 214-25

16 Fortes C et al; The effect of zinc and vitamin A supplementation on immune response in an older population. J Am Geriatr Soc, 1998 Jan, 46:1, 19-26

17 Sazawal S; Black RE; Bhan MK; Jalla S; Sinha A; Bhandari N. Efficacy of zinc supplementation in reducing the incidence and prevalence of acute diarrhea—a community-based, double-blind, controlled trial. Am J Clin Nutr, 1997 Aug, 66:2, 413-8

18 Garland ML; Hagmeyer KO The role of zinc lozenges in treatment of the common cold. Ann Pharmacother, 1998 Jan, 32:1, 63-9

19 Mossad SB; Macknin ML; Medendorp SV; Mason P. Zinc gluconate lzenges for treating the common cold. A randomized, double-blind, placebo-controlled study. Ann Intern Med, 1996 Jul, 125:2, 81-8

20 Eby GA Zinc ion availability—the determinant of efficacy in zinc lozenge treatment of common colds. J Antimicrob Chemother, 1997 Oct, 40:4, 483-93

21 Macknin ML et al. Zinc Gluconate Lozenges for Treating the Common Cold in Children. JAMA. 1998;279:1962-1967

22 Young B; Ott L; Kasarskis E; Rapp R; Moles K; Dempsey RJ; Tibbs PA; Kryscio R; McClain C. Zinc supplementation is associated with improved neurologic recovery rate and visceral protein levels of patients with severe closed head injury. J Neurotrauma, 1996 Jan, 13:1, 25-34

23 Mocchegiani E. Benefit of oral zinc supplementation as an adjunct to zidovudine (AZT) therapy against opportunistic infections in AIDS. Int J Immunopharmacol, 17: 9, 1995 Sep, 719-27

24 Goldenberg RL et al. The effect of zinc supplementation on pregnancy outcome. JAMA. 1995;274:463-468

25 Birmingham CL; Goldner EM; Bakan R Controlled trial of zinc supplementation in anorexia nervosa. Int J Eat Disord, 1994 Apr, 15:3, 251-5

26 Heyneman CA Zinc deficiency and taste disorders. Ann Pharmacother, 1996 Feb, 30:2, 186-7

27 Brun JF; Guintrand Hugret R; Fons C; Carvajal J; Fedou C; Fussellier M; Bardet L; Orsetti A Effects of oral zinc gluconate on glucose effectiveness and insulin sensitivity in humans. Biol Trace Elem Res, 1995 Jan, 47:1-3, 385-91

28 Leake A; Chisholm GD; Habib FK. The effect of zinc on the 5 alpha-reduction of testosterone by the hyperplastic human prostate gland. J Steroid Biochem, 1984 Feb, 20:2, 651-5

29 Leake A; Chisholm GD; Habib FK Interaction between prolactin and zinc in the human prostate gland. J Endocrinol, 1984 Jul, 102:1, 73-6

30 Newsome D A et al. Oral zinc in macular degeneration. Arch Opthalmol. 1988;106:192-198

31 Fortes C; Agabiti N; Fano V; Pacifici R; Forastiere F; Virgili F; Zuccaro P; Perruci CA; Ebrahim S Zinc supplementation and plasma lipid peroxides in an elderly population. Eur J Clin Nutr, 1997 Feb, 51:2, 97-101

32 Ochi K; Ohashi T; Kinoshita H; Akagi M; Kikuchi H; Mitsui M; Kaneko T; Kato I[The serum zinc level in patients with tinnitus and the effect of zinc treatment] Nippon Jibiinkoka Gakkai Kaiho, 1997 Sep, 100:9, 915-9

33 Walsh WJ; Isaacson HR; Rehman F; Hall A. Elevated blood copper/zinc ratios in assaultive young males. Physiol Behav, 1997 Aug, 62:2, 327-9

34 Wood RJ; Zheng JJ High dietary calcium intakes reduce zinc absorption and balance in humans. Am J Clin Nutr, 1997 Jun, 65:6, 1803-9

35 33 McKenna AA; Ilich JZ; Andon MB; Wang C; Matkovic V Zinc balance in adolescent females consuming a low- or high-calcium diet. Am J Clin Nutr, 1997 May, 65:5, 1460-4

36 Golik A; Zaidenstein R; Dishi V; Blatt A; Cohen N; Cotter G; Berman S; Weissgarten J. Effects of captopril and enalapril on zinc metabolism in hypertensive patients. J Am Coll Nutr, 1998 Feb, 17:1, 75-8

Essential fatty acids

1 Kromhout D; Bosschieter EB; de Lezenne Coulander C. The inverse relation between fish consumption and 20-year mortality from coronary heart disease. N Engl J Med, 1985 May 9, 312:19, 1205-9

2 Morris MC; Manson JE; Rosner B; Buring JE; Willett WC; Hennekens CH. Fish consumption and cardiovascular disease in the physicians' health study: a prospective study. Am J Epidemiol, 1995 Jul, 142:2, 166-75

3 Ascherio A; Rimm EB; Stampfer MJ; Giovannucci EL; Willett WC. Dietary intake of marine n-3 fatty acids, fish intake, and the risk of coronary disease among men. N Engl J Med, 1995 Apr, 332:15, 977-82

4 Burr ML et al. Effects of changes in fat, fish, and fibre intakes on death and myocardial reinfarction: diet and reinfarction trial (DART). Lancet, 1989 Sep 30, 2:8666, 757-61

5 Daviglus ML, Stamler J, Orencia AJ, et al. Fish consumption and the30-year risk of fatal myocardial infarction. N Engl J Med. 1997;336:1046-1053.

6 Albert CM; Hennekens CH; ODonnell CJ; Ajani UA; Carey VJ; Willett WC; Ruskin JN; Manson JE. Fish consumption and risk of sudden cardiac death. JAMA, 1998 Jan, 279:1, 23-8

7 Siscovick DS et al. Dietary intake and cell membrane levels of long-chain n-3 polyunsaturated fatty acids and the risk of primary cardiac arrest. JAMA, 1995 Nov, 274:17, 1363-7

8 Salonen JT, Seppaenen K, Nyyssoenen K, et al. Intake of mercury from fish, lipid peroxidation and the risk of myocardial infarction and coronary, cardiovascular, and any death in Eastern Finnish men. Circulation. 1995;91:645655.

9 Simon JA; Fong J; Bernert JT Jr; Browner WS. Serum fatty acids and the risk of stroke. Stroke, 1995 May, 26:5, 778-82

10 Rose DP Dietary fatty acids and prevention of hormone-responsive cancer. Proc Soc Exp Biol Med, 1997 Nov, 216:2, 224-33

11 Godley PA; Campbell MK; Gallagher P; Martinson FE; Mohler JL; Sandler RS. Biomarkers of essential fatty acid consumption and risk of prostatic carcinoma. Cancer Epidemiol Biomarkers Prev, 1996 Nov, 5:11, 889-95

12 Bougnoux P; Koscielny S; Chajès V; Descamps P; Couet C; Calais G. alpha-Linolenic acid content of adipose breast tissue: a host determinant of the risk of early metastasis in breast cancer. Br J Cancer, 1994 Aug, 70:2, 330-4

13 Simonsen N; vant Veer P; Strain JJ; Martin Moreno JM; Huttunen JK; Navajas JF; Martin BC; Thamm M; Kardinaal AF; Kok FJ; Kohlmeier L. Adipose tissue omega-3 and omega-6 fatty acid content and breast cancer in the EURAMIC study. European Community Multicenter Study on Antioxidants, Myocardial Infarction, and Breast Cancer. Am J Epidemiol, 1998 Feb, 147:4, 342-52

14 Caygill CP; Hill MJ. Fish, n-3 fatty acids and human colorectal and breast cancer mortality. Eur J Cancer Prev, 1995 Aug, 4:4, 329-32

15 Shapiro JA; Koepsell TD; Voigt LF; Dugowson CE; Kestin M; Nelson JL Diet and rheumatoid arthritis in women: a possible protective effect of fish consumption. Epidemiology, 1996 May, 7:3, 256-63

16 Sakai K; Okuyama H; Shimazaki H; Katagiri M; Torii S; Matsushita T; Baba S. Fatty acid compositions of plasma lipids in atopic dermatitis/asthma patients. Arerugi, 1994 Jan, 43:1, 37-43

17 Hodge L et al. Effect of dietary intake of omega-3 and omega-6 fatty acids on severity of asthma in children. Eur Respir J, 1998 Feb, 11:2, 361-5

18 Edwards R; Peet M; Shay J; Horrobin D. Omega-3 polyunsaturated fatty acid levels in the diet and in red blood cell membranes of depressed patients. J Affect Disord, 1998 Mar, 48:2-3, 149-55

19 Williams MA et al. Omega-3 fatty acids in maternal erythrocytes and risk of preeclampsia. Epidemiology, 6: 3, 1995 May, 232-7

20 Stevens LJ et al. Essential fatty acid metabolism in boys with attention-deficit hyperactivity disorder. Am J Clin Nutr, 62: 4, 1995 Oct, 761-8

21 Holman RT et al. Patients with anorexia nervosa demonstrate deficiencies of selected essential fatty acids, compensatory changes in nonessential fatty acids and decreased fluidity of plasma lipids. J Nutr, 125: 4, 1995 Apr, 901-7

22 Rose DP Effects of linoleic acid and gamma-linolenic acid on the growth and metastasis of a human breast cancer cell line in nude mice and on its growth and invasive capacity in vitro. Nutr Cancer, 24: 1, 1995, 33-45

23 Sacks FM et al. Short report: the effect of fish oil on blood pressure and high-density lipoprotein-cholesterol levels in phase I of the Trials of Hypertension Prevention. J Hypertens, 1994 Feb, 12:2, 209-13

24 Mori TA; Beilin LJ; Burke V; Morris J; Ritchie J. Interactions between dietary fat, fish, and fish oils and their effects on platelet function in men at risk of cardiovascular disease. Arterioscler Thromb Vasc Biol, 1997 Feb, 17:2, 279-86

25 Nestel PJ et al. Arterial compliance in obese subjects is improved with dietary plant n-3 fatty acid from flaxseed oil despite increased LDL oxidizability. Arterioscler Thromb Vasc Biol, 1997 Jun, 17:6, 1163-70

26 Toft I et al. Effects of n-3 polyunsaturated fatty acids on glucose homeostasis and blood pressure in essential hypertension. A randomized, controlled trial. Ann Intern Med, 123: 12, 1995 Dec 15, 911-8

27 Lungershausen YK; Abbey M; Nestel PJ; Howe PR Reduction of blood pressure and plasma triglycerides by omega-3 fatty acids in treated hypertensives. J Hypertens, 1994 Sep, 12:9, 1041-5

28 Gray DR; Gozzip CG; Eastham JH; Kashyap ML Fish oil as an adjuvant in the treatment of hypertension. Pharmacotherapy, 1996 Mar, 16:2, 295-300

29 Andreassen AK; Hartmann A; Offstad J; Geiran O; Kvernebo K; Simonsen S Hypertension prophylaxis with omega-3 fatty acids in heart transplant recipients. J Am Coll Cardiol, 1997 May, 29:6, 1324-31

30 Russo C et al. Omega-3 polyunsaturated fatty acid supplements and ambulatory blood pressure monitoring parameters in patients with mild essential hypertension. J Hypertens, 1995 Dec, 13:12 Pt 2, 1823-6

31 Rose DP; Connolly JM; Rayburn J; Coleman M. Influence of diets containing eicosapentaenoic or docosahexaenoic acid on growth and metastasis of breast cancer cells in nude mice. J Natl Cancer Inst, 1995 Apr, 87:8, 587-92

32 Veierod MB; Laake P; Thelle DS Dietary fat intake and risk of lung cancer: a prospective study of 51,452 Norwegian men and women. Eur J Cancer Prev, 1997 Dec, 6:6, 540-9

33 Gogos CA; Ginopoulos P; Salsa B; Apostolidou E; Zoumbos NC; Kalfarentzos F. Dietary omega-3 polyunsaturated fatty acids plus vitamin E restore immunodeficiency and prolong survival for severely ill patients with generalized malignancy: a randomized control trial. Cancer, 1998 Jan, 82:2, 395-402

34 Solomon LZ; Jennings AM; Hayes MC; Bass PS; Birch BR; Cooper AJ Is gamma-linolenic acid an effective intravesical agent for superficial bladder cancer? In vitro cytotoxicity and in vivo tolerance studies. Urol Res, 1998, 26:1, 11-5

35 Jiang WG et al. Inhibition of hepatocyte growth factor-induced motility and in vitro invasion of human colon cancer cells by gamma-linolenic acid. Br J Cancer, 71: 4, 1995 Apr, 744-52

36 Hrelia S; Bordoni A; Biagi P; Rossi CA; Bernardi L; Horrobin DF; Pession A gamma-Linolenic acid supplementation can affect cancer cell proliferation via modification of fatty acid composition. Biochem Biophys Res Commun, 1996 Aug, 225:2, 441-7

37 Lockwood K et al. Apparent partial remission of breast cancer in 'high risk' patients supplemented with nutritional antioxidants, essential fatty acids and coenzyme Q10. Mol Aspects Med. 1994; 15 Suppl: s231-40

38 Geusens P; Wouters C; Nijs J; Jiang Y; Dequeker J Long-term effect of omega-3 fatty acid supplementation in active rheumatoid arthritis. A 12-month, double-blind, controlled study. Arthritis Rheum, 1994 Jun, 37:6, 824-9

39 Zurier RB; Rossetti RG; Jacobson EW; DeMarco DM; Liu NY; Temming JE; White BM; Laposata M. gamma-Linolenic acid treatment of rheumatoid arthritis. A randomized, placebo-controlled trial. Arthritis Rheum, 1996 Nov, 39:11, 1808-17

40 Leventhal LJ; Boyce EG; Zurier RB Treatment of rheumatoid arthritis with blackcurrant seed oil. Br J Rheumatol, 1994 Sep, 33:9, 847-52

41 Hornstra G et al. Essential fatty acids in pregnancy and early human development. Eur J Obstet Gynecol Reprod Biol, 61: 1, 1995 Jul, 57-62

42 Uauy-Dagach R; Mena P. Nutritional role of omega-3 fatty acids during the perinatal period. Clin Perinatol, 22: 1, 1995 Mar, 157-75

43 Andreassi M; Forleo P; Di Lorio A; Masci S; Abate G; Amerio P Efficacy of gamma-linolenic acid in the treatment of patients with atopic dermatitis. J Int Med Res, 1997 Sep, 25:5, 266-74

44 Borrek S; Hildebrandt A; Forster J Gamma-linolenic-acid-rich borage seed oil capsules in children with atopic dermatitis. A placebo-controlled double-blind study. Klin Padiatr, 1997 May, 209:3, 100-4

45 Hederos CA; Berg A Epogam evening primrose oil treatment in atopic dermatitis and asthma. Arch Dis Child, 1996 Dec, 75:6, 494-7

46 Collier PM; Ursell A; Zaremba K; Payne CM; Staughton RC; Sanders T. Effect of regular consumption of oily fish compared with white fish on chronic plaque psoriasis. Eur J Clin Nutr, 1993 Apr, 47:4, 251-4

47 Mayser P et al. Omega-3 fatty acid-based lipid infusion in patients with chronic plaque psoriasis: results of a double-blind, randomized, placebo-controlled, multicenter trial. J Am Acad Dermatol, 1998 Apr, 38:4, 539-47

48 Escobar SO; Achenbach R; Iannantuono R; Torem V Topical fish oil in psoriasis—a controlled and blind study. Clin Exp Dermatol, 1992 May, 17:3, 159-62

49 Frati C; Bevilacqua L; Apostolico V. Association of etretinate and fish oil in psoriasis therapy. Inhibition of hypertriglyceridemia resulting from retinoid therapy after fish oil supplementation. Acta Derm Venereol Suppl (Stockh), 1994, 186:, 151-3

50 Harel, Z.; Biro, F., et al.Supplementation with omega-3 polyunsaturated fatty acids in the management of dysmenorrhea in adolescents. Am J Ob Gyn 1996;174:1335-1338

51 Sirtori CR; Paoletti R; Mancini M; Crepaldi G; Manzato E; Rivellese A; Pamparana F; Stragliotto E. N-3 fatty acids do not lead to an increased diabetic risk in patients with hyperlipidemia and abnormal glucose tolerance. Italian Fish Oil Multicenter Study. Am J Clin Nutr, 1997 Jun, 65:6, 1874-81

52 Keen H et al. Treatment of diabetic neuropathy with gamma-linolenic acid. The gamma-Linolenic Acid Multicenter Trial Group. Diabetes Care, 1993 Jan, 16:1, 8-15

53 Belluzzi A; Brignola C; Campieri M; Pera A; Boschi S; Miglioli M Effect of an enteric-coated fish-oil preparation on relapses in Crohn's disease. N Engl J Med, 1996 Jun, 334:24, 1557-60

54 Wagner W; Nootbaar Wagner U Prophylactic treatment of migraine with gamma-linolenic and alpha-linolenic acids. Cephalalgia, 1997 Apr, 17:2, 127-30; discussion 102

Choline

1 Zeisel SH; Da Costa KA; Franklin PD; Alexander EA; Lamont JT; Sheard NF; Beiser A Choline, an essential nutrient for humans. FASEB J, 1991 Apr, 5:7, 2093-8

2 Franco-Maside A; Caamaño J; Gómez MJ; Cacabelos R Brain mapping activity and mental performance after chronic treatment with CDP-choline in Alzheimer's disease. Methods Find Exp Clin Pharmacol, 16: 8, 1994 Oct, 597-607

3 Caamaño J; Gómez MJ; Franco A; Cacabelos R Effects of CDP-choline on cognition and cerebral hemodynamics in patients with Alzheimer's disease. Methods Find Exp Clin Pharmacol, 16: 3, 1994 Apr, 211-8

4 Wojcicki J et al. Clinical evaluation of lecithin as a lipid-lowering agent. Phytotherapy Res 1995, 9, 597-99

5 Stoll AL; Sachs GS; Cohen BM; Lafer B; Christensen JD; Renshaw PF. Choline in the treatment of rapid-cycling bipolar disorder: clinical and neurochemical findings in lithium-treated patients. Biol Psychiatry, 1996 Sep, 40:5, 382-8

6 Gupta SK; Gaur SN. A placebo controlled trial of two dosages of LPC antagonist—choline in the management of bronchial asthma. Indian J Chest Dis Allied Sci, 1997 Jul, 39:3, 149-56

7 Dodson WL; Sachan DS Choline supplementation reduces urinary carnitine excretion in humans. Am J Clin Nutr, 1996 Jun, 63:6, 904-10

Inositol

1 Levine J. Controlled trials of inositol in psychiatry. Eur Neuropsychopharmacol, 1997 May, 7:2, 147-55

2 Greene ND; Copp AJ Inositol prevents folate-resistant neural tube defects in the mouse. Nat Med, 1997 Jan, 3:1, 60-6

Laetrile

1 Moertel CG et al. A clinical trial of amygdalin (Laetrile) in the treatment of human cancer. N Engl J Med, 306: 4, 1982 Jan 28, 201-6

2 Beamer WC; Shealy RM; Prough DS. Acute cyanide poisoning from laetrile ingestion. Ann Emerg Med, 12: 7, 1983 Jul, 449-51

Greenberg DM The case against laetrile: the fraudulent cancer remedy. Cancer, 1980 Feb 15, 45:4, 799-807

Coenzyme Q10

1 Langsjoen H et al. Usefulness of coenzyme Q10 in clinical cardiology: a long-term study. Mol Aspects Med. 1994; 15 Suppl: s165-75

2 Baggio-E et al. Italian multicenter study on the safety and efficacy of coenzyme Q10 as adjunctive therapy in heart failure. CoQ10 Drug Surveillance Investigators. Mol Aspects Med. 1994; 15 Suppl: s287-94

3 Langsjoen P et al. Treatment of essential hypertension with coenzyme Q10. Mol Aspects Med. 1994; 15 Suppl: S265-72

4 Digiesi V et al. Coenzyme Q10 in essential hypertension. Mol Aspects Med. 1994; 15 Suppl: s257-63

5 Langsjoen PH; Langsjoen A; Willis R; Folkers K Treatment of hypertrophic cardiomyopathy with coenzyme Q10. Mol Aspects Med, 1997, 18 Suppl:, S145-51

6 Hanaki-Y et al. Coenzyme Q10 and coronary artery disease. Clin Investig. 1993; 71(8 Suppl): S112-5

7 Chello M et al. Protection by coenzyme Q10 of tissue reperfusion injury during abdominal aortic cross-clamping. J Cardiovasc Surg Torino. 1996 Jun; 37(3): 229-35

8 Kamikawa T et al. Effects of coenzyme Q10 on exercise tolerance in chronic stable angina pectoris. Am J Cardiol, 1985 Aug 1, 56:4, 247-51

9 Lockwood K et al. Apparent partial remission of breast cancer in 'high risk' patients supplemented with nutritional antioxidants, essential fatty acids and coenzyme Q10. Mol Aspects Med. 1994; 15 Suppl: s231-40

10 Folkers-K; Simonsen-R. Two successful double-blind trials with coenzyme Q10 (vitamin Q10) on muscular dystrophies and neurogenic atrophies. Biochim-Biophys-Acta. 1995 May 24; 1271(1): 281-6

11 Ylikoski T; Piirainen J; Hanninen O; Penttinen J. The effect of coenzyme Q10 on the exercise performance of cross-country skiers. Mol Aspects Med, 1997, 18 Suppl:, S283-90

12 Lewin A; Lavon H The effect of coenzyme Q10 on sperm motility and function. Mol Aspects Med, 1997, 18 Suppl:, S213-9

13 Mortensen SA; Leth A; Agner E; Rohde M Dose-related decrease of serum coenzyme Q10 during treatment with HMG-CoA reductase inhibitors. Mol Aspects Med, 1997, 18 Suppl:, S137-44

Flavonoids

1 Hertog MG; Feskens EJ; Hollman PC; Katan MB; Kromhout D. Dietary antioxidant flavonoids and risk of coronary heart disease: the Zutphen Elderly Study. Lancet, 1993 Oct 23, 342:8878, 1007-11

2 Rimm EB; Katan MB; Ascherio A; Stampfer MJ; Willett WC Relation between intake of flavonoids and risk for coronary heart disease in male health professionals. Ann Intern Med, 1996 Sep, 125:5, 384-9

3 Keli SO; Hertog MG; Feskens EJ; Kromhout D Dietary flavonoids, antioxidant vitamins, and incidence of stroke: the Zutphen study. Arch Intern Med, 1996 Mar, 156:6, 637-42

4 Hertog MG; Sweetnam PM; Fehily AM; Elwood PC; Kromhout D. Antioxidant flavonols and ischemic heart disease in a Welsh population of men: the Caerphilly Study. Am J Clin Nutr, 1997 May, 65:5, 1489-94

5 Imai K; Nakachi K Cross sectional study of effects of drinking green tea on cardiovascular and liver diseases. BMJ, 1995 Mar, 310:6981, 693-6

6 Knekt P; Järvinen R; Seppänen R; Hellövaara M; Teppo L; Pukkala E; Aromaa A. Dietary flavonoids and the risk of lung cancer and other malignant neoplasms. Am J Epidemiol, 1997 Aug, 146:3, 223-30

7 Zheng W; Doyle TJ; Kushi LH; Sellers TA; Hong CP; Folsom AR. Tea consumption and cancer incidence in a prospective cohort study of postmenopausal women. Am J Epidemiol, 1996 Jul, 144:2, 175-82

8 Dorant E; van den Brandt PA; Goldbohm RA; Sturmans F Consumption of onions and a reduced risk of stomach carcinoma. Gastroenterology, 1996 Jan, 110:1, 12-20

9 Imai K; Suga K; Nakachi K Cancer-preventive effects of drinking green tea among a Japanese population. Prev Med, 1997 Nov, 26:6, 769-75

10 Gao YT; McLaughlin JK; Blot WJ; Ji BT; Dai Q; Fraumeni JF Jr. Reduced risk of esophageal cancer associated with green tea consumption. J Natl Cancer Inst, 1994 Jun, 86:11, 855-8

11 Yu GP; Hsieh CC; Wang LY; Yu SZ; Li XL; Jin TH. Green-tea consumption and risk of stomach cancer: a population-based case-control study in Shanghai, China. Cancer Causes Control, 1995 Nov, 6:6, 532-8

12 Ji BT; Chow WH; Hsing AW; McLaughlin JK; Dai Q; Gao YT; Blot WJ; Fraumeni JF Jr. Green tea consumption and the risk of pancreatic and colorectal cancers. Int J Cancer, 1997 Jan, 70:3, 255-8

13 Shim JS; Kang MH; Kim YH; Roh JK; Roberts C; Lee IP Chemopreventive effect of green tea (Camellia sinensis) among cigarette smokers. Cancer Epidemiol Biomarkers Prev, 1995 Jun, 4:4, 387-91

14 Nakachi K; Suemasu K; Suga K; Takeo T; Imai K; Higashi Y Influence of drinking green tea on breast cancer malignancy among Japanese patients. Jpn J Cancer Res, 1998 Mar, 89:3, 254-61

15 Kurowska EM et al. Effects of substituting dietary soybean protein and oil for milk protein and fat in subjects with hypercholesterolemia. Clin Invest Med 1997 Jun;20(3):162-170

16 Goodman MT; Wilkens LR; Hankin JH; Lyu LC; Wu AH; Kolonel LN. Association of soy and fiber consumption with the risk of endometrial cancer. Am J Epidemiol, 1997 Aug, 146:4, 294-306

17 Wu AH; Ziegler RG; Horn Ross PL; Nomura AM; West DW; Kolonel LN; Rosenthal JF; Hoover RN; Pike MC. Tofu and risk of breast cancer in Asian-Americans. Cancer Epidemiol Biomarkers Prev, 1996 Nov, 5:11, 901-6

18 Albertazzi P; Pansini F; Bonaccorsi G; Zanotti L; Forini E; De Aloysio D The effect of dietary soy supplementation on hot flushes. Obstet Gynecol, 1998 Jan, 91:1, 6-11

Lipoic acid

1 Streeper RS; Henriksen EJ; Jacob S; Hokama JY; Fogt DL; Tritschler HJ Differential effects of lipoic acid stereoisomers on glucose metabolism in insulin-resistant skeletal muscle. Am J Physiol, 1997 Jul, 273:1 Pt 1, E185-91

2 Jacob S et al. Enhancement of glucose disposal in patients with type 2 diabetes by alpha-lipoic acid. Arzneimittelforschung, 45: 8, 1995 Aug, 872-4

3 Nagamatsu M et al. Lipoic acid improves nerve blood flow, reduces oxidative stress, and improves distal nerve conduction in experimental diabetic neuropathy. Diabetes Care, 18: 8, 1995 Aug, 1160-7

4 Ziegler D; Gries FA. Alpha-lipoic acid in the treatment of diabetic peripheral and cardiac autonomic neuropathy. Diabetes, 1997 Sep, 46 Suppl 2:, S62-63-61

5 Ou P; Tritschler HJ; Wolff SP. Thioctic (lipoic) acid: a therapeutic metal-chelating antioxidant? Biochem Pharmacol, 50: 1, 1995 Jun 29, 123-6

6 Kilic F; Handelman GJ; Serbinova E; Packer L; Trevithick JR. Modelling cortical cataractogenesis 17: in vitro effect of a-lipoic acid on glucose-induced lens membrane damage, a model of diabetic cataractogenesis. Biochem Mol Biol Int, 1995 Oct, 37:2, 361-70

Carnitine

1 Bartels GL; Remme WJ; Pillay M; Schönfeld DH; Kruijssen DA. Effects of L-propionylcarnitine on ischemia-induced myocardial dysfunction in men with angina pectoris. Am J Cardiol, 1994 Jul, 74:2, 125-30

2 Iliceto S; Scrutinio D; Bruzzi P; DAmbrosio G; Boni L; Di Biase M; Biasco G; Hugenholtz PG; Rizzon P. Effects of L-carnitine administration on left ventricular remodeling after acute anterior myocardial infarction: the L-Carnitine Ecocardiografia Digitalizzata Infarto Miocardico (CEDIM) Trial. J Am Coll Cardiol, 1995 Aug, 26:2, 380-7

3 Brevetti G; Perna S; Sabba C; Martone VD; Di Iorio A; Barletta G. Effect of propionyl-L-carnitine on quality of life in intermittent claudication. Am J Cardiol, 1997 Mar, 79:6, 777-80

4 Grandi M; Pederzoli S; Sacchetti C. Effect of acute carnitine administration on glucose insulin metabolism in healthy subjects. Int J Clin Pharmacol Res, 1997, 17:4, 143-7

5 Bowman BA Acetyl-carnitine and Alzheimer's disease. Nutr Rev, 1992 May, 50:5, 142-4

6 Pettegrew JW, et al. Clinical and neurochemical effects of acetyl-L-carnitine in Alzheimer's disease. Neurobiol Aging 1995;16:1-4.

7 Dodson WL; Sachan DS Choline supplementation reduces urinary carnitine excretion in humans. Am J Clin Nutr, 1996 Jun, 63:6, 904-10

Melatonin

1 Hughes RJ; Badia P. Sleep-promoting and hypothermic effects of daytime melatonin administration in humans. Sleep, 1997 Feb, 20:2, 124-31

2 Attenburrow ME; Cowen PJ; Sharpley AL Low dose melatonin improves sleep in healthy middle-aged subjects. Psychopharmacology (Berl), 1996 Jul, 126:2, 179-81

3 Petrie K; Dawson AG; Thompson L; Brook R. A double-blind trial of melatonin as a treatment for jet lag in international cabin crew. Biol Psychiatry, 1993 Apr 1, 33:7, 526-30

4 Neri B; de Leonardis V; Gemelli MT; di Loro F; Mottola A; Ponchietti R; Raugei A; Cini G. Melatonin as biological response modifier in cancer patients. Anticancer Res, 1998 Mar, 18:2B, 1329-32

Glucosamine

1 Gonarthrosis—current aspects of therapy with glucosamine sulfate. Fortschr Med Suppl, 1998, 183:, 1-12

2 da Camara CC; Dowless GV Glucosamine sulfate for osteoarthritis. Ann Pharmacother, 1998 May, 32:5, 580-7

3 McCarty MF Glucosamine for wound healing. Med Hypotheses, 1996 Oct, 47:4, 273-5

4 McCarty MF Glucosamine for psoriasis? Med Hypotheses, 1997 May, 48:5, 437-41

Shark cartilage

1 McGuire TR; Kazakoff PW; Hoie EB; Fienhold MA. Antiproliferative activity of shark cartilage with and without tumor necrosis factor-alpha in human umbilical vein endothelium. Pharmacotherapy, 1996 Mar, 16:2, 237-44

Digestive support

1 Kashtan H; Stern HS; Jenkins DJ; Jenkins AL; Hay K; Marcon N; Minkin S; Bruce WR. Wheat-bran and oat-bran supplements' effects on blood lipids and lipoproteins. Am J Clin Nutr, 1992 May, 55:5, 976-80

2 Cook IJ; Irvine EJ; Campbell D; Shannon S; Reddy SN; Collins SM. Effect of dietary fiber on symptoms and rectosigmoid motility in patients with irritable bowel syndrome. A controlled, crossover study. Gastroenterology, 1990 Jan, 98:1, 66-72

Immunity

1 Bogden JD; Bendich A; Kemp FW; Bruening KS; Shurnick JH; Denny T; Baker H; Louria DB. Daily micronutrient supplements enhance delayed-hypersensitivity skin test responses in older people. Am J Clin Nutr, 1994 Sep, 60:3, 437-47

2 Chandra RK. Effect of vitamin and trace-element supplementation on immune responses and infection in elderly subjects. Lancet, 1992 Nov 7, 340:8828, 1124-7

3 Bendich A Physiological role of antioxidants in the immune system. J Dairy Sci, 1993 Sep, 76:9, 2789-94

4 Penn ND; Purkins L; Kelleher J; Heatley RV; Mascie-Taylor BH; Belfield PW. The effect of dietary supplementation with vitamins A, C and E on cell-mediated immune function in elderly long-stay patients: a randomized controlled trial. Age Ageing, 1991 May, 20:3, 169-74

5 Arrieta AC; Zaleska M; Stutman HR; Marks MI. Vitamin A levels in children with measles in Long Beach, California. J Pediatr, 1992 Jul, 121:1, 75-8

6 Glasziou P, Mackerras D. Vitamin A supplementation in infectious diseases. Br Med J. 1993;306: 366-370

7 Hughes DA; Wright AJ; Finglas PM; Peerless AC; Bailey AL; Astley SB; Pinder AC; Southon S. The effect of beta-carotene supplementation on the immune function of blood monocytes from healthy male nonsmokers. J Lab Clin Med, 1997 Mar, 129:3, 309-17

8 Pfitzenmeyer P; Guilland JC; dAthis P. Vitamin B6 and vitamin C status in elderly patients with infections during hospitalization. Ann Nutr Metab, 1997, 41:6, 344-52

9 Hunt C; Chakravorty NK; Annan G; Habibzadeh N; Schorah CJ. The clinical effects of vitamin C supplementation in elderly hospitalised patients with acute respiratory infections. Int J Vitam Nutr Res, 1994, 64:3, 212-9

10 Heuser G; Vojdani A Enhancement of natural killer cell activity and T and B cell function by buffered vitamin C in patients exposed to toxic chemicals: the role of protein kinase-C. Immunopharmacol Immunotoxicol, 1997 Aug, 19:3, 291-312

11 Hemilä H Vitamin C supplementation and common cold symptoms: problems with inaccurate reviews. Nutrition, 1996 Nov, 12:11-12, 804-9

12 Meydani SN; Meydani M; Blumberg JB; Leka LS; Siber G; Loszewski R; Thompson C; Pedrosa MC; Diamond RD; Stollar BD Vitamin E supplementation and in vivo immune response in healthy elderly subjects. A randomized controlled trial. JAMA, 1997 May, 277:17, 1380-6

13 Rall LC; Meydani SN. Vitamin B6 and immune competence. Nutr Rev, 1993 Aug, 51:8, 217-25

14 Fata FT; Herzlich BC; Schiffman G; Ast AL. Impaired antibody responses to pneumococcal polysaccharide in elderly patients with low serum vitamin B12 levels. Ann Intern Med, 1996 Feb, 124:3, 299-304

15 Báez-Saldaña A; Diaz G; Espinoza B; and Ortega E. Biotin deficiency induces changes in subpopulations of spleen lymphocytes in mice. Am J Clin Nutr 1998;67:431-7

16 Komar VI The use of pantothenic acid preparations in treating patients with viral hepatitis A. Ter Arkh, 1991, 63:11, 58-60

17 Cakman I; Kirchner H; Rink L. Zinc supplementation reconstitutes the production of interferon-alpha by leukocytes from elderly persons. J Interferon Cytokine Res, 1997 Aug, 17:8, 469-72

18 Bogden JD; Oleske JM; Lavenhar MA; Munves EM; Kemp FW; Bruening KS; Holding KJ; Denny TN; Guarino MA; Holland BK. J Am Coll Nutr, 1990 Jun, 9:3, 214-25

19 Fortes C et al; The effect of zinc and vitamin A supplementation on immune response in an older population. J Am Geriatr Soc, 1998 Jan, 46:1, 19-26

20 Sazawal S; Black RE; Bhan MK; Jalla S; Sinha A; Bhandari N. Efficacy of zinc supplementation in reducing the incidence and prevalence of acute diarrhea—a community-based, double-blind, controlled trial. Am J Clin Nutr, 1997 Aug, 66:2, 413-8

21 Folkers K; Morita M; McRee J Jr. The activities of coenzyme Q10 and vitamin B6 for immune responses. Biochem Biophys Res Commun, 1993 May 28, 193:1, 88-92

Pregnancy

1 Rothman KJ; Moore LL; Singer MR; Nguyen US; Mannino S; Milunsky A Teratogenicity of high vitamin A intake. N Engl J Med, 1995 Nov, 333:21, 1369-73

2 Mills JL; Simpson JL; Cunningham GC; Conley MR; Rhoads GG. Vitamin A and birth defects. Am J Obstet Gynecol, 1997 Jul, 177:1, 31-6

3 Heiskanen K et al. Low vitamin B6 status associated with slow growth in healthy breast-fed infants. Pediatr Res, 38: 5, 1995 Nov, 740-6

4 Sahakian V; Rouse D; Sipes S; Rose N; Niebyl J Vitamin B6 is effective therapy for nausea and vomiting of pregnancy: a randomized, double-blind placebo-controlled study. Obstet Gynecol, 1991 Jul, 78:1, 33-6

5 Cuskelly GJ; McNulty H; Scott JM. Effect of increasing dietary folate on red-cell folate: implications for prevention of neural tube defects Lancet, 1996 Mar, 347:9002, 657-9

6 Czeizel AE; Dudás I Prevention of the first occurrence of neural-tube defects by periconceptional vitamin supplementation. N Engl J Med, 1992 Dec 24, 327:26, 1832-5

7 Mikhail MS; Anyaegbunam A; Garfinkel D; Palan PR; Basu J; Romney SL. Preeclampsia and antioxidant nutrients: decreased plasma levels of reduced ascorbic acid, alpha-tocopherol, and beta-carotene in women with preeclampsia. Am J Obstet Gynecol, 1994 Jul, 171:1, 150-7

8 Jain SK; Wise R. Relationship between elevated lipid peroxides, vitamin E deficiency and hypertension in preeclampsia. Mol Cell Biochem, 1995 Oct, 151:1, 33-8

9 Hansen KN; Ebbesen F. Neonatal vitamin K prophylaxis in Denmark: three years' experience with oral administration during the first three months of life compared with one oral administration at birth. Acta Paediatr, 1996 Oct, 85:10, 1137-9

10 Gulson BL; Mahaffey KR; Jameson CW; Mizon KJ; Korsch MJ; Cameron MA; Eisman JA Mobilization of lead from the skeleton during the postnatal period is larger than during pregnancy. J Lab Clin Med, 1998 Apr, 131:4, 324-9

11 Belizán JM; Villar J; Bergel E; del Pino A; Di Fulvio S; Galliano SV; Kattan C. Long-term effect of calcium supplementation during pregnancy on the blood pressure of offspring: follow up of a randomised controlled trial. BMJ, 1997 Aug, 315:7103, 281-5

12 Ritchie LD; Fung EB; Halloran BP; Turnlund JR; Van Loan MD; Cann CE; King JC. A longitudinal study of calcium homeostasis during human pregnancy and lactation and after resumption of menses. Am J Clin Nutr 1998;67:693-701.

13 Kalkwarf HJ, Specker BL, Bianchi DC, Ranz J, Ho M. The effect of calcium supplementation on bone density during lactation and after weaning. N Engl J Med 1997;337:523-8

14 Herrera JA; Arevalo Herrera M; Herrera S. Prevention of preeclampsia by linoleic acid and calcium supplementation: a randomized controlled trial. Obstet Gynecol, 1998 Apr, 91:4, 585-90

15 Bucher HC; Guyatt GH; Cook RJ; Hatala R; Cook DJ; Lang JD; Hunt D. Effect of calcium supplementation on pregnancy-induced hypertension and preeclampsia: a meta-analysis of randomized controlled trials. JAMA, 1996 Apr, 275:14, 1113-7

16 Levine RJ; Hauth JC; Curet LB; Sibai BM; Catalano PM; Morris CD; DerSimonian R; Esterlitz JR; Raymond EG; Bild DE; Clemens JD; Cutler JA. Trial of calcium to prevent preeclampsia. N Engl J Med, 1997 Jul, 337:2, 69-76

17 Richardson BE; Baird DD. A study of milk and calcium supplement intake and subsequent preeclampsia in a cohort of pregnant women. Am J Epidemiol, 1995 Apr, 141:7, 667-73

18 Chien PF; Khan KS; Arnott N. Magnesium sulphate in the treatment of eclampsia and pre-eclampsia: an overview of the evidence from randomised trials. Br J Obstet Gynaecol, 1996 Nov, 103:11, 1085-91

19 Schendel DE; Berg CJ; Yeargin Allsopp M; Boyle CA; Decoufle P Prenatal magnesium sulfate exposure and the risk for cerebral palsy or mental retardation among very low-birth-weight children aged 3 to 5 years. JAMA, 1996 Dec, 276:22, 1805-10

20 Dahle LO; Berg G; Hammar M; Hurtig M; Larsson L The effect of oral magnesium substitution on pregnancy-induced leg cramps. Am J Obstet Gynecol, 1995 Jul, 173:1, 175-80

21 Goldenberg RL et al. The effect of zinc supplementation on pregnancy outcome. JAMA. 1995;274:463-468

22 Greer FR; Marshall SP; Foley AL; Suttie JW. Improving the vitamin K status of breastfeeding infants with maternal vitamin K supplements. Pediatrics, 1997 Jan, 99:1, 88-92

23 Laskey MA; Prentice A; Hanratty LA; Jarjou LMA; Dibba B; Beavan SR; Cole TJ. Bone changes after 3 mo of lactation: influence of calcium intake, breast-milk output, and vitamin D—receptor genotype. Am J Clin Nutr 1998;67:685-92.

Vegetarians

1 Key TJ; Thorogood M; Appleby PN; Burr ML Dietary habits and mortality in 11,000 vegetarians and health conscious people: results of a 17 year follow up. BMJ, 1996 Sep, 313:7060, 775-9

2 Pauletto P et al. Blood pressure and atherogenic lipoprotein profiles of fish-diet and vegetarian villagers in Tanzania: the Lugalawa study. Lancet, 1996 Sep, 348:9030, 784-8

3 Dagnelie PC; van Staveren WA; van den Berg H. Vitamin B-12 from algae appears not to be bioavailable. Am J Clin Nutr, 1991 Mar, 53:3, 695-7

4 Uzel C; Conrad ME Absorption of heme iron. Semin Hematol, 1998 Jan, 35:1, 27-34

5 García Casal MN et al. Vitamin A and beta-carotene can improve nonheme iron absorption from rice, wheat and corn by humans. J Nutr, 1998 Mar, 128:3, 646-50

6 Chiu JF; Lan SJ; Yang CY; Wang PW; Yao WJ; Su LH; Hsieh CC Long-term vegetarian diet and bone mineral density in postmenopausal Taiwanese women. Calcif Tissue Int, 1997 Mar, 60:3, 245-9

7 Nathan I; Hackett AF; Kirby S A longitudinal study of the growth of matched pairs of vegetarian and omnivorous children, aged 7-11 years, in the north-west of England. Eur J Clin Nutr, 1997 Jan, 51:1, 20-5

8 Nathan I; Hackett AF; Kirby S. The dietary intake of a group of vegetarian children aged 7-11 years compared with matched omnivores. Br J Nutr, 1996 Apr, 75:4, 533-44

Older people

1 Lesourd BM Nutrition and immunity in the elderly: modification of immune responses with nutritional treatments. Am J Clin Nutr, 1997 Aug, 66:2, 478S-484S

2 Fisher GJ; Wang ZQ; Datta SC; Varani J; Kang S; Voorhees JJ. Pathophysiology of premature skin aging induced by ultraviolet light. N Engl J Med, 1997 Nov, 337:20, 1419-28

3 Wilkinson TJ; Hanger HC; Elmslie J; George PM; Sainsbury R. The response to treatment of subclinical thiamine deficiency in the elderly. Am J Clin Nutr, 1997 Oct, 66:4, 925-8

4 van der Wielen RP; Löwik MR; Haller J; van den Berg H; Ferry M; van Staveren WA Vitamin B-6 malnutrition among elderly Europeans: the SENECA study. J Gerontol A Biol Sci Med Sci, 1996 Nov, 51:6, B417-24

5 Quinn K; Basu TK. Folate and vitamin B12 status of the elderly. Eur J Clin Nutr, 1996 Jun, 50:6, 340-2

6 Ortega RM; Mañas LR; Andrés P; Gaspar MJ; Agudo FR; Jiménez A; Pascual T Functional and psychic deterioration in elderly people may be aggravated by folate deficiency. J Nutr, 1996 Aug, 126:8, 1992-9

7 Fata FT; Herzlich BC; Schiffman G; Ast AL. Impaired antibody responses to pneumococcal polysaccharide in elderly patients with low serum vitamin B12 levels. Ann Intern Med, 1996 Feb, 124:3, 299-304

8 Nilsson Ehle H Age-related changes in cobalamin (vitamin B12) handling. Implications for therapy. Drugs Aging, 1998 Apr, 12:4, 277-92

9 Thomas MK; Lloyd Jones DM; Thadhani RI; Shaw AC; Deraska DJ; Kitch BT; Vamvakas EC; Dick IM; Prince RL; Finkelstein JS. Hypovitaminosis D in medical inpatients. N Engl J Med, 1998 Mar, 338:12, 777-83

10 McAlindon TE; Felson DT; Zhang Y; Hannan MT; Aliabadi P; Weissman B; Rush D; Wilson PW. Relation of dietary intake and serum levels of vitamin D to progression of osteoarthritis of the knee among participants in the Framingham Study. Ann Intern Med, 1996 Sep, 125:5, 353-9

11 Dawson Hughes B; Harris SS; Krall EA; Dallal GE Effect of calcium and vitamin D supplementation on bone density in men and women 65 years of age or older. N Engl J Med, 1997 Sep, 337:10, 670-6

12 Lips P, Graafmans WC, Ooms ME, Bezemer PD, Bouter LM. Vitamin D supplementation and fracture incidence in elderly persons. A randomized, placebo-controlled clinical trial. Ann Intern Med 1996 Feb 15;124(4):400-406

13 Buckley et al.Calcium and vitamin D3 supplementation prevents bone loss in the spine secondary to low-dose corticosteroids in patients with rheumatoid arthritis. A randomized, double-blind, placebo-controlled trial. Ann Intern Med 1996 Dec 15;125(12):961-968

14 Jama JW; Launer LJ; Witteman JC; den Breeijen JH; Breteler MM; Grobbee DE; Hofman A. Dietary antioxidants and cognitive function in a population-based sample of older persons. The Am J Epidemiol, 1996 Aug, 144:3, 275-80

15 Perrig WJ; Perrig P; Stähelin HB The relation between antioxidants and memory performance in the old and very old. J Am Geriatr Soc, 1997 Jun, 45:6, 718-24

16 Pfitzenmeyer P; Guilland JC; dAthis P. Vitamin B6 and vitamin C status in elderly patients with infections during hospitalization. Ann Nutr Metab, 1997, 41:6, 344-52

17 Sahyoun NR; Jacques PF; Russell RM Carotenoids, vitamins C and E, and mortality in an elderly population. Am J Epidemiol, 1996 Sep, 144:5, 501-11

18 Losonczy KG; Harris TB; Havlik RJ Vitamin E and vitamin C supplement use and risk of all-cause and coronary heart disease mortality in older persons: the Established Populations for Epidemiologic Studies of the Elderly. Am J Clin Nutr, 1996 Aug, 64:2, 190-6

19 Martin A; Foxall T; Blumberg JB; Meydani M. Vitamin E inhibits low-density lipoprotein-induced adhesion of monocytes to human aortic endothelial cells in vitro. Arterioscler Thromb Vasc Biol, 1997 Mar, 17:3, 429-36

20 Barton DL et al. Prospective evaluation of vitamin E for hot flashes in breast cancer survivors. J Clin Oncol, 1998 Feb, 16:2, 495-500

21 Nieves JW, Komar L, Cosman F, Lindsay R. Calcium potentiates the effect of estrogen and calcitonin on bone mass: review and analysis. Am J Clin Nutr 1998;67:5-6, 18-24

22 Corti MC; Guralnik JM; Salive ME; Ferrucci L; Pahor M; Wallace RB; Hennekens CH. Serum iron level, coronary artery disease, and all-cause mortality in older men and women. Am J Cardiol, 1997 Jan, 79:2, 120-7

23 Cappuccio FP; Markandu ND; Carney C; Sagnella GA; MacGregor GA. Double-blind randomised trial of modest salt restriction in older people. Lancet, 1997 Sep, 350:9081, 850-4

24 Graudal NA et al. Effects of Sodium Restriction on Blood Pressure, Renin, Aldosterone, Catecholamines, Cholesterols, and Triglyceride. JAMA. 1998;279:1383-1391

Exercise

1 Nieman DC. Immune response to heavy exertion. J Appl Physiol, 1997 May, 82:5, 1385-94

2 Alessio HM; Goldfarb AH; Cao G Exercise-induced oxidative stress before and after vitamin C supplementation. Int J Sport Nutr, 1997 Mar, 7:1, 1-9

3 Hemilä H Vitamin C and common cold incidence: a review of studies with subjects under heavy physical stress. Int J Sports Med, 1996 Jul, 17:5, 379-83

4 McBride JM; Kraemer WJ; Triplett McBride T; Sebastianelli W Effect of resistance exercise on free radical production. Med Sci Sports Exerc, 1998 Jan, 30:1, 67-72

5 Suzuki M; Itokawa Y Effects of thiamine supplementation on exercise-induced fatigue. Metab Brain Dis, 1996 Mar, 11:1, 95-106

6 Klesges RC; Ward KD; Shelton ML; Applegate WB; Cantler ED; Palmieri GM; Harmon K; Davis J. Changes in bone mineral content in male athletes. Mechanisms of action and intervention effects. JAMA, 1996 Jul, 276:3, 226-30

7 J Am Coll Nutr 1998,17:124-27

8 Ylikoski T; Piirainen J; Hanninen O; Penttinen J. The effect of coenzyme Q10 on the exercise performance of cross-country skiers. Mol Aspects Med, 1997, 18 Suppl:, S283-90

Weight loss

1 Bahadori B; Wallner S; Schneider H; Wascher TC; Toplak H. Effect of chromium yeast and chromium picolinate on body composition of obese, non-diabetic patients during and after a formula diet. Acta Med Austriaca, 1997, 24:5, 185-7

2 Grant KE; Chandler RM; Castle AL; Ivy JL. Chromium and exercise training: effect on obese women. Med Sci Sports Exerc, 1997 Aug, 29:8, 992-8

Drug interactions

1 Volpi E; Lucidi P; Cruciani G; Monacchia F; Reboldi G; Brunetti P; Bolli GB; De Feo P Nicotinamide counteracts alcohol-induced impairment of hepatic protein metabolism in humans. J Nutr, 1997 Nov, 127:11, 2199-204

2 Lecomte E; Herbeth B; Pirollet P; Chancerelle Y; Arnaud J; Musse N; Paille F; Siest G; Artur Y. Am J Clin Nutr, 1994 Aug, 60:2, 255-61

3 Kitamura Y; Tanaka K; Kiyohara C; Hirohata T; Tomita Y; Ishibashi M; Kido K Relationship of alcohol use, physical activity and dietary habits with serum carotenoids, retinol and alpha-tocopherol among male Japanese smokers. Int J Epidemiol, 1997 Apr, 26:2, 307-14

4 Faizallah R et al. Alcohol enhances vitamin C excretion in the urine. Alcohol Alcohol, 21: 1, 1986, 81-4

5 Lloyd B; Lloyd RS; Clayton BE. Effect of smoking, alcohol, and other factors on the selenium status of a healthy population. J Epidemiol Community Health, 37: 3, 1983 Sep, 213-7

6 Abbott L; Nadler J; Rude RK. Magnesium deficiency in alcoholism: possible contribution to osteoporosis and cardiovascular disease in alcoholics. Alcohol Clin Exp Res, 18: 5, 1994 Oct, 1076-82

7 Embry CK; Lippmann S. Use of magnesium sulfate in alcohol withdrawal. Am Fam Physician, 35: 5, 1987 May, 167-70

8 Lehr HA; Weyrich AS; Saetzler RK; Jurek A; Arfors KE; Zimmerman GA; Prescott SM; McIntyre TM Vitamin C blocks inflammatory platelet-activating factor mimetics created by cigarette smoking. J Clin Invest, 1997 May, 99:10, 2358-64

9 Weber C; Erl W; Weber K; Weber PC Increased adhesiveness of isolated monocytes to endothelium is prevented by vitamin C intake in smokers. Circulation, 1996 Apr, 93:8, 1488-92

10 Motoyama T; Kawano H; Kugiyama K; Hirashima O; Ohgushi M; Yoshimura M; Ogawa H; Yasue H Endothelium-dependent vasodilation in the brachial artery is impaired in smokers: effect of vitamin C. Am J Physiol, 1997 Oct, 273:4 Pt 2, H1644-50

11 Journal of the American Chemical Society 1997;119:621-622

12 Saito M; Kato H; Tsuchida T; Konaka C Chemoprevention effects on bronchial squamous metaplasia by folate and vitamin B12 in heavy smokers. Chest, 1994 Aug, 106:2, 496-9

13 Buckley LM; Leib ES; Cartularo KS; Vacek PM; Cooper SM. Effects of low dose methotrexate on the bone mineral density of patients with rheumatoid arthritis. J Rheumatol, 1997 Aug, 24:8, 1489-94

14 Okunieff P. Interactions between ascorbic acid and the radiation of bone marrow, skin and tumor. Am J Clin Nutr 1991;54:1281S-1283S

15 Heyneman CA Zinc deficiency and taste disorders. Ann Pharmacother, 1996 Feb, 30:2, 186-7

16 Kim JM; White RH. Effect of vitamin E on the anticoagulant response to warfarin. Am J Cardiol, 1996 Mar, 77:7, 545-6

17 Fava M; Borus JS; Alpert JE; Nierenberg AA; Rosenbaum JF; Bottiglieri T Folate, vitamin B12, and homocysteine in major depressive disorder. Am J Psychiatry, 1997 Mar, 154:3, 426-8

18 Buckley LM; Leib ES; Cartularo KS; Vacek PM; Cooper SM. Calcium and vitamin D3 supplementation prevents bone loss in the spine secondary to low-dose corticosteroids in patients with rheumatoid arthritis. A randomized, double-blind, placebo-controlled trial. Ann Intern Med, 1996 Dec, 125:12, 961-8

19 Shimizu T; Maeda S; Arakawa H; Mochizuki H; Tokuyama K; Morikawa A. Relation between theophylline and circulating vitamin levels in children with asthma. Pharmacology, 1996 Dec, 53:6, 384-9

20 Berg G; Kohlmeier L; Brenner H. Use of oral contraceptives and serum beta-carotene. Eur J Clin Nutr, 1997 Mar, 51:3, 181-7

21 Harper JM; Levine AJ; Rosenthal DL; Wiesmeier E; Hunt IF; Swendseid ME; Haile RW. Acta Cytol, Erythrocyte folate levels, oral contraceptive use and abnormal cervical cytology. Author 1994 May, 38:3, 324-30

22 Massé PG; van den Berg H; Duguay C; Beaulieu G; Simard JM. Early effect of a low dose (30 micrograms) ethinyl estradiol-containing Triphasil on vitamin B6 status. A follow-up study on six menstrual cycles. Int J Vitam Nutr Res, 1996, 66:1, 46-54

Acne

1 Rasmussen JE Diet and Acne 1977 Int J Dermatol Jun - Aug 16:6 488-92

2 Allgood VE; Cidlowski JA. Vitamin B6 modulates transcriptional activation by multiple members of the steroid hormone receptor superfamily. J Biol Chem, 1992 Feb 25, 267:6, 3819-24

3 Shalita A R et al. Topical nicotinamide compared with clindamycin gel in the treatment of inflammatory acne vulgaris. In J Dermatol, 34: 6, 1995 Jun, 434-7

4 Michaëlsson G; Ljunghall K Patients with dermatitis herpetiformis, acne, psoriasis and Darier's disease have low epidermal zinc concentrations. Acta Derm Venereol, 1990, 70:4, 304-8

5 Dreno B; Amblard P; Agache P; Sirot S; Litoux P. Low doses of zinc gluconate for inflammatory acne. Acta Derm Venereol, 1989, 69:6, 541-3

6 Verma KC; Saini AS; Dhamija SK Oral zinc sulphate therapy in acne vulgaris: a double-blind trial. Acta Derm Venereol, 1980, 60:4, 337-40

7 McCarty M High-chromium yeast for acne? Med Hypotheses, 1984 Jul, 14:3, 307-10

8 Grattan C; Burton JL; Manku M; Stewart C; Horrobin DF Essential-fatty-acid metabolites in plasma phospholipids in patients with ichthyosis vulgaris, acne vulgaris and psoriasis. Clin Exp Dermatol, 1990 May, 15:3, 174-6

Alzheimer's disease

1 Ross GW; Abbott RD; Petrovitch H; Masaki KH; Murdaugh C; Trockman C; Curb JD; White LR. Frequency and characteristics of silent dementia among elderly Japanese-American men. The Honolulu-Asia Aging Study. JAMA, 1997 Mar, 277:10, 800-5

2 Breitner JC The role of anti-inflammatory drugs in the prevention and treatment of Alzheimer's disease. Annu Rev Med, 1996, 47:, 401-11

3 White L et al. Prevalence of dementia in older Japanese-American men in Hawaii: The Honolulu-Asia Aging Study. JAMA, 1996 Sep, 276:12, 955-60

4 Grant W B. Dietary links to Alzheimer's Disease. Alz Dis Rev 1997, 2; 47-55

5 Smith MA; Petot GJ; and Perry G. Diet and Oxidative Stress: A Novel Synthesis of Epidemiological Data on Alzheimer's Disease. Alz Dis Rev 1997, 2; 56-57

6 Beal MF. Aging, energy, and oxidative stress in neurodegenerative diseases. Ann Neurol, 1995 Sep, 38:3, 357-66

7 McIntosh LJ; Trush MA; Troncoso JC Increased susceptibility of Alzheimer's disease temporal cortex to oxygen free radical-mediated processes. Free Radic Biol Med, 1997, 23:2, 183-90

8 Zaman Z; Roche S; Fielden P; Frost PG; Niriella DC; Cayley AC. Plasma concentrations of vitamins A and E and carotenoids in Alzheimer's disease. Age Ageing, 21: 2, 1992 Mar, 91-4

9 Sano M et al. A controlled trial of selegiline, alpha-tocopherol, or both as treatment for Alzheimer's disease. The Alzheimer's Disease Cooperative Study. N Engl J Med, 1997 Apr, 336:17, 1216-22

10 Kristensen MO; Gulmann NC; Christensen JE; Ostergaard K; Rasmussen K. Serum cobalamin and methylmalonic acid in Alzheimer dementia. Acta Neurol Scand, 1993 Jun, 87:6, 475-81

11 Cole MG; Prchal JF Low serum vitamin B12 in Alzheimer-type dementia. Age Ageing, 1984 Mar, 13:2, 101-5

12 Levitt AJ; Karlinsky H Folate, vitamin B12 and cognitive impairment in patients with Alzheimer's disease. Acta Psychiatr Scand, 1992 Oct, 86:4, 301-5

13 Gold M; Chen MF; Johnson K. Plasma and red blood cell thiamine deficiency in patients with dementia of the Alzheimer's type. Arch Neurol, 1995 Nov, 52:11, 1081-6

14 Meador K; Loring D; Nichols M; Zamrini E; Rivner M; Posas H; Thompson E; Moore E Preliminary findings of high-dose thiamine in dementia of Alzheimer's type. J Geriatr Psychiatry Neurol, 1993 Oct-Dec, 6:4, 222-9

15 Licastro F; Davis LJ; Mocchegiani E; Fabris N. Impaired peripheral zinc metabolism in patients with senile dementia of probable Alzheimer's type as shown by low plasma concentrations of thymulin. Biol Trace Elem Res, 1996 Jan, 51:1, 55-62

16 Christine L. Tully MD, David A. Snowdon PhD, and William R. Markesbery Serum zinc, senile plaques, and neurofibrillary tangles: Findings from the Nun Study. NeuroReport 1995;6:2105-2108

17 Constantinidis J. Treatment of Alzheimer's disease by zinc compounds. Drug Develop Res 1992; 27, 1-14

18 Caamaño J; Gómez MJ; Franco A; Cacabelos R Effects of CDP-choline on cognition and cerebral hemodynamics in patients with Alzheimer's disease. Methods Find Exp Clin Pharmacol, 16: 3, 1994 Apr, 211-8

19 Franco-Maside A; Caamaño J; Gómez MJ; Cacabelos R Brain mapping activity and mental performance after chronic treatment with CDP-choline in Alzheimer's disease. Methods Find Exp Clin Pharmacol, 16: 8, 1994 Oct, 597-607

20 Bowman BA Acetyl-carnitine and Alzheimer's disease. Nutr Rev, 1992 May, 50:5, 142-4

21 Pettegrew JW, et al. Clinical and neurochemical effects of acetyl-L-carnitine in Alzheimer's disease. Neurobiol Aging 1995;16:1-4.

22 Le Bars PL; Katz MM; Berman N; Itil TM; Freedman AM; Schatzberg AF A placebo-controlled, double-blind, randomized trial of an extract of Ginkgo biloba for dementia. North American EGb Study Group. JAMA, 1997 Oct, 278:16, 1327-32

Anemia

1 Hash RB; Sargent MA; Katner H. Anemia secondary to combined deficiencies of iron and cobalamin. Arch Fam Med, 1996 Nov, 5:10, 585-8

2 Cook JD Iron-deficiency anaemia. Baillieres Clin Haematol, 7: 4, 1994 Dec, 787-804

3Casparis D; Del Carlo P; Branconi F; Grossi A; Merante D; Gafforio L[Effectiveness and tolerability of oral liquid ferrous gluconate in iron-deficiency anemia in pregnancy and in the immediate post-partum period: comparison with other liquid or solid formulations containing bivalent or trivalent iron] Minerva Ginecol, 1996 Nov, 48:11, 511-8

4 Lozoff B; Wolf AW; Jimenez E. Iron-deficiency anemia and infant development: effects of extended oral iron therapy. J Pediatr, 1996 Sep, 129:3, 382-9

5 Carmel R Prevalence of undiagnosed pernicious anemia in the elderly. Arch Intern Med, 1996 May, 156:10, 1097-100

6 Fairweather-Tait SJ; Powers HJ; Minski MJ; Whitehead J; Downes R Riboflavin deficiency and iron absorption in adult Gambian men. Ann Nutr Metab, 1992, 36:1, 34-40

7 Machlin LJ Clinical uses of vitamin E. Acta Vitaminol Enzymol, 1985, 7 Suppl:, 33-43

8 Phelps DL The role of vitamin E therapy in high-risk neonates. Clin Perinatol, 1988 Dec, 15:4, 955-63

9 Gyorffy EJ; Chan H. Copper deficiency and microcytic anemia resulting from prolonged ingestion of over-the-counter zinc. Am J Gastroenterol, 1992 Aug, 87:8, 1054-5

10 Sanchez A Jr; Sanchez B; Blair-West; JR; et al Selenium deficiency in cattle associated with Heinz bodies and anemia. Science, 1984 Feb 3, 223:4635, 491-3

11 Prasad AS; Kaplan J; Brewer GJ; Dardenne M. Immunological effects of zinc deficiency in sickle cell anemia (SCA). Prog Clin Biol Res, 1989, 319:, 629-47; discussion 648-9

Arthritis

1 Spector TD; Harris PA; Hart DJ; Cicuttini FM; Nandra D; Etherington J; Wolman RL; Doyle DV. Risk of osteoarthritis associated with long-term weight-bearing sports: a radiologic survey of the hips and knees in female ex-athletes and population controls. Arthritis Rheum, 1996 Jun, 39:6, 988-95

2 Spector TD; Nandra D; Hart DJ; Doyle DV. Is hormone replacement therapy protective for hand and knee osteoarthritis in women?: The Chingford Study. Ann Rheum Dis, 1997 Jul, 56: 432-44

3 McAlindon TE; Felson DT; Zhang Y; Hannan MT; Aliabadi P; Weissman B; Rush D; Wilson PW; Jacques P. Relation of dietary intake and serum levels of vitamin D to progression of osteoarthritis of the knee among participants in the Framingham Study. Ann Intern Med, 1996 Sep, 125:5, 353-9

4 McAlindon TE; Jacques P; Zhang Y; Hannan MT; Aliabadi P; Weissman B; Rush D; Levy D; Felson DT Do antioxidant micronutrients protect against the development and progression of knee osteoarthritis? Arthritis Rheum, 1996 Apr, 39:4, 648-56

5 Flynn MA; Irvin W; Krause G. The effect of folate and cobalamin on osteoarthritic hands. J Am Coll Nutr, 1994 Aug, 13:4, 351-6

6 12 Newnham RE Essentiality of boron for healthy bones and joints. Environ Health Perspect, 1994 Nov, 102 Suppl 7:, 83-5

7 da Camara CC; Dowless GV Glucosamine sulfate for osteoarthritis. Ann Pharmacother, 1998 May, 32:5, 580-7

8 Mulherin DM; Struthers GR; Situnayake RD Do gold rings protect against articular erosion in rheumatoid arthritis? Ann Rheum Dis, 1997 Aug, 56:8, 497-9

9 Parker JC; Smarr KL; Buckelew SP; Stucky Ropp RC; Hewett JE; Johnson JC; Wright GE; Irvin WS; Walker SE Effects of stress management on clinical outcomes in rheumatoid arthritis. Arthritis Rheum, 1995 Dec, 38:12, 1807-18

10 Shapiro JA; Koepsell TD; Voigt LF; Dugowson CE; Kestin M; Nelson JL. Diet and rheumatoid arthritis in women: a possible protective effect of fish consumption. Epidemiology, 1996 May, 7:3, 256-63

11 Kjeldsen-Kragh J; Haugen M; Borchgrevink CF; Laerum E; Eek M; Mowinkel P; Hovi K; Forre O. Controlled trial of fasting and one-year vegetarian diet in rheumatoid arthritis. Lancet, 1991 Oct 12, 338:8772, 899-902

12 Kjeldsen-Kragh J; Haugen M; Borchgrevink CF; Forre O. Vegetarian diet for patients with rheumatoid arthritis – status: two years after the introduction of the diet. Clin Rheumatol, 1994 Sep, 13:3 475-82

13 Kaur H; Edmonds SE; Blake DR; Halliwell B Hydroxyl radical generation by rheumatoid blood and knee joint synovial fluid. Ann Rheum Dis, 1996 Dec, 55:12, 915-20

14 Comstock GW; Burke AE; Hoffman SC; Helzlsouer KJ; Bendich A; Masi AT; Norkus EP; Malamet RL; Gershwin ME. Serum concentrations of alpha tocopherol, beta carotene, and retinol preceding the diagnosis of rheumatoid arthritis and systemic lupus erythematosus. Ann Rheum Dis, 1997 May, 56:5, 323-5

15 Oldroyd KG; Dawes PT. Clinically significant vitamin C deficiency in rheumatoid arthritis. Br J Rheumatol, 24: 4, 1985 Nov, 362-3

16 Edmonds SE et al. Putative analgesic activity of repeated oral doses of vitamin E in the treatment of rheumatoid arthritis. Results of a prospective placebo controlled double blind trial. Ann Rheum Dis, 1997 Nov, 56:11, 649-55

17 Morgan SL et al. Supplementation with folic acid during methotrexate therapy for rheumatoid arthritis. A double-blind, placebo-controlled trial. Ann Intern Med, 1994 Dec, 121:11, 833-41

18 Mulherin DM; Thurnham DI; Situnayake RD Glutathione reductase activity, riboflavin status, and disease activity in rheumatoid arthritis. Ann Rheum Dis, 1996 Nov, 55:11, 837-40

19 Oelzner P; Müller A; Deschner F; Hüller M; Abendroth K; Hein G; Stein G. Relationship between disease activity and serum levels of vitamin D metabolites and PTH in rheumatoid arthritis. Calcif Tissue Int, 1998 Mar, 62:3, 193-8

20 Buckley LM; Leib ES; Cartularo KS; Vacek PM; Cooper SM. Calcium and vitamin D3 supplementation prevents bone loss in the spine secondary to low-dose corticosteroids in patients with rheumatoid arthritis. A randomized, double-blind, placebo-controlled trial. Ann Intern Med, 1996 Dec, 125:12, 961-8

21 Serum copper/zinc superoxide dismutase levels in patients with rheumatoid arthritis. Mazzetti I; Grigolo B; Borzì RM; Meliconi R; Facchini A. Int J Clin Lab Res, 1996, 26:4, 245-9

22 Weber J. Decreased iron absorption in patients with active rheumatoid arthritis, with and without iron deficiency. Ann Rheum Dis, 47: 5, 1988 May, 404-9

23 Pasquier C et al. Manganese containing superoxide dismutase deficiency in polymorphonuclear lymphocytes in rheumatoid arthritis. Inflammation. 1984;8:27-32

24 Heinle K; Adam A; Gradl M; Wiseman M; Adam O. Selenium concentration in erythrocytes of patients with rheumatoid arthritis. Clinical and laboratory chemistry infection markers during administration of selenium. Med Klin, 1997 Sep, 92 Suppl 3:, 29-31

25 Geusens P; Wouters C; Nijs J; Jiang Y; Dequeker J Long-term effect of omega-3 fatty acid supplementation in active rheumatoid arthritis. A 12-month, double-blind, controlled study. Arthritis Rheum, 1994 Jun, 37:6, 824-9

26 Leventhal LJ; Boyce EG; Zurier RB Treatment of rheumatoid arthritis with blackcurrant seed oil. Br J Rheumatol, 1994 Sep, 33:9, 847-52

Asthma

1 Buckley et al.Calcium and vitamin D3 supplementation prevents bone loss in the spine secondary to low-dose corticosteroids in patients with rheumatoid arthritis. A randomized, double-blind, placebo-controlled trial. Ann Intern Med 1996 Dec 15;125(12):961-968

2 Shimizu T; Maeda S; Arakawa H; Mochizuki H; Tokuyama K; Morikawa A. Relation between theophylline and circulating vitamin levels in children with asthma. Pharmacology, 1996 Dec, 53:6, 384-9

3 Carey OJ; Cookson JB; Britton J; Tattersfield AE The effect of lifestyle on wheeze, atopy, and bronchial hyperreactivity in Asian and white children. Am J Respir Crit Care Med, 1996 Aug, 154:2 Pt 1, 537-40

4 Troisi RJ; Willett WC; Weiss ST; Trichopoulos D; Rosner B; Speizer FE A prospective study of diet and adult-onset asthma. Am J Respir Crit Care Med, 1995 May, 151:5, 1401-8

5 Pletsityi KD; Vasipa SB; Davydova TV; Fomina VG. Vitamin E: immunocorrecting effect in bronchial asthma patients. Vopr Med Khim, 1995 Jul, 41:4, 33-6

6 Hatch GE Asthma, inhaled oxidants, and dietary antioxidants. Am J Clin Nutr, 1995 Mar, 61:3 Suppl, 625S-630S

7 Soutar A; Seaton A; Brown K Bronchial reactivity and dietary antioxidants. Thorax, 1997 Feb, 52:2, 166-70

8 Bielory L; Gandhi R Asthma and vitamin C. Ann Allergy, 1994 Aug, 73:2, 89-96; quiz 96-100

9 Cohen HA; Neuman I; Nahum H Blocking effect of vitamin C in exercise-induced asthma. Vitamin C supplements can also help to reduce exercise induced asthma by reducing airway hyperreactivity. Arch Pediatr Adolesc Med, 1997 Apr, 151:4, 367-70

10 Collipp PJ; Goldzier S 3d; Weiss N; Soleymani Y; Snyder R. Pyridoxine treatment of childhood bronchial asthma. Ann Allergy, 1975 Aug, 35:2, 93-7

11 Reynolds RD; Natta CL. Depressed plasma pyridoxal phosphate concentrations in adult asthmatics. Am J Clin Nutr, 1985 Apr, 41:4, 684-8

12 Sur S; Camara M; Buchmeier A; Morgan S; Nelson HS. Double-blind trial of pyridoxine (vitamin B6) in the treatment of steroid-dependent asthma. Ann Allergy, 1993 Feb, 70:2, 147-52

13 Ciarallo L; Sauer AH; Shannon MW a Intravenous magnesium therapy for moderate to severe pediatric asthma: results of a randomized, placebo-controlled trial. J Pediatr, 1996 Dec, 129:6, 809-14

14 Emelianova AV; Goncharova VA; Sinitsina TM. Magnesium sulfate in management of bronchial asthma. Klin Med (Mosk), 1996, 74:8, 55-8

15 Hill J; Micklewright A; Lewis S; Britton J Investigation of the effect of short-term change in dietary magnesium intake in asthma. Eur Respir J, 1997 Oct, 10:10, 2225-9

16 Britton J et al. Dietary Magnesium, Lung Function, Wheezing, And Airway Hyperreactivity In a Random Adult Population Sample. Lancet. 1994; 344: 357-361.

17 Shaw R, Woodman K, Crane J, Moyes C, Kennedy J, Pearce N. Risk factors for asthma symptoms in Kawerau children. N Z Med J. 1994;107:387-391.

18 Flatt A, Pearce N, Thomson CD, Sears MR, Robinson MF, Beasley R. Reduced selenium in asthmatic subjects in New Zealand. Thorax. 1990;45:95-99

19 Hasselmark L, Malmgren R, Zetterstrom O, Unge G. Selenium supplementation in intrinsic asthma. Allergy. 1993;48:3026.

20 Carey OJ; Locke C; Cookson JB Effect of alterations of dietary sodium on the severity of asthma in men. Thorax, 1993 Jul, 48:7, 714-8

21 Sakai K; Okuyama H; Shimazaki H; Katagiri M; Torii S; Matsushita T; Baba S. Fatty acid compositions of plasma lipids in atopic dermatitis/asthma patients. Arerugi, 1994 Jan, 43:1, 37-43

22 Hodge L et al. Effect of dietary intake of omega-3 and omega-6 fatty acids on severity of asthma in children. Eur Respir J, 1998 Feb, 11:2, 361-5

Cancer

1 Zhang S; Tang G; Russell RM; Mayzel KA; Stampfer MJ; Willett WC; Hunter DJ. Measurement of retinoids and carotenoids in breast adipose tissue and a comparison of concentrations in breast cancer cases and control subjects. Am J Clin Nutr, 1997 Sep, 66:3, 626-32

2 Xu XC; Sozzi G; Lee JS; Lee JJ; Pastorino U; Pilotti S; Kurie JM; Hong WK; Lotan R. Suppression of retinoic acid receptor beta in non-small-cell lung cancer in vivo: implications for lung cancer development. J Natl Cancer Inst, 1997 May, 89:9, 624-9

3 10 Smith AH; Waller KD. Serum beta-carotene in persons with cancer and their immediate families. Am J Epidemiol, 1991 Apr 1, 133:7, 661-71

4 Comstock GW; Alberg AJ; Huang HY; Wu K; Burke AE; Hoffman SC; Norkus EP; Gross M; Cutler RG; Morris JS; Spate VL; Helzlsouer KJ. The risk of developing lung cancer associated with antioxidants in the blood: ascorbic acid, carotenoids, alpha-tocopherol, selenium, and total peroxyl radical absorbing capacity. Cancer Epidemiol Biomarkers Prev, 1997 Nov, 6:11, 907-16

5 Mayne ST; Janerich DT; Greenwald P; Chorost S; Tucci C; Zaman MB; Melamed MR; Kiely M; McKneally MF Dietary beta carotene and lung cancer risk in U.S. nonsmokers. J Natl Cancer Inst, 1994 Jan, 86:1, 33-8

6 Dorgan JF; Sowell A; Swanson CA; Potischman N; Miller R; Schussler N; Stephenson HE Jr Relationships of serum carotenoids, retinol, alpha-tocopherol, and selenium with breast cancer risk: results from a prospective study in Columbia, Missouri (United States) Cancer Causes Control, 1998 Jan, 9:1, 89-97

7 Negri E; La Vecchia C; Franceschi S; DAvanzo B; Talamini R; Parpinel M; Ferraroni M; Filiberti R; Montella M; Falcini F; Conti E; Decarli A. Intake of selected micronutrients and the risk of breast cancer. Int J Cancer, 1996 Jan, 65:2, 140-4

8 Ingram D. Diet and subsequent survival in women with breast cancer. Br J Cancer, 1994 Mar, 69:3, 592-5

9 Freudenheim JL; Marshall JR; Vena JE; Laughlin R; Brasure JR; Swanson MK; Nemoto T; Graham S. Premenopausal breast cancer risk and intake of vegetables, fruits, and related nutrients. J Natl Cancer Inst, 1996 Mar, 88:6, 340-

10 Daviglus ML; Dyer AR; Persky V; Chavez N; Drum M; Goldberg J; Liu K; Morris DK; Shekelle RB; Stamler J Dietary beta-carotene, vitamin C, and risk of prostate cancer: results from the Western Electric Study. Epidemiology, 1996 Sep, 7:5, 472-7

11 Giovannucci E; Ascherio A; Rimm EB; Stampfer MJ; Colditz GA; Willett WC. Intake of carotenoids and retinol in relation to risk of prostate cancer. J Natl Cancer Inst, 1995 Dec, 87:23, 1767-76

12 Pappalardo G; Maiani G; Mobarhan S; Guadalaxara A; Azzini E; Raguzzini A; Salucci M; Serafini M; Trifero M; Illomei G; Ferro Luzzi A. Plasma (carotenoids, retinol, alpha-tocopherol) and tissue (carotenoids) levels after supplementation with beta-carotene in subjects with precancerous and cancerous lesions of sigmoid colon. Eur J Clin Nutr, 1997 Oct, 51:10, 661-6

13 Batieha AM; Armenian HK; Norkus EP; Morris JS; Spate VE; Comstock GW. Serum micronutrients and the subsequent risk of cervical cancer in a population-based nested case-control study. Cancer Epidemiol Biomarkers Prev, 1993 Jul-Aug, 2:4, 335-9

14 Muto Y; Fujii J; Shidoji Y; Moriwaki H; Kawaguchi T; Noda T Growth retardation in human cervical dysplasia-derived cell lines by beta-carotene through down-regulation of epidermal growth factor receptor. Am J Clin Nutr, 1995 Dec, 62:6 Suppl, 1535S-1540S

15 Palan PR; Mikhail MS; Basu J; Romney SL Beta-carotene levels in exfoliated cervicovaginal epithelial cells in cervical intraepithelial neoplasia and cervical cancer. Am J Obstet Gynecol, 1992 Dec, 167:6, 1899-903

16 Block G Vitamin C and cancer prevention: the epidemiologic evidence. Am J Clin Nutr, 1991 Jan, 53:1 Suppl, 270S-282S

17 Pandey DK; Shekelle R; Selwyn BJ; Tangney C; Stamler J. Dietary vitamin C and beta-carotene and risk of death in middle-aged men. The Western Electric Study. Am J Epidemiol, 1995 Dec, 142:12, 1269-78

18 Daviglus ML; Dyer AR; Persky V; Chavez N; Drum M; Goldberg J; Liu K; Morris DK; Shekelle RB; Stamler J Dietary beta-carotene, vitamin C, and risk of prostate cancer: results from the Western Electric Study. Epidemiology, 1996 Sep, 7:5, 472-7

19 Ocké MC; Bueno de Mesquita HB; Feskens EJ; van Staveren WA; Kromhout D Repeated measurements of vegetables, fruits, beta-carotene, and vitamins C and E in relation to lung cancer. The Zutphen Study. Am J Epidemiol, 1997 Feb, 145:4, 358-65

20 Ocké MC; Kromhout D; Menotti A; Aravanis C; Blackburn H; Buzina R; Fidanza F; Jansen A; Nedeljkovic S; Nissienen A; et al. Average intake of anti-oxidant (pro)vitamins and subsequent cancer mortality in the 16 cohorts of the Seven Countries Study. Int J Cancer, 1995 May, 61:4, 480-4

21 La Vecchia C; Ferraroni M; DAvanzo B; Decarli A; Franceschi S Selected micronutrient intake and the risk of gastric cancer. Cancer Epidemiol Biomarkers Prev, 1994 Jul, 3:5, 393-8

22 Shibata A; Paganini-Hill A; Ross RK; Henderson BE Intake of vegetables, fruits, beta-carotene, vitamin C and vitamin supplements and cancer incidence among the elderly: a prospective study. Br J Cancer, 1992 Oct, 66:4, 673-9

23 Ferraroni M; La Vecchia C; DAvanzo B; Negri E; Franceschi S; Decarli A Selected micronutrient intake and the risk of colorectal cancer. Br J Cancer, 1994 Dec, 70:6, 1150-5

24 Jain M; Miller AB; To T. Premorbid diet and the prognosis of women with breast cancer. J Natl Cancer Inst, 1994 Sep, 86:18, 1390-7

25 Hunter DJ; Manson JE; Colditz GA; Stampfer MJ; Rosner B; Hennekens CH; Speizer FE; Willett WC A prospective study of the intake of vitamins C, E, and A and the risk of breast cancer. N Engl J Med, 1993 Jul 22, 329:4, 234-40

26 Zheng W; Sellers TA; Doyle TJ; Kushi LH; Potter JD; Folsom AR Retinol, antioxidant vitamins, and cancers of the upper digestive tract in a prospective cohort study of postmenopausal women. Am J Epidemiol, 1995 Nov, 142:9, 955-60

27 Bostick RM; Potter JD; McKenzie DR; Sellers TA; Kushi LH; Steinmetz KA; Folsom AR. Reduced risk of colon cancer with high intake of vitamin E: the Iowa Women's Health Study. Cancer Res, 1993 Sep 15, 53:18, 4230-7

28 London SJ; Stein EA; Henderson IC; Stampfer MJ; Wood WC; Remine S; Dmochowski JR; Robert NJ; Willett WC. Carotenoids, retinol, and vitamin E and risk of proliferative benign breast disease and breast cancer. Cancer Causes Control, 1992 Nov, 3:6, 503-12

29 Hunter DJ; Manson JE; Colditz GA; Stampfer MJ; Rosner B; Hennekens CH; Speizer FE; Willett WC. A prospective study of the intake of vitamins C, E, and A and the risk of breast cancer. N Engl J Med, 1993 Jul 22, 329:4, 234-40

30 Slattery ML; Abbott TM; Overall JC Jr; Robison LM; French TK; Jolles C; Gardner JW; West DW. Dietary vitamins A, C, and E and selenium as risk factors for cervical cancer. Epidemiology, 1990 Jan, 1:1, 8-15

31 Palan PR; Mikhail MS; Basu J; Romney SL. Plasma levels of antioxidant beta-carotene and alpha-tocopherol in uterine cervix dysplasias and cancer. Nutr Cancer, 1991, 15:1, 13-20

32 Comstock GW; Helzlsouer KJ; Bush TL. Prediagnostic serum levels of carotenoids and vitamin E as related to subsequent cancer in Washington County, Maryland. Am J Clin Nutr, 1991 Jan, 53:1 Suppl, 260S-264S

33 Russo MW; Murray SC; Wurzelmann JI; Woosley JT; Sandler RS Plasma selenium levels and the risk of colorectal adenomas. Nutr Cancer, 1997, 28:2, 125-9

34 Psathakis D; Wedemeyer N; Oevermann E; Krug F; Siegers CP; Bruch HP Blood selenium and glutathione peroxidase status in patients with colorectal cancer. Dis Colon Rectum, 1998 Mar, 41:3, 328-35

35 van den Brandt PA; Goldbohm RA; van 't Veer P; Bode P; Dorant E; Hermus RJ; Sturmans F A prospective cohort study on selenium status and the risk of lung cancer. Cancer Res, 1993 Oct 15, 53:20, 4860-5

36 Blot WJ et al. Nutrition intervention trials in Linxian, China: supplementation with specific vitamin/mineral combinations, cancer incidence, and disease-specific mortality in the general population. J Natl Cancer Inst, 1993 Sep 15, 85:18, 1483-92

37 Pastorino U; Infante M; Maioli M; Chiesa G; Buyse M; Firket P; Rosmentz N; Clerici M; Soresi E; Valente M; et al Adjuvant treatment of stage I lung cancer with high-dose vitamin A. J Clin Oncol, 1993 Jul, 11:7, 1216-22

38 de Klerk NH; Musk AW; Ambrosini GL; Eccles JL; Hansen J; Olsen N; Watts VL; Lund HG; Pang SC; Beilby J; Hobbs MS. Vitamin A and cancer prevention II: comparison of the effects of retinol and beta-carotene. Int J Cancer, 1998 Jan, 75:3, 362-7

39 Musk AW; de Klerk NH; Ambrosini GL; Eccles JL; Hansen J; Olsen NJ; Watts VL; Lund HG; Pang SC; Beilby J; Hobbs MS. Vitamin A and cancer prevention I: observations in workers previously exposed to asbestos at Wittenoom, Western Australia. Int J Cancer, 1998 Jan, 75:3, 355-61

40 Issing WJ; Struck R; Naumann A. Positive impact of retinyl palmitate in leukoplakia of the larynx. Eur Arch Otorhinolaryngol Suppl, 1997, 1:, S105-9

41 Albanes D et al; Alpha-Tocopherol and beta-carotene supplements and lung cancer incidence in the alpha-tocopherol, beta-carotene cancer prevention study: effects of base-line characteristics and study compliance J Natl Cancer Inst, 1996 Nov, 88:21, 1560-70

42 Omenn G et al. Effects of a combination of beta carotene and vitamin A on lung cancer and cardiovascular disease. N Engl J Med. 1996;334: 1150-5

43 Hennekens C H et al. Lack of effect of long term supplementation with beta carotene on the incidence of malignant neoplasms and cardiovascular disease. N Engl J Med. 1996;334: 1145-9 and 1189-90

44 Handelman GJ, Packer L and Cross C E. Destruction of tocopherols, carotenoids and retinol in human plasma by cigarette smoke. Am J Clin Nutr. 1996;63: 559-65

45 Journal of the American Chemical Society 1997;119:621-622

46 Waring AJ; Drake IM; Schorah CJ; White KL; Lynch DA; Axon AT; Dixon MF Ascorbic acid and total vitamin C concentrations in plasma, gastric juice, and gastrointestinal mucosa: effects of gastritis and oral supplementation. Gut, 1996 Feb, 38:2, 171-6

47 Zhang HM; Wakisaka N; Maeda O; Yamamoto T. Vitamin C inhibits the growth of a bacterial risk factor for gastric carcinoma: *Helicobacter pylori*. Cancer, 1997 Nov, 80:10, 1897-903

48 Paganelli GM; Biasco G; Brandi G; Santucci R; Gizzi G; Villani V; Cianci M; Miglioli M; Barbara L Effect of vitamin A, C, and E supplementation on rectal cell proliferation in patients with colorectal adenomas. J Natl Cancer Inst, 1992 Jan 1, 84:1, 47-51

49 Maramag C; Menon M; Balaji KC; Reddy PG; Laxmanan S Effect of vitamin C on prostate cancer cells in vitro: effect on cell number, viability, and DNA synthesis. Prostate, 1997 Aug, 32:3, 188-95

50 Okunieff P. Interactions between ascorbic acid and the radiation of bone marrow, skin and tumor. Am J Clin Nutr 1991;54:1281S-1283S

51 Losonczy KG; Harris TB; Havlik RJ. Vitamin E and vitamin C supplement use and risk of all-cause and coronary heart disease mortality in older persons: the Established Populations for Epidemiologic Studies of the Elderly. Am J Clin Nutr, 1996 Aug, 64:2, 190-6

52 Heinonen OP et al. Prostate cancer and supplementation with alpha-tocopherol and beta-carotene: incidence and mortality in a controlled trial. J Natl Cancer Inst, 1998 Mar, 90:6, 440-6

53 Wang GQ et al. Effects of vitamin/mineral supplementation on the prevalence of histological dysplasia and early cancer of the esophagus and stomach: results from the General Population Trial in Linxian, China. Cancer Epidemiol Biomarkers Prev, 1994 Mar, 3:2, 161-6

54 Clark LC et al. Effects of selenium supplementation for cancer prevention in patients with carcinoma of the skin. A randomized controlled trial. Nutritional Prevention of Cancer Study Group. JAMA, 1996 Dec, 276:24, 1957-63

55 Feldman D; Skowronski RJ; Peehl DM Vitamin D and prostate cancer. Adv Exp Med Biol, 1995, 375:, 53-63

56 Brenner RV; Shabahang M; Schumaker LM; Nauta RJ; Uskokovic MR; Evans SR; Buras RR The antiproliferative effect of vitamin D analogs on MCF-7 human breast cancer cells. Cancer Lett, 1995 May, 92:1, 77-82

57 Colston KW; James SY; Ofori Kuragu EA; Binderup L; Grant AG. Vitamin D receptors and anti-proliferative effects of vitamin D derivatives in human pancreatic carcinoma cells in vivo and in vitro. Br J Cancer, 1997, 76:8, 1017-20

58 Lefkowitz ES; Garland CF Sunlight, vitamin D, and ovarian cancer mortality rates in US women. Int J Epidemiol, 1994 Dec, 23:6, 1133-6

59 Pritchard RS; Baron JA; Gerhardsson de Verdier M. Dietary calcium, vitamin D, and the risk of colorectal cancer in Stockholm, Sweden. Cancer Epidemiol Biomarkers Prev, 1996 Nov, 5:11, 897-900

60 Martínez ME; Giovannucci EL; Colditz GA; Stampfer MJ; Hunter DJ; Speizer FE; Wing A; Willett WC Calcium, vitamin D, and the occurrence of colorectal cancer among women. J Natl Cancer Inst, 1996 Oct, 88:19, 1375-82

61 Gann PH; Ma J; Hennekens CH; Hollis BW; Haddad JG; Stampfer MJ Circulating vitamin D metabolites in relation to subsequent development of prostate cancer. Cancer Epidemiol Biomarkers Prev, 1996 Feb, 5:2, 121-6

62 Taylor JA; Hirvonen A; Watson M; Pittman G; Mohler JL; Bell DA Association of prostate cancer with vitamin D receptor gene polymorphism. Cancer Res, 1996 Sep, 56:18, 4108-10

63 Kim YI; Pogribny IP; Basnakian AG; Miller JW; Selhub J; James SJ; Mason JB Folate deficiency in rats induces DNA strand breaks and hypomethylation within the p53 tumor suppressor gene. Am J Clin Nutr, 1997 Jan, 65:1, 46-52

64 Glynn SA; Albanes D; Pietinen P; Brown CC; Rautalahti M; Tangrea JA; Gunter EW; Barrett MJ; Virtamo J; Taylor PR. Colorectal cancer and folate status: a nested case-control study among male smokers. Cancer Epidemiol Biomarkers Prev, 1996 Jul, 5:7, 487-94

65 Butterworth CE Jr; Hatch KD; Macaluso M; Cole P; Sauberlich HE; Soong SJ; Borst M; Baker VV. Folate deficiency and cervical dysplasia. JAMA, 1992 Jan 22-29, 267:4, 528-33

66 Lashner BA; Provencher KS; Seidner DL; Knesebeck A; Brzezinski A The effect of folic acid supplementation on the risk for cancer or dysplasia in ulcerative colitis. Gastroenterology, 1997 Jan, 112:1, 29-32

67 Biasco G et al. Folic acid supplementation and cell kinetics of rectal mucosa in patients with ulcerative colitis. Cancer Epidemiol Biomarkers Prev, 1997 Jun, 6:6, 469-71

68 Saito M; Kato H; Tsuchida T; Konaka C Chemoprevention effects on bronchial squamous metaplasia by folate and vitamin B12 in heavy smokers. Chest, 1994 Aug, 106:2, 496-9

69 Butterworth CE Jr; Hatch KD; Soong SJ; Cole P; Tamura T; Sauberlich HE; Borst M; Macaluso M; Baker V. Oral folic acid supplementation for cervical dysplasia: a clinical intervention trial. Am J Obstet Gynecol, 1992 Mar, 166:3, 803-9

70 Harper JM; Levine AJ; Rosenthal DL; Wiesmeier E; Hunt IF; Swendseid ME; Haile RW. Acta Cytol, Erythrocyte folate levels, oral contraceptive use and abnormal cervical cytology. Author 1994 May, 38:3, 324-30

71 Kearney J; Giovannucci E; Rimm EB; Ascherio A; Stampfer MJ; Colditz GA; Wing A; Kampman E; Willett WC. Calcium, vitamin D, and dairy foods and the occurrence of colon cancer in men. Am J Epidemiol, 1996 May, 143:9, 907-17

72 Martínez ME; Giovannucci EL; Colditz GA; Stampfer MJ; Hunter DJ; Speizer FE; Wing A; Willett WC. Calcium, vitamin D, and the occurrence of colorectal cancer among women. J Natl Cancer Inst, 1996 Oct, 88:19, 1375-82

73 Zheng W; Anderson KE; Kushi LH; Sellers TA; Greenstein J; Hong CP; Cerhan JR; Bostick RM; Folsom AR. A prospective cohort study of intake of calcium, vitamin D, and other micronutrients in relation to incidence of rectal cancer among postmenopausal women. Cancer Epidemiol Biomarkers Prev, 1998 Mar, 7:3, 221-5

74 Tohyama E. Relationship between fluoride concentration in drinking water and mortality rate from uterine cancer in Okinawa prefecture, Japan. Epidemiol, 1996 Dec, 6:4, 184-91

75 Tseng M; Sandler RS; Greenberg ER; Mandel JS; Haile RW; Baron JA. Dietary iron and recurrence of colorectal adenomas. Cancer Epidemiol Biomarkers Prev, 1997 Dec, 6:12, 1029-32

76 Stevens R et al. Moderate elevation of body iron level and increased risk of cancer occurrence and death. Int J Cancer 1994;56:364-369

77 Heyneman CA Zinc deficiency and taste disorders. Ann Pharmacother, 1996 Feb, 30:2, 186-7

78 Rose DP Dietary fatty acids and prevention of hormone-responsive cancer. Proc Soc Exp Biol Med, 1997 Nov, 216:2, 224-33

79 Godley PA; Campbell MK; Gallagher P; Martinson FE; Mohler JL; Sandler RS. Biomarkers of essential fatty acid consumption and risk of prostatic carcinoma. Cancer Epidemiol Biomarkers Prev, 1996 Nov, 5:11, 889-95

80 Simonsen N; vant Veer P; Strain JJ; Martin Moreno JM; Huttunen JK; Navajas JF; Martin BC; Thamm M; Kardinaal AF; Kok FJ; Kohlmeier L. Adipose tissue omega-3 and omega-6 fatty acid content and breast cancer in the EURAMIC study. European Community Multicenter Study on Antioxidants, Myocardial Infarction, and Breast Cancer. Am J Epidemiol, 1998 Feb, 147:4, 342-52

81 Caygill CP; Hill MJ. Fish, n-3 fatty acids and human colorectal and breast cancer mortality. Eur J Cancer Prev, 1995 Aug, 4:4, 329-32

82 Rose DP; Connolly JM; Rayburn J; Coleman M. Influence of diets containing eicosapentaenoic or docosahexaenoic acid on growth and metastasis of breast cancer cells in nude mice. J Natl Cancer Inst, 1995 Apr, 87:8, 587-92

83 Veierod MB; Laake P; Thelle DS Dietary fat intake and risk of lung cancer: a prospective study of 51,452 Norwegian men and women. Eur J Cancer Prev, 1997 Dec, 6:6, 540-9

84 Gogos CA; Ginopoulos P; Salsa B; Apostolidou E; Zoumbos NC; Kalfarentzos F. Dietary omega-3 polyunsaturated fatty acids plus vitamin E restore immunodeficiency and prolong survival for severely ill patients with generalized malignancy: a randomized control trial. Cancer, 1998 Jan, 82:2, 395-402

85 Solomon LZ; Jennings AM; Hayes MC; Bass PS; Birch BR; Cooper AJ Is gamma-linolenic acid an effective intravesical agent for superficial bladder cancer? In vitro cytotoxicity and in vivo tolerance studies. Urol Res, 1998, 26:1, 11-5

86 Jiang WG et al. Inhibition of hepatocyte growth factor-induced motility and in vitro invasion of human colon cancer cells by gamma-linolenic acid. Br J Cancer, 71: 4, 1995 Apr, 744-52

Cardiovascular disease

1 Rimm EB; Ascherio A; Giovannucci E; Spiegelman D; Stampfer MJ; Willett WC. Vegetable, fruit, and cereal fiber intake and risk of coronary heart disease among men. JAMA, 1996 Feb, 275:6, 447-51

2 Hu FB; Stampfer MJ; Manson JE; Rimm E; Colditz GA; Rosner BA; Hennekens CH; Willett WC Dietary fat intake and the risk of coronary heart disease in women. N Engl J Med, 1997 Nov, 337:21, 1491-9

3 Gaziano JM; Manson JE; Branch LG; Colditz GA; Willett WC; Buring JE. A prospective study of consumption of carotenoids in fruits and vegetables and decreased cardiovascular mortality in the elderly. Ann Epidemiol, 1995 Jul, 5:4, 255-60

4 Kohlmeier L et al; Lycopene and myocardial infarction risk in the EURAMIC Study. Am J Epidemiol, 1997 Oct, 146:8, 618-26

5 Tavani A; Negri E; DAvanzo B; La Vecchia C. Beta-carotene intake and risk of nonfatal acute myocardial infarction in women. Eur J Epidemiol, 1997 Sep, 13:6, 631-7

6 Daviglus ML; Orencia AJ; Dyer AR; Liu K; Morris DK; Persky V; Chavez N; Goldberg J; Drum M; Shekelle RB; Stamler J Dietary vitamin C, beta-carotene and 30-year risk of stroke: results from the Western Electric Study. Neuroepidemiology, 1997, 16:2, 69-77

7 Albanes D et al; Alpha-Tocopherol and beta-carotene supplements and lung cancer incidence in the alpha-tocopherol, beta-carotene cancer prevention study: effects of base-line characteristics and study compliance J Natl Cancer Inst, 1996 Nov, 88:21, 1560-70

8 Omenn G et al. Effects of a combination of beta carotene and vitamin A on lung cancer and cardiovascular disease. N Engl J Med. 1996;334: 1150-5

9 Journal of the American Chemical Society 1997;119:621-622

10 Sahyoun NR; Jacques PF; Russell RM Carotenoids, vitamins C and E, and mortality in an elderly population. Am J Epidemiol, 1996 Sep, 144:5, 501-11

11 Gale CR; Martyn CN; Winter PD; Cooper C Vitamin C and risk of death from stroke and coronary heart disease in cohort of elderly people. BMJ, 1995 Jun, 310:6994, 1563-6

12 Nyyssönen K; Parviainen MT; Salonen R; Tuomilehto J; Salonen JT. Vitamin C deficiency and risk of myocardial infarction: prospective population study of men from eastern Finland. BMJ, 1997 Mar, 314:7081, 634-8

13 Rimm EB; Stampfer MJ; Ascherio A; Giovannucci E; Colditz GA; Willett WC Vitamin E consumption and the risk of coronary heart disease in men. N Engl J Med, 1993 May 20, 328:20, 1450-6

14 Stampfer MJ; Hennekens CH; Manson JE; Colditz GA; Rosner B; Willett WC Vitamin E consumption and the risk of coronary disease in women. N Engl J Med, 1993 May 20, 328:20, 1444-9

15 Ness AR; Khaw KT; Bingham S; Day NE Vitamin C status and undiagnosed angina. J Cardiovasc Risk, 1996 Aug, 3:4, 373-7

16 Ness AR; Khaw KT; Bingham S; Day NE Vitamin C status and serum lipids. Eur J Clin Nutr, 1996 Nov, 50:11, 724-9

17 Losonczy KG; Harris TB; Havlik RJ Vitamin E and vitamin C supplement use and risk of all-cause and coronary heart disease mortality in older persons: the Established Populations for Epidemiologic Studies of the Elderly. Am J Clin Nutr, 1996 Aug, 64:2, 190-6

18 Plotnick GD; Corretti MC; Vogel RA Effect of antioxidant vitamins on the transient impairment of endothelium-dependent brachial artery vasoactivity following a single high-fat meal. JAMA 1997;278:1682-1686

19 Levine GN; Frei B; Koulouris SN; Gerhard MD; Keaney JF Jr; Vita JA Ascorbic acid reverses endothelial vasomotor dysfunction in patients with coronary artery disease. Circulation, 1996 Mar, 93:6, 1107-13

20 Ting HH; Timimi FK; Haley EA; Roddy MA; Ganz P; Creager MA Vitamin C improves endothelium-dependent vasodilation in forearm resistance vessels of humans with hypercholesterolemia. Circulation, 1997 Jun, 95:12, 2617-22

21 Hornig B; Arakawa N; Kohler C; Drexler H Vitamin C improves endothelial function of conduit arteries in patients with chronic heart failure. Circulation, 1998 Feb, 97:4, 363-8

22 Dingchao H; Zhiduan Q; Liye H; Xiaodong F The protective effects of high-dose ascorbic acid on myocardium against reperfusion injury during and after cardiopulmonary bypass. Thorac Cardiovasc Surg, 1994 Oct, 42:5, 276-8

23 Motoyama T; Kawano H; Kugiyama K; Hirashima O; Ohgushi M; Yoshimura M; Ogawa H; Yasue H Endothelium-dependent vasodilation in the brachial artery is impaired in smokers: effect of vitamin C. Am J Physiol, 1997 Oct, 273:4 Pt 2, H1644-50

24 Kushi LH; Fee RM; Sellers TA; Zheng W; Folsom AR. Intake of vitamins A, C, and E and postmenopausal breast cancer. The Iowa Women's Health Study. Am J Epidemiol, 1996 Jul, 144:2, 165-74

25 Rimm EB. Vitamin E consumption and the risk of coronary heart disease in men. N Engl J Med, 328: 20, 1993 May 20, 1450-6

26 Miwa K; Miyagi Y; Igawa A; Nakagawa K; Inoue H Vitamin E deficiency in variant angina. Circulation, 1996 Jul, 94:1, 14-8

27 Rapola JM; Virtamo J; Haukka JK; Heinonen OP; Albanes D; Taylor PR; Huttunen JK Effect of vitamin E and beta carotene on the incidence of angina pectoris. A randomized, double-blind, controlled trial. JAMA, 1996 Mar, 275:9, 693-8

28 Stampfer M et al. Vitamin E consumption and the risk of coronary disease in women. N Engl J Med. 1993;328:1450-1456

29 Stephens N G et al. Randomised controlled trial of vitamin E in patients with coronary disease: Cambridge Heart Antioxidant Study (CHAOS). Lancet, 347: 9004, 1996 Mar 23, 781-6

30 5 Vitoux D; Chappuis P; Arnaud J; Bost M; Accominotti M; Roussel AM Selenium, glutathione peroxidase, peroxides and platelet functions. Ann Biol Clin (Paris), 1996, 54:5, 181-7

31 Kok FJ; Hofman A; Witteman JC; de Bruijn AM; Kruyssen DH; de Bruin M; Valkenburg HA. Decreased selenium levels in acute myocardial infarction. JAMA, 1989 Feb 24, 261:8, 1161-4

32 Salvini S; Hennekens CH; Morris JS; Willett WC; Stampfer MJ. Plasma levels of the antioxidant selenium and risk of myocardial infarction among U.S. physicians. Am J Cardiol, 1995 Dec, 76:17, 1218-21

33 Korpela H; Kumpulainen J; Jussila E; Kemilä S; Kääriäinen M; Kääriäinen T; Sotaniemi EA Effect of selenium supplementation after acute myocardial infarction. Res Commun Chem Pathol Pharmacol, 1989 Aug, 65:2, 249-52

34 Thiele R; Wagner D; Gassel M; Winnefeld K; Pleissner J; Pfeifer R Selenium substitution in acute myocardial infarct. Med Klin, 1997 Sep, 92 Suppl 3:, 26-8

35 O'Connor PJ; Rush WA; Trence DL. Relative effectiveness of niacin and lovastatin for treatment of dyslipidemias in a health maintenance organization. J Fam Pract, 1997 May, 44:5, 462-7

36 Gardner SF; Schneider EF; Granberry MC; Carter IR. Combination therapy with low-dose lovastatin and niacin is as effective as higher-dose lovastatin. Pharmacotherapy, 1996 May, 16:3, 419-23

37 Johansson JO; Egberg N; Asplund Carlson A; Carlson LA. Nicotinic acid treatment shifts the fibrinolytic balance favourably and decreases plasma fibrinogen in hypertriglyceridaemic men. J Cardiovasc Risk, 1997 Jun, 4:3, 165-71

38 Robinson K; Arheart K; Refsum H; Brattström L; Boers G; Ueland P; Rubba P; Palma Reis R; Meleady R; Daly L; Witteman J; Graham I. Low circulating folate and vitamin B6 concentrations: risk factors for stroke, peripheral vascular disease, and coronary artery disease. European COMAC Group. Circulation, 1998 Feb, 97:5, 437-43

39 Selhub J; Jacques PF; Bostom AG; DAgostino RB; Wilson PW; Belanger AJ; OLeary DH; Wolf PA; Rush D; Schaefer EJ; Rosenberg IH. Relationship between plasma homocysteine, vitamin status and extracranial carotid-artery stenosis in the Framingham Study population. J Nutr, 1996 Apr, 126:4 Suppl, 1258S-65S

40 Rimm EB; Willett WC; Hu FB; Sampson L; Colditz GA; Manson JE; Hennekens C; Stampfer MJ Folate and vitamin B6 from diet and supplements in relation to risk of coronary heart disease among women. JAMA, 1998 Feb, 279:5, 359-64

41 Woodside JV et al. Effect of B-group vitamins and antioxidant vitamins on hyperhomocysteinemia: a double-blind, randomized, factorial-design, controlled trial. Am J Clin Nutr, 1998 May, 67:5, 858-66

42 Sermet A; Aybak M; Ulak G; Güzel C; Denli O Effect of oral pyridoxine hydrochloride supplementation on in vitro platelet sensitivity to different agonists.

43 Brattström L; Stavenow L; Galvard H; Nilsson-Ehle P; Berntorp E; Jerntorp P; Elmståhl S; Pessah-Rasmussen H. Pyridoxine reduces cholesterol and low-density lipoprotein and increases antithrombin III activity in 80-year-old men with low plasma pyridoxal 5-phosphate. Scand J Clin Lab Invest, 1990 Dec, 50:8, 873-7

44 Robinson K; Arheart K; Refsum H; Brattström L; Boers G; Ueland P; Rubba P; Palma Reis R; Meleady R; Daly L; Witteman J; Graham I Low circulating folate and vitamin B6 concentrations: risk factors for stroke, peripheral vascular disease, and coronary artery disease. European COMAC Group. Circulation, 1998 Feb, 97:5, 437-43

45 Morrison HI; Schaubel D; Desmeules M; Wigle DT Serum folate and risk of fatal coronary heart disease. JAMA, 1996 Jun, 275:24, 1893-6

46 Schwartz SM et al. Myocardial infarction in young women in relation to plasma total homocysteine, folate, and a common variant in the methylenetetrahydrofolate reductase gene. Circulation, 1997 Jul, 96:2, 412-7

47 Lowering blood homocysteine with folic acid based supplements: meta-analysis of randomised trials. Homocysteine Lowering Trialists' Collaboration. BMJ, 1998 Mar, 316:7135, 894-8

48 Ward M, McNulty H, McPartlin J, Strain JJ, Weir DG, Scott JM. Plasma homocysteine, a risk factor for cardiovascular disease, is lowered by physiological doses of folic acid. QJM 1997;90:519-24.

49 Chadefaux B; Cooper BA; Gilfix BM; Lue Shing H; Carson W; Gavsie A; Rosenblatt DS. Homocysteine: relationship to serum cobalamin, serum folate, erythrocyte folate, and lobation of neutrophils. Clin Invest Med, 1994 Dec, 17:6, 540-50

50 Watson KE; Abrolat ML; Malone LL; Hoeg JM; Doherty T; Detrano R; Demer LL Active serum vitamin D levels are inversely correlated with coronary calcification. Circulation, 1997 Sep, 96:6, 1755-60

51 Thomas VL; Gropper SS. Effect of chromium nicotinic acid supplementation on selected cardiovascular disease risk factors. Biol Trace Elem Res, 1996 Dec, 55:3, 297-305

52 Jones AA; DiSilvestro RA; Coleman M; Wagner TL Copper supplementation of adult men: effects on blood copper enzyme activities and indicators of cardiovascular disease risk. Metabolism, 1997 Dec, 46:12, 1380-3

53 Tzonou A; Lagiou P; Trichopoulou A; Tsoutsos V; Trichopoulos D. Dietary iron and coronary heart disease risk: a study from Greece. Am J Epidemiol, 1998 Jan, 147:2, 161-6

54 Tuomainen TP; Punnonen K; Nyyssönen K; Salonen JT Association between body iron stores and the risk of acute myocardial infarction in men. Circulation, 1998 Apr, 97:15, 1461-6

55 Corti MC; Guralnik JM; Salive ME; Ferrucci L; Pahor M; Wallace RB; Hennekens CH. Serum iron level, coronary artery disease, and all-cause mortality in older men and women. Am J Cardiol, 1997 Jan, 79:2, 120-7

56 Rubenowitz E; Axelsson G; Rylander R. Magnesium in drinking water and death from acute myocardial infarction. Am J Epidemiol, 1996 Mar, 143:5, 456-62

57 Ma J et al. Associations of serum and dietary magnesium with cardiovascular disease, hypertension, diabetes, insulin, and carotid arterial wall thickness: the ARIC study. Atherosclerosis Risk in Communities. J Clin Epidemiol, 1995 Jul, 48:7, 927-40

58 Goto K; Yasue H; Okumura K; Matsuyama K; Kugiyama K; Miyagi H; Higashi T Magnesium deficiency detected by intravenous loading test in variant angina pectoris. Am J Cardiol, 1990 Mar 15, 65:11, 709-12

59 Satake K; Lee JD; Shimizu H; Ueda T; Nakamura T Relation between severity of magnesium deficiency and frequency of anginal attacks in men with variant angina. J Am Coll Cardiol, 1996 Oct, 28:4, 897-902

60 Rabbani LE; Antman EM The role of magnesium therapy in acute myocardial infarction. Clin Cardiol, 1996 Nov, 19:11, 841-4

61 Woods KL; Fletcher S Long-term outcome after intravenous magnesium sulphate in suspected acute

myocardial infarction: the second Leicester Intravenous Magnesium Intervention Trial (LIMIT-2). Lancet, 1994 Apr, 343:8901, 816-9

62 ISIS-4: a randomised factorial trial assessing early oral captopril, oral mononitrate, and intravenous magnesium sulphate in 58,050 patients with suspected acute myocardial infarction. ISIS-4 (Fourth International Study of Infarct Survival) Collaborative Group Lancet, 1995 Mar, 345:8951, 669-85

63 26 Redwood SR; Bashir Y; Huang J; Leatham EW; Kaski JC; Camm AJ Effect of magnesium sulphate in patients with unstable angina. A double blind, randomized, placebo-controlled study. Eur Heart J, 1997 Aug, 18:8, 1269-77

64 Lichodziejewska B; K et al. Clinical symptoms of mitral valve prolapse are related to hypomagnesemia and attenuated by magnesium supplementation. Am J Cardiol, 1997 Mar, 79:6, 768-72

65 Young DB, Lin H, McCabe RD. Potassium's cardiovascular protective mechanisms. Am J Physiol 1995 Apr;268(4 Pt 2):R825-R837

66 Reunanen A; Knekt P; Marniemi J; Mäki J; Maatela J; Aromaa A Serum calcium, magnesium, copper and zinc and risk of cardiovascular death. Eur J Clin Nutr, 1996 Jul, 50:7, 431-7

67 Hennig B; Toborek M; Mcclain CJ Antiatherogenic properties of zinc: implications in endothelial cell metabolism. Nutrition, 1996 Oct, 12:10, 711-7

68 Fortes C; Agabiti N; Fano V; Pacifici R; Forastiere F; Virgili F; Zuccaro P; Perruci CA; Ebrahim S Zinc supplementation and plasma lipid peroxides in an elderly population. Eur J Clin Nutr, 1997 Feb, 51:2, 97-101

69 Kromhout D; Bosschieter EB; de Lezenne Coulander C. The inverse relation between fish consumption and 20-year mortality from coronary heart disease. N Engl J Med, 1985 May 9, 312:19, 1205-9

70 Burr ML et al. Effects of changes in fat, fish, and fibre intakes on death and myocardial reinfarction: diet and reinfarction trial (DART). Lancet, 1989 Sep 30, 2:8666, 757-61

71 Albert CM; Hennekens CH; ODonnell CJ; Ajani UA; Carey VJ; Willett WC; Ruskin JN; Manson JE. Fish consumption and risk of sudden cardiac death. JAMA, 1998 Jan, 279:1, 23-8

72 Siscovick DS et al. Dietary intake and cell membrane levels of long-chain n-3 polyunsaturated fatty acids and the risk of primary cardiac arrest. JAMA, 1995 Nov, 274:17, 1363-7

73 Sacks FM et al. Short report: the effect of fish oil on blood pressure and high-density lipoprotein-cholesterol levels in phase I of the Trials of Hypertension Prevention. J Hypertens, 1994 Feb, 12:2, 209-13

74 Mori TA; Beilin LJ; Burke V; Morris J; Ritchie J. Interactions between dietary fat, fish, and fish oils and their effects on platelet function in men at risk of cardiovascular disease. Arterioscler Thromb Vasc Biol, 1997 Feb, 17:2, 279-86

75 Nestel PJ et al. Arterial compliance in obese subjects is improved with dietary plant n-3 fatty acid from flaxseed oil despite increased LDL oxidizability. Arterioscler Thromb Vasc Biol, 1997 Jun, 17:6, 1163-70

76 Wojcicki J et al. Clinical evaluation of lecithin as a lipid-lowering agent. Phytotherapy Res 1995, 9, 597-99

77 Hanaki-Y et al. Coenzyme Q10 and coronary artery disease. Clin Investig. 1993; 71(8 Suppl): S112-5

78 Langsjoen H et al. Usefulness of coenzyme Q10 in clinical cardiology: a long-term study. Mol Aspects Med. 1994; 15 Suppl: s165-75

Carpal tunnel syndrome

1 Fuhr JE; Farrow A; Nelson HS Jr Vitamin B6 levels in patients with carpal tunnel syndrome. Arch Surg, 1989 Nov, 124:11, 1329-30

2 Ellis JM; Folkers K; Levy M; Shizukuishi S; Lewandowski J; Nishii S; Schubert HA; Ulrich R. Response of vitamin B-6 deficiency and the carpal tunnel syndrome to pyridoxine. Proc Natl Acad Sci U S A, 1982 Dec, 79:23, 7494-8

3 Franzblau A; Rock CL; Werner RA; Albers JW; Kelly MP; Johnston EC . The relationship of vitamin B6 status to median nerve function and carpal tunnel syndrome among active industrial workers. J Occup Environ Med, 1996 May, 38:5, 485-91

4 Folkers K; Ellis J Successful therapy with vitamin B6 and vitamin B2 of the carpal tunnel syndrome and need for determination of the RDAs for vitamins B6 and B2 for disease states. Ann N Y Acad Sci, 1990, 585:, 295-301

5 Folkers K; Wolaniuk A; Vadhanavikit S. Enzymology of the response of the carpal tunnel syndrome to riboflavin and to combined riboflavin and pyridoxine. Proc Natl Acad Sci U S A, 1984 Nov, 81:22, 7076-8

Cervical dysplasia

1 Liu T; Soong SJ; Wilson NP; Craig CB; Cole P; Macaluso M; Butterworth CE Jr. A case control study of nutritional factors and cervical dysplasia. Cancer Epidemiol Biomarkers Prev, 1993 Nov-Dec, 2:6, 525-30

2 Harper JM; Levine AJ; Rosenthal DL; Wiesmeier E; Hunt IF; Swendseid ME; Haile RW. Acta Cytol, Erythrocyte folate levels, oral contraceptive use and abnormal cervical cytology. Author 1994 May, 38:3, 324-30

3 Butterworth CE Jr; Hatch KD; Macaluso M; Cole P; Sauberlich HE; Soong SJ; Borst M; Baker VV. Folate deficiency and cervical dysplasia. JAMA, 1992 Jan 22-29, 267:4, 528-33

4 Butterworth CE Jr; Hatch KD; Soong SJ; Cole P; Tamura T; Sauberlich HE; Borst M; Macaluso M; Baker V. Oral folic acid supplementation for cervical dysplasia: a clinical intervention trial. Am J Obstet Gynecol, 1992 Mar, 166:3, 803-9

5 Giuliano AR; Papenfuss M; Nour M; Canfield LM; Schneider A; Hatch K. Antioxidant nutrients: associations with persistent human papillomavirus infection. Cancer Epidemiol Biomarkers Prev, 1997 Nov, 6:11, 917-23

6 VanEenwyk J; Davis FG; Bowen PE. Dietary and serum carotenoids and cervical intraepithelial neoplasia. Int J Cancer, 1991 Apr 22, 48:1, 34-8

7 Kwasniewska A; Tukendorf A; Semczuk M Content of alpha-tocopherol in blood serum of human Papillomavirus-infected women with cervical dysplasias. Nutr Cancer, 1997, 28:3, 248-51

8 Shimizu H; Nagata C; Komatsu S; Morita N; Higashiiwai H; Sugahara N; Hisamichi S. Decreased serum retinol levels in women with cervical dysplasia. Br J Cancer, 1996 Jun, 73:12, 1600-4

9 Meyskens FL Jr et al. Enhancement of regression of cervical intraepithelial neoplasia II (moderate dysplasia) with

topically applied all-trans-retinoic acid: a randomized trial. J Natl Cancer Inst, 1994 Apr, 86:7, 539-43

10 Wassertheil-Smoller S et al. Dietary vitamin C and uterine cervical dysplasia. Am J Epidemiol, 114: 5, 1981 Nov, 714-24

11 Grail A; Norval M Copper and zinc levels in serum from patients with abnormalities of the uterine cervix. Acta Obstet Gynecol Scand, 1986, 65:5, 443-7

12 Liu T; Soong SJ; Alvarez RD; Butterworth CE Jr A longitudinal analysis of human papillomavirus 16 infection, nutritional status, and cervical dysplasia progression. Cancer Epidemiol Biomarkers Prev, 1995 Jun, 4:4, 373-80

Common cold

1 Hemilä H Vitamin C supplementation and common cold symptoms: problems with inaccurate reviews. Nutrition, 1996 Nov, 12:11-12, 804-9

2 Hemilä H Vitamin C intake and susceptibility to the common cold. Br J Nutr, 1997 Jan, 77:1, 59-72

3 Hemilä H Vitamin C and common cold incidence: a review of studies with subjects under heavy physical stress. Int J Sports Med, 1996 Jul, 17:5, 379-83

4 Garland ML; Hagmeyer KO The role of zinc lozenges in treatment of the common cold. Ann Pharmacother, 1998 Jan, 32:1, 63-9

5 Mossad SB; Macknin ML; Medendorp SV; Mason P. Zinc gluconate lzenges for treating the common cold. A randomized, double-blind, placebo-controlled study. Ann Intern Med, 1996 Jul, 125:2, 81-8

6 Eby GA Zinc ion availability—the determinant of efficacy in zinc lozenge treatment of common colds. J Antimicrob Chemother, 1997 Oct, 40:4, 483-93

7 Macknin ML et al. Zinc Gluconate Lozenges for Treating the Common Cold in Children. JAMA. 1998;279:1962-1967

Diabetes

1 Atkinson MA; Ellis TM. Infants diets and insulin-dependent diabetes: evaluating the "cows' milk hypothesis" and a role for anti-bovine serum albumin immunity. J Am Coll Nutr, 1997 Aug, 16:4, 334-4

2 Huang B; Rodriguez BL; Burchfiel CM; Chyou PH; Curb JD; Yano K. Acculturation and prevalence of diabetes among Japanese-American men in Hawaii. Am J Epidemiol, 1996 Oct, 144:7, 674-81

3 Salmerón J; Manson JE; Stampfer MJ; Colditz GA; Wing AL; Willett WC. Dietary fiber, glycemic load, and risk of non-insulin-dependent diabetes mellitus in women. JAMA, 1997 Feb, 277:6, 472-7

4 Salmerón J; Ascherio A; Rimm EB; Colditz GA; Spiegelman D; Jenkins DJ; Stampfer MJ; Wing AL; Willett WC Dietary fiber, glycemic load, and risk of NIDDM in men. Diabetes Care, 1997 Apr, 20:4, 545-50

5 Maxwell SR; Thomason H; Sandler D; Leguen C; Baxter MA; Thorpe GH; Jones AF; Barnett AH. Antioxidant status in patients with uncomplicated insulin-dependent and non-insulin-dependent diabetes mellitus. Eur J Clin Invest, 1997 Jun, 27:6, 484-90

6 Holecek V; Racek J; Jerábek Z. Administration of multivitamin combinations and trace elements in diabetes. Cas Lek Cesk, 1995 Feb, 134:3, 80-3

7 Sinclair AJ; Taylor PB; Lunec J; Girling AJ; Barnett AH Low plasma ascorbate levels in patients with type 2 diabetes mellitus consuming adequate dietary vitamin C. Diabet Med, 1994 Nov, 11:9, 893-8

8 Eriksson J; Kohvakka A Magnesium and ascorbic acid supplementation in diabetes mellitus. Ann Nutr Metab, 1995, 39:4, 217-23

9 Cunningham JJ; Mearkle PL; Brown RG Vitamin C: an aldose reductase inhibitor that normalizes erythrocyte sorbitol in insulin-dependent diabetes mellitus. J Am Coll Nutr, 1994 Aug, 13:4, 344-5

10 Timimi FK; Ting HH; Haley EA; Roddy MA; Ganz P; Creager MA Vitamin C improves endothelium-dependent vasodilation in patients with insulin-dependent diabetes mellitus. J Am Coll Cardiol, 1998 Mar, 31:3, 552-7

11 Jain SK; McVie R; Jaramillo JJ; Palmer M; Smith T. Effect of modest vitamin E supplementation on blood glycated hemoglobin and triglyceride levels and red cell indices in type I diabetic patients. J Am Coll Nutr, 1996 Oct, 15:5, 458-61

12 Jain SK; McVie R; Jaramillo JJ; Palmer M; Smith T; Meachum ZD; Little RL The effect of modest vitamin E supplementation on lipid peroxidation products and other cardiovascular risk factors in diabetic patients. Lipids, 1996 Mar, 31 Suppl:, S87-90

13 Pozzilli P et al. Vitamin E and nicotinamide have similar effects in maintaining residual beta cell function in recent onset insulin-dependent diabetes (the IMDIAB IV study). Eur J Endocrinol, 1997 Sep, 137:3, 234-9

14 Elliott RB; Chase HP. Prevention or delay of type 1 (insulin-dependent) diabetes mellitus in children using nicotinamide. Diabetologia, 1991 May, 34:5, 362-5

15 Elliott RB; Pilcher CC; Fergusson DM; Stewart AW A population based strategy to prevent insulin-dependent diabetes using nicotinamide. Pediatr Endocrinol Metab, 1996 Sep, 9:5, 501-9

16 Koutsikos D et al. Oral glucose tolerance test after high-dose i.v. biotin administration in normoglucemic hemodialysis patients. Ren Fail, 1996 Jan, 18:1, 131-7

17 Koutsikos D et al. Biotin for diabetic peripheral neuropathy. Biomed Pharmacother. 1990; 44: 511-514

18 Boucher BJ; Mannan N; Noonan K; Hales CN; Evans SJ Glucose intolerance and impairment of insulin secretion in relation to vitamin D deficiency in east London Asians. Diabetologia, 1995 Oct, 38:10, 1239-45

19 Baynes KC; Boucher BJ; Feskens EJ; Kromhout D Vitamin D, glucose tolerance and insulinaemia in elderly men. Diabetologia, 1997 Mar, 40:3, 344-7

20 Ma J et al. Associations of serum and dietary magnesium with cardiovascular disease, hypertension, diabetes, insulin, and carotid arterial wall thickness: the ARIC study. Atherosclerosis Risk in Communities. J Clin Epidemiol, 1995 Jul, 48:7, 927-40

21 Paolisso G; Barbagallo M Hypertension, diabetes mellitus, and insulin resistance: the role of intracellular magnesium. Am J Hypertens, 1997 Mar, 10:3, 346-55

22 Paolisso G et al. Changes in glucose turnover parameters and improvement of glucose oxidation after 4-week magnesium administration in elderly noninsulin-dependent (type II) diabetic patients. J Clin Endocrinol Metab, 1994 Jun, 78:6, 1510-4

23 Gilleran G; OLeary M; Bartlett WA; Vinall H; Jones AF; Dodson PM Effects of dietary sodium substitution with potassium and magnesium in hypertensive type II diabetics: a randomised blind controlled parallel study. J Hum Hypertens, 1996 Aug, 10:8, 517-21

24 Aharoni A; Tesler B; Paltieli Y; Tal J; Dori Z; Sharf M Hair chromium content of women with gestational diabetes compared with nondiabetic pregnant women. Am J Clin Nutr, 1992 Jan, 55:1, 104-7

25 Anderson RA Nutritional factors influencing the glucose/insulin system: chromium. J Am Coll Nutr, 1997 Oct, 16:5, 404-10

26 Anderson RA; Cheng N; Bryden NA; Polansky MM; Cheng N; Chi J; Feng J. Elevated intakes of supplemental chromium improve glucose and insulin variables in individuals with type 2 diabetes. Diabetes, 1997 Nov, 46:11, 1786-91

27 Thomas VL; Gropper SS. Effect of chromium nicotinic acid supplementation on selected cardiovascular disease risk factors. Biol Trace Elem Res, 1996 Dec, 55:3, 297-305

28 Verma S; Cam MC; McNeill JH. Nutritional factors that can favorably influence the glucose/insulin system: vanadium. J Am Coll Nutr, 1998 Feb, 17:1, 11-8

29 Halberstam M; Cohen N; Shlimovich P; Rossetti L; Shamoon H Oral vanadyl sulfate improves insulin sensitivity in NIDDM but not in obese nondiabetic subjects. Diabetes, 1996 May, 45:5, 659-66

30 Haglund B; Ryckenberg K; Selinus O; Dahlquist G Evidence of a relationship between childhood-onset type I diabetes and low groundwater concentration of zinc. Diabetes Care, 1996 Aug, 19:8, 873-5

31 Brun JF; Guintrand Hugret R; Fons C; Carvajal J; Fedou C; Fussellier M; Bardet L; Orsetti A Effects of oral zinc gluconate on glucose effectiveness and insulin sensitivity in humans. Biol Trace Elem Res, 1995 Jan, 47:1-3, 385-91

32 Collier PM; Ursell A; Zaremba K; Payne CM; Staughton RC; Sanders T. Effect of regular consumption of oily fish compared with white fish on chronic plaque psoriasis. Eur J Clin Nutr, 1993 Apr, 47:4, 251-4

33 Mayser P et al. Omega-3 fatty acid-based lipid infusion in patients with chronic plaque psoriasis: results of a double-blind, randomized, placebo-controlled, multicenter trial. J Am Acad Dermatol, 1998 Apr, 38:4, 539-47

34 Streeper RS; Henriksen EJ; Jacob S; Hokama JY; Fogt DL; Tritschler HJ Differential effects of lipoic acid stereoisomers on glucose metabolism in insulin-resistant skeletal muscle. Am J Physiol, 1997 Jul, 273:1 Pt 1, E185-91

35 Jacob S et al. Enhancement of glucose disposal in patients with type 2 diabetes by alpha-lipoic acid. Arzneimittelforschung, 45: 8, 1995 Aug, 872-4

36 Nagamatsu M et al. Lipoic acid improves nerve blood flow, reduces oxidative stress, and improves distal nerve conduction in experimental diabetic neuropathy. Diabetes Care, 18: 8, 1995 Aug, 1160-7

37 Ziegler D; Gries FA. Alpha-lipoic acid in the treatment of diabetic peripheral and cardiac autonomic neuropathy. Diabetes, 1997 Sep, 46 Suppl 2:, S62-63-61

Eye disorders

1 Hankinson SE; Stampfer MJ; Seddon JM; Colditz GA; Rosner B; Speizer FE; Willett WC Nutrient intake and cataract extraction in women: a prospective study. BMJ, 1992 Aug 8, 305:6849, 335-9

2 Knekt P; Heliövaara M; Rissanen A; Aromaa A; Aaran RK. Serum antioxidant vitamins and risk of cataract. BMJ, 1992 Dec 5, 305:6866, 1392-4

3 Hammond BR Jr; Wooten BR; Snodderly DM. Density of the human crystalline lens is related to the macular pigment carotenoids, lutein and zeaxanthin. Optom Vis Sci, 1997 Jul, 74:7, 499-504

4 Mares Perlman JA; Brady WE; Klein BE; Klein R; Haus GJ; Palta M; Ritter LL; Shoff SM. Diet and nuclear lens opacities. Am J Epidemiol, 1995 Feb, 141:4, 322-34

5 Jacques PF; Taylor A; Hankinson SE; Willett WC; Mahnken B; Lee Y; Vaid K; Lahav M. Long-term vitamin C supplement use and prevalence of early age-related lens opacities. Am J Clin Nutr, 1997 Oct, 66:4, 911-6

6 Rouhiainen P; Rouhiainen H; Salonen JT. Association between low plasma vitamin E concentration and progression of early cortical lens opacities. Am J Epidemiol, 1996 Sep, 144:5, 496-500

7 Leske MC et al; Biochemical factors in the lens opacities. Case-control study. The Lens Opacities Case-Control Study Group. Arch Ophthalmol, 1995 Sep, 113:9, 1113-9

8 Antioxidant status and neovascular age-related macular degeneration. Eye Disease Case-Control Study. Arch Ophthalmol, 1993 Jan, 111:1, 104-9

9 Landrum JT; Bone RA; Joa H; Kilburn MD; Moore LL; Sprague KE A one year study of the macular pigment: the effect of 140 days of a lutein supplement. Exp Eye Res, 1997 Jul, 65:1, 57-62

10 Mares Perlman JA; Klein R; Klein BE; Greger JL; Brady WE; Palta M; Ritter LL. Association of zinc and antioxidant nutrients with age-related maculopathy. Arch Ophthalmol, 1996 Aug, 114:8, 991-7

11 Tsang NC; Penfold PL; Snitch PJ; Billson F. Serum levels of antioxidants and age-related macular degeneration. Doc Ophthalmol, 1992, 81:4, 387-400

Fibrocystic breast disease

1 Band PR et al. Treatment of benign breast disease with vitamin A. Prev Med, 13: 5, 1984 Sep, 549-54

2 London RS; Sundaram GS; Murphy L; Goldstein PJ. The effect of alpha-tocopherol on premenstrual symptomatology: a double-blind study. J Am Coll Nutr, 1983, 2:2, 115-22

3 Sundaram GS; London R; Margolis S; Wenk R; Lustgarten J; Nair PP; Goldstein P. Serum hormones and lipoproteins in benign breast disease. Cancer Res, 1981 Sep, 41:9 Pt 2, 3814-6

4 London RS; Sundaram GS; Schultz M; Nair PP; Goldstein PJ. Endocrine parameters and alpha-tocopherol therapy of patients with mammary dysplasia. Cancer Res, 1981 Sep, 41:9 Pt 2, 3811-3

5 Meyer EC et al. Vitamin E and benign breast disease. Surgery, 107: 5, 1990 May, 549-51

6 Ghent W R et al. Iodine replacement in fibrocystic disease of the breast. Can J Surg 36, 453-460, 1993

7 Gateley CA; Maddox PR; Pritchard GA; Sheridan W; Harrison BJ; Pye JK; Webster DJ; Hughes LE; Mansel RE Plasma fatty acid profiles in benign breast disorders. Br J Surg, 1992 May, 79:5, 407-9

Headache and migraine

1 Schoenen J; Jacquy J; Lenaerts M. Effectiveness of high-dose riboflavin in migraine prophylaxis. A randomized controlled trial. Neurology, 1998 Feb, 50:2, 466-70

2 Gallai V; Sarchielli P; Morucci P; Abbritti G. Red blood cell magnesium levels in migraine patients. Cephalalgia, 1993 Apr, 13:2, 94-81; discussion 73

3 Peikert A; Wilimzig C; Köhne Volland R Prophylaxis of migraine with oral magnesium: results from a prospective, multi-center, placebo-controlled and double-blind randomized study. Cephalalgia, 1996 Jun, 16:4, 257-63

4 Facchinetti F; Sances G; Borella P; Genazzani AR; Nappi G Magnesium prophylaxis of menstrual migraine: effects on intracellular magnesium. Headache, 1991 May, 31:5, 298-301

5 Thys-Jacobs S. Vitamin D and calcium in menstrual migraine. Headache, 34: 9, 1994 Oct, 544-6

6 Thys-Jacobs S. Alleviation of migraines with therapeutic vitamin D and calcium. Headache, 34: 10, 1994 Nov-Dec, 590-2

7 Wagner W; Nootbaar Wagner U Prophylactic treatment of migraine with gamma-linolenic and alpha-linolenic acids. Cephalalgia, 1997 Apr, 17:2, 127-30; discussion 102

HIV/AIDS

1 Am J Psychiatry 1997; 154: 630-634

2 Am J Epidemiology 1998; 147: 289-301

3 Skurnick JH; Bogden JD; Baker H; Kemp FW; Sheffet A; Quattrone G; Louria DB. Micronutrient profiles in HIV-1-infected heterosexual adults. J Acquir Immune Defic Syndr Hum Retrovirol, 1996 May 1, 12:1, 75-83

4 Baker D. Cellular antioxidant status and human immunodeficiency virus replication. Nutr Rev 1992;50:15-17

5 Karter DL et al. Vitamin A deficiency in non-vitamin-supplemented patients with AIDS: a cross-sectional study. J Acquir Immune Defic Syndr Hum Retrovirol, 8: 2, 1995 Feb 1, 199-203

6 Cimoch PJ; Hoppe JB Correlation of vitamin-A deficiency with body composition, nutrient intake and immune competence in HIV/AIDS patients. Int Conf AIDS, 1996 Jul 7-12, 11:2, 103 (abstract no. We.B.3270

7 Semba RD et al. Vitamin A deficiency and wasting as predictors of mortality in human immunodeficiency virus-infected injection drug users. J Infect Dis, 171: 5, 1995 May, 1196-202

8 Baum MK et al. Micronutrients and HIV-1 disease progression. AIDS, 9: 9, 1995 Sep, 1051-6

9 Greenberg BL; Semba RD; Vink PE; Farley JJ; Sivapalasingam M; Steketee RW; Thea DM; Schoenbaum EE. Vitamin A deficiency and maternal-infant transmissions of HIV in two metropolitan areas in the United States. AIDS, 1997 Mar, 11:3, 325-32

10 Semba RD. Overview of the potential role of vitamin A in mother-to-child transmission of HIV-1. Acta Paediatr Suppl, 1997 Jun, 421:, 107-12

11 Burger H; Kovacs A; Weiser B; Grimson R; Nachman S; Tropper P; van Bennekum A; Elie M; Blaner W. Maternal serum vitamin-A levels are not associated with mother-to-child transmission of HIV-1 in the United States. J Acquir Immune Defic Syndr Hum Retrovirol, 1997 Apr 1, 14:4, 321-6

12 Omene JA, Easington CR, Glew RH, Prosper M, Ledlie S. Serum beta-carotene deficiency in HIV-infected children. J Natl Med Assoc 1996 Dec;88(12):789-793

13 Sappey C et al. Vitamin, trace element and peroxide status in HIV seropositive patients: asymptomatic patients present a severe beta-carotene deficiency. Clin Chim Acta, 230: 1, 1994 Oct 14, 35-42

14 Fryburg DA, Mark RJ, Griffith BP, Askenase PW, Patterson TF. The effect of supplemental beta-carotene on immunologic indices in patients with AIDS: a pilot study. Yale J Biol Med 1995 Jan;68(1-2):19-23

15 Coodley GO; Coodley MK; Lusk R; Green TR; Bakke AC; Wilson D; Wachenheim D; Sexton G; Salveson C. Beta-carotene in HIV infection: an extended evaluation. AIDS, 1996 Aug, 10:9, 967-73

16 Rivas CI; Vera JC; Guaiquil VH; Velásquez FV; Bórquez-Ojeda OA; Cárcamo JG; Concha II; Golde DW Increased uptake and accumulation of vitamin C in human immunodeficiency virus 1-infected hematopoietic cell lines. J Biol Chem, 1997 Feb 28, 272:9, 5814-20

17 Pacht ER; Diaz P; Clanton T; Hart J; Gadek JE. Serum vitamin E decreases in HIV-seropositive subjects over time. J Lab Clin Med, 1997 Sep, 130:3, 293-6

18 Tang AM; Graham NM; Semba RD; Saah AJ. Association between serum vitamin A and E levels and HIV-1 disease progression. AIDS, 1997 Apr, 11:5, 613-20

19 Tang et al. Vitamin B supplements may improve survival in HIV-positive individuals. Am J Epidemiol, 143, 1996, Jun, 1244-1256

20 Tang AM; Graham NM; Chandra RK; Saah AJ. Low serum vitamin B-12 concentrations are associated with faster human immunodeficiency virus type 1 (HIV-1) disease progression. J Nutr, 1997 Feb, 127:2, 345-51

21 Kieburtz KD; Giang DW; Schiffer RB; Vakil N. Abnormal vitamin B12 metabolism in human immunodeficiency virus infection. Association with neurological dysfunction. Arch Neurol, 1991 Mar, 48:3, 312-4

22 Baum MK; Beach R; Morgan R; Mantero-Atienza A; Wilke F; Eisdorfer C. Vitamin B12 and cognitive function in HIV infection. Int Conf AIDS, 1990 Jun 20-23, 6:2, 97 (abstract no. F.B.32)

23 Baum MK; Mantero-Atienza E; Shor-Posner G; Fletcher MA; Morgan R; Eisdorfer C; Sauberlich HE; Cornwell PE; Beach RS. Association of vitamin B6 status with parameters of immune function in early HIV-1 infection. J Acquir Immune Defic Syndr, 1991, 4:11, 1122-32

24 Look MP; Rockstroh JK; Rao GS; Kreuzer KA; Barton S; Lemoch H; Sudhop T; Hoch J; Stockinger K; Spengler U; Sauerbruch T Serum selenium, plasma glutathione (GSH) and erythrocyte glutathione peroxidase (GSH-Px)-levels in asymptomatic versus symptomatic human immunodeficiency virus-1 (HIV-1)-infection. Eur J Clin Nutr, 1997 Apr, 51:4, 266-72

25 Look MP; Rockstroh JK; Rao GS; Kreuzer KA; Spengler U; Sauerbruch T Serum selenium versus lymphocyte subsets and markers of disease progression and inflammatory

response in human immunodeficiency virus-1 infection. Biol Trace Elem Res, 1997 Jan, 56:1, 31-41

26 Baum MK; Shor Posner G; Lai S; Zhang G; Lai H; Fletcher MA; Sauberlich H; Page JB High risk of HIV-related mortality is associated with selenium deficiency. J Acquir Immune Defic Syndr Hum Retrovirol, 1997 Aug, 15:5, 370-4

27 Cowgill UM The distribution of selenium and mortality owing to acquired immune deficiency syndrome in the continental United States. Biol Trace Elem Res, 1997 Jan, 56:1, 43-61

28 Boelaert JR; Weinberg GA; Weinberg ED. Altered iron metabolism in HIV infection: mechanisms, possible consequences, and proposals for management. Infect Agents Dis, 1996 Jan, 5:1, 36-46

29 Edeas M; Peltier E; Claise C; Khalfoun Y; Lindenbaum A. Protective effects of exogenous copper-zinc superoxide dismutase on the TNF-alpha induced oxidative stress and HIV replication. Int Conf AIDS, 1996 Jul 7-12, 11:1, 59 (abstract no. Mo.A.1024)

30 Mocchegiani E. Benefit of oral zinc supplementation as an adjunct to zidovudine (AZT) therapy against opportunistic infections in AIDS. Int J Immunopharmacol, 17: 9, 1995 Sep, 719-27.

31 Koch J; Neal EA; Schlott MJ; Garcia-Shelton YL; Chan MF; Weaver KE; Cello JP. Zinc levels and infections in hospitalized patients with AIDS. Nutrition, 1996 Jul-Aug, 12:7-8, 515-8

Hypertension

1 Mark SD; Wang W; Fraumeni JF Jr; Li JY; Taylor PR; Wang GQ; Guo W; Dawsey SM; Li B; Blot WJ. Lowered risks of hypertension and cerebrovascular disease after vitamin/mineral supplementation: the Linxian Nutrition Intervention Trial. Am J Epidemiol, 1996 Apr, 143:7, 658-64

2 Stamler J The INTERSALT Study: background, methods, findings, and implications. Am J Clin Nutr, 1997 Feb, 65:2 Suppl, 626S-642S

3 McCarron DA Role of adequate dietary calcium intake in the prevention and management of salt-sensitive hypertension. Am J Clin Nutr, 1997 Feb, 65:2 Suppl, 712S-716S

4 Beard TC; Blizzard L; OBrien DJ; Dwyer T. Association between blood pressure and dietary factors in the dietary and nutritional survey of British adults. Arch Intern Med 1997;157:234-238

5 Cappuccio FP; Markandu ND; Carney C; Sagnella GA; MacGregor GA. Double-blind randomised trial of modest salt restriction in older people. Lancet, 1997 Sep, 350:9081, 850-4

6 Graudal NA et al. Effects of Sodium Restriction on Blood Pressure, Renin, Aldosterone, Catecholamines, Cholesterols, and Triglyceride. JAMA. 1998;279:1383-1391

7 Geleijnse JM; Hofman A; Witteman JC; Hazebroek AA; Valkenburg HA; Grobbee DE. Long-term effects of neonatal sodium restriction on blood pressure. Hypertension, 1997 Apr, 29:4, 913-7

8 Rollnik JD; Mills PJ; Dimsdale JE. Characteristics of individuals who excrete versus retain sodium under stress. J Psychosom Res, 1995 May, 39:4, 499-505

9 Whelton P K et al. Effects of oral potassium on blood pressure. JAMA 1997;277:1624-1632

10 Sacks FM, Willett WC, Smith A, Brown LE, Rosner B, Moore TJ. Effect on blood pressure of potassium, calcium, and magnesium in women with low habitual intake. Hypertension 1998 Jan;31(1):131-138

11 McCarron DA Calcium and magnesium nutrition in human hypertension. Ann Intern Med, 1983 May, 98:5 Pt 2, 800-5

12 Grobbee DE et al. Calcium metabolism and familial risk of hypertension. Semin Nephrol, 15: 6, 1995 Nov, 512-8

13 McCarron DA; Morris CD Blood pressure response to oral calcium in persons with mild to moderate hypertension. A randomized, double-blind, placebo-controlled, crossover trial. Ann Intern Med, 1985 Dec, 103:6 (Pt 1), 825-31

14 Yamamoto ME; Applegate WB; Klag MJ; Borhani NO; Cohen JD; Kirchner KA; Lakatos E; Sacks FM; Taylor JO; Hennekens CH Lack of blood pressure effect with calcium and magnesium supplementation in adults with high-normal blood pressure. Results from Phase I of the Trials of Hypertension Prevention (TOHP). Trials of Hypertension Prevention (TOHP) Collaborative Research Group. Ann Epidemiol, 1995 Mar, 5:2, 96-107

15 Belizán JM; Villar J; Bergel E; del Pino A; Di Fulvio S; Galliano SV; Kattan C. Long-term effect of calcium supplementation during pregnancy on the blood pressure of offspring: follow up of a randomised controlled trial. BMJ, 1997 Aug, 315:7103, 281-5

16 Herrera JA; Arevalo Herrera M; Herrera S. Prevention of preeclampsia by linoleic acid and calcium supplementation: a randomized controlled trial. Obstet Gynecol, 1998 Apr, 91:4, 585-90

17 Bucher HC; Guyatt GH; Cook RJ; Hatala R; Cook DJ; Lang JD; Hunt D. Effect of calcium supplementation on pregnancy-induced hypertension and preeclampsia: a meta-analysis of randomized controlled trials. JAMA, 1996 Apr, 275:14, 1113-7

18 Levine RJ; Hauth JC; Curet LB; Sibai BM; Catalano PM; Morris CD; DerSimonian R; Esterlitz JR; Raymond EG; Bild DE; Clemens JD; Cutler JA. Trial of calcium to prevent preeclampsia. N Engl J Med, 1997 Jul, 337:2, 69-76

19 Joffres MR; Reed DM; Yano K. Relationship of magnesium intake and other dietary factors to blood pressure: the Honolulu heart study. Am J Clin Nutr, 1987 Feb, 45:2, 469-75

20 Witteman JC et al. A prospective study of nutritional factors and hypertension among US women. Circulation, 1989 Nov, 80:5, 1320-7

21 Ascherio A et al. A prospective study of nutritional factors and hypertension among US men. Circulation, 1992 Nov, 86:5, 1475-84

22 Itoh K; Kawasaka T; Nakamura M The effects of high oral magnesium supplementation on blood pressure, serum lipids and related variables in apparently healthy Japanese subjects. Br J Nutr, 1997 Nov, 78:5, 737-50

23 Witteman J et al. Reduction of blood pressure with oral magnesium supplementation in women with mild to moderate hypertension. Am J Clin Nutr. 1994;60:129-135

24 Ness AR; Khaw KT; Bingham S; Day NE Vitamin C status and blood pressure. J Hypertens, 1996 Apr, 14:4, 503-8

25 Ness AR; Chee D; Elliott P Vitamin C and blood pressure—an overview. J Hum Hypertens, 1997 Jun, 11:6, 343-50

26 Solzbach U; Hornig B; Jeserich M; Just H Vitamin C improves endothelial dysfunction of epicardial coronary arteries in hypertensive patients. Circulation, 1997 Sep, 96:5, 1513-9

27 Toft I et al. Effects of n-3 polyunsaturated fatty acids on glucose homeostasis and blood pressure in essential hypertension. A randomized, controlled trial. Ann Intern Med, 123: 12, 1995 Dec 15, 911-8

28 Lungershausen YK; Abbey M; Nestel PJ; Howe PR Reduction of blood pressure and plasma triglycerides by omega-3 fatty acids in treated hypertensives. J Hypertens, 1994 Sep, 12:9, 1041-5

29 Gray DR; Gozzip CG; Eastham JH; Kashyap ML Fish oil as an adjuvant in the treatment of hypertension. Pharmacotherapy, 1996 Mar, 16:2, 295-300

30 Andreassen AK; Hartmann A; Offstad J; Geiran O; Kvernebo K; Simonsen S Hypertension prophylaxis with omega-3 fatty acids in heart transplant recipients. J Am Coll Cardiol, 1997 May, 29:6, 1324-31

31 Russo C et al. Omega-3 polyunsaturated fatty acid supplements and ambulatory blood pressure monitoring parameters in patients with mild essential hypertension. J Hypertens, 1995 Dec, 13:12 Pt 2, 1823-6

Inflammatory bowel disease

1 Reif S; Klein I; Lubin F; Farbstein M; Hallak A; Gilat. T Pre-illness dietary factors in inflammatory bowel disease. Gut, 1997 Jun, 40:6, 754-60

2 Geerling BJ; Badart Smook A; Stockbrügger RW; Brummer RJ. Comprehensive nutritional status in patients with long-standing Crohn disease currently in remission. Am J Clin Nutr, 1998 May, 67:5, 919-26

3 Hunter JO. Nutritional factors in inflammatory bowel disease. Eur J Gastroenterol Hepatol, 1998 Mar, 10:3, 235-7

4 Siguel EN; Lerman RH. Prevalence of essential fatty acid deficiency in patients with chronic gastrointestinal disorders. Metabolism, 1996 Jan, 45:1, 12-23

5 Hoffenberg EJ; Deutsch J; Smith S; Sokol RJ Circulating antioxidant concentrations in children with inflammatory bowel disease. Am J Clin Nutr, 1997 May, 65:5, 1482-8

6 Bousvaros A; Zurakowski D; Duggan C; Law T; Rifai N; Goldberg NE; Leichtner AM. Vitamins A and E serum levels in children and young adults with inflammatory bowel disease: effect of disease activity. J Pediatr Gastroenterol Nutr, 1998 Feb, 26:2, 129-35

7 Bayat M; Brynskov J; Dige Petersen H; Hippe E; L‡nborg Jensen H Direct and quantitative vitamin B12 absorption measurement in patients with disorders in the distal part of the bowel. Comparison of stool spot test [SST] with whole body counting in patients with ileal pelvic reservoir, ileostomy or Crohn's disease. Int J Colorectal Dis, 1994 May, 9:2, 68-72

8 Fernández-Bañares F et al. Serum zinc, copper, and selenium levels in inflammatory bowel disease: effect of total enteral nutrition on trace element status. Am J Gastroenterol, 1990 Dec, 85:12, 1584-9

9 Belluzzi A; Brignola C; Campieri M; Pera A; Boschi S; Miglioli M Effect of an enteric-coated fish-oil preparation on relapses in Crohn's disease. N Engl J Med, 1996 Jun, 334:24, 1557-60

10 Favier C; Neut C; Mizon C; Cortot A; Colombel JF; Mizon J. Fecal beta-D-galactosidase production and Bifidobacteria are decreased in Crohn's disease. Dig Dis Sci, 1997 Apr, 42:4, 817-22

11 Malin M; Suomalainen H; Saxelin M; Isolauri E. Promotion of IgA immune response in patients with Crohn's disease by oral bacteriotherapy with Lactobacillus GG. Ann Nutr Metab, 1996, 40:3, 137-45

Insomnia

1 Bohr KC. Effect of vitamin B12 on sleep quality and performance of shift workers. Wien Med Wochenschr, 1996, 146:13-14, 289-91

2 Hughes RJ; Badia P. Sleep-promoting and hypothermic effects of daytime melatonin administration in humans. Sleep, 1997 Feb, 20:2, 124-31

3 Attenburrow ME; Cowen PJ; Sharpley AL Low dose melatonin improves sleep in healthy middle-aged subjects. Psychopharmacology (Berl), 1996 Jul, 126:2, 179-81

4 Petrie K; Dawson AG; Thompson L; Brook R. A double-blind trial of melatonin as a treatment for jet lag in international cabin crew. Biol Psychiatry, 1993 Apr 1, 33:7, 526-30

5 Neri B; de Leonardis V; Gemelli MT; di Loro F; Mottola A; Ponchietti R; Raugei A; Cini G. Melatonin as biological response modifier in cancer patients. Anticancer Res, 1998 Mar, 18:2B, 1329-32

Kidney stones

1 Jaeger P; Portmann L; Jacquet AF; Burckhardt P. Pyridoxine can normalize oxaluria in idiopathic renal lithiasis. Schweiz Med Wochenschr, 1986 Dec 13, 116:50, 1783-6

2 Curhan GC; Willett WC; Rimm EB; Stampfer MJ. A prospective study of the intake of vitamins C and B6, and the risk of kidney stones in men. J Urol, 1996 Jun, 155:6, 1847-51

3 Vermeer C; Soute BA; Ulrich MM; van de Loo PG. Vitamin K and the urogenital tract. Haemostasis, 1986, 16:3-4, 246-57

4 Ettinger B et al. Potassium magnesium citrate is an effective prophylaxis against recurrent calcium oxalate nephrolithiasis. Journal of Urology 1997;158:2069-73

Mood disorders

1 Bell IR et al. B complex vitamin patterns in geriatric and young adult inpatients with major depression. J Am Geriatr Soc, 39: 3, 1991 Mar, 252-7

2 Bell IR; Edman JS; Morrow FD; Marby DW; Perrone G; Kayne HL; Greenwald M; Cole JO Brief communication. Vitamin B1, B2, and B6 augmentation of tricyclic antidepressant treatment in geriatric depression with cognitive dysfunction. J Am Coll Nutr, 1992 Apr, 11:2, 159-63

3 4 Benton D; Griffiths R; Haller J Thiamine supplementation mood and cognitive functioning. Psychopharmacology (Berl), 1997 Jan, 129:1, 66-71

4 Bell IR; Morrow FD; Read M; Berkes S; Perrone G. Low thyroxine levels in female psychiatric inpatients with riboflavin deficiency: implications for folate-dependent methylation. Acta Psychiatr Scand, 1992 May, 85:5, 360-3

5 Alpert JE; Fava M Nutrition and depression: the role of folate. Nutr Rev, 1997 May, 55:5, 145-9

6 Fava M; Borus JS; Alpert JE; Nierenberg AA; Rosenbaum JF; Bottiglieri T Folate, vitamin B12, and homocysteine in major depressive disorder. Am J Psychiatry, 1997 Mar, 154:3, 426-8

7 Hawkes WC; Hornbostel L Effects of dietary selenium on mood in healthy men living in a metabolic research unit. Biol Psychiatry, 1996 Jan, 39:2, 121-8

8 Linde K et al. St John's wort for depression—an overview and meta-analysis of randomised clinical trials. BMJ, 1996 Aug 3, 313:7052, 253-8

Osteoporosis

1 Devine A; Criddle RA; Dick IM; Kerr DA; Prince RL. A longitudinal study of the effect of sodium and calcium intakes on regional bone density in postmenopausal women. Am J Clin Nutr, 1995 Oct, 62:4, 740-5

2 Feskanich D; Willett WC; Stampfer MJ; Colditz GA Milk, dietary calcium, and bone fractures in women: a 12-year prospective study. Am J Public Health, 1997 Jun, 87:6, 992-7

3 Graafmans WC; Lips P; Ooms ME; van Leeuwen JP; Pols HA; Uitterlinden AG. The effect of vitamin D supplementation on the bone mineral density of the femoral neck is associated with vitamin D receptor genotype. J Bone Miner Res, 1997 Aug, 12:8, 1241-5

4 Dawson-Hughes B, Harris SS, Krall EA, Dallal GE. Effect of calcium and vitamin D supplementation on bone density in men and women 65 years of age or older. N Engl J Med 1997 Sep 4;337(10):670-676

5 Buckley et al.Calcium and vitamin D3 supplementation prevents bone loss in the spine secondary to low-dose corticosteroids in patients with rheumatoid arthritis. A randomized, double-blind, placebo-controlled trial. Ann Intern Med 1996 Dec 15;125(12):961-968

6 21 Lips P, Graafmans WC, Ooms ME, Bezemer PD, Bouter LM. Vitamin D supplementation and fracture incidence in elderly persons. A randomized, placebo-controlled clinical trial. Ann Intern Med 1996 Feb 15;124(4):400-406

7 Kanai T; Takagi T; Masuhiro K; Nakamura M; Iwata M; Saji F Serum vitamin K level and bone mineral density in post-menopausal women. Int J Gynaecol Obstet, 1997 Jan, 56:1, 25-30

8 Tamatani M; Morimoto S; Nakajima M; Fukuo K; Onishi T; Kitano S; Niinobu T; Ogihara T. Decreased circulating levels of vitamin K and 25-hydroxyvitamin D in osteopenic elderly men. Metabolism, 1998 Feb, 47:2, 195-9

9 Nielsen FH. Biochemical and physiologic consequences of boron deprivation in humans. Environ Health Perspect, 1994 Nov, 102 Suppl 7:, 59-63

10 Nielsen FH Studies on the relationship between boron and magnesium which possibly affects the formation and maintenance of bones. Magnes Trace Elem, 1990, 9:2, 61-9

11 Nielsen FH; Hunt CD; Mullen LM; Hunt JR. Effect of dietary boron on mineral, estrogen, and testosterone metabolism in postmenopausal women. FASEB J, 1987 Nov, 1:5, 394-7

12 Meacham SL; Taper LJ; Volpe SL Effects of boron supplementation on bone mineral density and dietary, blood, and urinary calcium, phosphorus, magnesium, and boron in female athletes. Environ Health Perspect, 1994 Nov, 102 Suppl 7:, 79-82

13 Abrams SA; Stuff JE Calcium metabolism in girls: current dietary intakes lead to low rates of calcium absorption and retention during puberty. Am J Clin Nutr, 1994 Nov, 60:5, 739-43

14 Lloyd T et al. Calcium supplementation and bone mineral density in adolescent girls. JAMA, 1993 Aug 18, 270:7, 841-4

15 Suleiman S, Nelson M, Li F, Buxton-Thomas M, Moniz C. Effect of calcium intake and physical activity level on bone mass and turnover in healthy, white, postmenopausal women. Am J Clin Nutr 1997 Oct;66(4):937-943

16 Burger H et al Risk Factors for Increased Bone Loss in an Elderly Population The Rotterdam Study. Am J Epidemiol 1998;147:871-9

17 Nieves JW, Komar L, Cosman F, Lindsay R. Calcium potentiates the effect of estrogen and calcitonin on bone mass: review and analysis. Am J Clin Nutr 1998;67:5-6, 18-24

18 Ann Int Med 1998;129:1-8

19 Pak CYC, et. al. Treatment of postmenopausal osteoporosis with slow-release sodium fluoride. Annals of Internal Medicine 1995 September 15;123(6):401-408.

20 Talbot JR; Fischer MM; Farley SM; Libanati C; Farley J; Tabuenca A; Baylink DJ. The increase in spinal bone density that occurs in response to fluoride therapy for osteoporosis is not maintained after the therapy is discontinued. Osteoporos Int, 1996, 6:6, 442-7

21 Sowers MF; Clark MK; Jannausch ML; Wallace RB A prospective study of bone mineral content and fracture in communities with differential fluoride exposure. Am J Epidemiol, 1991 Apr 1, 133:7, 649-60

22 Tucker K et al. Magnesium intake is associated with bone mineral density (BMD) in elderly women. J Bone Miner Res, 1995, 10S:466

23 Rude RK et al. Low serum concentrations of 1,25-dihydroxyvitamin D in human magnesium deficiency. J Clin Endocrinol Metab, 1985 Nov, 61:5, 933-40

24 Fatemi S; Ryzen E; Flores J; Endres DB; Rude RK. Effect of experimental human magnesium depletion on parathyroid hormone secretion and 1,25-dihydroxyvitamin D metabolism. J Clin Endocrinol Metab, 1991 Nov, 73:5, 1067-72

25 Zofková I; Kancheva RL. The relationship between magnesium and calciotropic hormones. Magnes Res, 1995 Mar, 8:1, 77-84

26 Abraham GE; Grewal H A total dietary program emphasizing magnesium instead of calcium. Effect on the mineral density of calcaneous bone in postmenopausal women on hormonal therapy. J Reprod Med, 1990 May, 35:5, 503-7

27 Stendig-Lindberg G; Tepper R; Leichter I. Trabecular bone density in a two year controlled trial of peroral magnesium in osteoporosis. Magnes Res, 1993 Jun, 6:2, 155-63

28 Golub MS; Keen CL; Gershwin ME; Styne DM; Takeuchi PT; Ontell F; Walter RM; and Hendrickx AG. Adolescent growth and maturation in zinc-deprived rhesus monkeys. Am J Clin Nutr 1996;64:274-82.

29 McCarty MF Anabolic effects of insulin on bone suggest a role for chromium picolinate in preservation of bone density. Med Hypotheses, 1995 Sep, 45:3, 241-6

Periodontal disease

1 Rubinoff AB et al. Vitamin C and oral health. J Can Dent Assoc, 55: 9, 1989 Sep, 705-7

2 Eklund SA; Burt BA. Risk factors for total tooth loss in the United States; longitudinal analysis of national data. J Public Health Dent, 1994 Win, 54:1, 5-14

3 Väänänen MK; Markkanen HA; Tuovinen VJ; Kullaa AM; Karinpää AM; Kumpusalo EA. Periodontal health related to plasma ascorbic acid. Proc Finn Dent Soc, 1993, 89:1-2, 51-9

4 Pack AR. Folate mouthwash: effects on established gingivitis in periodontal patients. J Clin Periodontol, 1984 Oct, 11:9, 619-28

5 Paine ML; Slots J; Rich SK. Fluoride use in periodontal therapy: a review of the literature. J Am Dent Assoc, 1998 Jan, 129:1, 69-77

Premenstrual syndrome

1 London RS et al. Effect of a nutritional supplement on premenstrual symptomatology in women with premenstrual syndrome: a double-blind longitudinal study. J Am Coll Nutr, 10: 5, 1991 Oct, 494-9

2 Doll H; Brown S; Thurston A; Vessey M. Pyridoxine (vitamin B6) and the premenstrual syndrome: a randomized crossover trial. J R Coll Gen Pract, 1989 Sep, 39:326, 364-8

3 Muneyvirci Delale O; Nacharaju VL; Altura BM; Altura BT. Sex steroid hormones modulate serum ionized magnesium and calcium levels throughout the menstrual cycle in women. Fertil Steril, 1998 May, 69:5, 958-62

4 Facchinetti F; Borella P; Sances G; Fioroni L; Nappi RE; Genazzani AR Oral magnesium successfully relieves premenstrual mood changes. Obstet Gynecol, 1991 Aug, 78:2, 177-81

5Thys-Jacobs S, Starkey P, Bernstein D, Tian J. Calcium carbonate and the premenstrual syndrome: effects on premenstrual and menstrual symptoms. Am J Obstet Gynecol 1998 Aug;179(2):444-52

6 London RS; Sundaram GS; Murphy L; Goldstein PJ The effect of alpha-tocopherol on premenstrual symptomatology: a double-blind study. J Am Coll Nutr, 1983, 2:2, 115-22

7 Chuong CJ; Dawson EB Zinc and copper levels in premenstrual syndrome. Fertil Steril, 1994 Aug, 62:2, 313-20

8 Harel, Z.; Biro, F., et al.Supplementation with omega-3 polyunsaturated fatty acids in the management of dysmenorrhea in adolescents. Am J Ob Gyn 1996;174:1335-1338

Skin disorders

1 Eberlein König B; Placzek M; Przybilla B Protective effect against sunburn of combined systemic ascorbic acid (vitamin C) and d-alpha-tocopherol (vitamin E). Am Acad Dermatol, 1998 Jan, 38:1, 45-8

2 16 Fisher GJ; Wang ZQ; Datta SC; Varani J; Kang S; Voorhees JJ. Pathophysiology of premature skin aging induced by ultraviolet light. N Engl J Med, 1997 Nov, 337:20, 1419-28

3 Hayakawa R et al. Effects of combination treatment with vitamins E and E on chloasma and pigmented contact dermatitis. A double blind controlled clinical trial. Acta Vitaminol Enzymol 1981;3(1):31-38

4 David TJ, Wells FE, Sharpe TC, Gibbs. Low serum zinc in children with atopic eczema. Br J Dermatol 1984 Nov;111(5):597-601

5 Ewing CI, Gibbs AC, Ashcroft C, David TJ. Failure of oral zinc supplementation in atopic eczema. Eur J Clin Nutr 1991 Oct;45 (10):507-510

6 Fairris GM, Perkins PJ, Lloyd B, Hinks L, Clayton BE. The effect on atopic dermatitis of supplementation with selenium and vitamin E. Acta Derm Venereol 1989;69(4):359-362

7 Andreassi M; Forleo P; Di Lorio A; Masci S; Abate G; Amerio P Efficacy of gamma-linolenic acid in the treatment of patients with atopic dermatitis. J Int Med Res, 1997 Sep, 25:5, 266-74

8 Borrek S; Hildebrandt A; Forster J Gamma-linolenic-acid-rich borage seed oil capsules in children with atopic dermatitis. A placebo-controlled double-blind study. Klin Padiatr, 1997 May, 209:3, 100-4

9 Hederos CA; Berg A Epogam evening primrose oil treatment in atopic dermatitis and asthma. Arch Dis Child, 1996 Dec, 75:6, 494-7

10 Berth-Jones J; Hutchinson PE. Vitamin D analogues and psoriasis. Br J Dermatol, 127: 2, 1992 Aug, 71-8

11 McMillan EM; Rowe D. Plasma zinc in psoriasis: relation to surface area involvement. Br J Dermatol, 108: 3, 1983 Mar, 301-5

12 Frigo A, Tambalo C, Bambara LM, Biasi D, Marrella M, Milanino R, Moretti U, Velo G, De Sandre G. Zinc sulfate in the treatment of psoriatic arthritis. Recenti Prog Med 1989 Nov;80(11):577-581

13 Harvima RJ et al. Screening of effects of selenomethionine-enriched yeast supplementation on various immunological and chemical parameters of skin and blood in psoriatic patients. Acta Derm Venereol, 1993 Apr, 73:2, 88-91

14 Juhlin L et al. Blood glutathione-peroxidase levels in skin diseases: effect of selenium and vitamin E treatment. Acta Derm Venereol, 62: 3, 1982, 211-4

15 Fairris GM et al. The effect of supplementation with selenium and vitamin E in psoriasis. Ann Clin Biochem, 26 (Pt 1):1989 Jan, 83-8

16 Vahlquist C; Berne B; Boberg M; Michaëlsson G; Vessby B. The fatty-acid spectrum in plasma and adipose tissue in patients with psoriasis. Arch Dermatol Res, 1985, 278:2, 114-9

17 Collier PM; Ursell A; Zaremba K; Payne CM; Staughton RC; Sanders T. Effect of regular consumption of oily fish compared with white fish on chronic plaque psoriasis. Eur J Clin Nutr, 1993 Apr, 47:4, 251-4

18 Mayser P et al. Omega-3 fatty acid-based lipid infusion in patients with chronic plaque psoriasis: results of a double-blind, randomized, placebo-controlled, multicenter trial. J Am Acad Dermatol, 1998 Apr, 38:4, 539-47

19 Escobar SO; Achenbach R; Iannantuono R; Torem V Topical fish oil in psoriasis—a controlled and blind study. Clin Exp Dermatol, 1992 May, 17:3, 159-62

20 Frati C; Bevilacqua L; Apostolico V. Association of etretinate and fish oil in psoriasis therapy. Inhibition of hypertriglyceridemia resulting from retinoid therapy after fish oil supplementation. Acta Derm Venereol Suppl (Stockh), 1994, 186:, 151-3

Index

A

B

C

D

F

G

O

Q

R

U

V

W